Atlas of Thyroid Cytopathology on Liquid-Based Preparations

Rana S. Hoda • Rema Rao
Theresa Scognamiglio
Editors

Atlas of Thyroid Cytopathology on Liquid-Based Preparations

Correlation with Clinical, Radiological, Molecular Tests and Histopathology

Springer

Editors
Rana S. Hoda
CBLPath
Rye Brook, NY
USA

Rema Rao
Weill Cornell Medical College
NewYork–Presbyterian Hospital
New York, NY
USA

Theresa Scognamiglio
Weill Cornell Medical College
NewYork–Presbyterian Hospital
New York, NY
USA

ISBN 978-3-030-25065-2 ISBN 978-3-030-25066-9 (eBook)
https://doi.org/10.1007/978-3-030-25066-9

This Springer imprint is published by the registered company Springer Nature Switzerland AG
The registered company address is: Gewerbestrasse 11, 6330 Cham, Switzerland

"In memory of my loving parents, Atiqa and Shafiq Ismail; for my dear husband, Syed; my dear son, Raza; and my beloved daughter-in-law, Sehyr."

Dr. Rana S. Hoda

"To my daughter Ananya Rao, my biggest cheerleader."

Dr. Rema Rao

"To my family, friends, and colleagues; thanks for the support and encouragement."

Dr. Theresa Scognamiglio

Preface

Fine-needle aspiration (FNA) cytology of the thyroid is the initial diagnostic procedure for the evaluation of nodules and triage thereof to either observation or surgery. Traditionally, thyroid FNAs have been prepared as conventional smears (CS), but these presented certain drawbacks that led to the use of liquid-based preparations (LBP) in thyroid cytology, either as the sole preparation or in combination with CS. Although both methods are useful, the cytomorphologic differences require familiarity for accurate interpretation and avoidance of diagnostic pitfalls. This Atlas was inspired by the increasing use of LBP as a processing method for thyroid FNA.

The second edition of the *Bethesda System for Reporting Thyroid Cytopathology* (TBSRTC) has been widely accepted by pathologists and endorsed by major endocrine clinical organizations including the American Thyroid Association (ATA) for the management of thyroid nodules. It has also received global recognition. This Atlas emphasizes the use of LBP based on TBSRTC diagnostic categories.

The Atlas of Thyroid Cytopathology on Liquid-Based Preparations serves as a handy guide to diagnostic cytology on LBP. It is intended to be a ready resource to accurately diagnose thyroid lesions on LBP using key cytomorphologic features. Key cytologic differential diagnosis, gross, and histopathological correlations accompany the cytological findings.

The Atlas is lavishly illustrated with color images of various thyroid diseases that should familiarize pathologists with the differences between CS and LBP and between the two commonly used LBPs. The authors have done their best to provide clear, concise, and practical guidance pertaining to cytomorphology and the implications of thyroid FNA diagnoses for patient care in this era of precision medicine.

Rye Brook, NY, USA — Rana S. Hoda
New York, NY, USA — Rema Rao
New York, NY, USA — Theresa Scognamiglio

Acknowledgments

The inspiration imparted to the authors by their many beloved teachers, peers, and trainees is gratefully acknowledged.

Dr. Rana Shafiq-Hoda would especially like to gratefully acknowledge the constant support of Dr. Carlos Urmacher, Chief Executive Officer and Chief Medical Officer, as well as the pathologists and staff of CBLPath, Rye Brook, NY.

Contents

Contributors

Elizabeth Austin CBLPath, Rye Brook, NY, USA

Sumita Gokhale Department of Cytology, Winchester Hospital, Winchester, MA, USA

Rana S. Hoda CBLPath, Rye Brook, NY, USA

Megha Joshi Winchester Hospital, Winchester, MA, USA

Christina M. Narick Interpace Diagnostics, Pittsburgh, PA, USA

Yuri E. Nikiforov Department of Pathology, Division of Molecular and Genomic Pathology, University of Pittsburgh, Pittsburgh, PA, USA

Rema Rao Department of Pathology and Laboratory Medicine, New York Presbyterian Hospital, Weill Cornell Medical College, New York, NY, USA

Theresa Scognamiglio Department of Pathology and Laboratory Medicine, New York Presbyterian Hospital, Weill Cornell Medical College, New York, NY, USA

1 Liquid-Based Preparations in Thyroid Fine Needle Aspiration

Rana S. Hoda

Thyroid Nodules

- Estimated annual incidence of thyroid nodules in the United States is 0.1%, which translates to 300,000 new nodules every year.
- Up to 50% of the general population may have sonographically detectable thyroid nodules, although only up to 5% of these harbor a malignancy.
- The high incidence of thyroid nodules and low rate of cancer among nodules pose a clinical dilemma.
- The necessity for fine needle aspiration (FNA) is assessed by clinical and ultrasound (US) risk factors for malignant disease.

Thyroid Cancer

- Thyroid cancer is the eighth most common cancer in the United States.
- In 2019, the American Cancer Society project that there will be approximately 52,070 new cases of thyroid cancer in the United States (37,810 in women and 14,260 in men), with 2170 deaths from the disease (1150 women and 1020 men). Nearly 3 out of 4 cases are found in women. Thyroid cancer is commonly diagnosed at a younger age than most other adult cancers.
- Thyroid cancer currently makes up just 5% of newly diagnosed cancers.
- The incidence rates of thyroid cancer in both women and men increased at a rate of about 4% a year from 2005 to 2014, according to the latest available data. Thyroid cancer is the most rapidly increasing cancer in the United States, and by 2030 it will become the fourth most prevalent cancer in the United States [2].
- The rise in the detection of thyroid cancer can be attributed to the increasing use of US, which can detect small, nonpalpable thyroid nodules that were not detected in the past.

Fine Needle Aspiration of Thyroid Nodules

- FNA is the standard test for initial assessment of thyroid nodules.
- The sensitivity of FNA is 80–98% and specificity is 58–100% in the triage of patients to observation or surgery. FNA performed under US guidance is much more sensitive.
- FNA diagnoses are reported based on The Bethesda System for Reporting Thyroid Cytopathology (TBSRTC), the second edition of which was released in 2017.
- Overall, thyroid FNA shows malignancy in about 5–10% of cases; another 10–25% are indeterminate or suspicious for cancer. Findings are benign in 60–70%. Patients with nodules that are malignant or suspicious for cancer by FNA usually undergo thyroid surgery.
- Malignancy is found in more than 50% of excised thyroid nodules.
- The American Thyroid Association (ATA) recommends FNA of all thyroid nodules larger than 1 cm.
- Nodules smaller than 1 cm are aspirated if they have high-risk US features:
  - Solid or hypoechoic
  - Irregular margins
  - Height taller than width
  - Microcalcifications
  - Disrupted rim calcifications
- Molecular testing in conjunction with indeterminate cytology on FNA aids in the preoperative detection of neoplastic and malignant thyroid nodules.

R. S. Hoda (✉)
CBLPath, Rye Brook, NY, USA
e-mail: rhoda@cblpath.com

R. S. Hoda et al. (eds.), *Atlas of Thyroid Cytopathology on Liquid-Based Preparations*,
https://doi.org/10.1007/978-3-030-25066-9_1

The Principal Indications for FNA in Thyroid Nodules

- Initial assessment of a newly discovered nodule
- Follow-up of benign nodules after initial assessment
- Follow-up of patients with a history of thyroid cancer for the early detection of recurrences. The current standard for follow-up consists of US and FNA every 3–6 months or as clinically indicated.

Comparison of Liquid-Based Preparations and Conventional Smears

- Traditionally, thyroid FNA has been prepared as conventional smears (CS), but liquid-based preparations (LBP) are increasingly being used, because of major technical limitations of CS (Fig. 1.1)
- The following tables list advantages and disadvantages of CS and LBP (Table 1.1), a technical comparison (Table 1.2), a morphologic comparison (Table 1.3), and cytological features of commonly encountered thyroid lesions as seen in CS and LBP (Table 1.4).

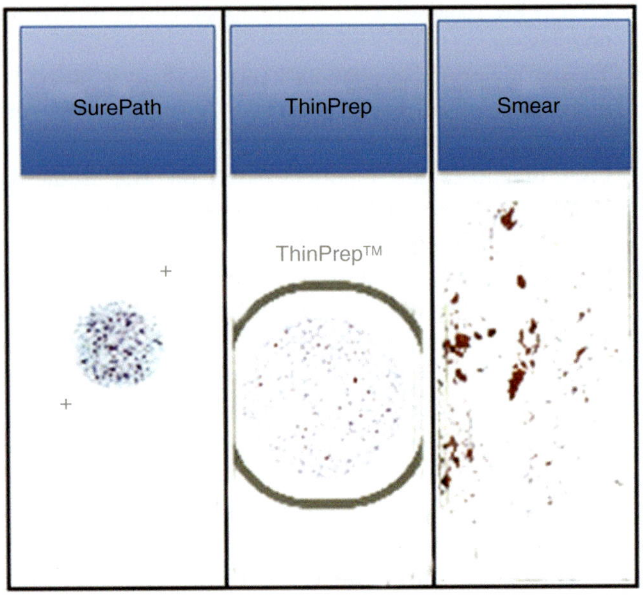

Fig. 1.1 SurePath™ (SP), ThinPrep® (TP) and conventional smear (CS). For the SP slide, the diameter of the circle is 13 mm and the specimen collection preservative medium is ethanol-based. For the TP slide, the circle where the cytologic material is deposited has a diameter of 20 mm. The specimen collection preservative medium is methanol-based. The Papanicolaou (Pap)-stained CS shows material deposited unevenly along the entire slide surface

Table 1.1 Principal advantages and disadvantages of conventional smears and liquid-based preparations

Method	Advantages	Disadvantages
Conventional smears	Inexpensive; no special preparation or staining equipment needed; simple; good cellularity; larger-sized clusters; better preserved architecture; good morphology	Multiple slides with variable cell deposition; smear-related artifacts including air-drying artifact, thick cellular areas, obscuring blood; tedious to screen
ThinPrep®[a]	Standardized and easy preparation; monolayer; less/good cellularity; better preservation; decrease in unsatisfactory specimens; uniform cell distribution; clean background; fast and easy screening; multiple slides can be prepared; additional cost is offset by improved specimen quality	Some alteration of key nuclear features and background elements; fragmentation of cell clusters; cell shrinkage; more expensive than conventional preparations
SurePath™[b]	Standardized preparation; stained on the processor; good cell yield and preservation of morphology; relative ease of screening; multiple slides can be prepared	Cells are in various planes of focus, making screening and focusing at high magnification tedious

[a]BD Diagnostics, Burlington, NC, USA
[b]Hologic, Marlborough, MA, USA

The Limitations and Artifacts of Conventional Smears

- Technical limitations of CS impair cell details and adequate assessment of cytology.
- The many limitations and artifacts result from the preparatory method and fixation:
  - *Slide labeling*: Labeling the slides (putting at least two patient identifiers) and packing them can be tedious and time-consuming.
  - *Uneven smearing of cells on slides*: The smearing of the collected sample on the slides is uneven and non-uniform (Fig. 1.2), with interindividual and intraindividual variations in smear preparation.
  - *Thick and overcrowded cellular areas*: These are fairly common and result from uneven smearing (Fig. 1.2).

Table 1.2 Technical comparison of conventional smears and liquid-based preparations

Features	Conventional smears	Liquid-based preparations
Slide Preparation	Less easy; slides are manually prepared and labeled with two patient identifiers	Easy, fully automated (TP) or semi-automated (SP)
Instrument	No special instrument required	Special instruments required
Glass slides	Ordinary glass slides	Manufacturer provides specially made & marked slides
Cost	Less expensive; no special requirements	Expensive due to costs of special instrument, solution, and slides
Specimen handling and transport	More handling, less easy transport. Air-dried slides transported in cardboard boxes; ethanol-fixed slides transported in Coplin jars	Less handling, easy transport. Specimen rinsed in tubes with proprietary collection medium, capped, and transported
Method of preparation	Time-consuming: specimen is smeared on glass slides, resulting in nonuniform and variable slides	Fast, automated, uniform, standardized preparations
Number of slides	Usually four or more	One
Cell deposition	Nonuniform deposition on the entire 5 × 2.5 cm area	Cells deposited within a well-defined marked area, a circle 20 mm (TP) or 13 mm (SP) in diameter
Fixative	Ethanol	Methanol (TP) or ethanol (SP)
Fixation and air-drying	Variable, usually 5–10 seconds; potential for air-drying artifact	Immediate, prevents air-drying artifact
Staining	Both Romanowsky & Pap stains	Only Pap stain
Obscuring elements	Present: Blood, inflammation	None or reduced
Cell distribution	Nonuniform; cell distribution in thick cellular areas with overlap	Uniform; thick cell distribution and overlap absent or reduced
Screening and time	Screening is time-consuming, tedious: many slides, cells unevenly deposited on the entire slide; obscuring elements	Screening is easy: one slide, cells deposited uniformly in a marked area with limited fields of view; obscuring elements reduced or absent
On-site evaluation	Can be performed with Romanowsky stains, such as Diff Quik (DQ) stain	Not possible

SP SurePath, *TP* ThinPrep

Table 1.3 Cytological differences between conventional smears and liquid-based preparations

Features	Conventional smears	Liquid-based preparations
Inadequate rate	Variable 15–30%	<15%
Obscuring elements	Yes	No
Background elements	Present	Reduced
Thick cellular areas	Yes	No
Colloid	Diffusely present, allows evaluation of amount	Thin colloid appears as "wrinkled tissue paper" or clumped, and thick colloid as globules; does not allow accurate quantification
Retention of large cell clusters	Yes	Inconsistent and smaller
Complex 3D fragments	Retained, easy to interpret	Fragmented, smaller, difficult to interpret due to thickness, especially in SP
Papillary structures	Easy to interpret	Difficult to interpret due to thickness, especially in SP
Follicular cells	Retain size and shape	Cells become smaller
Nuclei of papillary thyroid carcinoma (PTC)	Retain all features	Retain all features. Intranuclear pseudoinclusions (INPI) may be reduced or less apparent, especially in TP
Hürthle cells	Smooth nuclear membranes	Sometimes irregular nuclear membranes, smaller size
Aggregation of lymphocytes	No	Yes

SP SurePath, *TP* ThinPrep

Uneven staining: Because Diff Quik (DQ) staining is performed manually, overstaining is usual, due to nonuniform and thick and overcrowded cell distribution and cells partially obscured by blood (Figs. 1.2 and 1.3).

Partially obscuring blood: This artifact is fairly common and because cells cannot clearly be assessed, it usually results in overdiagnosis for fear of missing a significant lesion. In LBP, even though some blood is retained, it does not obscure cell detail (Figs. 1.4a–e and 1.5a–d).

– *Crush artifact*: Cells are fragile; if more pressure is used for smearing, the nuclei crush and smear, and cytoplasm is disrupted. This artifact is more pronounced in lesions with a lymphoid component (Fig. 1.6).

Table 1.4 Cytologic criteria for interpretation of thyroid lesions on conventional smears and liquid-based preparations

Diagnosis	Conventional smears	Liquid-based preparations
TBS II, Benign Follicular Nodule	Abundant watery colloid, honeycomb and ordered sheets and macrofollicles of small follicular cells, small uniform nuclei, clear to granular cytoplasm ± hemorrhage with hemosiderin-laden histiocytes & abundant thin colloid	All features present, single cells, bare nuclei, sheets are smaller, with smaller cells and nuclei, less watery colloid appears as "wrinkled tissue paper–like"
TBS II, Lymphocytic Thyroiditis	Mostly mature lymphocytes, few plasma cells, epithelioid histiocytes, lymphoid tangles, lymphoepithelial aggregates, sheets and clusters of Hürthle cells ± atypia, scant colloid	All features present, lymphocytes may be reduced, aggregate and may mimic follicular cells
TBS III, AUS/FLUS	Enlarged nuclei with subtle and few of the nuclear features of PTC, cells present in clusters/microfollicles. Follicular-patterned lesions may not always show PTC nuclear features if they represent FA/FC	All features present, cell clusters and microfollicles may appear tighter and cells and nuclei may appear smaller
TBS IV, Follicular Neoplasm (FN)/ Suspicious for FN	Scant or absent colloid; microfollicles or small clusters of larger (medium-sized) follicular cells arranged in honeycomb sheets with altered polarity, rounded, overlapping nuclei, ± slight nuclear irregularity, nucleoli, vascular fragments, diffuse or globules of thick colloid, usually in association with follicular cells. Nuclear clearing, grooves represent follicular-patterned PTC.	All features present, cells appear small, microfollicles may be tighter, scattered and isolated, colloid globules may be few and dispersed, or associated with follicular cells. In SP, microfollicle lumens are visualized in different planes of focus.
TBS IV, Follicular Neoplasm (FN)/ Suspicious for FN, Oncocytic Type	All features of FN as described above are present; cells are exclusively oncocytes with enlarged, monotonous nuclei, bi-nucleation, small or prominent nucleoli, dense or granular pinkish cytoplasm with distinct outline, low to high N:C, transgressing vessels or vascular fragments	All features present; oncocytes are smaller, nuclear chromatin appears more condensed, nucleoli may be more prominent
TBS V, Suspicious for Papillary Thyroid Carcinoma (PTC)	Colloid less and thick, ± dense globules "bubble gum" or thick "ropy" strands, syncytial fragments, clusters or papillary-like structures of medium- to large-sized nuclei with moderate nuclear pleomorphism, overlap, and crowding, irregular membrane, clearing and grooves (none/few INPI and absent true papillary fragments with fibrovascular core and psammoma bodies)	All features present; cells appear small; syncytial fragments, clusters or papillary-like structures are smaller with more disruption
TBS VI, Malignant, Papillary Thyroid Carcinoma (PTC)	Colloid less, hard and thick, forms dense globules "bubble gum" or "ropy" strands, large syncytial fragments, clusters, papillary fragments with fibrovascular cores of medium- to large-sized follicular cells with nuclear pleomorphism, overlap, and crowding, irregular membrane, clearing, grooves, INPI, nucleoli, ± psammoma bodies, ± cystic degeneration and histiocytes	All features present; cells appear small, ± elongated, many single cells, syncytial fragments, clusters and papillary fragments are smaller, thinner with more disruption; INPI may be reduced, smaller, and difficult to find
TBS VI, Malignant, Medullary Thyroid Carcinoma (MTC)	Cellular, small clusters of round to spindled cells with round or ovoid, slightly pleomorphic plasmacytoid (eccentrically placed) nuclei, "salt & pepper" neuroendocrine chromatin, fragments of hyaline material (amyloid); scant colloid	All features present; cells appear small, many isolated and dispersed cells, syncytial fragments; "salt & pepper" neuroendocrine chromatin retained, amyloid can be seen

FA follicular adenoma, *FC* follicular carcinoma, *FN* follicular neoplasm, *FVPTC* follicular variant of papillary thyroid carcinoma, *MTC* medullary thyroid carcinoma, *N:C* nucleus to cytoplasmic ratio, *PTC* papillary thyroid carcinoma, *SP* SurePath, *TBS* The Bethesda System

– *Nuclear features*: Evaluation of nuclear features is important in the diagnosis of thyroid lesions, particularly papillary thyroid carcinoma (PTC), so most pathologists prefer to examine specimens using the Pap stain. However, such material must be immediately fixed in alcohol to prevent air-drying artifact. Clinicians often do not appreciate how quickly the air-drying artifact occurs and do not see the impact of poor preparation. In a busy office, the clinician may unintentionally allow the slides to air-dry prior to placement in alcohol. This results in a

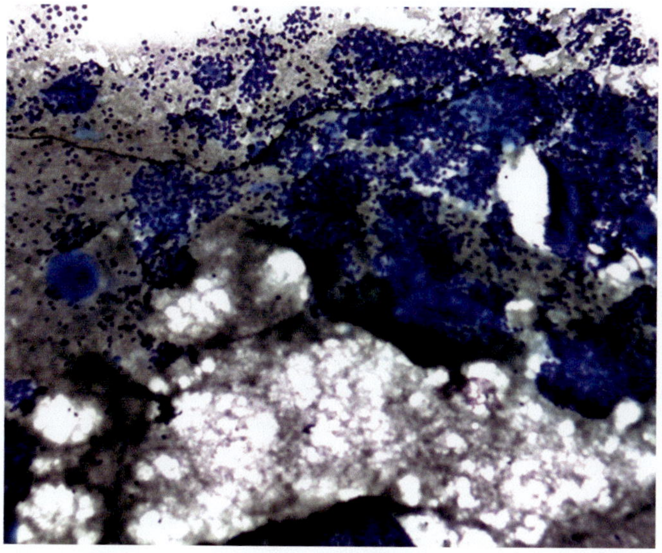

Fig. 1.2 Artifacts of CS. The smearing of the collected sample on the slides is uneven and non-uniform. Note thick and overcrowded cellular areas concentrated on the top of the slide (Diff-Quik [DQ] stain, CS)

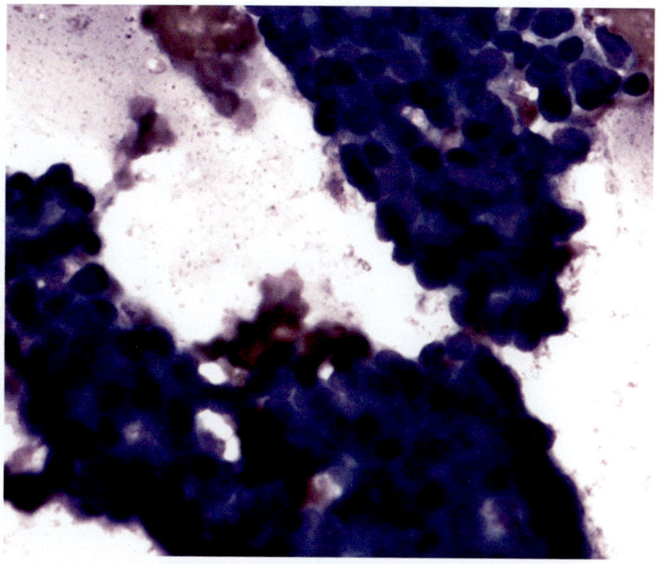

Fig. 1.3 Artifacts of CS. DQ staining in CS is uneven and overstained due to nonuniform and thick cell distribution

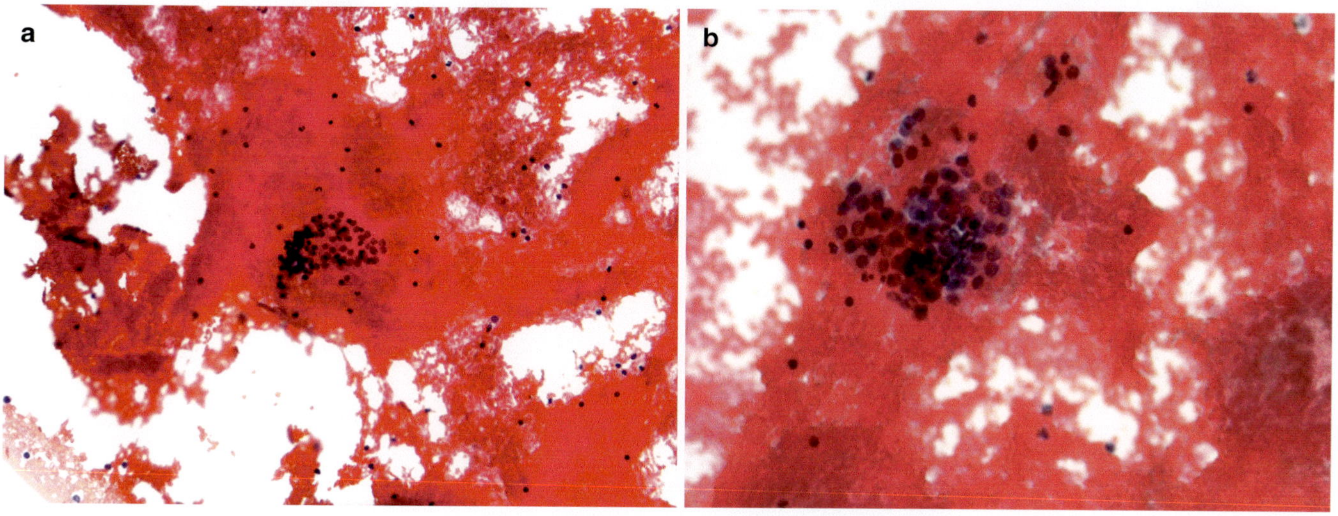

Fig. 1.4 (**a**–**e**) Artifacts of CS. (**a**, **b**) CS slide shows abundant blood, which partially obscures follicular cell detail. These are benign follicular cells. (**c**, **d**) Same case processed as TP shows background blood, but the follicular cells are not obscured. (**e**) Same case processed as a SP shows follicular cells within blood. Cell details are not obscured. Note macrophage in a different plane of focus. (**a**, **b**, Pap stain CS; **c**, **d**, Pap stain TP; e, Pap stain SP)

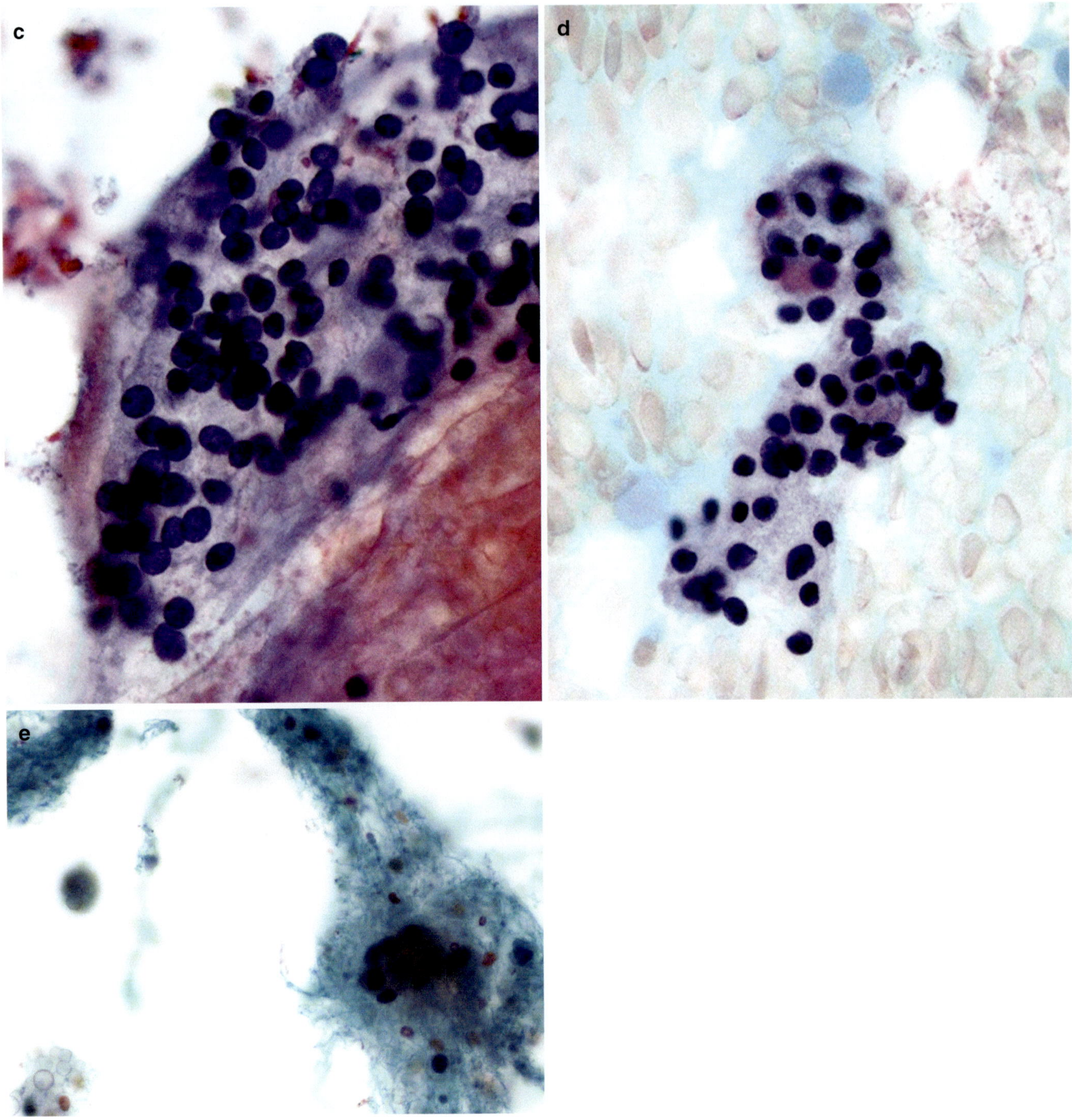

Fig. 1.4 (continued)

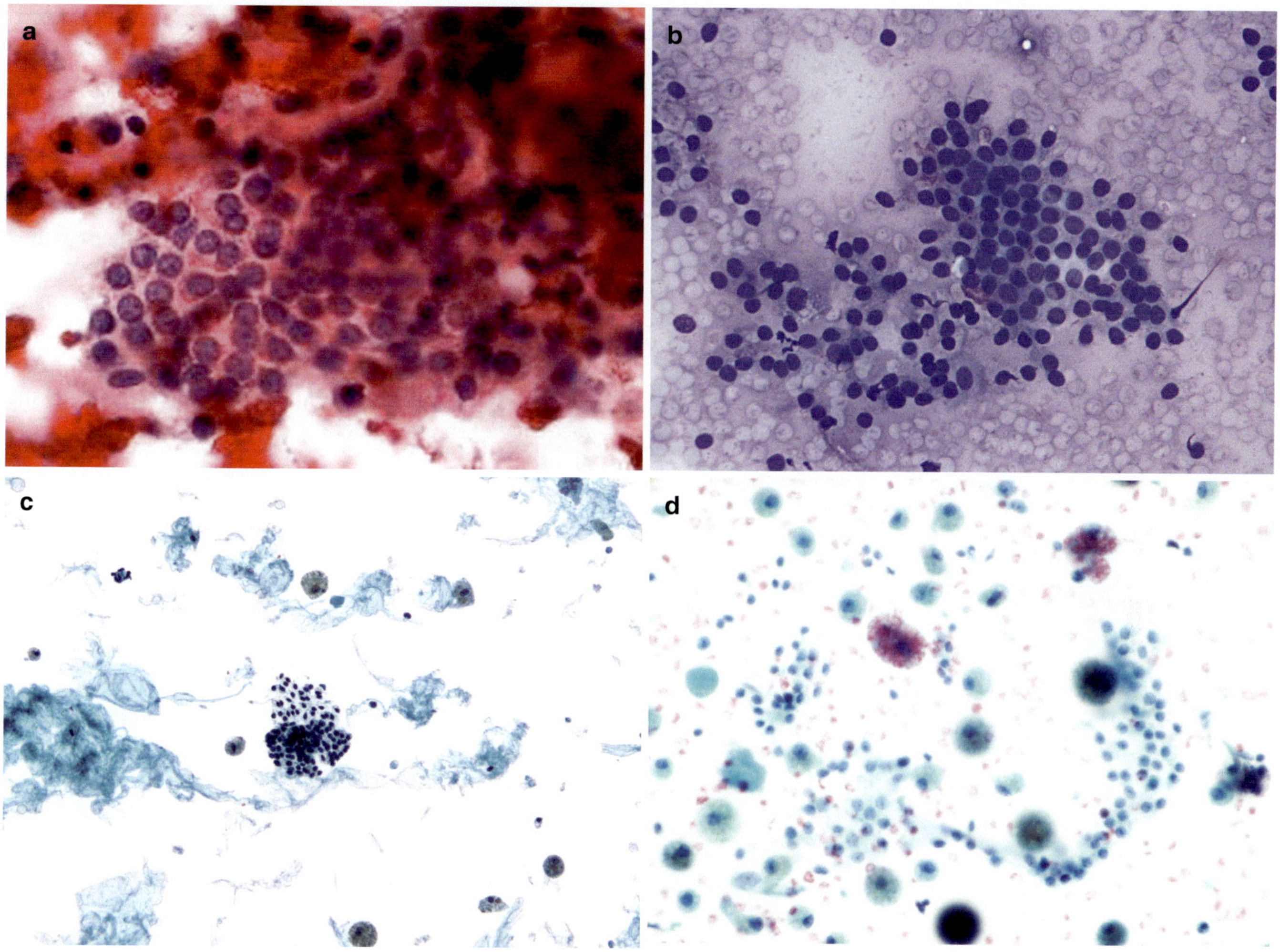

Fig. 1.5 (**a–d**) Blood and Colloid in CS and LBP. (**a**, **b**) Blood and thin colloid in CS. Note blood obscures cell detail as seen in (**a**) and thin colloid forms a diffuse film as seen in (**b**). (**a**, Pap stain CS; **b**, DQ stain CS). (**c**) Same case processed TP shows a clean background without blood. Thin colloid as is retained and appears like wrinkled tissue paper or a folded napkin. (**d**) Same case processed SP shows some blood in the background. Thin colloid is not as clearly evident as in the TP slide (**c**, **d**, Pap stain)

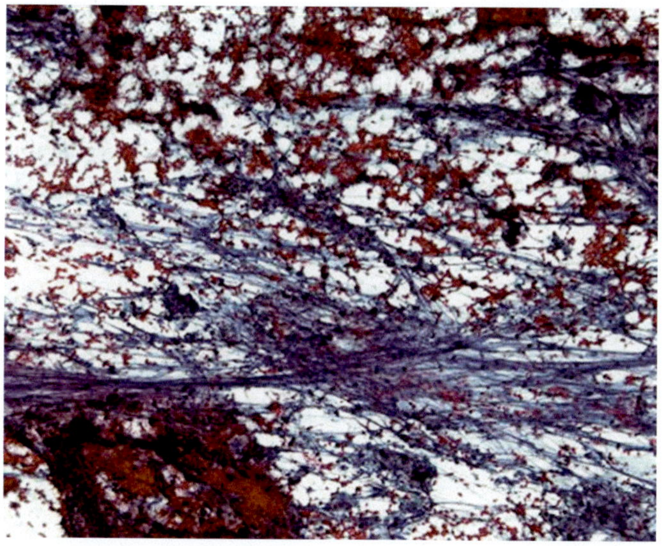

Fig. 1.6 Artifacts of CS. CS slide shows "crush artifact" with crushed nuclei and disrupted cytoplasm from a case of lymphocytic thyroiditis (Pap stain, CS)

suboptimal or even nondiagnostic specimen, owing to loss of nuclear details (Fig. 1.7a–c).

– *Contamination*: There is also a potential for contamination from cellular samples during staining.

Liquid-Based Preparations (LBP) for Thyroid FNA

- FNA is used to triage thyroid nodules to a specific management—surgery (either total or subtotal) or observation.
- The most common malignancy of the thyroid is PTC. Because of its multifocal nature, a diagnosis of malignancy on FNA typically results in a total thyroidectomy. A benign diagnosis is reassuring and allows the patient to avoid surgery and undergo periodic observation. These diagnoses require well-preserved nuclei.

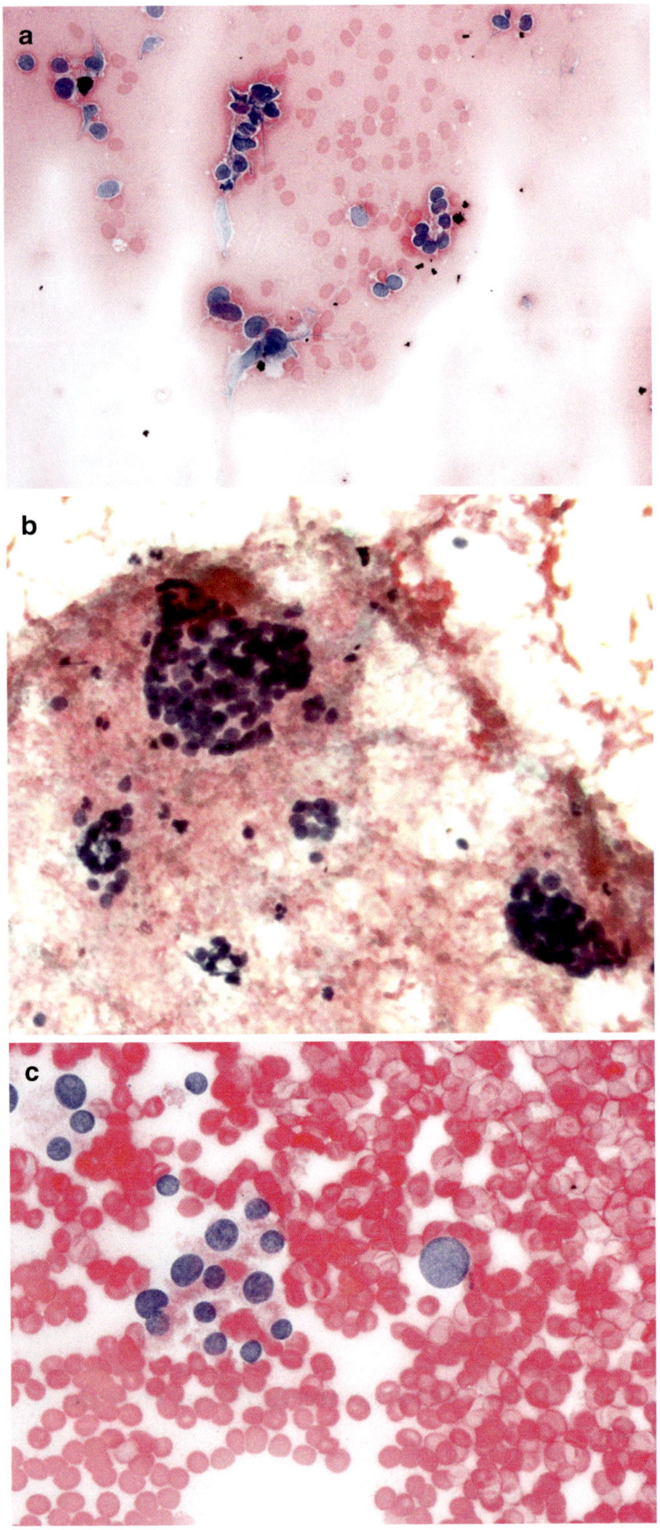

Fig. 1.7 (**a–c**) Artifacts of CS. (**a, b**) Slides show air-drying artifact. Note poor nuclear details and larger cell and nuclear size. (**c**) Case shows benign Hürthle cells that appeared much larger and were interpreted as atypical (Pap stain, CS)

- Most laboratories report thyroid FNA diagnoses according to TBSRTC, which has retained six diagnostic categories, each with their own risk of malignancy and recommended clinical management. (*See* Chap. 2, Tables 2.1 and 2.2.)
- Usually multiple CS slides are prepared from each FNA pass. If rapid on-site specimen evaluation (ROSE) is performed, a few slides are air-dried and stained with a Romanowski-type stain such as the Diff Quik (DQ) stain and reviewed. A few slides are fixed in alcohol for later Papanicolaou (Pap) staining.
- Many clinicians also perform thyroid FNA in their clinics without ROSE, and make multiple CS slides to ensure the adequacy of the sample.

Types of LBP and Preparatory Techniques for LBP

- The popularity of LBP is increasing, as these techniques can improve the quality of thyroid specimens and reduce the number of slides per specimen.
- Two types of LBP currently in use are ThinPrep® (TP) (Hologic, Marlborough, MA, USA) and SurePath™ (SP) (BD Diagnostics, Burlington, NC, USA).
- Both reduce the variations and artifacts of CS and produce uniform, standardized preparations by an automated process that is representative of the entire collected sample.
- Details of the LBP collection and processing techniques, technical differences, general cytologic and specific cellular features for the two types of LBP, and comparison with CS have previously been published [15].
- LBP techniques are automated to avoid contamination during manual processes and to reduce labor time for batch sample preparation (Fig. 1.8).
- The TP method, in brief:
  - The specimen is collected in a methanol-based solution (Cytolyt™), then filtered and transferred onto a positively charged slide with a gentle positive pressure and stained with Pap stain.
  - All the steps prior to staining occur in automated systems, TP2000™ or TP5000™ processors. TP 2000 processes one slide at a time, whereas TP5000 can batch-process 20 samples at one time.
  - The TP method is based on membrane filtration, in which the cells of interest are separated when the liquid collection medium is drawn through a filter using negative pressure pulse. Thus, the cells appear in a true monolayer.

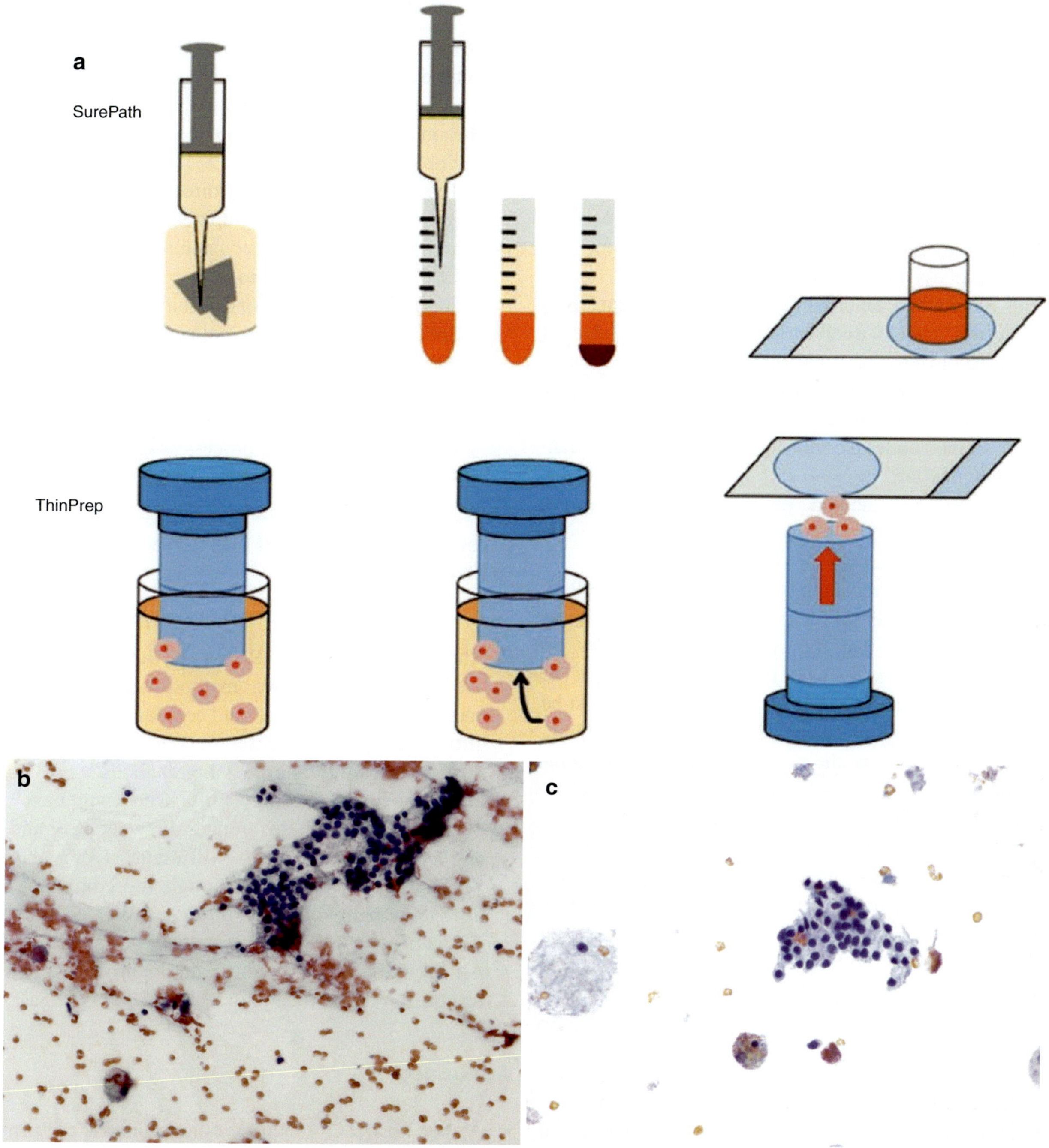

Fig. 1.8 (**a–c**) LBP Processing Techniques and Background. (**a**) *SurePath™ Technique*: The sample is collected in CytoRich®, an ethanol-based proprietary preservative fluid which is vortexed prior to preparation. A syringe is used to disaggregate larger cell fragments. The specimen is then dispersed onto a density gradient reagent, a polysaccharide solution that acts to trap small particles and debris. The specimen is centrifuged and then the cell pellet is resuspended. The PrepStain™ processor transfers the fluid to a settling chamber that rests on a positively charged glass slide. Cells are allowed to settle on the slide under the influence of gravity. The PrepStain™ processor also automatically stains the slides. *ThinPrep™ Technique*: A cylinder with a polycarbonate filter attached to one end is introduced into the specimen vial and gently rotated creating a current that disaggregates mucus, blood, colloid and other background material, breaks up large cell clusters, and mixes and homogenizes the cell suspension. A gentle vacuum is then applied to the cylinder, most of the broken erythrocytes, thin mucus, thin colloid, and other debris pass through the filter pores, while the cells of interest adhere to the filter. The instrument monitors the cell density across the filter and the flow rate decreases when cells are evenly distributed on the filter with minimal overlap. The cylinder then moves out of the specimen and is lightly pressed against a positively charged slide. A whiff of positive air pressure is applied to transfer the cells to the slide. The slide is immediately dropped into 95% ethanol fixative. The prepared slide is removed from the processor and either stained manually or on an automatic slide stainer (From Hoda RS, VandenBussche C, Hoda SA. Liquid-based specimen collection, preparation, and morphology. In: Diagnostic liquid-based cytology. Hoda RS, VandenBussche C, Hoda SA, editors. New York: Springer; 2017; with permission). (**b**) CS shows abundant thin colloid which stains light blue-green (Pap stain). (**c**) In TP, the amount of colloid is diminished, compared with CS and appears as droplets, as seen here, or like wrinkled tissue paper or a folded napkin as seen in Fig. 1.5C (Pap stain)

 - Colloid, lymphocytes, and large tissue fragments are reduced in TP, however, and the large tissue fragments are more fragmented than in CS.
- The SP method, in brief:
  - The specimen is collected in an ethanol-based solution (CytoRich™), cells are transferred onto one poly-l-lysine coated slide, and they are stained with Pap stain.
  - All the steps, including the staining, occur in an automated system, PrepStain™ (BD Diagnostics, Burlington, NC, USA). The PrepStain system can batch-process 48 specimens per run.
  - The SP method employs density gradient separation and centrifugation, a cell enrichment process producing cells devoid of blood and other obscuring materials. The cells of interest are separated as a result of the simple sedimentation of cells and allowed to settle on the slide surface under the influence of gravity rather than applied pressure.
  - Thus, the SP method produces a more three-dimensional (3-D) configuration for both single cells and clusters than does CS.
- Use of liquid-based technology allows for only one Pap-stained slide to be created for screening, and greatly minimizes the chances that the specimen will air-dry. In addition, it minimizes the work required on the part of the clinician performing the FNA, as no glass slides must be prepared. Needle passes can be taken in quick succession, minimizing the time of the procedure for both the clinician and the patient.
- Overall, the diagnostic accuracy of CS and LBP is comparable with sensitivities of 79% and 76%, specificities of 64% and 55%, positive predictive values (PPV) of 92% and 94%, and negative predictive values (NPV) of 90% and 82% for CS and LBP respectively. Correlation between CS and LBP is 90%.
- There are, however, cytomorphologic differences between CS and LBP with regard to background elements such as blood and the amount and character of colloid, architectural features, and nuclear and cytoplasmic details.
- Familiarity and experience with the cytomorphological appearance on LBP is required for correct interpretation, and to avoid diagnostic pitfalls. Studies have shown that LBP morphology differs from that seen on CS [10, 11, 24]. Most importantly, colloid often has a delicate "tissue paper" appearance on LBP that is not seen on CS. Thyroid follicular cells often shrink, giving them a smaller appearance than what is seen on Pap-stained CS. Details of these and other differences are described below and on Tables 1.3 and 1.4.

Methods for LBP Triage

- LBP can be prepared by two methods, the "split-sample" method and the "direct to vial" method.
- *"Split-sample" method:* Both CS and LBP are prepared. This method is usually employed when a cytologist is available to render ROSE.
  - The first pass is expelled directly onto the slides, and two or more slides are prepared from each pass for DQ and Pap staining. Residual material is rinsed in the LBP collection medium.
  - DQ stain is assessed for adequacy from each pass.
  - Specimens may also be collected for molecular tests. (*See* Chap. 14.)
- *"Direct to vial" method*: Only LBP is used.
  - Two or more dedicated passes are rinsed directly in the LB collection fluid to process as one LBP.

Alterations in General Features in LBP in Thyroid FNA

- Although both TP and SP are LBP, there are subtle differences between the two methods *vis-a-vis* cellularity, background, architecture, and cellular morphology. These differences are due to different collection media and fixation and the different processing methods.
- Practitioners of cytology only need awareness of the cytomorphological differences between CS and LBP and between the two different LBP, TP, and SP. Diagnostic features, although altered in appearance in LBP, remain similar to those seen in CS (Tables 1.5, 1.6, and 1.7).
- All background and cellular alterations in the two LBP result from their processing techniques (Fig. 1.8a).

Adequacy

- As per TBSRTC, adequacy criteria in LBP are similar to those for CS. (*See* Chap. 3.)
- Cellularity is usually high or adequately high in LBP.
- An additional LBP slide may help decrease the number of inadequate results.
- Ultrasound gel must be wiped from the needle insertion site. Excess gel can obscure the cellular component in both LBP and CS. In TP, the filter may become clogged by the gel, preventing cells from being transferred to the slide.

Table 1.5 Technical differences between LBP preparations

Features	ThinPrep	SurePath
Cost	Expensive	Less expensive
Sample collection	Uniform	Uniform
Sample transfer	Entire	Entire
Fixation	Immediate	Immediate
Transport	Easy	Easy
Slide preparation	Fully automated	Partial automation
Slide evaluation	Easier	Easy
Cells deposition	Well-defined 20 mm diameter area	Well-defined 13 mm diameter area
Cell preservation	Good	Good
Obscuring factors	None	None
Air-drying	None	None
Screening time	Reduced	Reduced
Reproducibility	Yes	Yes
Ancillary studies	Possible	Possible

Adapted from Hoda RS, VandenBussche C, Hoda SA. Liquid-based specimen collection, preparation, and morphology. In: Diagnostic liquid-based cytology. Hoda RS, Van den Bussche C, Hoda SA, editors. New York: Springer; 2017. p. 1–12; with permission

Table 1.6 General cytologic features on LBP preparations

Features	ThinPrep	SurePath
Quality	Enhanced	Enhanced
Background		
Clean	Yes	Yes
RBCs	More reduced	Reduced
Neutrophils	Reduced	Reduced
Necrosis	Clumped	Clumped
Cellularity	Lower	Higher
Cell Distribution	Uniform, one plane of focus	Uniform, thick, different planes of focus
Cell size	Smaller	Small
Architecture	Less well-preserved	Better preserved
Cytomorphology	Preserved	Preserved
[a]Extracellular material		
Quantity	Reduced	Less reduced
Appearance	Altered	Less altered

Adapted from Hoda RS, VandenBussche C, Hoda SA. Liquid-based specimen collection, preparation, and morphology. In: Diagnostic liquid-based cytology. Hoda RS, Van den Bussche C, Hoda SA, editors. New York: Springer; 2017. p. 1–12; with permission

[a]Extracellular material including necrosis, mucin, lubricant are altered in quality

Background

- The background in LBP is clean and has less or no obscuring elements. The TP and SP collection media, PreservCyt and CytoRich Red, contain mucolytic and hemolytic agents that reduce blood, polymorphonuclear leucocytes

Table 1.7 Specific cellular features LBP preparations

Features	ThinPrep	SurePath
Architecture		
Fragmentation	Present ++	Present +
Monolayer cells	+	–
Cell clusters	Present, 3D, flat, smaller cohesive, minimal overlap	Present, thick, 3-D > depth of focus, cohesive, more overlap
Flattening	More	Less
Cellular morphology		
Shape	More rounded	Rounded/elongated
Nucleus		
Detail	Enhanced	Enhanced
Nucleoli	More prominent	Preserved
Inclusions	Less apparent	Preserved
Cytoplasm		
Detail	May be denser	May be denser
Shape	Retained	Retained
Elements[a]	Preserved	Preserved

Adapted from Hoda RS, VandenBussche C, Hoda SA. Liquid-based specimen collection, preparation, and morphology. In: Diagnostic liquid-based cytology. Hoda RS, Van den Bussche C, Hoda SA, editors. New York: Springer; 2017. p. 1–12; with permission

+ *indicates* present, – *indicates* not present

[a]Cytoplasmic elements include: vacuolations, pigment, PMNs

(PMNs), and cystic and necrotic debris. Even if excess blood and other background elements are present, they do not obscure the cells (Fig. 1.4c–e).

- The amount of colloid may be diminished, compared with CS (Fig. 1.8b, c).
- Thin colloid may resemble delicate tissue paper or a folded napkin, or may be granular rather than in a film as in CS (Figs. 1.5c, 1.8b and 1.9a–c); thick colloid appears as small, dense droplets or globules, rather than the thicker sheets seen in CS (Fig. 1.9d, e).
- In chronic lymphocytic thyroiditis (CLT) or Hashimoto's thyroiditis, lymphocytes may be reduced in TP and may affect the diagnosis (Fig. 1.10a, b). (*See also* Chap. 4.)
- The number of lymphocytes is slightly increased in SP slides; the difference may represent lymphocytes from peripheral blood contamination.
- In TP, necrosis forms granular clumps and clings to tumor cells ("clinging" diathesis). This feature makes tumor cells stand out (Fig. 1.11a, b).

Cellularity and Cell Distribution

- LBP shows higher cellularity.
- Cells are generally distributed singly and in thin layers with less overlap in LBP, particularly in TP, which consistently

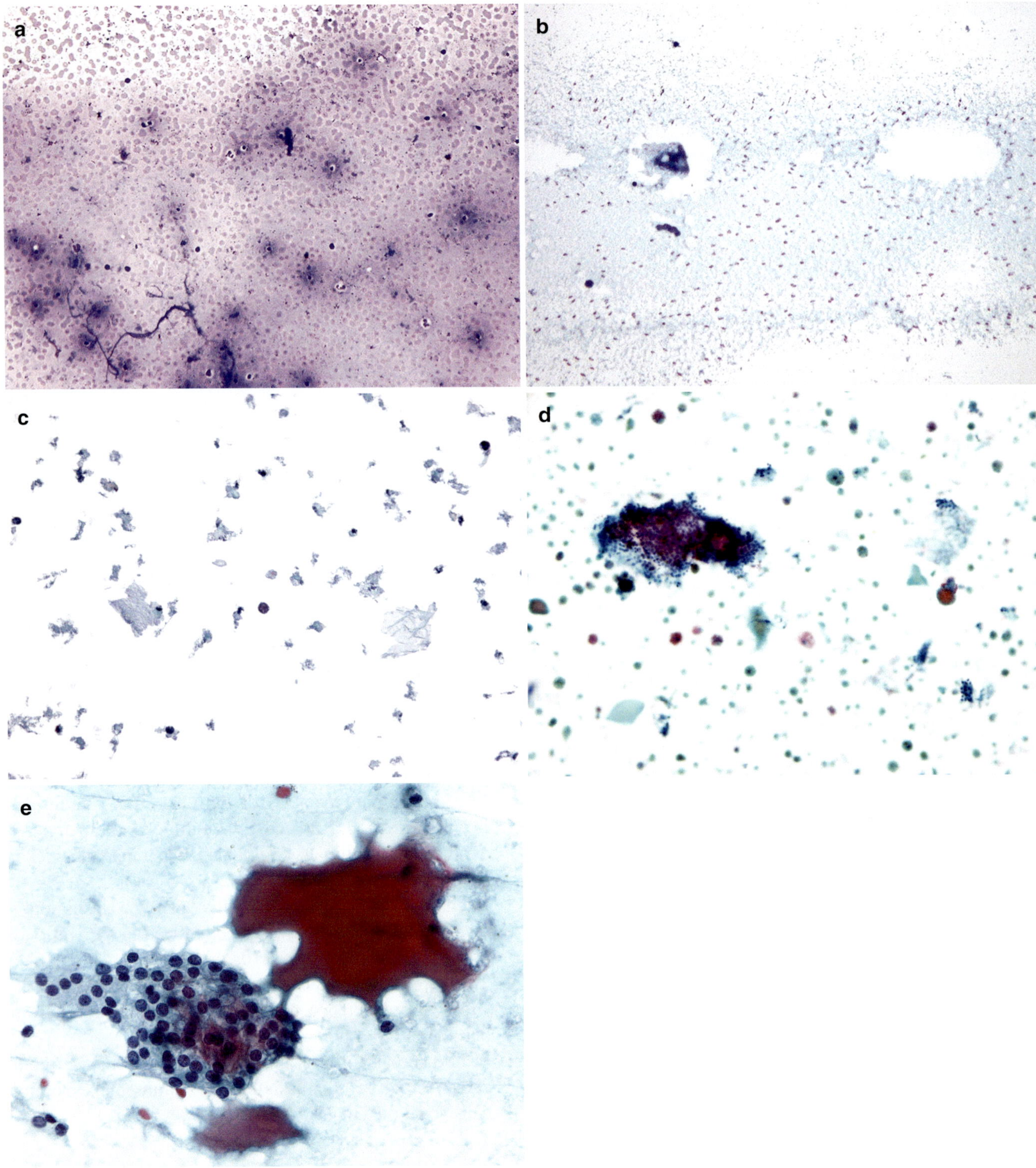

Fig. 1.9 (**a**–**e**) Background. Identifying the amount and nature of colloid is important for proper interpretation of thyroid nodules. (**a**, **b**) This cystic lesion on CS show a diffuse thin film of thin watery colloid (**a**, DQ stain, CS; **b**, Pap stain CS). **c**, Same case processed as TP shows the fragmented colloid which appears as delicate wrinkled sheets and granular material rather than in a film as in CS (Pap stain). (**d**) In SP, thick colloid appears as small, dense droplets or globules, rather than the thick sheets of colloid seen in CS (Pap stain). (**e**) Thick colloid forms a dense irregular thick sheet in CS (Pap stain)

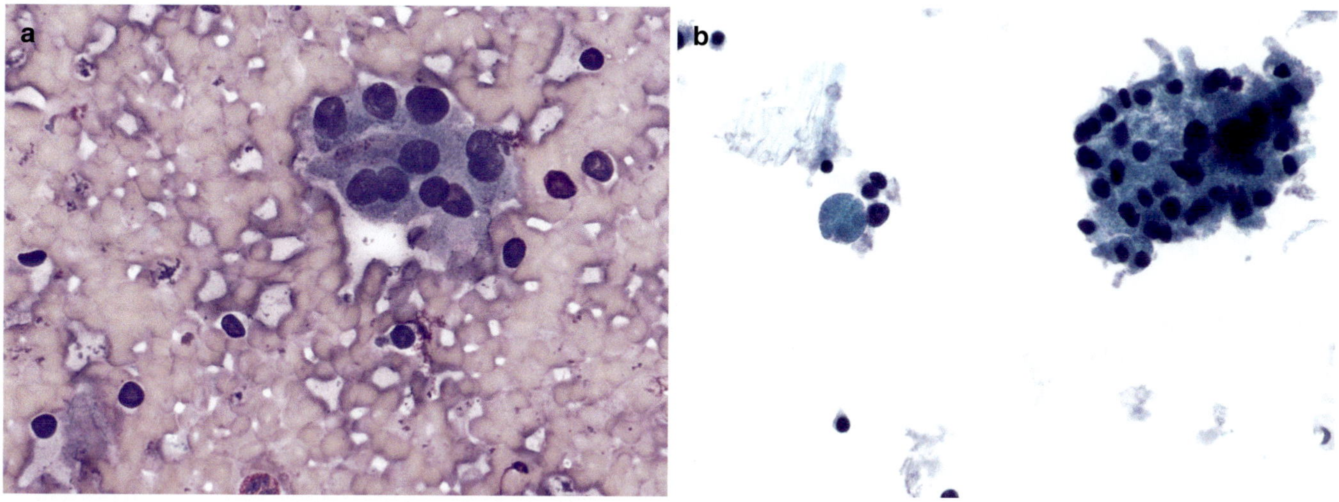

Fig. 1.10 (**a**, **b**) Background. Chronic lymphocytic thyroiditis (CLT) shows Hurthle cells and scattered lymphocytes (DQ stain, CS). (**b**) CLT shows a similar appearance in TP from the same case. Lymphocytes may be reduced in TP (Pap stain)

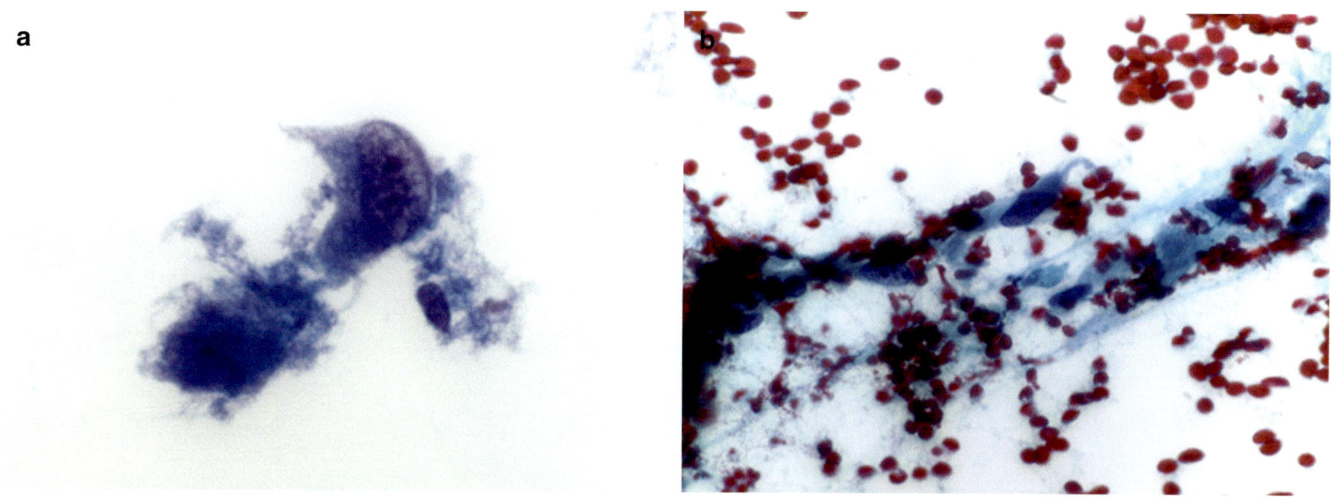

Fig. 1.11 (**a**, **b**) Background. (**a**) A case of anaplastic carcinoma of thyroid shows "clinging" diathesis in TP. The necrosis forms granular clumps and clings to tumor cells which makes tumor cells stand out. (**b**) In the CS from the same case, the tumor cells are embedded in the necrosis which compromises cell detail (**a**, **b**, Pap stain)

produces thinner monolayered preparations. More 3-D configuration is noticeable in SP. LBP shows all cell distribution patterns as seen in CS (Fig. 1.12a, b).

Architectural Features

- Honeycomb sheets, macrofollicles, microfollicles, syncytial fragments, three-dimensional (3-D) clusters, branching sheets, and papillary formations are all retained in LBP (Figs. 1.13a–d and 1.14a, b).
- Smaller macrofollicles may be seen.
- 3-D clusters are present and are easy to evaluate (Fig. 1.14c).
- Fragmentation of large sheets occurs (particularly in TP), especially branching sheets and complex papillary groups. See examples of fragmentation of sheets in benign follicular nodules in TP and PTC in SP. This increased fragmentation may be beneficial for observing the nuclear features of PTC, without affecting proper interpretation (Figs. 1.15a–e and 1.16a–d).
- 3-D cellular fragments are flatter in TP and allow for better observation of nuclear and cytoplasmic characteristics of follicular cell clusters. The flattening of cells clusters may be the result of the positive air-pressure applied during transfer of cells to the glass slide.
- In SP, balling up of cells with greater depth of focus, smaller strips of cells, more complex 3-D and branch-

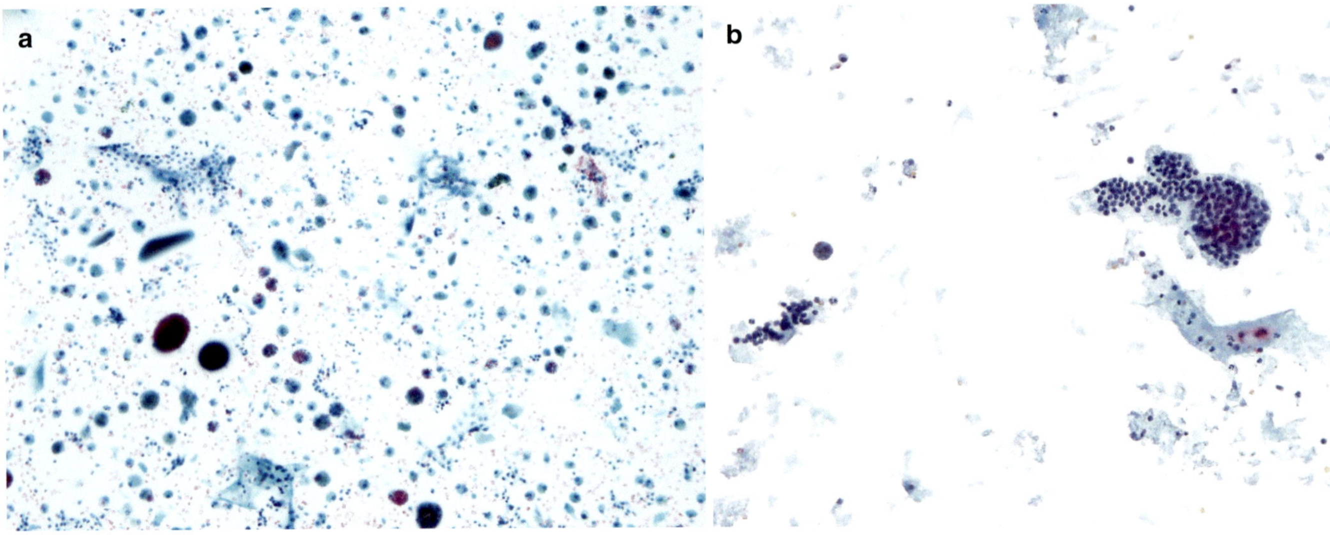

Fig. 1.12 (**a**, **b**) Cellularity and cell distribution. (**a**) Nodular goiter processed as SP shows small flat sheets of follicular cells, cyst-lining cells, hemosiderin-laden macrophages and thick and thin colloid. Note that cells appear in different planes of focus. (**b**) Same case processed as TP shows similar features to SP, except the preparation is more monolayered (**a**, **b**, Pap stain)

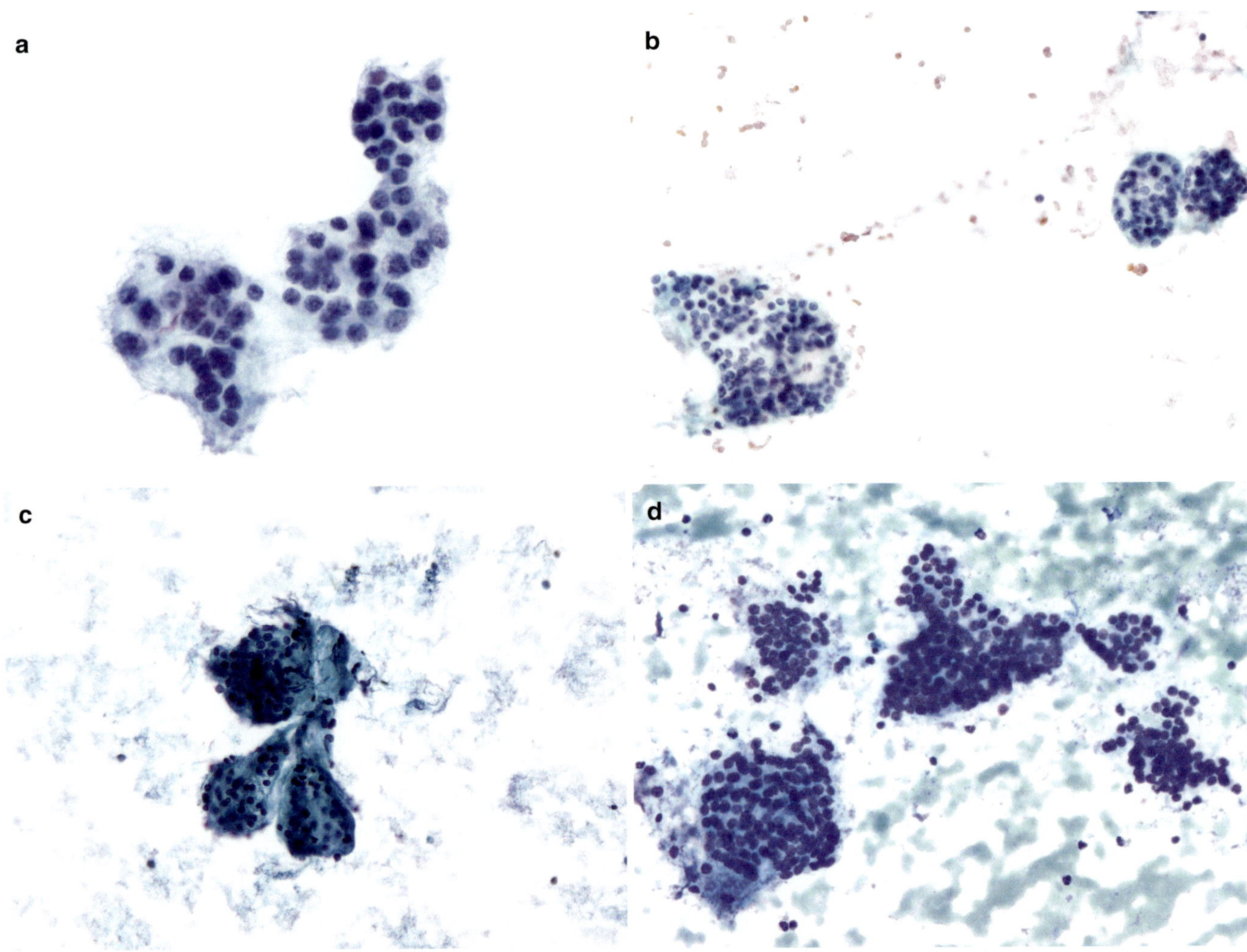

Fig. 1.13 (**a–d**) Architectural features. (**a**, **b**) TP shows aggregates and single macrofollicles in two different cases of benign thyroid nodules. Note uniform small and round nuclei and low N:C ratio. (**c**) Aggregates of macrofollicles in SP from a benign thyroid nodule. Background shows abundant colloid. Nuclear morphology is well-preserved and similar to TP (**a–c**, Pap stain). (**d**) CS from same case as the SP shows similar morphology of follicular cells (DQ stain)

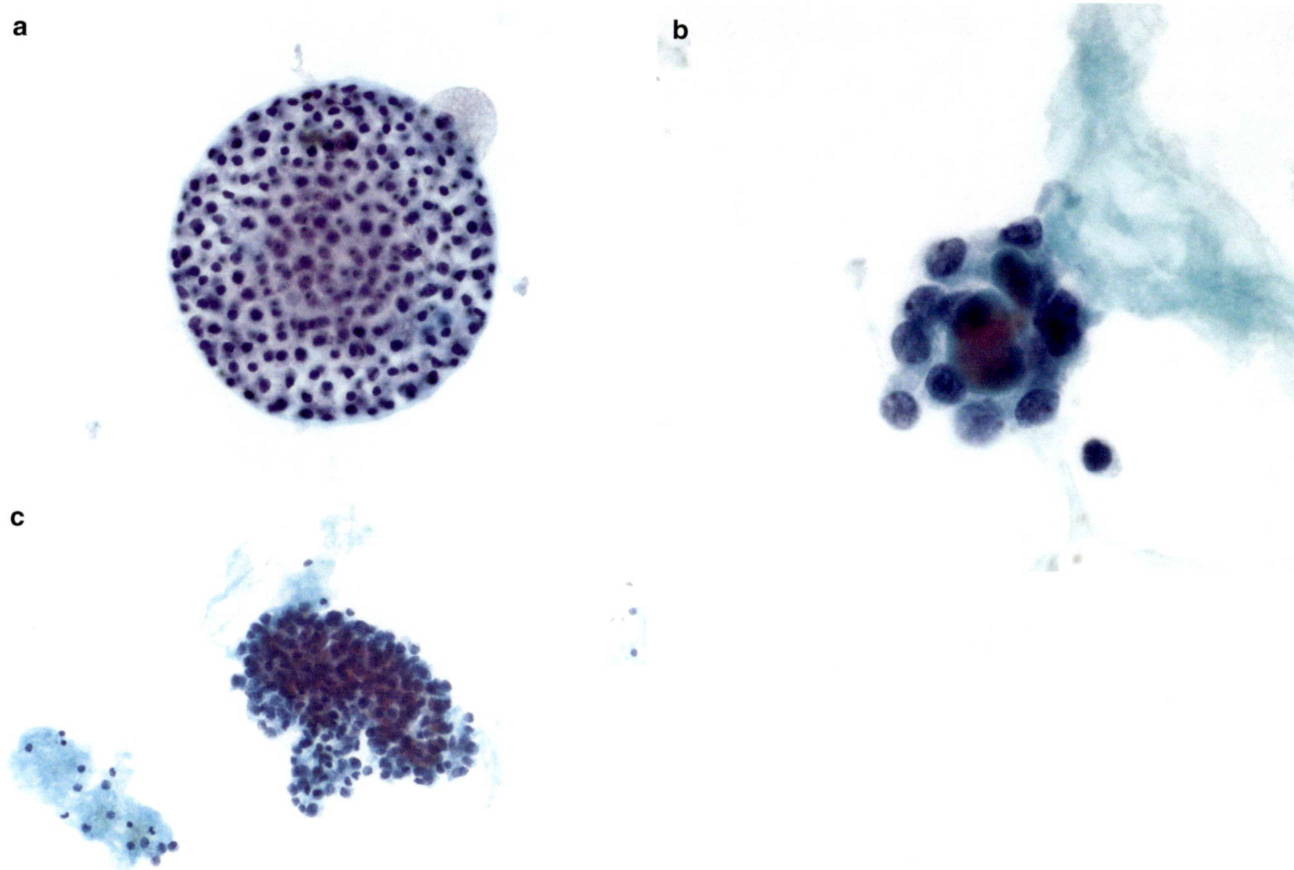

Fig. 1.14 (**a–c**) Architectural features. (**a**) Perfectly round macrofollicle commonly seen in TP from a benign thyroid nodule. (**b**) Microfollicle in TP from a case diagnosed as FLUS. Note nuclear enlargement, slight overlap, irregularity and nucleoli. (**c**) TP shows a 3D cluster from a case diagnosed as SFCN. Even though the cells are crowded, morphology is easy to evaluate (**a–c**, Pap stain)

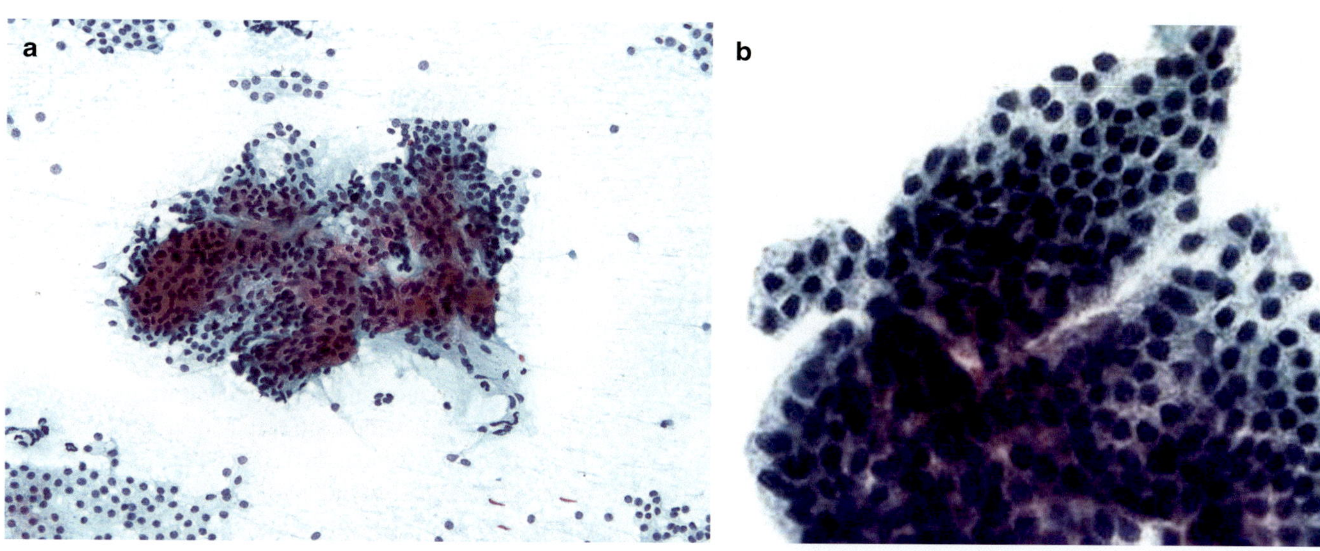

Fig. 1.15 (**a–e**) Architectural features. (**a**) Nodular hyperplasia showing a large flat and branching sheet in a CS. (**b–e**) Same case processed as a TP has retained large flat and branching sheets and also shows fragmentation of large sheets. The latter is more common in LBP (particularly in TP) (**a–e**, Pap stain)

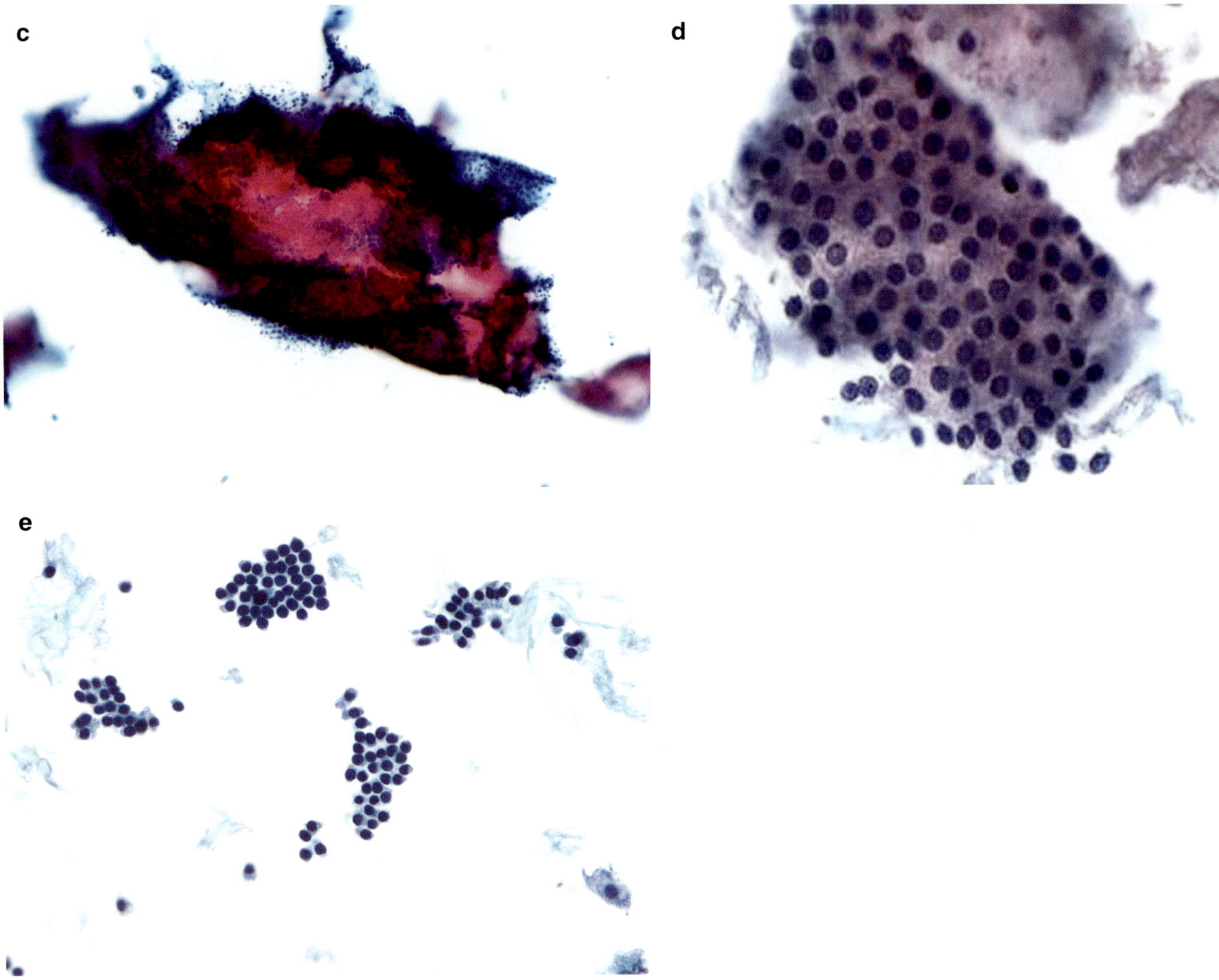

Fig. 1.15 (continued)

ing fragments, more single cells, and apparent cellular elongation are seen. SP slides tend to retain large tissue fragments, colloid, and lymphocytes. Cell clusters appear more three-dimensional and may be difficult to assess at higher magnification. Moreover, in SP, both single cells and clusters are present in different planes of focus, which requires constant focus adjustment during slide review at higher magnification. These alterations probably result from multiple centrifugation steps and from allowing the cells to settle under the influence of gravity during SP processing (*see* Figs. 1.13c and 1.17).

Cytology

- Cellular and nuclear details are better preserved and enhanced in LBP.
- Cytoplasmic quality and intracytoplasmic structures and material are retained, including pigment, vacuoles, and other elements.
- Nuclei tend to appear smaller in LBP, but the nuclear details, including the nuclear membrane irregularity, chromatin texture, and nucleoli, are more accentuated and easily observed. The nuclear size may be larger in SP than in TP.
- Nucleoli appear prominent and cherry-red in neoplastic lesions and may even be prominent in benign cells. To avoid misinterpretation, it is best to evaluate other nuclear features of malignancy, including nuclear irregularity and chromatin changes, which are retained in LBP. Nuclear membrane irregularity may be less obvious in SP.
- In cases of benign thyroid nodule, large colloid fragments, thin tissue paper–like colloid, cystic change, and monolayered sheets of follicular cells are retained in LBP. Nuclear membranes are uniform, and chromatin is fine, uniform, and pale.

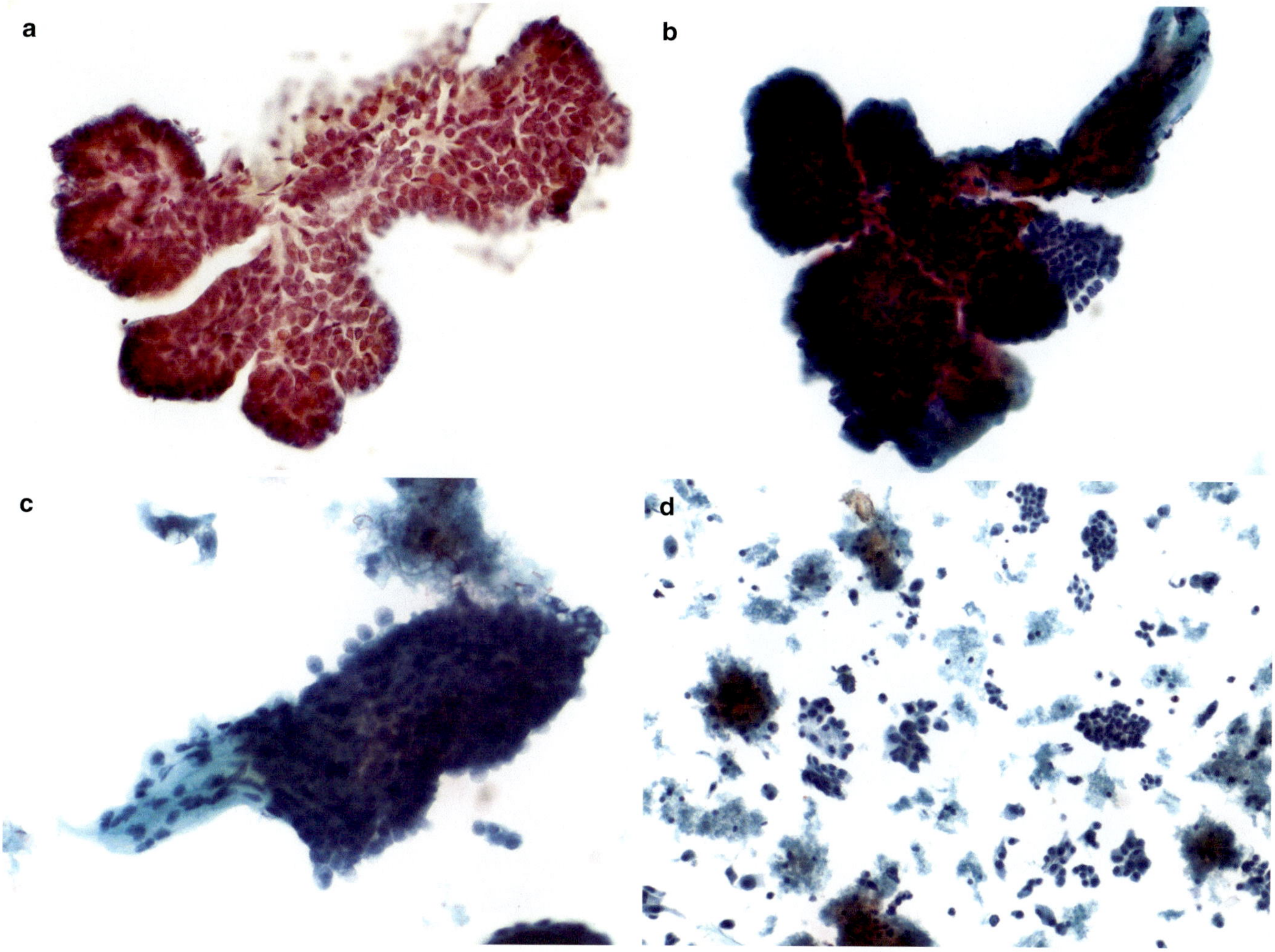

Fig. 1.16 (**a–d**) Architectural features. (**a**) PTC in a CS showing a well-formed papillary structure with a fibrovascular core. Nuclear features of PTC can be appreciated. (**b**) Same case of PTC processed a TP has retained a complex papillary structure. (**c**, **d**) Few other papillary structures were fragmentated into smaller, less complex forms and into smaller sheets and single cells. This case was cellular and basically showed mixed architectural patterns of PTC (**a–d**, Pap stain)

- Diagnosis of Hashimoto's thyroiditis may be more difficult than on CS (particularly in TP), because of the limited number of lymphocytes.
- In cases of PTC, all nuclear features of PTC are preserved, including nuclear irregularity, grooves, and ground-glass nuclei. Intranuclear pseudoinclusions (INPI), although easily identified, may be reduced. In SP, nuclear membrane irregularity and grooves may be less obvious (Fig. 1.18a, b).
- Hobnail features in PTC are often associated with well-defined cytoplasmic border and vacuole, and background macrophages (Fig. 1.18c).
- In cases of follicular neoplasm, the nucleus appears regular with nucleoli (Fig. 1.18d).
- Large oncocytic cells with a dyscohesive or isolated cell pattern are more common in malignant oncocytic/Hürthle cell neoplasms. The cytoplasm may appear pale, with fine pale granules, or rarified or dense (Figs. 1.18e, f). The granules are more blue on CS.
- Psammoma bodies are retained (Fig. 1.18g).

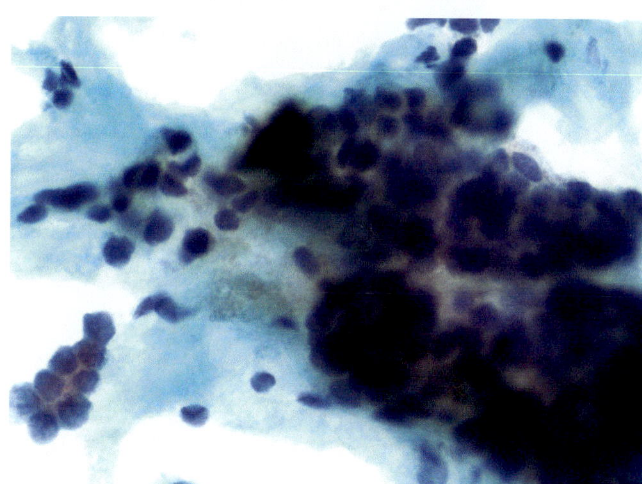

Fig. 1.17 Architectural features. SP from a case of PTC shows a large tissue fragment with balling up of cells with greater depth of focus, smaller strips of cells, more complex 3-D and branching fragments single cells, and apparent cellular elongation. Cell clusters appear more 3D and are present in different planes of focus (Pap stain)

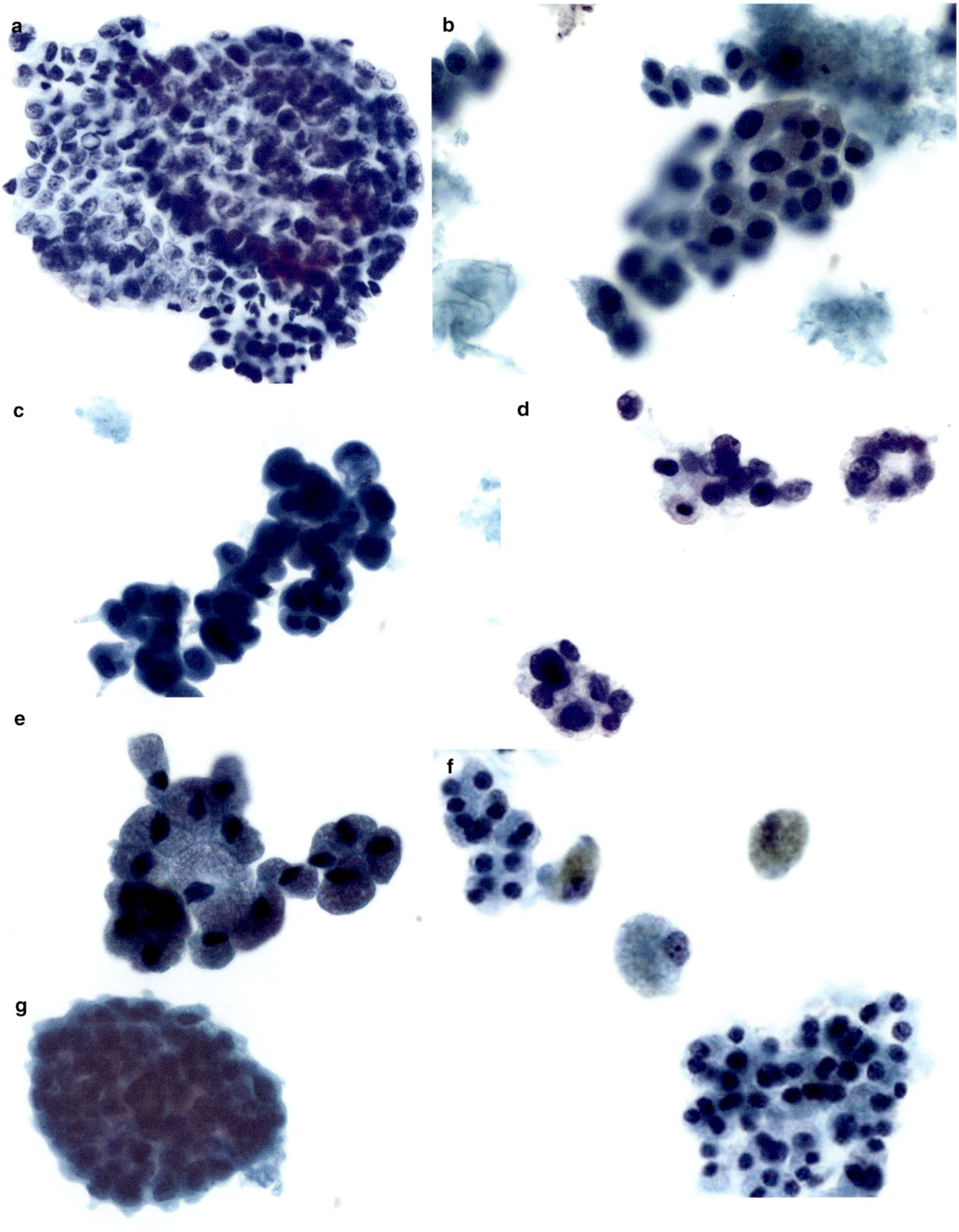

Fig. 1.18 (**a–g**) Cytology**.** TP (**a**) and SP (**b**) from a case of PTC, all nuclear features of PTC are preserved, including nuclear irregularity, grooves, and ground-glass nuclei. Intranuclear pseudoinclusions (INPI). In SP, the nuclear membrane irregularity and grooves are less obvious (**a**, **b**, Pap stain). (**c**) SP from a case of PTC with Hobnail features show well-defined cytoplasmic borders and vacuoles (Pap stain). (**d**) TP from a case of follicular neoplasm, shows regular and overlapping nuclei with nucleoli (Pap stain). (**e**, **f**) TP from two cases of Hürthle cell neoplasms show large oncocytic cells with a dyscohesive or isolated cell pattern. Nuclei are small to enlarged with small to prominent nucleoli. The cytoplasm appears pale, with fine pink granules, or rarified or dense (Pap stain). (**g**) Psammoma body within a cluster of PTC cells (TP, Pap stain)

Salient Differences in Cytomorphology Between SP and TP

- SP retains more background elements such as blood and colloid.
- In SP, cells are deposited in different planes of focus, so constant focusing is required for evaluation of cells at high magnification. In TP, cells are in a monolayer and in one plane.
- In SP, clusters of cells are more three-dimensional and round up. All cells in a group may not be focused. Cells may also become elongated, owing to multiple vortex steps during preparation. In TP, the clusters of cells appear flattened; all cells are in focus but retain a 3-D appearance.
- SP may show higher cellularity than TP.
- Large sheets, complex branching fragments, and papillary structures do become fragmented in LBP, but they are retained and are easily visible. SP may show less fragmentation.
- In SP, the lumens of microfollicular structures may not be visible, or they may become visible only after focusing in a different plane. In TP, lumens of microfollicles are easily visualized.

Summary of Cytomorphological Alterations in LBP

- Background material is reduced or altered.
- Well-preserved cells are evenly distributed.
- Smaller cell clusters and more single cells are seen.
- Cells are generally smaller, with occasional elongation.
- Chromatin detail may be attenuated.
- Nucleoli are prominent even in benign lesions.
- Intranuclear pseudoinclusions (INPI) may be reduced or difficult to visualize.

Residual LBP Specimen

- Residual sample in LBP vials can be stored at room temperature for up to 6 months for TP and 3 months for SP.
- Residual sample can be used for processing additional slides for review and for immunocytochemistry. Laboratories need to validate immunocytochemistry on LBP.
- Residual sample can also be processed as a cell block. Cellient (Hologic, Marlborough, MA) is a new automated cell block processing machine based on centrifugation and filtration, which can capture cells from low-cellularity specimens. (*See* Chap. 3.)

Advantages of LBP

- No significant differences between LBP and CS in any quality indicators
- Low false-negative rate. An accurate preoperative cytologic diagnosis of thyroid nodules allows for better selection of patients for surgery and reduces the number of unnecessary thyroidectomies.
- Ease of sample submission by the clinician, as the aspirated sample is directly rinsed in liquid collection medium with decreased needle handling, no slide labeling, and no triage of specimen for smears and cell block
- Uniform specimen collection, with theoretical collection of 100% of the sample
- Preferred methods of preparation when a cytologist is not present at FNA for rendering ROSE. Yet ROSE can be performed with part of the sample. (*See* Chap. 3.)
- Convenient transportation from all locations
- Standardized, automated processing techniques, which produce a homogenized sample with uniform and even cell distribution, with minimal thick areas and cellular overlap. TP preparation technique is simple and less labor-intensive.
- Reproducibility, with less variability in specimen preservation, staining, and quality
- Less cell loss than with cytospins, which require multiple slides to counter the loss of cells during preparation
- Reduced labor cost because one slide is easier to screen and there are few or no artifacts
- Increased productivity because of screening of one slide rather than two to 10 with CS
- Cost-effective because of decreased screening time due to smaller and well-defined screening area (TP, 20 mm; SP, 13 mm)
- Adequate cell preservation and better visualization of cells owing to rapid fixation
- Good preservation of cell types and cellular arrangements
- Better appreciation of cytomorphology because obscuring background is reduced
- Clean background leads to better appreciation of cytomorphology and fewer inadequate or unsatisfactory specimens because obscuring background elements are reduced. Blood is the most common obscuring element and CytoRich™ for SP collection is more effective in reducing blood than CytoLyt® for TP collection. These features also make LBP more cost-effective as repeat FNA is avoided.
- Better nuclear preservation due to immediate liquid fixation, resulting in high diagnostic accuracy
- Cytologic features of malignancy are retained.

- Ability to perform ancillary testing, immunocytohistochemistry (ICC), and molecular testing by processing additional slides from the residual material

Disadvantages of LBP

- Requirement for special collection media and processing equipment
- Experience and learning curve required for interpretation
- Slightly longer specimen processing time than with CS
- Reduction or alteration of background material. The cleaner background may remove abundant thin colloid, necrosis and other materials that may be helpful in diagnosis.
- Colloid film and the lymphocytic component are more easily evaluated on CS. In TP, lymphocytes are reduced. In SP, neutrophils and lymphocytes from the lysed blood may give a false assessment of inflammatory lesions.
- Quantity of colloid and ratio of follicular cells to colloid cannot be assessed. Generally, the cytologic assessment of follicular lesions of the thyroid is based on evaluation of the amount of colloid and the number of follicular cells. Usually, more colloid and fewer follicular cells favor a benign lesion; more cells and less colloid favor a neoplastic lesion. This approach may not be applicable when using LBP, necessitating a closer evaluation of cytologic and architectural features of the lesion.
- A potential pitfall is the presence of thin, watery colloid as "tissue paper–like material," which can be missed by a pathologist unfamiliar with it.
- More unsatisfactory samples in cystic lesions.
- Morphological artifacts, including decreased presence of colloid and disaggregation of larger fragments, clusters, and macrofollicles.
- Reduction in well-formed papillary structures. Fragmentation of papillae may be seen, resulting in smaller/rudimentary papillae, cell groups, and slightly more dyscohesion of cells.
- Cells appear more shrunken, crowded, three-dimensional, and as tight clusters with loss of cellular preservation within the center of the larger aggregates, increased disruption of the cytoplasm of the follicular cells, and more naked nuclei. In SP, multiple processing steps and settling of cells under the influence of gravity results in cellular elongation, cells in different planes of focus, and increased 3-D appearance.
- Lymphocytes may be seen without other features of chronic thyroiditis (such as Hürthle cell metaplasia, plasma cells, and histiocytes). This appears to be a result of lysis of red blood cells in bloody samples, leaving many lymphocytes without follicular cells. This may be a diagnostic pitfall.
- In TP, peripheral rim artifact occasionally compresses cells at the periphery and can potentially influence cell morphology. The size of the nucleus and cytoplasm may be overestimated and misinterpreted as atypical large cells; the nuclei may appear more indistinct and hypochromatic, and nucleoli may appear less distinct or larger and more prominent.

Summary

- Based on the review of existing literature, LBP are a valid alternative to CS. A learning curve is essential to become familiar with the altered cytomorphology in the LBP, but indeterminate diagnoses and workload are both reduced, while accuracy is maintained.
- Although LBP are more expensive than CS, the sample adequacy of LBP is statistically superior to CS because the LBP slide is representative of the entire aspirated sample. In CS, part of the diagnostic sample may be discarded with the collection device. This feature also makes LBP more cost-effective, as a repeat FNA is not needed.
- LBP are superior to CS with regard to cleaner background, standardized preparation, and cell preservation.
- LBP—particularly TP—has the potential to be used as the sole preparation for FNA of thyroid. Currently, the SP method can supplement CS but cannot replace it.
- LBP are easier and less time-consuming to screen because the cells are concentrated in a smaller area without obscuring elements.
- Artifacts of CS are not present in LBP.
- Background elements, although retained in LBP, do not obscure cell detail.
- The sensitivity and specificity of LBP are similar to CS.
- Apart from slight morphologic differences between CS and LBP, the typical features of benign, neoplastic, and malignant lesions can be clearly evaluated with LBP.
- Additional LBP from the residual material in collection media can be used for further slides for review and for adjunctive testing such as immunocytochemistry.
- Because of the differing preparatory techniques involved and the morphologic differences between CS and LBP, the LBP require a learning period and experience for correct interpretation. Familiarity with the morphologic differences is important, to avoid diagnostic pitfalls.
- Once familiarity with the different diagnostic criteria for benign and malignant lesions on LBP has been achieved, the diagnostic accuracy in diagnosing thyroid cytology is enhanced.
- The advantages of LBP make them worth the effort.

Suggested Reading

1. Ali SZ, Cibas ES. The Bethesda system for reporting thyroid cytopathology; definitions, criteria, and explanatory notes. 2nd ed. Cham: Springer International Publishing AG; 2018.
2. American Cancer Society. Key statistics for thyroid cancer. 2019. https://www.cancer.org/cancer/thyroid-cancer/about/key-statistics.html. Accessed 14 Mar 2019.
3. Bessey LJ, Lai NBK, Coorough NE, Chen H, Sippel RS. The incidence of thyroid cancer by FNA varies by age and gender. J Surg Res. 2013;184:761–5. https://doi.org/10.1016/j.jss.2013.03.086.
4. Chang H, Lee E, Lee H, Choi J, Kim A, Kim BH. Comparison of diagnostic values of thyroid aspiration samples using liquid-based preparation and conventional smear: one-year experience in a single institution. APMIS. 2013;121:139–45. https://doi.org/10.1111/j.1600-0463.2012.02944.x.
5. Chong Y, Ji SJ, Kang CS, Lee EJ. Can liquid-based preparation substitute for conventional smear in thyroid fine-needle aspiration? A systematic review based on meta-analysis. Endocr Connect. 2017;6:817–29. https://doi.org/10.1530/EC-17-0165.
6. Cibas ES, Ali SZ. The 2017 Bethesda system for reporting thyroid cytopathology. Thyroid. 2017;27:1341–6. https://doi.org/10.1089/thy.2017.0500.
7. Cochand-Priollet B, Prat JJ, Polivka M, Thienpont L, Dahan H, Wassef M, et al. Thyroid fine needle aspiration: the morphological features on ThinPrep slide preparations. Eighty cases with histological control. Cytopathology. 2003;14:343–9.
8. Duncan LD, Forrest L, Law WM Jr, Hubbard E, Stewart LE. Evaluation of thyroid fine-needle aspirations: can ThinPrep be used exclusively to appropriately triage patients having a thyroid nodule? Diagn Cytopathol. 2011;39:341–8. https://doi.org/10.1002/dc.21392.
9. Fischer AH, Clayton AC, Bentz JS, Wasserman PG, Henry MR, Souers RJ, et al. Performance differences between conventional smears and liquid-based preparations of thyroid fine-needle aspiration samples: analysis of 47,076 responses in the College of American Pathologists Interlaboratory Comparison Program in Non-Gynecologic Cytology. Arch Pathol Lab Med. 2013;137:26–31. https://doi.org/10.5858/arpa.2012-0009-CP.
10. Geers C, Bourgain C. Liquid-based FNAC of the thyroid: a 4-year survey with SurePath. Cancer Cytopathol. 2011;119:58–67. https://doi.org/10.1002/cncy.20125.
11. Hoda RS. Non-gynecologic cytology on liquid-based preparations: a morphologic review of facts and artifacts. Diagn Cytopathol. 2007;35:621–34.
12. Hoda RS, VandenBussche C, Hoda SA. Diagnostic liquid-based cytology. New York: Springer; 2017.
13. Isik A, Firat D, Yilmaz I, Peker K, Idiz O, Yilmaz B, et al. A survey of current approaches to thyroid nodules and thyroid operations. Int J Surg. 2018;28:100–4. https://doi.org/10.1016/j.ijsu.2018.04.037.
14. Kim SY, Kim EK, Moon HJ, Yoon JH, Kwon HJ, Song MK, et al. Combined use of conventional smear and liquid-based preparation versus conventional smear for thyroid fine-needle aspiration. Endocrine. 2016;53:157–65. https://doi.org/10.1007/s12020-015-0835-z.
15. Langer JE, Baloch ZW, McGrath C, Loevner LA, Mandel SJ. Thyroid nodule fine-needle aspiration. Semin Ultrasound CT MR. 2012;33:158–65. https://doi.org/10.1053/j.sult.2011.12.002.
16. Luu MH, Fischer AH, Pisharodi L, Owens CL. Improved preoperative definitive diagnosis of papillary thyroid carcinoma in FNAs prepared with both ThinPrep and conventional smears compared with FNAs prepared with ThinPrep alone. Cancer Cytopathol. 2011;119:68–73. https://doi.org/10.1002/cncy.20124.
17. Michael CW, Hunter B. Interpretation of fine-needle aspirates processed by the ThinPrep technique: Cytologic artifacts and diagnostic pitfalls. Diagn Cytopathol. 2000;23:6–13.
18. Michael CW, McConnel J, Pecott J, Afify AM, Al-Khafaji B. Comparison of ThinPrep and TriPath PREP liquid-based preparations in nongynecologic specimens: a pilot study. Diagn Cytopathol. 2001;25:177–84.
19. Moss W, Finegersh A, Pang J, Califano JA, Coffey CS, Orosco R, et al. Needle biopsy of routine thyroid nodules should be performed using a capillary action technique with 24-27 gauge needles: a systematic review and meta-analysis. Thyroid. 2018;28:857–63. https://doi.org/10.1089/thy.2017.0643.
20. Nasuti JF, Tam D, Gupta PK. Diagnostic value of liquid-based (ThinPrep) preparations in nongynecologic cases. Diagn Cytopathol 2001;24:137–141.
21. Nagarajan N, Schneider EB, Ali SZ, Zeiger MA, Olson MT. How do liquid-based preparations of thyroid fine-needle aspiration compare with conventional smears? An analysis of 5475 specimens. Thyroid. 2015;25:308–13. https://doi.org/10.1089/thy.2014.0394.
22. Rosa M. Cytologic features of subacute granulomatous thyroiditis can mimic malignancy in liquid-based preparations. Diagn Cytopathol. 2016;44:682–4. https://doi.org/10.1002/dc.23495.
23. Rossi ED, Morassi F, Santeusanio G, Zannoni GF, Fadda G. Thyroid fine needle aspiration cytology processed by ThinPrep: an additional slide decreased the number of inadequate results. Cytopathology. 2010;21:97–102. https://doi.org/10.1111/j.1365-2303.2009.00659.x.
24. Rossi ED, Raffaelli M, Zannoni GF, Pontecorvi A, Mulè A, Callà C, et al. Diagnostic efficacy of conventional as compared to liquid-based cytology in thyroid lesions: evaluation of 10,360 fine needle aspiration cytology cases. Acta Cytol. 2009;53:659–66.
25. Rossi ED, Schmitt F. When morphology meets somatic mutations: the new possible scenario in thyroid fine-needle aspiration. Acta Cytol. 2016;60:93–6. https://doi.org/10.1159/000446796.
26. Suzuki A, Hirokawa M, Higuchi M, Takada N, Yamao N, Kuma S, et al. Differentiating between benign follicular nodules and follicular neoplasms in thyroid liquid-based cytology preparations. Diagn Cytopathol. 2016;44:659–64. https://doi.org/10.1002/dc.23500.
27. Tulecke MA, Wang HH. ThinPrep for cytologic evaluation of follicular thyroid lesions: correlation with histologic findings. Diagn Cytopathol. 2004;30:7–13.
28. Weeks KS, Kahl AR, Lynch CF, Charlton ME. Racial/ethnic differences in thyroid cancer incidence in the United States, 2007-2014. Cancer. 2018;124:1483–91. https://doi.org/10.1002/cncr.31229.
29. Yassa L, Cibas ES, Benson CB, Frates MC, Doubilet PM, Gawande AA, et al. Long-term assessment of a multidisciplinary approach to thyroid nodule diagnostic evaluation. Cancer. 2007;111:508–16.

The Second Edition Bethesda System for Reporting Thyroid Cytopathology

2

Rana S. Hoda

The Bethesda System for Reporting Thyroid Cytopathology (TBSRTC)

- The Bethesda System for Reporting Thyroid Cytopathology (TBSRTC), a uniform and standardized reporting system for thyroid fine needle aspiration (FNA), was originally established in 2009 and updated in 2017. The system is widely accepted in the United States and globally.
- It is specifically designed for the reporting of thyroid follicular and C-cell–derived lesions based on clearly outlined diagnostic criteria.
- The succinct and unambiguous reports and clarity of communication allows clinicians to manage their patients based on recommended clinical management guidelines.
- The 2nd Edition of TBSRTC retained the original six diagnostic categories, which span the spectrum of benign and malignant thyroid lesions and the indeterminate diagnoses (Table 2.1). (From this point, "TBSRTC" in this atlas refers to the 2nd Edition.)
- Three categories are "indeterminate for malignancy":
  - Atypia of Undetermined Significance or Follicular Lesion of Undetermined Significance (AUS/FLUS)
  - Follicular Neoplasm or Suspicious for a Follicular Neoplasm (FN/SFN)
  - Suspicious for Malignancy (SM)
- FN/SFN includes a category of Hürthle cell (oncocytic) lesions, entitled FNHCT or SFNHCT.
- A non-thyroid entity presenting as a thyroid nodule, such as a parathyroid gland, is also reported using TBSRTC categories.
- Each TBSRTC diagnostic category is associated with an implied risk of malignancy (ROM) based on an analysis of the available literature, and each translates directly into a clinical management algorithm (Table 2.2).

R. S. Hoda (✉)
CBLPath, Rye Brook, NY, USA
e-mail: rhoda@cblpath.com

Table 2.1 Recommended diagnostic categories for the second edition Bethesda system for reporting thyroid cytopathology

I.	Nondiagnostic or Unsatisfactory[a, b]
II.	Benign
III.	Atypia of Undetermined Significance or Follicular Lesion of Undetermined Significance[b]
IV.	Follicular Neoplasm or Suspicious for a Follicular Neoplasm[a] (Specify if Hürthle cell [oncocytic] type)
V.	Suspicious for Malignancy
VI.	Malignant

Modified from Ali and Cibas [1]; with permission
[a]Adequacy criteria are the same for conventional smears (CS) and LBP
[b]The two terms for these categories are synonymous. A laboratory should choose the one it prefers and use it exclusively for that category

Updates in TBSRTC

- The 2nd edition of TBSRTC was unveiled in light of many recent advances and developments in the field of thyroid disease:
  - The category of Noninvasive Follicular Thyroid Neoplasm with Papillary-like Nuclear Features (NIFTP) was introduced and has led to an increased use of the indeterminate categories and changes in the TBSRTC-implied ROM for various categories.
  - In 2015, the American Thyroid Association (ATA) updated the management guidelines for adult patients with thyroid nodules and differentiated thyroid cancer and incorporated the role of molecular testing for management [10]. The ATA has endorsed TBSRTC
  - Ultrasound (US)–based risk stratification systems for thyroid nodules have been improved, including 2015 ATA guidelines [9], 2016 Korean Thyroid Association (KTA)/Korean Society of Thyroid Radiology (KSThR) guidelines [21], and the new 2017 American College of Radiology (ACR) guidelines [23].
  - The use of liquid-based preparations (LBP) for thyroid cytology has increased.

R. S. Hoda et al. (eds.), *Atlas of Thyroid Cytopathology on Liquid-Based Preparations*,
https://doi.org/10.1007/978-3-030-25066-9_2

Table 2.2 TBSRTC: updates in the implied risk of malignancy (ROM) and recommended clinical management

Diagnostic category	2009 ROM, %	2017 ROM, %	2017 ROM with NIFTP, %	Usual management,[c] 2017	Optional note, 2017
Nondiagnostic or Unsatisfactory (ND/Unsat)	1–4	5–10	No significant change	Solid nodules, repeat FNA with US; cystic nodules correlated with US. Re-aspiration, if clinically indicated	None
Benign	0–3	0–3	No significant change	Clinical & US follow-up at intervals of 6–18 mon for 3–5 y	None
Atypia of Undetermined Significance or Follicular Lesion of Undetermined Significance (AUS/FLUS)	~5–15	10–30	6–18	Repeat FNA or molecular test	None
Follicular Neoplasm or Suspicious for a Follicular Neoplasm (FN/SFN)	15–30	25–40	10–40	Molecular test or lobectomy	Histopathologic follow-up usually show follicular adenoma, follicular carcinoma, and follicular variant of papillary thyroid carcinoma (FVPTC), including its recently described indolent counterpart, NIFTP.
Suspicious for Malignancy (SM)	60–75	50–75	45–60	Total thyroidectomy or lobectomy[a,b]	Suspicious for FVPTC and NIFTP; definitive distinction not possible on cytological material
Malignant (PMC)	97–99	97–99	94–96	Surgical consultation for-total thyroidectomy[b]	About 3–4% of cases diagnosed as PTC may prove to be NIFTP on histopathological examination, reducing the PPV of the Malignant category from 99% to about 94–96%.

Modified from Ali and Cibas [1]; with permission

NIFTP noninvasive follicular thyroid neoplasm with papillary-like nuclear features, *PMC* positive for malignant cells, *PPV* positive predictive value, *US* ultrasound

[a]Some studies recommend molecular analysis to assess the type of surgical procedure

[b]Management decision may vary for metastatic and lymphoid tumors

[c]Actual management may depend on other factors (e.g., clinical, sonographic) besides the FNA interpretation

  - Information and knowledge of molecular pathology of thyroid disease has vastly increased in the past few years. Thyroid molecular testing is increasingly being used in conjunction with indeterminate cytologic diagnoses. Molecular testing enhances the sensitivity of cytologic diagnosis and leads to more informed and better patient management.
- Specific updates in the TBSRTC reflect many of these advances:
  - Proper use of diagnostic category terminology
    - Three TBSRTC categories have two names each: ND/Unsat, AUS/FLUS, and FN/SFN. These terms are synonymous and should not be used interchangeably or to denote two distinct interpretations.
    - TBSRTC recommends that only one term should be applied to each category.
  - Nondiagnostic or Unsatisfactory (ND/Unsat) category with "Cyst fluid (macrophages) only"
    - These cases should be reported as ND/Unsat with an explanatory note.
    - The 2015 ATA guidelines has updated the management recommendation for ND/Unsat samples including cystic lesions. They recommend that if a nodule shows an initial ND/Unsat cytology result, FNA should be repeated with US guidance and, if available, with rapid on-site evaluation (ROSE).
  - Recommended interval to repeat FNA for ND/Unsat cases
    - Originally, the recommendation was to wait for >3 months to repeat FNA, to allow biopsy-related reactive changes to subside.
    - TBSRTC permits shorter interval times, though the potential for reactive atypia and cellular changes remains.
  - Increasing use of LBP
    - TBSRTC acknowledges the increasing use of LBP for processing of thyroid FNA specimens, and provides more examples of LBP cases and comparison with conventional smears (CS) for various entities.
  - AUS/FLUS category, with subcategorization of AUS/FLUS
    - AUS and FLUS are synonymous terms; each laboratory should use only one term.
    - The use of *AUS* for cases with nuclear atypia, *FLUS* for cases with architectural atypia, and *AUS/FLUS*

to denote that both types of atypia are present is discouraged.
    - Subcategorization for the AUS/FLUS category is recommended to help guide management. (*See* Chap. 5)
- Risk of malignancy (ROM)
    - Implied ROM in TBSRTC is based upon a selected group of studies that included large cohorts of cases or meta-analyses (*see* Table 2.2).
    - The introduction of NIFTP has had the most significant impact on ROM.
- Inclusion of newly described entities, including mammary secretory analogue of thyroid gland, which is a primary thyroid carcinoma harboring *ETV6-NTRK3* fusion.
- Expanded differential diagnoses for various lesions (as covered in later chapters)
- Optional notes, comments, and recommendation can be given for some categories such as FN/SFN, SM, or Malignant. (*See* Table 2.2.)
    - A note would be most useful in cases with cytologic features of papillary thyroid carcinoma (PTC) but a follicular architecture, indicating that the differential diagnosis includes follicular variant of papillary thyroid carcinoma (FVPTC) or its indolent counterpart, NIFTP. The cytologic diagnosis alone or in conjunction with molecular testing will help guide clinical management.
    - An optional note is also recommended for metastatic tumors and lymphomas.
- Molecular testing (*See* Chap. 15)
    - Currently, three molecular tests are commercially available for use as an adjunct to cytology: ThyGenX®/ThyraMIR™ combination test (Interpace Diagnostics Group, Parsippany, NJ); Afirma® Genomic Sequencing Classifier (GSC), (Veracyte, South San Francisco, CA); and ThyroSeq® v3 genomic classifier (CBLPath, Rye Brook, NY, and University of Pittsburgh Medical Center, Pittsburgh, PA).
    - The tests, when used for the 15–30% of samples of indeterminate cytology, further enhance the accuracy of the preoperative cytologic diagnosis and can be recommended for management.
    - Tests are also useful in follicular-patterned lesions such as NIFTP.
- Intra-laboratory quality control monitoring
    - TBSRTC recommends regular quality assurance (QA) monitoring for laboratories, to prevent overuse of the AUS/FLUS category, which should not exceed 10%.
    - Continuous cytohistologic correlation is also essential to maintain quality.
    - Continuous correlation of cytology and molecular test results also should be instituted.

Modifications in TBSRTC

- Use "oncocytic" instead of "Hürthle cell" in FN/SFN category.
- Suggests to diagnose PTC only when the following features of classic PTC are present:
    - True papillae
    - Psammoma bodies
    - Frequent inclusions; Krane et al. [14] recommend >3 intranuclear pseudoinclusions (INPI) to establish a diagnosis of PTC.

Ultrasonographic Patterns for Risk Stratification of Thyroid Nodules for FNA

- Certain sonographic features of a thyroid nodule are associated with an increased ROM, but no single predictor has been found to have a high positive predictive value (PPV) for cancer.
- Many professional societies have published guidelines to aid in the selection of thyroid nodules for US-guided FNA (USGFNA), including the 2015 ATA guidelines [9], 2016 Korean Thyroid Association (KTA)/Korean Society of Thyroid Radiology (KSThR) guidelines [21], and the new 2017 American College of Radiology (ACR) guidelines [23].
- These guidelines recommend that only nodules with suspicious or high-risk US characteristics be aspirated.
- High-risk characteristics of a thyroid nodule on US include a solid or hypoechoic nodule or a solid and hypoechoic component of a partially cystic nodule with one or more of the following features: irregular margins, taller-than-wide morphology, microcalcifications, disrupted rim calcifications, and extra-thyroidal extension (ETE).

Suggested Reading

1. Ali SZ, Cibas ES. The Bethesda system for reporting thyroid cytopathology; definitions, criteria, and explanatory notes. 2nd ed. Cham: Springer International Publishing AG; 2018.
2. Ali SZ, Cibas ES. The Bethesda system for reporting thyroid cytopathology II. Acta Cytol. 2016;60:397–8.
3. Bychkov A, Keelawat S, Agarwal S, Jain D, Jung CK, Hong S, et al. Impact of non-invasive follicular thyroid neoplasm with papillary-like nuclear features on the Bethesda system for reporting thyroid cytopathology: a multi-institutional study in five Asian countries. Pathology. 2018;50:411–7. https://doi.org/10.1016/j.pathol.2017.11.088.

4. Cibas ES, Ali SZ. The 2017 Bethesda system for reporting thyroid cytopathology. Thyroid. 2017;27:1341–6. https://doi.org/10.1089/thy.2017.0500.
5. Cibas ES, Ali SZ. The Bethesda system for reporting thyroid cytopathology. Thyroid. 2009;19:1159–65. https://doi.org/10.1089/thy.2009.0274.
6. Crippa S, Mazzucchelli L, Cibas ES, Ali SZ. The Bethesda system for reporting thyroid fine-needle aspiration specimens. Am J Clin Pathol. 2010;134:343–4.; author reply 345. https://doi.org/10.1309/AJCPXM9WIRQ8JZBJ.
7. Faquin WC, Wong LQ, Afrogheh AH, Ali SZ, Bishop JA, Bongiovanni M, et al. Impact of reclassifying noninvasive follicular variant of papillary thyroid carcinoma on the risk of malignancy in the Bethesda system for reporting thyroid cytopathology. Cancer Cytopathol. 2016;124:181–7.
8. Guo A, Kaminoh Y, Forward T, Schwartz FL, Jenkinson S. Fine needle aspiration of thyroid nodules using the Bethesda system for reporting thyroid cytopathology: an institutional experience in a rural setting. Int J Endocrinol. 2017;2017:9601735. https://doi.org/10.1155/2017/9601735.
9. Ha EJ, Na DG, Moon WJ, Lee YH, Choi N. Diagnostic performance of ultrasound-based risk-stratification systems for thyroid nodules: comparison of the 2015 American Thyroid Association Guidelines with the 2016 Korean Thyroid Association/Korean Society of Thyroid Radiology and 2017 American Congress of Radiology Guidelines. Thyroid. 2018;28:1532–7. https://doi.org/10.1089/thy.2018.0094. Erratum in: Thyroid. 2019;29:159.
10. Haugen BR, Alexander EK, Bible KC, Doherty GM, Mandel SJ, Nikiforov YE, et al. American Thyroid Association management guidelines for adult patients with thyroid nodules and differentiated thyroid cancer: the American Thyroid Association Guidelines Task Force on Thyroid Nodules and Differentiated Thyroid Cancer. Thyroid. 2016;26:1–133. https://doi.org/10.1002/cncr.30360.
11. Hoda RS. Non-gynecologic cytology on liquid-based preparations: a morphologic review of facts and artifacts. Diagn Cytopathol. 2007;35:621–34.
12. Hoda RS, VandenBussche C, Hoda SA. Diagnostic liquid-based cytology. New York: Springer; 2017.
13. Kim SD, Han SH, Jeong WJ, Kim H, Ahn SH. Differences in clinical features between subcategories of "atypia/follicular lesion of undetermined significance". Endocr Pathol. 2017;28:247–52. https://doi.org/10.1007/s12022-017-9486-3.
14. Krane JF, Alexander EK, Cibas ES, Barletta JA. Coming to terms with NIFTP: a provisional approach for cytologists. Cancer Cytopathol. 2016;124:767–72. https://doi.org/10.1002/cncy.21769.
15. Lau RP, Paulsen JD, Brandler TC, Liu CZ, Simsir A, Zhou F. Impact of the reclassification of "noninvasive encapsulated follicular variant of papillary thyroid carcinoma" to "noninvasive follicular thyroid neoplasm with papillary-like nuclear features" on the Bethesda system for reporting thyroid cytopathology: a large academic institution's experience. Am J Clin Pathol. 2017;149:50–4. https://doi.org/10.1093/ajcp/aqx136.
16. Legesse T, Parker L, Heath J, Staats PN. Distinguishing noninvasive follicular thyroid neoplasm with papillary-like nuclear features (NIFTP) from classic and follicular variant of papillary thyroid carcinomas based on cytologic features. J Am Soc Cytopathol. 2019;8:11–7. https://doi.org/10.1016/j.jasc.2018.07.004.
17. Nikiforov YE, Seethala RR, Tallini G, Baloch ZW, Basolo F, Thompson LD, et al. Nomenclature revision for encapsulated follicular variant of papillary thyroid carcinoma: a paradigm shift to reduce overtreatment of indolent tumors. JAMA Oncol. 2016;2:1023–9.
18. Nusztaszeri M, Rossi ED, Auger M, Baloch Z, Bishop J, Bongiovanni M, et al. The Bethesda system for reporting thyroid cytopathology: proposed modifications and updates for the second edition from an international panel. Acta Cytol. 2016;60:399–405.
19. Park VY, Lee HS, Kim EK, Kwak JY, Yoon JH, Moon HJ. Frequencies and malignancy rates of 6-tiered Bethesda categories of thyroid nodules according to ultrasound assessment and nodule size. Head Neck. 2018;40:1947–54. https://doi.org/10.1002/hed.25179.
20. Poller DN, Baloch ZW, Fadda G, Johnson SJ, Bongiovanni M, Pontecorvi A, et al. Thyroid FNA: new classifications and new interpretations. Cancer Cytopathol. 2016;124:457–66. https://doi.org/10.1002/cncy.21703.
21. Shin JH, Baek JH, Chung J, Ha EJ, Kim JH, Lee YH, et al. Ultrasonography diagnosis and imaging-based management of thyroid nodules: revised Korean Society of Thyroid Radiology consensus statement and recommendations. Korean J Radiol. 2016;17:370–95. https://doi.org/10.3348/kjr.2016.17.3.370.
22. Strickland KC, Howitt BE, Marqusee E, Alexander EK, Cibas ES, Krane JF, et al. The impact of noninvasive follicular variant of papillary thyroid carcinoma on rates of malignancy for fine-needle aspiration diagnostic categories. Thyroid. 2015;25:987–92. https://doi.org/10.1089/thy.2014.0612.
23. Tessler FN, Middleton WD, Grant EG, Hoang JK, Berland LL, Teefey SA, et al. ACR thyroid imaging, reporting and data system (TI-RADS): white paper of the ACR TI-RADS Committee. J Am Coll Radiol. 2017;14:587–95. https://doi.org/10.1016/j.jacr.2017.01.046.
24. Vivero M, Renshaw AA, Krane JF. Adequacy criteria for thyroid FNA evaluated by ThinPrep slides only. Cancer. 2017;125:534–43. https://doi.org/10.1002/cncy.21858.

Nondiagnostic/Unsatisfactory Thyroid Fine Needle Aspiration on Liquid-Based Preparations

3

Rana S. Hoda

Introduction to Adequacy Criteria for Thyroid FNA Specimen

- Thyroid fine needle aspiration (FNA) is well established as a first-line diagnostic procedure in patients with thyroid nodules, but despite improved FNA techniques and increase use of ultrasound (US) guidance, about 20% of initial FNA specimens may be nondiagnostic or unsatisfactory (ND/Unsat).
- Nondiagnostic FNA of thyroid nodules presents a clinical dilemma, as the nature of the nodule is not clear and the nodule must be re-aspirated for a diagnosis.
- An adequate FNA specimen, representative of the lesion, is necessary to make an accurate cytopathologic interpretation for proper patient management.
- Adequacy encompasses adequate specimen cellularity and satisfactory specimen quality (thickness, fixation, and staining).

TBSRTC Criteria for Adequate Thyroid FNA Specimen and Application to LBP

- In The Bethesda System for Reporting Thyroid Cytopathology (TBSRTC) [2], a thyroid FNA is defined as "Adequate" when it contains six well-preserved, well-stained follicular cell groups with 10 cells each or 60 follicular cells (Fig. 3.1a, b).

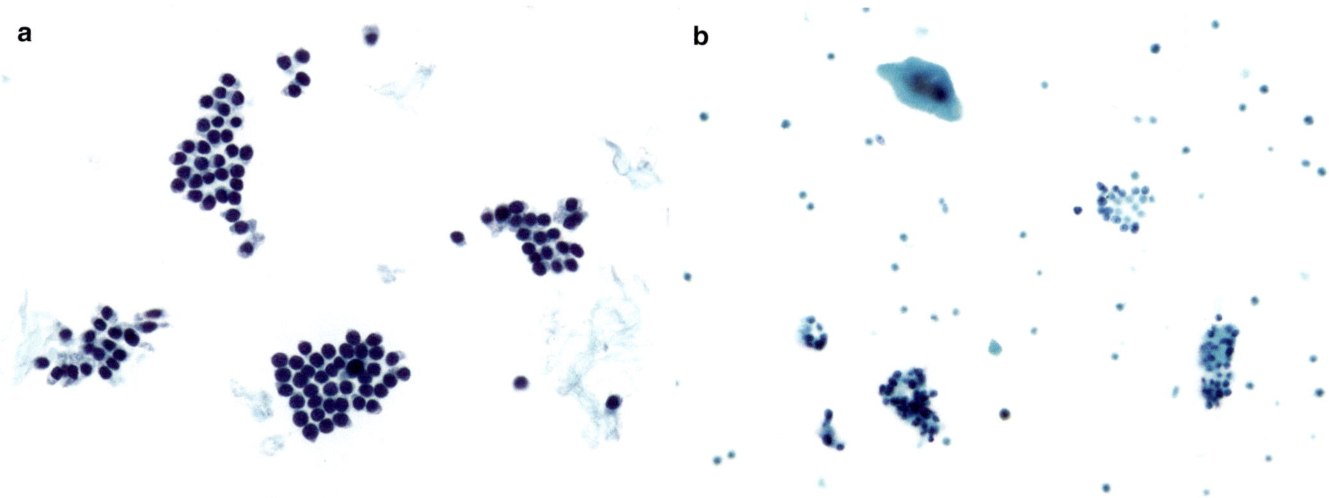

Fig. 3.1 Adequate thyroid FNA. (**a**, **b**) The case showed the required number of six groups of follicular cells with at least 10 cells each. The follicular cell groups are well preserved, well stained, and not covered by any background factors obscuring their features. Benign features are indicated by small, flat sheets of polarized, uniform follicular cells with regular, small, round nuclei and intact cytoplasm. A few small groups and single follicular cells are also present. Note the thin colloid appearance of "wrinkled tissue paper" (**a**, Papanicolaou [Pap] stain ThinPrep® [TP] and **b**, Pap stain, SurePath [SP])

R. S. Hoda (✉)
CBLPath, Rye Brook, NY, USA
e-mail: rhoda@cblpath.com

R. S. Hoda et al. (eds.), *Atlas of Thyroid Cytopathology on Liquid-Based Preparations*,
https://doi.org/10.1007/978-3-030-25066-9_3

- A benign diagnosis with 60 benign follicular cells has 97% sensitivity and 42% specificity.
- Adequacy criteria on liquid-based preparations (LBP) are the same as those for conventional smears (CS).
- Use of these well-defined criteria for adequacy is helpful, as they improve the diagnostic efficiency of thyroid FNA.
- The overall risk of malignancy (ROM) in this category is 5–10%.
- On surgical resection, the malignancy rate for a nodule initially reported as ND/Unsat is 9–32%.

TBSRTC Criteria for ND/Unsat Thyroid FNA Specimen and Application to LBP

- In TBSRTC, ND/Unsat cytologic diagnoses are synonymous.
- The following are examples of thyroid FNA that are considered "ND/Unsat"
  - Cases with fewer than six well-preserved, well-stained follicular cell groups with 10 cells each, or <60 follicular cells. The same criteria apply to LBP (Fig. 3.2).
  - Cases with smear-related artifacts that compromise cell detail and interfere with accurate interpretation (Fig. 3.3a). Artifacts include air-drying, which is seen in alcohol-fixed slides stained with Pap stain and results from a delay in slide fixation. Other artifacts include obscuring of cells by blood (Fig. 3.3b)., ultrasound gel, or thick cellular areas. Because of the processing techniques in LBP, the background elements are reduced, and even if they are present, they do not obscure cells (Figs. 3.3c and 3.4a, b).
  - Cases with cyst fluid, with or without histiocytes, and fewer than six groups of 10 benign follicular cells. Cystic lesions are most commonly responsible for ND/Unsat cases (Fig. 3.5a–c).

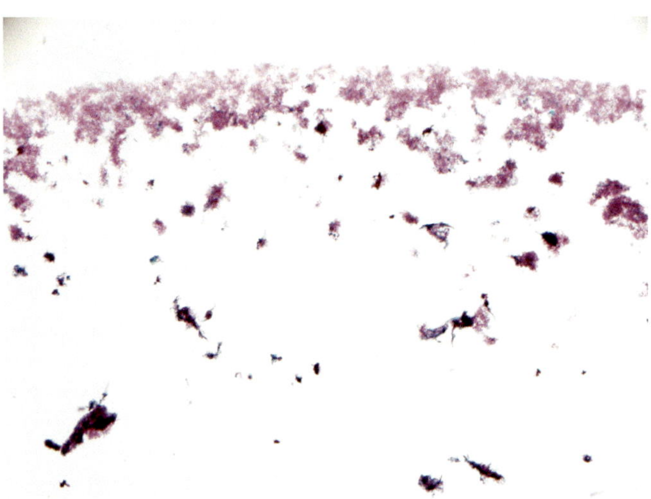

Fig. 3.2 Nondiagnostic/Unsatisfactory (ND/Unsat) in LBP. ND/Unsat TP case showing abundant blood only. TP is more likely to be ND/Unsat due to excess blood (Pap stain, TP)

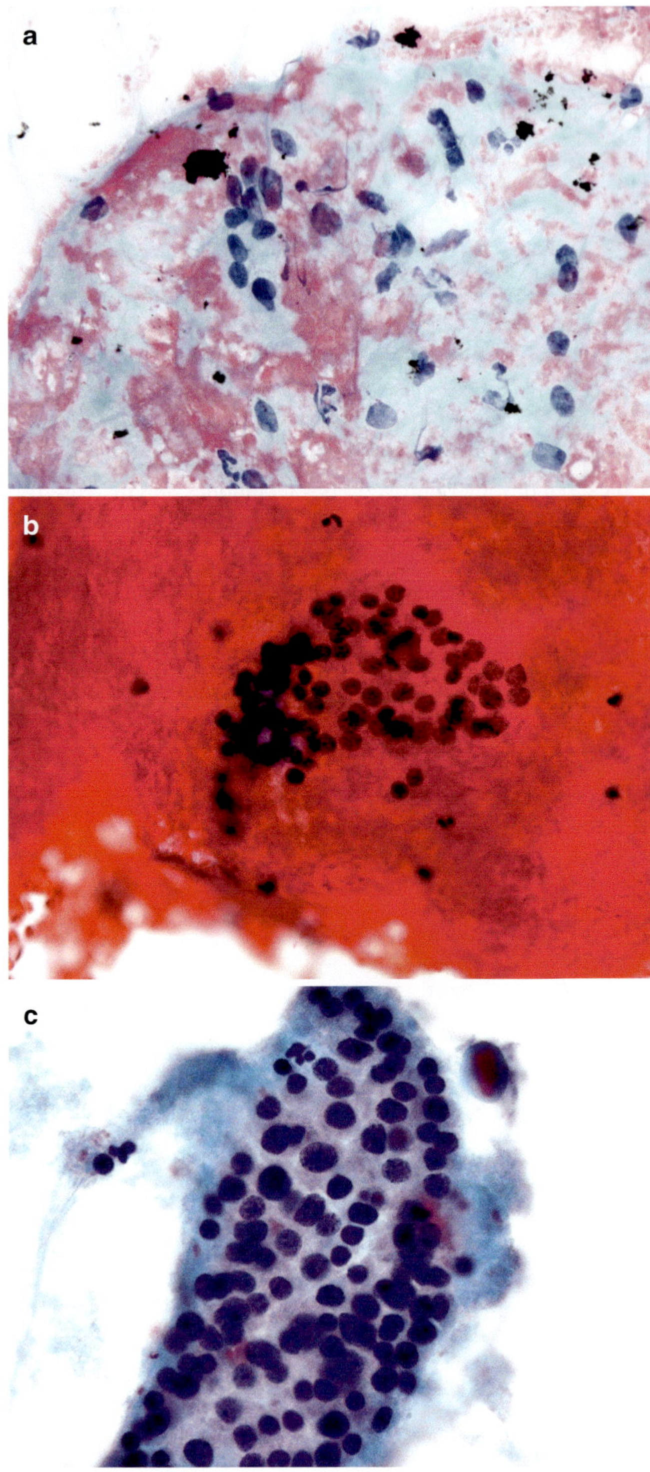

Fig. 3.3 ND/Unsat due to Smear-related Artifacts. (**a**) In a CS case, air-drying distorts cells and prevents a definitive diagnosis. (**b**) Excess blood in a CS case obscures cell detail; even though the cells look benign, it may be difficult to render a definitive diagnosis. (**c**) TP, a liquid-based preparation (LBP), shows abundant blood with no obscuring (**a**–**c**, Pap stain)

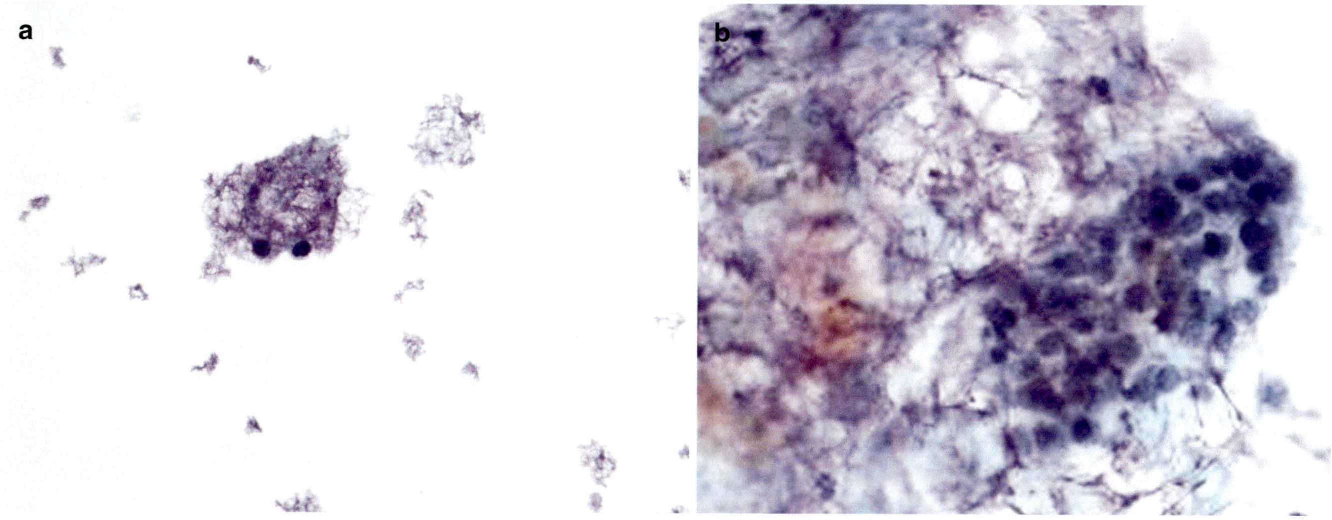

Fig. 3.4 ND/Unsat with Ultrasound Gel Only. (**a**) In LBP, the ultrasound (US) gel stains purple with a lacy or weblike texture. (**b**) The case showed follicular cells surrounded by US gel, but the cytology of benign follicular cells in a macrofollicle is not obscured (**a**, **b**, Pap stain, TP)

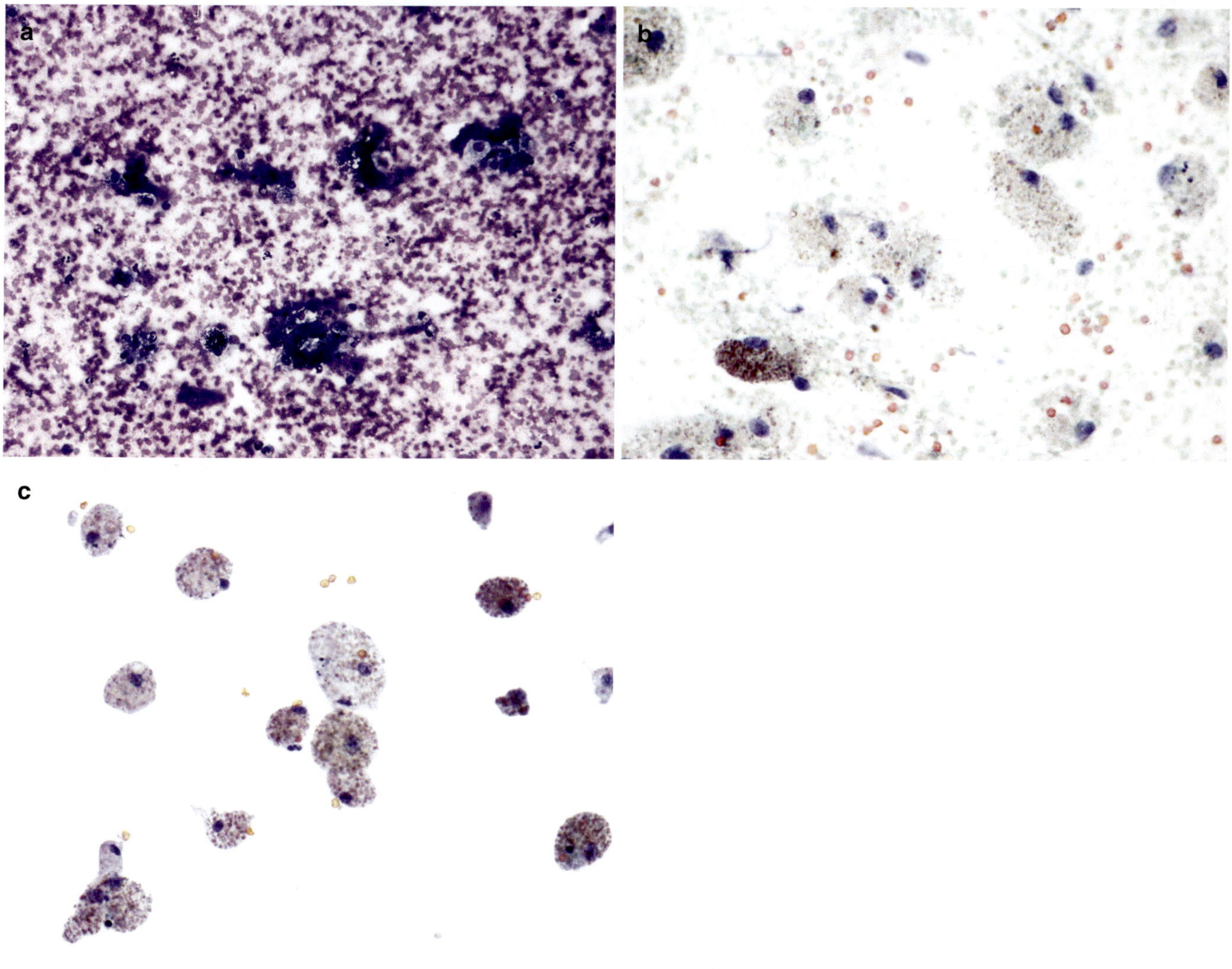

Fig. 3.5 ND/Unsat, Cyst Fluid Only. (a) On Diff-Quik (DQ)-stained CS, a cystic nodule shows non-cohesive macrophages with ill-defined cell walls and cytoplasmic hemosiderin pigment, which appears dark blue. (**b**) Pap-stained CS from the same case shows golden brown cytoplasmic hemosiderin pigment and red blood cells (RBCs) and cystic debris in the background. (**c**) When processed with TP, cystic fluid from the same case showed hemosiderin-laden macrophages with distinct cytoplasmic contours in a clean background. LBP retain all cytoplasmic elements. Nuclear morphology is crisp, with round, oval, and reniform shape, pale chromatin, and small nucleolus. Note RBCs in the background (Pap stain)

TBSRTC Exceptions to Adequacy Criteria, and Application to LBP

- There are exceptions to the ND/Unsat criteria:
  - *Colloid nodule:* This is composed of variably sized dilated follicles filled with colloid, which produce a specimen composed entirely of colloid (Fig. 3.6). Such a nodule contains abundant colloid, and the minimum number of follicular cells is not required, but this standard can only be reliably applied to CS. In LBP, the amount of thin colloid may be reduced and cannot be quantified accurately, so this diagnosis is not recommended for LBP. Moreover, the quality of colloid also changes; it may be mistaken for serum. Thyroglobulin immunostain can be performed, if needed, as colloid stains with thyroglobulin.
  - *Solid nodule with thyroiditis:* Thyroiditis is a diverse group of disorders with different etiologies that are characterized by thyroid inflammation. It is categorized as acute, subacute, or chronic forms. The latter, chronic lymphocytic thyroiditis (CLT) or Hashimoto's thyroiditis (Fig. 3.7a–c) is the most common form of thyroiditis. FNA cytology shows increased background lymphocytes, lymphocytic infiltration of Hürthle cells, and/or follicular cell clusters and lymphohistiocytic aggregates. In ThinPrep® (TP), the diagnosis of CLL or Hashimoto's thyroiditis sometimes may be challenging because of low cellularity and fewer lymphocytes or clumped lymphocytes. The latter may be mistaken for follicular cells. (*See* Chap. 4 for details on HT.)
  - *Solid nodule with any cytologic atypia:* This feature is applied regardless of the number of follicular cells; it is seen in LBP (Fig. 3.8a–c).

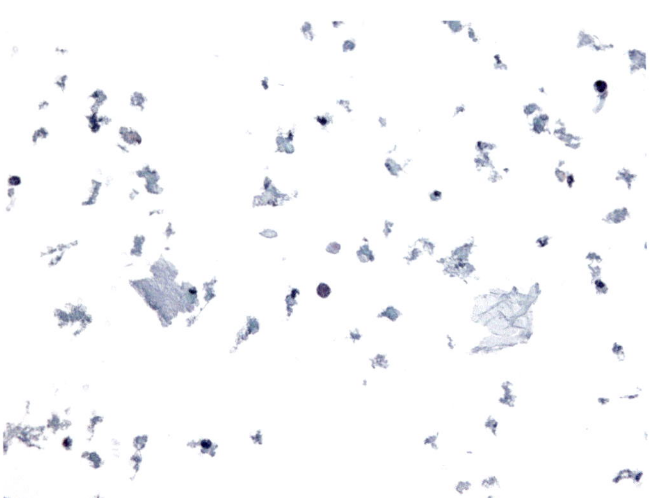

Fig. 3.6 ND/Unsat, Colloid Only in LBP. In CS a diagnosis of colloid nodule can be rendered if abundant colloid is present and the minimum number of follicular cells is not required. This standard can only be reliably applied to CS. In LBP, the amount of thin colloid may be reduced and cannot be quantified accurately. In this case, the TP shows only thin colloid only and is best considered ND/Unsat (Pap stain)

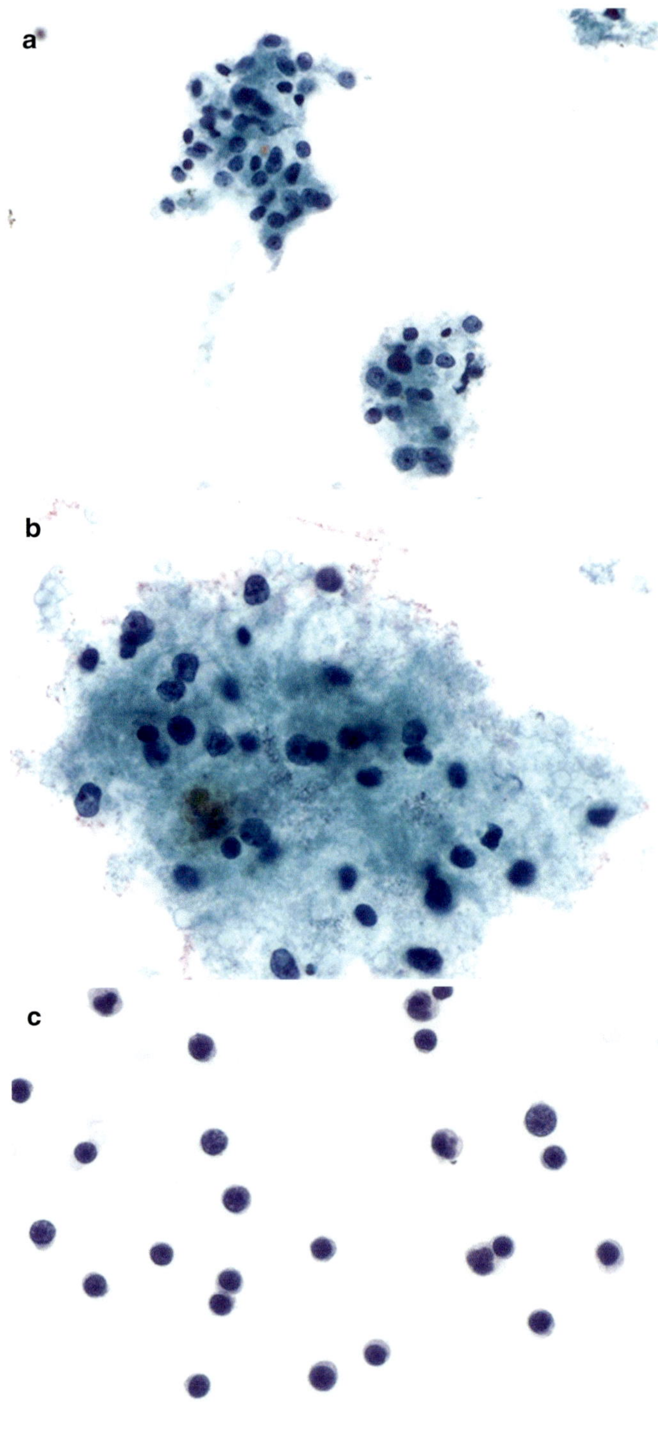

Fig. 3.7 Adequate, Hashimoto's Thyroiditis (HT). (**a–c**), Specimen shows lymphohistiocytic aggregates and dispersed polymorphous lymphocytes. No follicular cells were identified. (**a–c**, Pap stain TP). In TBSRTC, a minimum number of follicular cells is not required in these cases, but ancillary studies such as flow cytometry can be helpful for lymphocyte-only aspirates if the lymphoid population appears monoclonal

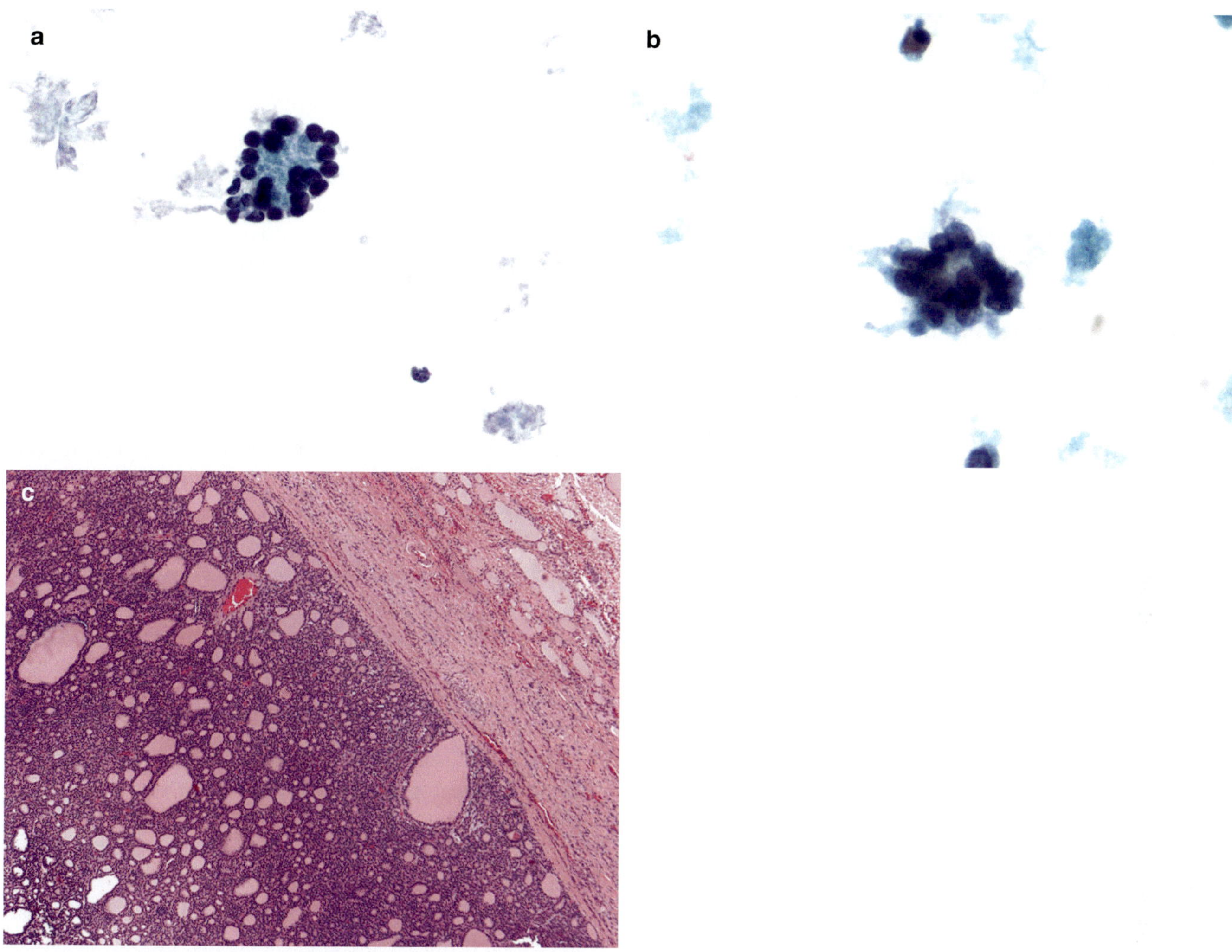

Fig. 3.8 Adequate, AUS/FLUS. (**a**, **b**) Specimen shows few atypical follicular cells (<60), with both nuclear and architectural atypia. The enlarged nuclei (compare with scattered RBCs in both images) are round and hyperchromatic, with occasional small nucleoli, and present in a microfollicular structure. Nuclear features of papillary thyroid carcinoma (PTC) are not seen (**a**, TP; **b**, SP; Pap stain). The thyroid molecular test showed a *NRAS* mutation in both cases. (**c**) On subsequent lobectomy, a histologic section from the nodule seen in (**a**) proved to be a follicular adenoma (hematoxylin & eosin [H&E] stain)

TBSRTC Updates for ND/Unsat Specimens

- Repeat FNA for a ND/Unsat can be performed at an interval of less than 3 months, but the potential for reactive/reparative atypia remains. The American Thyroid Association (ATA) 2015 guidelines [17] also state that a waiting period is probably not necessary.
- Repeat FNA after an ND/Unsat aspirate is often successful and results in a diagnostic sample in 60–80% of cases. This should be the standard approach to ND/Unsat nodules, given the ROM [1, 29]. Ultrasound-guided FNA (USGFNA) is preferred for repeat FNA.
- Patients with repeatedly ND/Unsat nodules should be closely observed or undergo surgical excision, especially if nodule size increases and sonographic findings are suspicious.

Causes for ND/Unsat Thyroid FNA and Application to LBP

- The most common pitfalls for false negative diagnoses in thyroid FNA result from rendering an interpretation on an inadequate sample from a solid nodule, or underdiagnoses of papillary thyroid carcinoma (PTC) due to cystic degeneration. A ND/Unsat sample should not be regarded as negative [29].
- Inadequate sampling of a solid nodule could be due to small nodule size, location in the thyroid, fibrosis, calcification, and excessive blood in the sample. The problem of excessive blood does not apply to LBP.
- The majority of ND/Unsat FNA results are due to cystic lesions. In such cases, the sample may consist solely of histiocytes and/or hemosiderin-laden macrophages. These

cases should be evaluated cautiously, with clinical and imaging correlation. A descriptive ND/Unsat diagnosis can be rendered, and the clinician can be alerted to the possibility of an underlying unsampled lesion such as PTC with cystic degeneration. In a review of 927 consecutive aspirations, García-Pascual et al. [14] reported an 11.1% malignancy rate among partially cystic thyroid nodules with ND/Unsat FNA cytology.

ND/Unsat Specimens in LBP

- Details of ND/Unsat cytology have been published in the Second Edition of the Bethesda System for Reporting Thyroid Cytopathology; the emphasis here is on ND/Unsat cases on LBP.
- Adequacy criteria for thyroid FNA in the TBSRTC were developed on CS, but they are also being applied to FNA evaluated with LBP alone.
- It remains controversial whether LBP should be the sole preparation used for thyroid FNA (direct-to-vial) or if LBP should be used in conjunction with CS (split sample). Each method has its proponents and opponents, and advantages and disadvantages.
- The inadequacy rate for LBP alone without CS is generally less than 15%, but the rate in LBP is higher if the split-sample technique is used. In this technique, cellular material is first smeared on slides and the residual specimen is then rinsed in liquid-based collection medium for LBP.
- In a study by Rossi et al. [26], three parameters of efficacy (rate of inadequate, indeterminate, and malignant) were evaluated in a series of 10,360 thyroid FNAs. The use of TP alone was as effective as CS in decreasing both inadequate and indeterminate cases. Most problems occurred when a split-sample method was used, with a resultant high rate of inadequate and false negative diagnoses.
- The sole use of LBP reduces the unsatisfactory rate and false negative diagnosis because of specific advantages that include a clean background, proper fixation, and increased cellularity (which occurs because the liquid-based slide is representative of the entire procured sample, unlike the split-sample method). See the study by Rossi et al. [26] for details of the two specimen collection techniques.
- The adequacy criteria in thyroid FNA evaluated with LBP alone have not been widely assessed. Vivero et al. [33] showed that in thyroid FNA examined with TP only, lowering the adequacy threshold and eliminating the requirement of six groups of 10 cells each does not significantly affect test performance if cytological features associated with malignancy are absent. Nevertheless, TBSRTC has retained similar adequacy criteria for both CS and LBP.
- A meta-analysis by Chong et al. [10] of studies on both LBP and CS published between 2000 and 2013 showed that sample adequacy for the two mainstream LBP methods (TP and SurePath™ [SP]) was significantly superior to CS for most sampling methods. Average sample inadequacy in TP studies (24.0%) was significantly lower than in CS (33.4%; $P < 0.01$). Likewise, average sample inadequacy in SP studies (7.1%) was significantly lower than in CS (13.2%; $P < 0.02$). In the same study, the sensitivity and specificity of LBP were similar or slightly better than for CS.
- When an LBP specimen does not contain an adequate number of cells, a second slide can be prepared with the residual material to help meet the adequacy criteria. Tulecke and Wang [31] and Rossi et al. [27] found good results with this technique. In the study by Rossi et al., this procedure led to an 18.5% increase in the overall diagnostic rate, especially in cases classified as benign and follicular lesions. Rossi et al. [27] and Tulecke and Wang [31] concluded that the making of a second slide for an ND/Unsat case with inadequate cellularity may improve the diagnostic efficacy of the technique and may avoid either a repeat FNA or more aggressive treatment.
- However, Hasteh et al. [16] found only a 3% adequacy retrieval rate for a second slide, which was regarded as insufficient for processing of an additional slide.
- Additional liquid-based slides can also be used for immunocytochemistry or molecular tests.
- A cell block (CB) can also be attempted from the residual specimen if the sample appears cloudy, bloody, or blood-tinged. Traditional CB sections not only serve as an important diagnostic adjunct to LBP or cytologic smears but also are used for immunohistochemical (IHC) studies.
- There are many ways to prepare a CB and the methods continue to be revised. Our group compared the traditional CB with CBs processed on the Cellient™ automated cell block system (Hologic, Toronto, Canada) [34]. The Cellient™ system, the first fully automated CB system, improves cell recovery when compared with traditional methods. The vacuum-assisted filtration concentrates available cells within the block, resulting in consistently high quality and a diagnostic CB in less than 1 hour, which can be used for IHC.
- Horton et al. [19] studied the utility of Cellient™ CBs in the evaluation of thyroid FNAs submitted in Cytolyt, with an emphasis on low-cellularity specimens. TP slides were first prepared from thyroid FNA. After assessment using TBSRTC criteria, Cellient™CBs were requested on samples with residual FNA material and an initial cytologic impression of ND/Unsat or AUS/FLUS, and on apparently benign samples with marginally adequate cellularity. Overall, the CB findings resulted in a

change of the initial TP impression in 15% of cases, the vast majority of which were initially ND/Unsat. Moreover, 31% of the ND/Unsat TP samples became diagnostic with a CB. The CB findings contributed to a change in diagnosis in 8% of AUS/FLUS cases. The low-cellularity benign samples gained very little additional information from the CB.

- Currently, TP is being used more often than SP for nongynecological cytology, including FNA, so more representations of TP cases will be seen. The choice of LBP depends on individual laboratory preferences and needs, however.
- Cytomorphological appearance is comparable with TP and SP, with subtle differences, as listed in Chap. 1 and mentioned elsewhere. A learning curve is essential for adapting to the cytomorphologic features of the LBP technique, and it is hoped that this volume will educate cytologists in the differences between CS and LBP and the subtle differences between TP and SP.

The Role of Rapid On-Site Evaluation for Adequacy Assessment and Application to LBP

- Air-dried Diff-Quik (DQ)–stained smears are prepared for rapid on-site adequacy evaluation (ROSE).
- ROSE of thyroid FNA reduces the ND/Unsat rate. This assessment provides a preliminary diagnosis, ensures that the sample is adequate, limits the number of passes, allows for appropriate specimen triage for ancillary studies including molecular tests, and often facilitates clinical decision-making. It is cost-saving, as a repeat FNA is avoided [35].
- ROSE cannot be performed for LBP, as the collected sample is immediately rinsed in the collection medium, but ROSE can be performed if LBP are used in conjunction with DQ-stained smears. Cytologists or clinicians who perform ROSE can make one or two DQ-stained smears per pass and if the specimen is adequate, the remaining sample can be rinsed in the liquid-based collection medium.
- The gauge of the FNA needle and FNA technique also influence the ND/Unsat rate. For solid and mixed nodules, the non-aspiration FNA method using a 25G needle with multiple (≥3) passes results in a higher diagnostic rate for thyroid FNA than does a single pass with a 22G needle, with or without aspiration.
- The study by Zhu et al. [35] revealed that when the number of needle passes was fewer than three, the nondiagnostic rate could be 25% or more, but it was significantly reduced to 11% with four passes performed per thyroid lesion. The authors concluded that, with ROSE, four to six passes per thyroid nodule is the optimal number to maximize diagnostic certainty.

The Role of Ultrasound-Guided FNA

- Ultrasound-guided FNA (USGFNA) is preferred over palpation-guided FNA (PGFNA).
- Although the rate of ND/Unsat FNA is reported to be lower with USGFNA, 10% to 35% of cases continue to be nondiagnostic. This rate includes both CS and LBP.
- USGFNA is more advantageous in nonpalpable, predominantly cystic nodules or nodules with previous ND/Unsat FNA.
- The 2015 ATA guidelines for management of adult patients with thyroid nodules and differentiated thyroid cancer indicate that PGFNA remains an acceptable alternative for FNA of a palpable thyroid nodule that meets sonographic criteria for biopsy [17].

Suggested Reading

1. Alexander EK, Heering JP, Benson CB, Frates MC, Doubilet PM, Cibas ES, et al. Assessment of nondiagnostic ultrasound-guided fine needle aspirations of thyroid nodules. J Clin Endocrinol Metab. 2002;87:4924–7.
2. Ali SZ, Cibas ES. The Bethesda system for reporting thyroid cytopathology; definitions, criteria, and explanatory notes. 2nd ed. Cham: Springer International Publishing AG; 2018.
3. Bongiovanni M, Papadakis GE, Rouiller N, Marino L, Lamine F, Bisig B, et al. The Bethesda system for reporting thyroid cytopathology explained for practitioners: frequently asked questions. Thyroid. 2018;28:556–65. https://doi.org/10.1089/thy.2017.0685.
4. Brito JP, Castro MR, Dean DS, Fatourechi V, Stan M. Survey of current approaches to non-diagnostic fine-needle aspiration from solid thyroid nodules. Endocrine. 2015;49:745–51. https://doi.org/10.1007/s12020-015-0539-4.
5. Chandanwale SS, Nair R, Gambhir A, Kaur S, Pandey A, Shetty A, et al. Cytomorphological spectrum of thyroiditis: a review of 110 cases. J Thyroid Res. 2018;2018:5246516. https://doi.org/10.1155/2018/5246516.
6. Chang H, Lee E, Lee H, Choi J, Kim A, Kim BH. Comparison of diagnostic values of thyroid aspiration samples using liquid-based preparation and conventional smear: one-year experience in a single institution. APMIS. 2013;121:139–45. https://doi.org/10.1111/j.16000463.2012.02944.x.
7. Cibas ES, Ali SZ. The 2017 Bethesda system for reporting thyroid cytopathology. Thyroid. 2017;27:1341–6. https://doi.org/10.1089/thy.2017.0500.
8. Clark DP, Faquin WC. Thyroid cytopathology. 2nd ed. New York: Springer; 2010.
9. Chong Y, Baek KH, Kim JY, Kim TJ, Lee EJ, Kang CS. Comparison of EASYPREP and SurePath in thyroid fine-needle aspiration. Diagn Cytopathol. 2016;44:283–90. https://doi.org/10.1002/dc.23438.
10. Chong Y, Ji SJ, Kang CS, Lee EJ. Can liquid-based preparation substitute for conventional smear in thyroid fine-needle aspiration? A systematic review based on meta-analysis. Endocr Connect. 2017;6:817–29. https://doi.org/10.1530/EC-17-0165.
11. Choong KC, Khiyami A, Tamarkin SW, McHenry CR. Fine-needle aspiration biopsy of thyroid nodules: is routine ultrasound-guidance necessary? Surgery. 2018;164:789–94. https://doi.org/10.1016/j.surg.2018.04.047.

12. Duncan LD, Forrest L, Law WM Jr, Hubbard E, Stewart LE. Evaluation of thyroid fine-needle aspirations: can ThinPrep be used exclusively to appropriately triage patients having a thyroid nodule? Diagn Cytopathol. 2011;39:341–8. https://doi.org/10.1002/dc.21392.
13. Ferreira MA, Gerhard R, Schmitt F. Analysis of nondiagnostic results in a large series of thyroid fine-needle aspiration cytology performed over 9 years in a single center. Acta Cytol. 2014;58:229–34. https://doi.org/10.1159/000360066.
14. García-Pascual L, Barahona MJ, Balsells M, del Pozo C, Anglada-Barceló J, Casalots-Casado J, et al. Complex thyroid nodules with nondiagnostic fine needle aspiration cytology: histopathologic outcomes and comparison of the cytologic variants (cystic vs. acellular). Endocrine. 2011;39:33–40. https://doi.org/10.1007/s12020-010-9409-2.
15. Geers C, Bourgain C. Liquid-based FNAC of the thyroid: a 4-year survey with SurePath. Cancer Cytopathol. 2011;119:58–67. https://doi.org/10.1002/cncy.20125.
16. Hasteh F, Pang Y, Pu R, Michael CW. Do we need more than one ThinPrep to obtain adequate cellularity in fine needle aspiration? Diagn Cytopathol. 2007;35:740–3.
17. Haugen BR, Alexander EK, Bible KC, Doherty GM, Mandel SJ, Nikiforov YE, et al. 2015 American Thyroid Association management guidelines for adult patients with thyroid nodules and differentiated thyroid cancer: the American Thyroid Association Guidelines Task Force on Thyroid Nodules and Differentiated Thyroid Cancer. Thyroid. 2016;26:1–133. https://doi.org/10.1089/thy.2015.0020.
18. Hoda RS, VandenBussche C, Hoda SA. Diagnostic liquid-based cytology. New York: Springer; 2017.
19. Horton M, Been L, Starling C, Traweek ST. The utility of Cellient cell blocks in low-cellularity thyroid fine needle aspiration biopsies. Diagn Cytopathol. 2016;44:737–41. https://doi.org/10.1002/dc.23522.
20. Jung CK, Lee A, Jung ES, Choi YJ, Jung SL, Lee KY. Split sample comparison of a liquid-based method and conventional smears in thyroid fine needle aspiration. Acta Cytol. 2008;52:313–9.
21. Lee HY, Baek JH, Yoo H, Kim JK, Lim MK, Chu YC, et al. Repeat fine-needle aspiration biopsy within a short interval does not increase the atypical cytologic results for thyroid nodules with previously nondiagnostic results. Acta Cytol. 2014;58:330–4. https://doi.org/10.1159/000363277.
22. Liu X, Zhu L, Wang Z, Cui D, Chen H, Wei L, et al. Comparison of two different standards of care in detecting malignant thyroid nodules using thyroid fine-needle aspiration. Mol Clin Oncol. 2015;3:682–6.
23. Ljung BM. Thyroid fine-needle aspiration: smears versus liquid-based preparations. Cancer. 2008;114:144–8. https://doi.org/10.1002/cncr.23541.
24. Pitman MB, Abele J, Ali SZ, Duick D, Elsheikh TM, Jeffrey RB, et al. Techniques for thyroid FNA: a synopsis of the National Cancer Institute Thyroid Fine-Needle Aspiration State of the Science Conference. Diagn Cytopathol. 2008;36:407–24. https://doi.org/10.1002/dc.20829.
25. Renshaw AA. Histologic follow-up of nondiagnostic thyroid fine needle aspirations: implications for adequacy criteria. Diagn Cytopathol. 2012;40(Suppl 1):E13–5. https://doi.org/10.1002/dc.21492.
26. Rossi ED, Raffaelli M, Zannoni GF, Pontecorvi A, Mulè A, Callà C, et al. Diagnostic efficacy of conventional as compared to liquid-based cytology in thyroid lesions: evaluation of 10,360 fine needle aspiration cytology cases. Acta Cytol. 2009;53:659–66.
27. Rossi ED, Morassi F, Santeusanio G, Zannoni GF, Fadda G. Thyroid fine needle aspiration cytology processed by ThinPrep: an additional slide decreased the number of inadequate results. Cytopathology. 2010;21:97–102. https://doi.org/10.1111/j.1365-2303.2009.00659.x.
28. Sahin D, Yilmazbayhan D, Firat P, Hacisalihoglu UP, Kirimlioglu SH, Celenk E, et al. Comparison of conventional cytology and SurePath in split thyroid fine needle aspiration materials. Cytopathology. 2017;28:291–8. https://doi.org/10.1111/cyt.12430.
29. Saieg MA, Barbosa B, Nishi J, Ferrari A, Costa F. The impact of repeat FNA in non-diagnostic and indeterminate thyroid nodules: a 5-year single-centre experience. Cytopathology. 2018;29:196–200. https://doi.org/10.1111/cyt.12508.
30. Sharma S, Agarwal S, Jain M, Singh GB, Andley M. Cytomorphological differences between liquid-based cytology and conventional smears in fine-needle aspirates of thyroid lesions. J Cytol. 2018;35:208–11. https://doi.org/10.4103/JOC.JOC_150_17.
31. Tulecke MA, Wang HH. ThinPrep for cytologic evaluation of follicular thyroid lesions: correlation with histologic findings. Diagn Cytopathol. 2004;30:7–13.
32. Upadhyaya P, Dhakal S, Adhikari P, Adhikari B, Khadka D, Niraula SR. Histopathological review of diagnostic categories of the Bethesda system for reporting thyroid cytopathology – an institutional experience of 5 years. J Cytol. 2019;36:48–52. https://doi.org/10.4103/JOC.JOC_64_18.
33. Vivero M, Renshaw AA, Krane JF. Adequacy criteria for thyroid FNA evaluated by ThinPrep slides only. Cancer Cytopathol. 2017;125:534–43. https://doi.org/10.1002/cncy.21858.
34. Wagner DG, Russell DK, Benson JM, Schneider AE, Hoda RS, Bonfiglio TA. Cellient™ automated cell block versus traditional cell block preparation: a comparison of morphologic features and immunohistochemical staining. Diagn Cytopathol. 2011;39:730–6. https://doi.org/10.1002/dc.21457.
35. Zhu W, Michael CW. How important is on-site adequacy assessment for thyroid FNA? An evaluation of 883 cases. Diagn Cytopathol. 2007;35:183–6.

4 Fine Needle Aspiration of Benign Thyroid Nodules

Rana S. Hoda and Elizabeth Austin

Introduction to Benign Thyroid Lesions

- The prevalence of thyroid nodules in the general population ranges from 2% to 6%, but only 10–20% of these nodules are malignant. The clinical challenge is to identify those nodules requiring surgical management.
- In this clinical setting, fine needle aspiration (FNA) represents an invaluable diagnostic tool for characterizing thyroid nodules. FNA aids in identifying nodules that require surgery and decreases the overall incidence of thyroidectomy in patients with benign disease. It has found worldwide application because of its simplicity, safety, cost-effectiveness, and accuracy, with a reported sensitivity of 80–98% and specificity of 58–100%.
- Benign cytology is the most common diagnostic result of FNA, with a reported negative predictive value (NPV) greater than 95%.
- The Bethesda System for Reporting Thyroid Cytopathology (TBSRTC) predicts that the risk of malignancy (ROM) of a solitary thyroid nodule with a benign cytology on FNA is 0–3%. However, a meta-analysis of 14 studies encompassing over 43,000 patients reported a significantly higher ROM of 3–5%, when resection was used as the gold standard [35].
- The overall false-negative (FN) rate depends on four important parameters: sampling error, poor specimen quality, scant specimen, and cytologic interpretation.
  - Sampling errors can result from multiple factors, including the nature of the nodules, multiple suspicious nodules, the use of palpation-guided FNA (PGFNA) vs. ultrasound-guided FNA (USGFNA), the FNA technique, and the skill of the operator.
  - Poor specimen quality, usually encountered with conventional smears (CS), includes poor cellular preservation due to multiple smear-related artifacts such as air-drying artifact, overlapping and thick cellular areas, and abundant blood and ultrasound gel. All these elements partially or completely obscure cell details. In such cases, identifying benign or neoplastic cells can be a challenge.
  - Scant specimen can be due to the nature of the lesion, inadequate sampling, or the discarding of diagnostic sample with the needle and syringe after CS have been made.
  - Cytologic interpretation errors occur most commonly in nodules with focal features of papillary thyroid carcinoma (PTC) or microPTC.
- The cytologic criteria for FNA of thyroid lesions were devised on conventional smears, which have been the preparation of choice, especially in settings where rapid onsite specimen evaluation (ROSE) is available.

Liquid-Based Preparations (LBP) in Benign Thyroid FNA

- Despite the initial controversy regarding the efficacy of the use of LBP alone, good results have been achieved in recent years [9, 14, 18, 36, 41]. Studies have shown that ThinPrep® (TP) has diagnostic equivalence to CS, but one should acknowledge the cytologic differences between the two preparations with regard to the amount and character of colloid, architectural features, background elements, and nuclear and cytoplasmic details.
- Details of the LBP collection and processing techniques and cellular morphology have previously been published [25].
- For a reliable diagnosis on LBP, features of thyroid FNA as seen on CS need to be slightly modified.
- Accurate recognition of benign lesions on LBP requires familiarity with the alterations in the amount and character of colloid, architecture, and cytomorphology (Tables 4.1 and 4.2).

R. S. Hoda (✉) · E. Austin
CBLPath, Rye Brook, NY, USA
e-mail: rhoda@cblpath.com

R. S. Hoda et al. (eds.), *Atlas of Thyroid Cytopathology on Liquid-Based Preparations*,
https://doi.org/10.1007/978-3-030-25066-9_4

Table 4.1 Features of benign lesions in LBP and conventional smears

Cytological features	SurePath (SP)	ThinPrep (TP)	Conventional smears (CS)
Cellularity	Increased, allows assessment of overall specimen cellularity but not individual passes	Increased, allows assessment of overall specimen cellularity but not individual passes	Variable, allows assessment of cellularity for each pass with ROSE
Macrofollicles	3-D, cells in orderly honeycomb	Flat monolayer, may be smaller; cells in orderly honeycomb	Large to medium-sized, cells in orderly honeycomb
Clusters	More clustered, with cellular overlap	Tighter, crowded with cellular overlap	Loose aggregates of cells, may be crowded
3-D Configuration	Present, more 3-D, difficult to interpret, requires continuous focusing at higher magnification	May be seen, easy to interpret, loss of cellular preservation may be seen in the large aggregates	May be seen, easy to interpret
Single Cells and Cell Shrinkage	Increased, cell shrinkage apparent	Increased, cell shrinkage apparent	Not increased; no cell shrinkage
Cytoplasm	Fewer details, fragile, fragmented, lipofuscin pigment visible	May be disrupted, with naked nuclei, lipofuscin pigment visible	May be disrupted with naked nuclei, lipofuscin pigment visible
Nuclei	Fewer details, shrunken, round, regular with dense chromatin; PTC nuclear features retained	Shrunken, round, regular with dense chromatin, PTC nuclear features retained with few INPI	Maintained size and all diagnostic features
Amount of Colloid	Reduced and different	Reduced and different	Abundant watery colloid
Thin Colloid	Wrinkled tissue paper, napkin fold, granular	Wrinkled tissue paper, napkin fold, granular	Diffuse thin layer or coalescing "broken glass" pieces
Thick Colloid	Dense, in chunks, round to oval aggregates or dense droplets	Fragmented chunks, round to oval aggregates or dense droplets	Diffuse dried and cracked "desert sand" or diffuse thick bands
Number of Macrophages	Present, hemosiderin pigment retained	Increased, hemosiderin pigment retained	Present, hemosiderin pigment retained
Stroma	Reduced	Reduced and fragmented	Retained as large fragments
Lymphocytes in LT	Increased, evenly dispersed; fewer lymphohistiocytic aggregates	Increased, evenly dispersed; fewer lymphohistiocytic aggregates	Increased, dispersed, and lymphohistiocytic aggregates
Obscuring Elements (blood, US gel)	Reduced, clean background, less/no obscuring elements	Reduced, clean background, less/no obscuring elements	Present; background usually bloody, with obscured cells
Artifacts	Reduced; 3-D clusters, cells in different planes of focus and cellular overlap present	None/reduced; cells in one plane, no cellular overlap, cells in the periphery appear distorted	Several due to technique, including air-drying, thick cellular areas, overlapping cell clusters
Additional Slides	Processed from residual specimen	Processed from residual specimen	Cannot be prepared
Sensitivity and Accuracy	Currently recommended use with CS	91.0% sensitivity; 89.4% accuracy; similar to CS; can be used as a sole preparation	Similar to LBP, can be used with LBP

3-D three-dimensional, *FN* false negative, *INPI* intranuclear pseudoinclusions, *LBP* liquid-based preparations, *LT* lymphocytic thyroiditis, *PTC* papillary thyroid carcinoma, *ROSE* rapid onsite specimen evaluation, *US* ultrasound

Table 4.2 Morphologic criteria for benign thyroid lesions on LBP and CS

Histological Diagnosis	SurePath (SP)	ThinPrep (TP)	Conventional Smears (CS)
MNG/BFN	Small sheets, clusters, and macrofollicles of small, monomorphic follicular cells with clear or granular cytoplasm, wrinkled tissue paper–like thin colloid, or small clumps or globules of dense colloid, histiocytes	Small sheets, clusters, and macrofollicles of small, monomorphic follicular cells with clear or granular cytoplasm, wrinkled tissue paper–like thin colloid, or small clumps or globules of dense colloid, histiocytes	Abundant, diffuse thin or thick colloid; large sheets and macrofollicles of small follicular cells, histiocytes
Colloid Nodule	Small clumps of dense colloid (colloid globules)	Small clumps of dense colloid (colloid globules)	Abundant and clumped
Lymphocytic (Hashimoto's) Thyroiditis	Mixture of small clusters of follicular cells and/or Hürthle cells, lymphocytes; small clumps of colloid. Multinucleated histiocytes may or may not be present.	Mixture of small clusters of follicular cells and/or Hürthle cells, lymphocytes; small clumps of colloid. Multinucleated histiocytes may or may not be present (diagnosed less frequently on TP slides than on CS).	Inflammatory cells (mostly mature lymphocytes, few plasma cells), epithelioid histiocytes; lymphohistiocytic aggregates, small clusters of follicular cells, sometimes with Hürthle cell metaplasia; scant colloid. Multinucleated histiocytes are diagnosed more frequently on CS than on TP.

MNG/BFN multinodular goiter/benign follicular nodule

- In addition, although TP and SurePath™ (SP) are both LBP, one must also be aware of the subtle differences between the two methods (Table 4.3).
- A study by the College of American Pathologists, as part of their Interlaboratory Comparison Program in Non-Gynecologic Cytology [19], concluded that LBPs performed better than CS for cases with a benign reference diagnosis. Cytopathologists also seemed to have the highest concordance for this diagnosis.
- The benign entities discussed in this chapter are those most commonly encountered in thyroid FNA practice. For less common benign entities, readers are referred to specialty textbooks.

Multinodular Goiter/Benign Follicular Nodule (MNG/BFN)

- Goiter is thyroid enlargement. A simple goiter can become multinodular through repeated episodes of hyperplasia and involution (degeneration) of follicular epithelium with colloid accumulation within dilated follicles. Grossly, the thyroid gland shows asymmetric diffuse or nodular enlargement. The nodules are irregular and variable in size. Histology reveals multiple irregularly dilated and variably sized microfollicles and macrofollicles, lined by flattened to hyperplastic epithelium, with or without degenerative cystic and hemorrhagic change (Fig. 4.1a, b).

Table 4.3 Morphological criteria for benign thyroid lesions on SP and TP

Technical and Cytological Features	SurePath (SP)	ThinPrep (TP)
Technique	Method employs density gradient separation and centrifugation, a cell enrichment process producing cells devoid of blood and other obscuring materials. The cells of interest are separated as a result of the simple sedimentation of cells on the slide surface without any applied pressure, and the SP method produces a more 3-D configuration for both single cells and clusters than CS and TP.	Membrane filtration method; the cells of interest are separated when the liquid collection medium is drawn through a filter using negative pressure pulse.
Cells	Tends to retain large tissue fragments, cellular elongation	More cellular dyscohesion and fragmentation
Lymphocytes	Number of lymphocytes is slightly increased; infiltrate follicular cells, lymphocytes are evenly dispersed, with fewer lymphohistiocytic aggregates than CS	Number of lymphocytes increased but less than in SP; infiltrate follicular cells, lymphocytes are evenly dispersed, with fewer lymphohistiocytic aggregates than CS
Peripheral Blood Contamination	Lymphocytes from the lysed blood may give a false assessment of lymphocytic thyroiditis	Lymphocytes from the lysed blood may give a false assessment of lymphocytic thyroiditis
Diagnosis	Easier method for diagnosis of lymphocytic thyroiditis than the TP method	Less easy than SP and CS
Experience for Interpretation	Required to avoid diagnostic pitfalls	Required to avoid diagnostic pitfalls

CS conventional smears

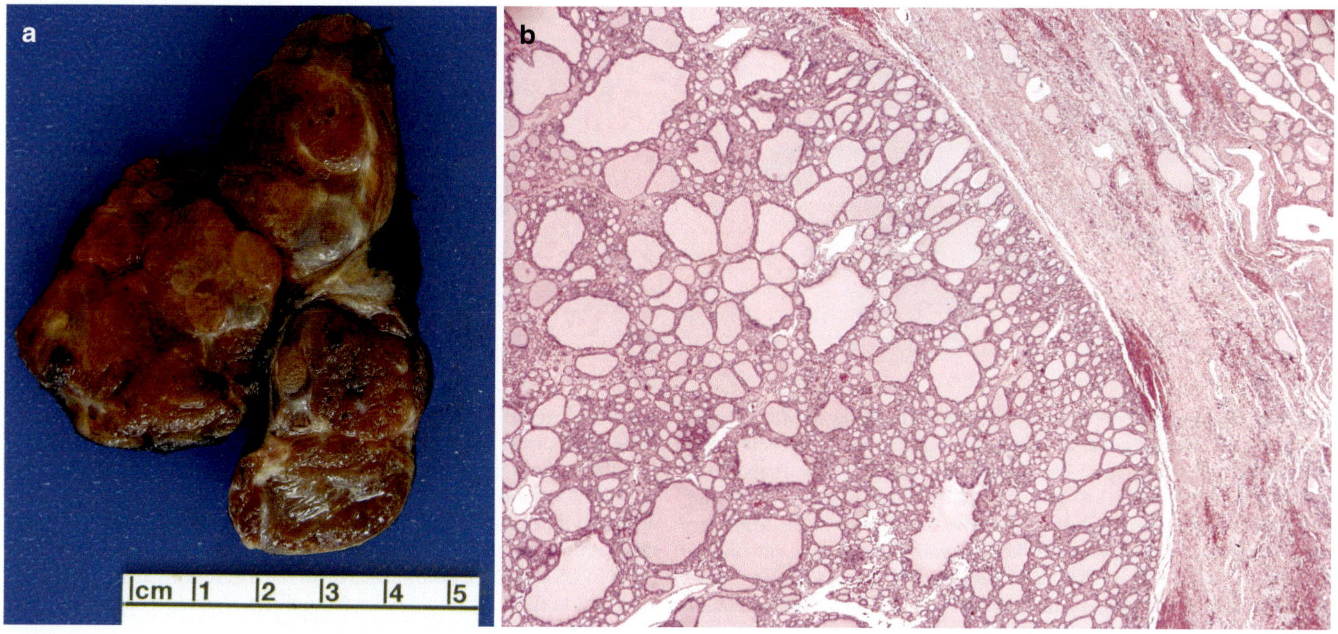

Fig. 4.1 Multinodular goiter (MNG). (**a**) MNG of the thyroid gland with asymmetric nodular enlargement. The nodules are irregular, brown, and variable in size. (**b**) Histology of MNG with multiple irregularly dilated follicles of variable sizes, including both microfollicles and macrofollicles (H&E stain)

- MNG/BNF reflects morphologic changes of the different stages of the disease, which include early follicular hyperplasia, cycles of involution/regeneration, and nodule formation. Hürthle cell metaplasia, hemorrhage, cystic degeneration, and calcification may occur in all stages.

Cytology of MNG/BFN on LBP

- Typical features of MNG/BFN are easily identified on the two LBP, TP and SP, with subtle differences from and similarities to the features seen on CS (*see* Table 4.2).
- The main overall differences between LBP and CS are that architecture is more disrupted in LBP: sheets, macrofollicles and microfollicles appear smaller and tighter and follicular cells may reveal more cell shrinkage, with smaller nuclear size, lower nuclear-cytoplasmic (N:C) ratio, more disruption of the cytoplasm, an increase in the number of naked nuclei, and a prominence of nucleoli. Thick and thin colloid appears more clumped than on CS (Fig. 4.2a–i).
- In TP, uniform follicular cells form small, flat, orderly sheets with cells arranged in a "honeycomb" configuration, with macrofollicles (spheres or balls), cell clusters, a few microfollicles, and singly dispersed cells with colloid, histiocytes, and other degenerative changes in the background (*see* Fig. 4.2a–d).
- In SP, follicular cells also appear as both flat, orderly sheets in a "honeycomb" arrangement and as macrofol-

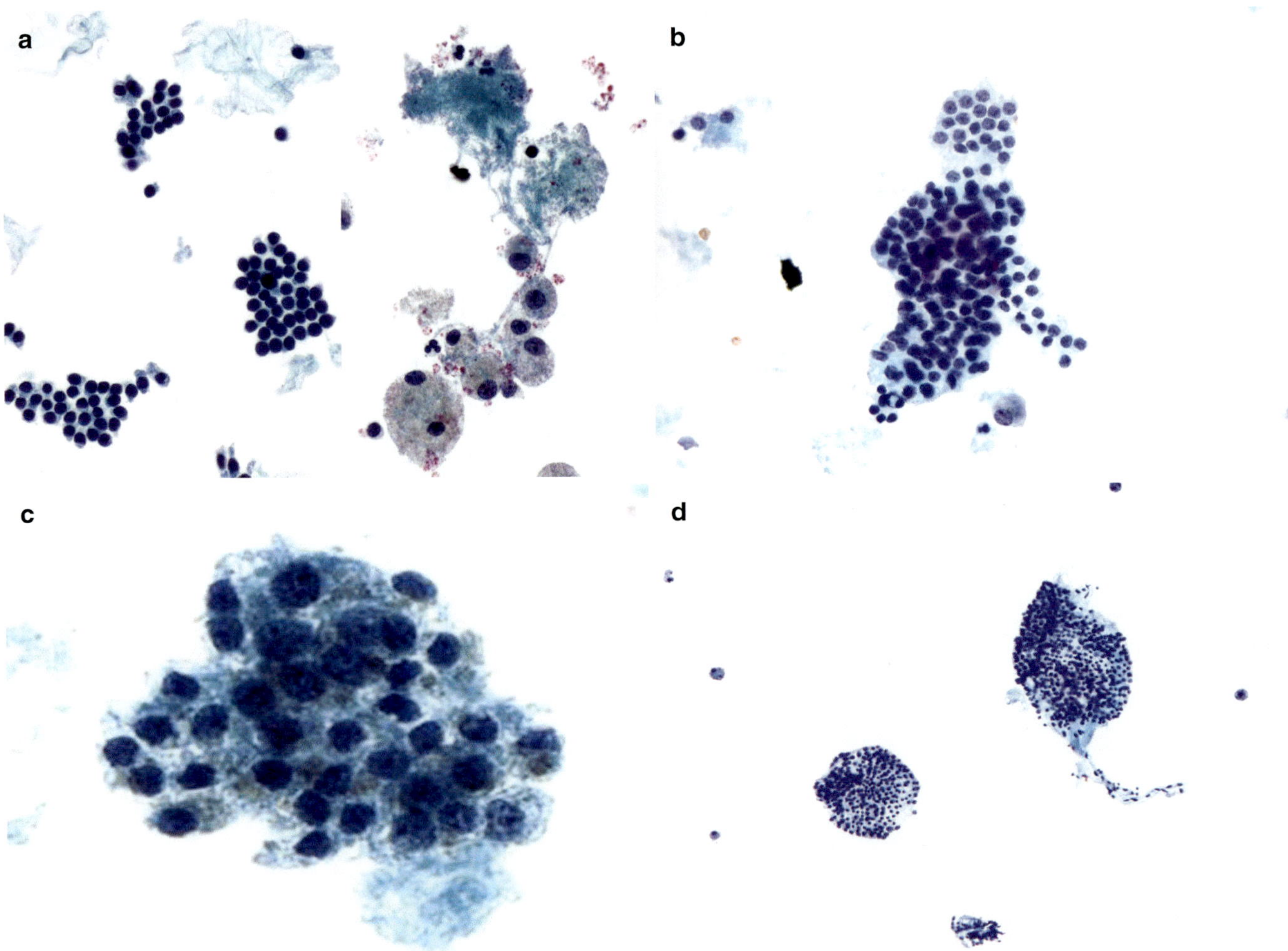

Fig. 4.2 Cytology of MNG. (**a–d**) Typical field of view in MNG showing benign follicular cells, hemosiderin pigment-laden macrophages, and colloid in the two liquid-based preparations (LBP), ThinPrep® (TP, **a–d**) and SurePath™ (SP, **e–g**), and in conventional smears (CS, **h** and **i**). Note subtle differences between the two LBP. (**a–c**) In TP, follicular cells form small, flat sheets with "honeycomb" arrangement of benign-appearing, uniform follicular cells with coarsely textured chromatin. Note the granular clumps of thin colloid and green-black granules of lipofuscin pigment (**c**). (**d**) Macrofollicles (spheres or balls) with oval and round configuration of benign-appearing follicular cells. (**a–d**, Pap stain, TP). (**e–g**) SP shows large, flat, and orderly sheets of follicular cells. Cell sheets are usually bigger and less fragmented than with TP, but the various sheets of follicular cells and background elements appear at various planes of focus. A macrofollicle (**g**) appears evenly spaced with round, uniform nuclei and low nuclear-cytoplasmic (N:C) ratio. All intracytoplasmic pigments are retained (**e–g**, Pap stain, SP). (**h, i**) In CS of MNG, note similarity in the macrofollicular architecture with that in **d**. Thin colloid has a faint, diffuse, cracked appearance. (**h**, Diff-Quik (DQ) stain, CS; **i**, Pap stain, CS)

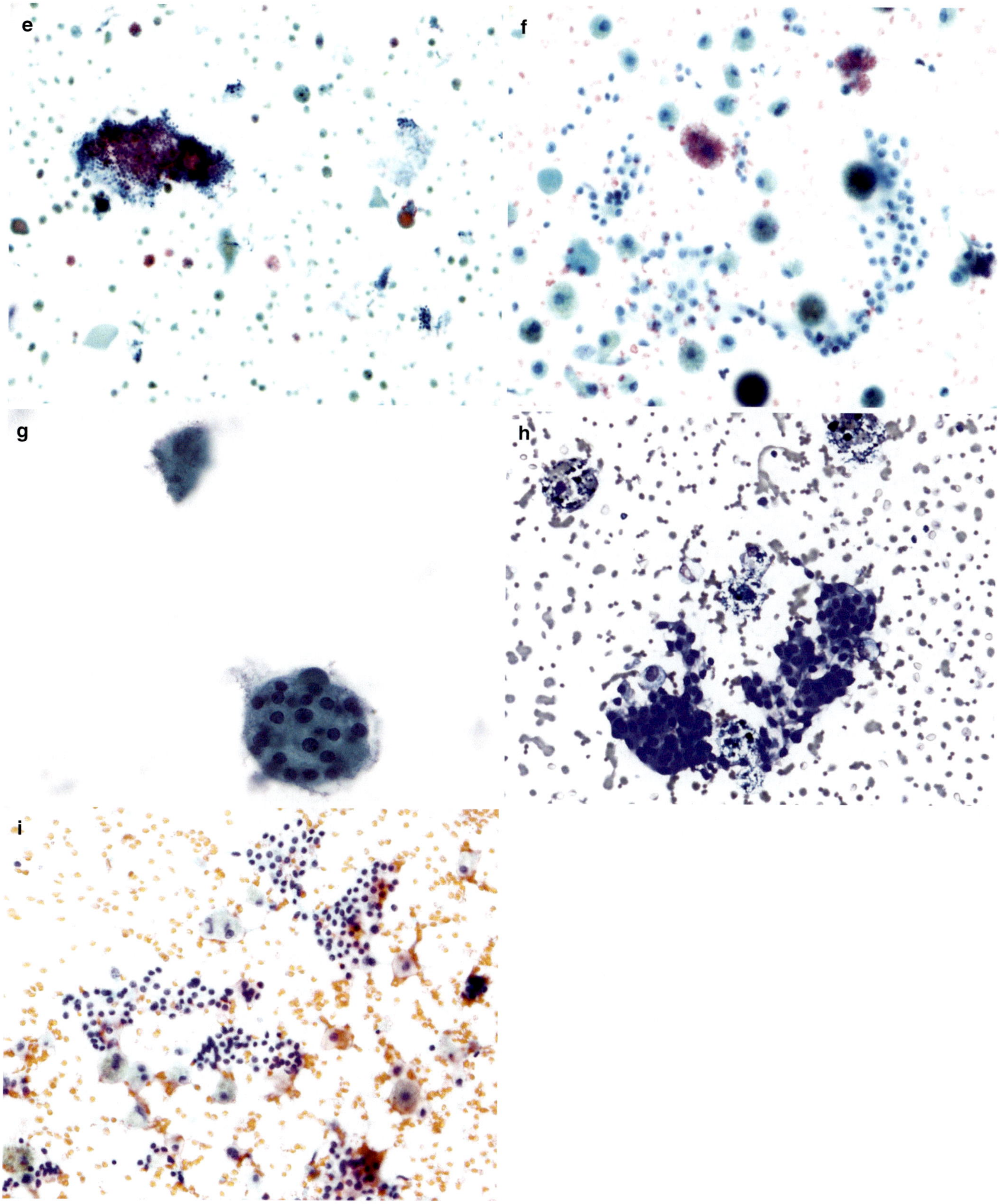

Fig. 4.2 (continued)

licles, cell clusters, a few microfollicles, and singly dispersed cells. Cell sheets are usually bigger and less fragmented than on TP. The follicular cells appear smaller and at various planes of focus, revealing a more three-dimensional (3-D) appearance of cell clusters, which may be difficult to interpret and require constant focusing at higher magnifications. Background elements of colloid, histiocytes, and other degenerative changes are retained and may also appear in different planes of focus (*see* Fig. 4.2e–g).

- On CS, follicular cells form small and large flat and folded sheets and large and medium-sized macrofollicles. Cytology correlates well with histology and LBP, with subtle differences (*see* Fig. 4.2h, i).
- On LBP, macrofollicles may appear smaller, but they remain intact and maintain similar features to CS. Unlike CS, where blood may obscure cell detail, the cells are clearly visible as benign on LBP (Figs. 4.3a–e and 4.4a, b).
- Colloid is readily identified on LBP (*see* Figs. 4.2a, b, e and 4.3a).
- Thin and thick colloid has a unique appearance:
  - Thin, watery colloid appears diffuse or as aggregates of granular deposits, napkin-folds, and sheets of wrinkled tissue paper (Fig. 4.5a–d). Watery colloid appears more clumped in TP than in SP, where it may be more diffuse in distribution. On CS, this type of colloid forms a diffuse, thin layer or appears as coalescing "broken glass" pieces (Fig. 4.5e, f).
  - In LBP, thick colloid appears as markedly fragmented chunks, round to oval aggregates, or dense droplets (globules), which show a dual staining pattern with a blue-staining periphery and central eosinophilia on Pap stain (Figs. 4.6a, b). On CS, this type of colloid appears as diffuse, dried and cracked desert sand, as diffuse thick bands, or as bigger globules (Figs. 4.6c, d).
- Cytoplasmic pigments are retained, including hemosiderin (*see* Figs. 4.2a, e and 4.5a, d) and green-black granules of lipofuscin pigment (Fig. 4.2c).
- Hürthle cell metaplasia is commonly observed in MNG/BFN, appearing similar to CS with subtle differences. The cells are polarized, with round nuclei, granular cytoplasm, and a low N:C ratio. In LBP, nuclei may appear smaller, and cytoplasm can either retain the granular quality or have a soft, lacy appearance with distinct boundaries (Fig. 4.7a–d).

Salient Points for LBP in MNG/BFN

- In LBP, collection of specimens in an alcohol-based preservative solution eliminates air-drying artifacts.
- Immediate cell fixation in LBP allows for better visualization of cytomorphology of follicular cell clusters.
- In LBP, the background is clean, as the collection medium also disintegrates red blood cells and mucus that may interfere with cytologic interpretation.
- Cells in each LBP slide are representative of all the material that is collected in the vial.
- Preparation of two LBP -based slides will improve specimen adequacy.
- In LBP, alterations in background, architecture, and cytomorphology can be understood to be a result of the fixation, homogenizing, and filtration process. These steps explain the cell shrinkage, appearance of colloid, fragmentation of cell sheets and macrofollicles, and follicular cell morphology.
- In the TP method, the cells of interest are separated when the liquid collection medium is drawn through a filter using negative pressure pulse. Thus, the cells appear in a true monolayer, but colloid, lymphocytes, and large tissue fragments are reduced, and the tissue fragments are more fragmented than on CS.
- In the SP method, the cells of interest are separated as a result of simple sedimentation and are transferred onto the slide surface without any applied pressure, so both single cells and clusters have a more 3-D configuration than on CS or TP.
- Various types of metaplasia, including Hürthle cell and squamous metaplasia, are often seen in MNG/BFN. These are seen as flat sheets, 3-D clusters, or single cells.
- The approach to diagnosis of MNG/BNF involves assessment of two elements, the amount of colloid and the number of follicular cells. Generally, the more colloid, the more likely the lesion is benign, and the more cells, the more likely the lesion is neoplastic. In TP, the amount of thin colloid may be diminished and is therefore difficult to quantify, requiring a closer evaluation of architectural and cytological features.
- However, a large study by the College of American Pathologists [19] found that LBP perform better than CS for MNG/BFN. The key diagnostic features of MNG/BFN, including watery colloid and follicular cells in macrofollicles and as large tissue fragments, are easily identified and better preserved in LBP than in CS.
- Features favoring MNG/BFN include variation in cytologic features between follicular cell groups in nuclear size, chromatin compaction, and amount of cytoplasm; focal marked nuclear pleomorphism as part of benign endocrine atypia; and the presence of macrophages (after cystic PTC is excluded).
- Follicular cells at the peripheral edge of the TP slide commonly appear distorted, blurred, and poorly-stained, an artifact associated with the TP technique.
- Ultrasound gel may mimic colloid. It appears as blue-purple, lace-like material, which may be closely associated with follicular cells (*see* Fig. 3.4). Lack of thyroglobulin staining confirms ultrasound gel.

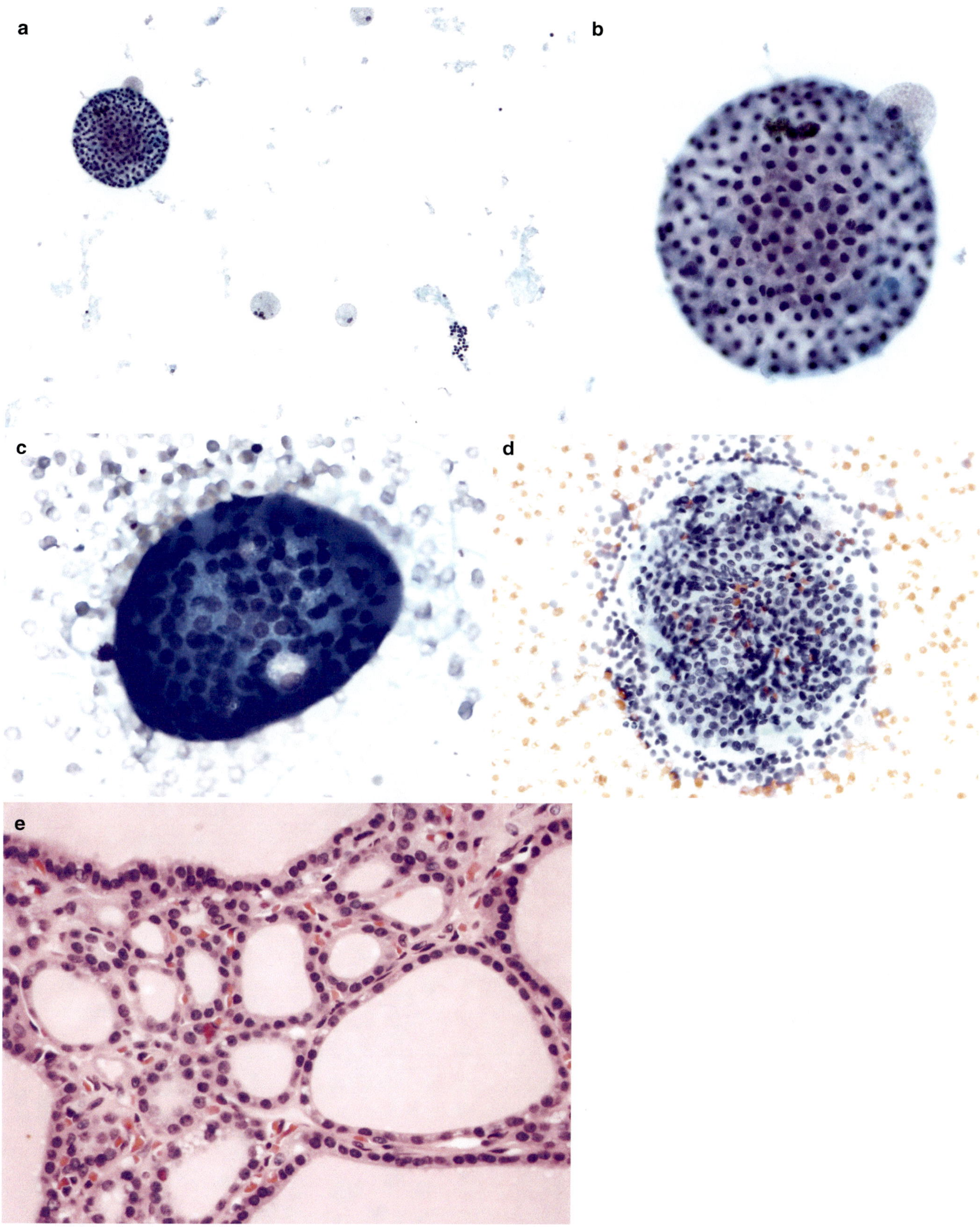

Fig. 4.3 Macrofollicles. (**a**, **b**) Macrofollicle in TP with oval and round configuration of benign follicular cells. Although this is a 3-D structure it retains a monolayer appearance of evenly spaced follicular cells in the same plane of focus, and all cells are visible in one plane. Note the thin colloid (Pap stain, TP). (**c**, **d**) Macrofollicle in CS with similar appearance (**c**, DQ stain, CS; **d**, Pap stain, CS). (**e**) Histology of MNG with microfollicles and macrofollicles, lined by flattened to hyperplastic epithelium (H&E stain)

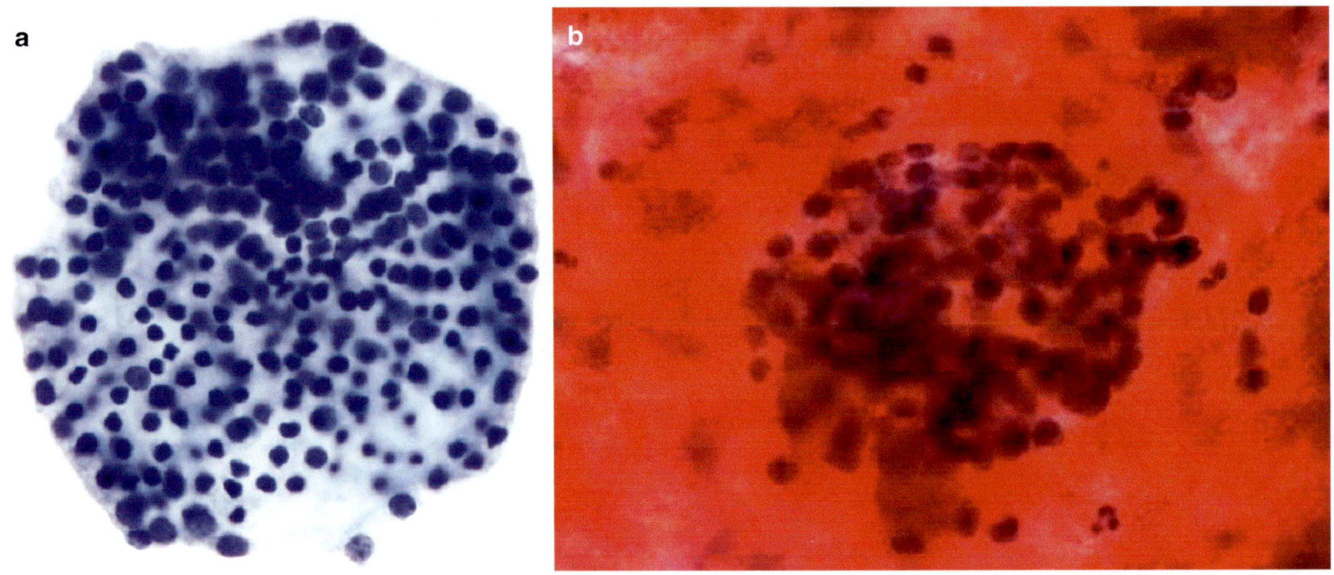

Fig. 4.4 Macrofollicles in LBP and CS. The appearance of MNG/BFN in TP (**a**) and SP is similar to the features seen in CS (**b**), with subtle differences. Note the similarities between the macrofollicular appearance in CS and that seen in Figs. 4.2d, g and 4.3a, b, except that abundant blood partially obscures cell detail in CS. (**a**, Pap stain, TP; **b**, Pap stain, CS)

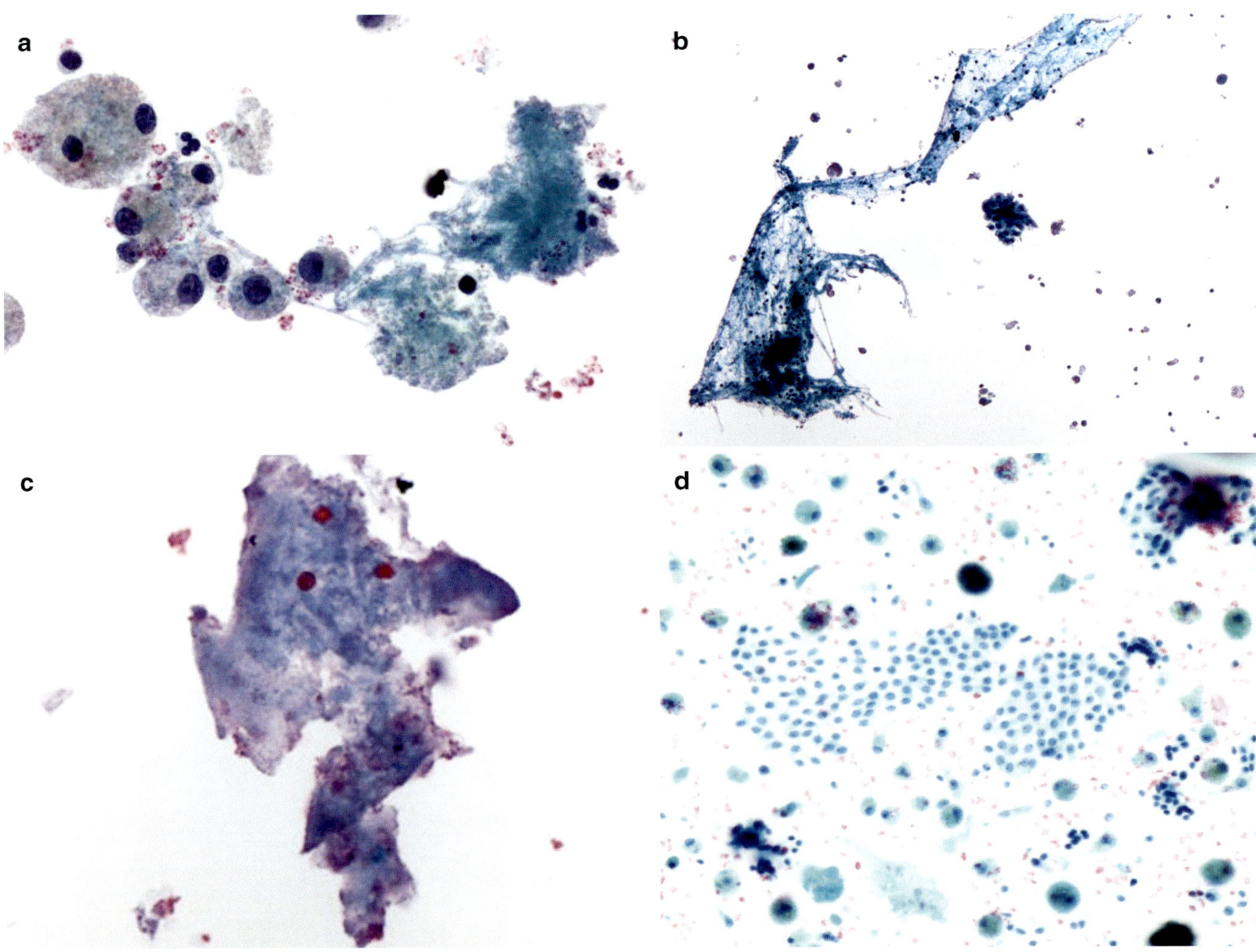

Fig. 4.5 Thin colloid in LBP and CS. Colloid is readily identified on LBP with a unique appearance of thin and thick colloid. (**a–d**) Thin, watery colloid appears as diffuse or aggregates of granular deposits, napkin-folds, and sheets of wrinkled tissue paper. Note the retained cytoplasmic hemosiderin pigment (**a–c**, Pap stain, TP; **d**, Pap stain, SP.) (**e**, **f**) On CS, this type of colloid forms a diffuse, thin layer or coalescing "broken glass" pieces. (**e**, DQ stain, CS; **f**, Pap stain, CS)

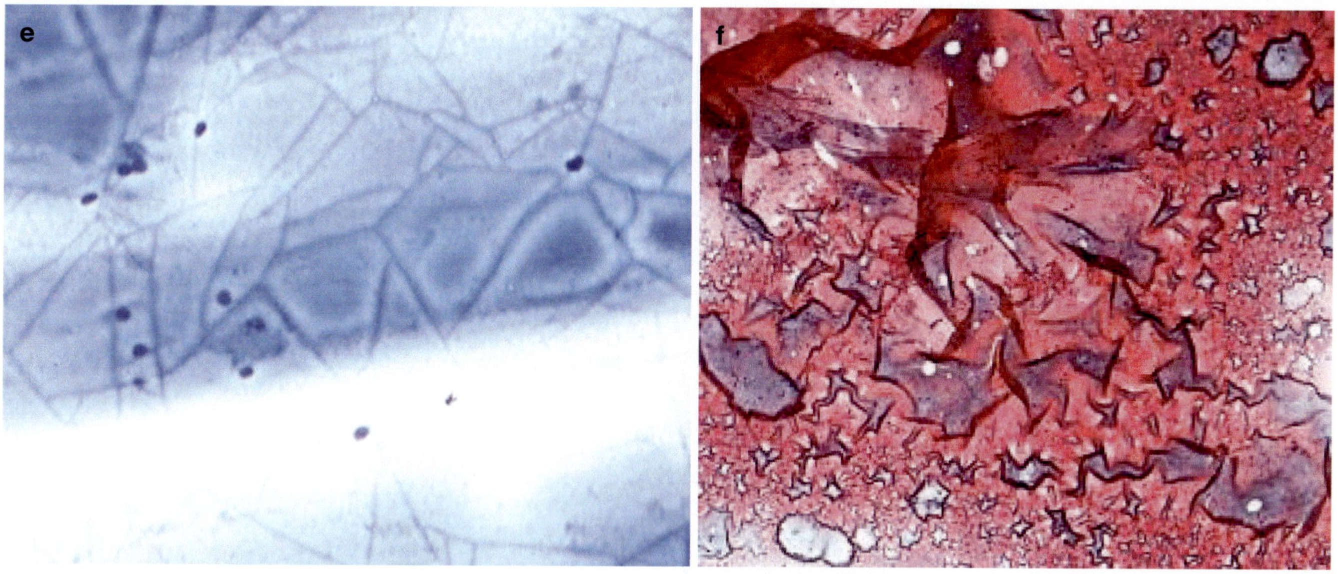

Fig. 4.5 (continued)

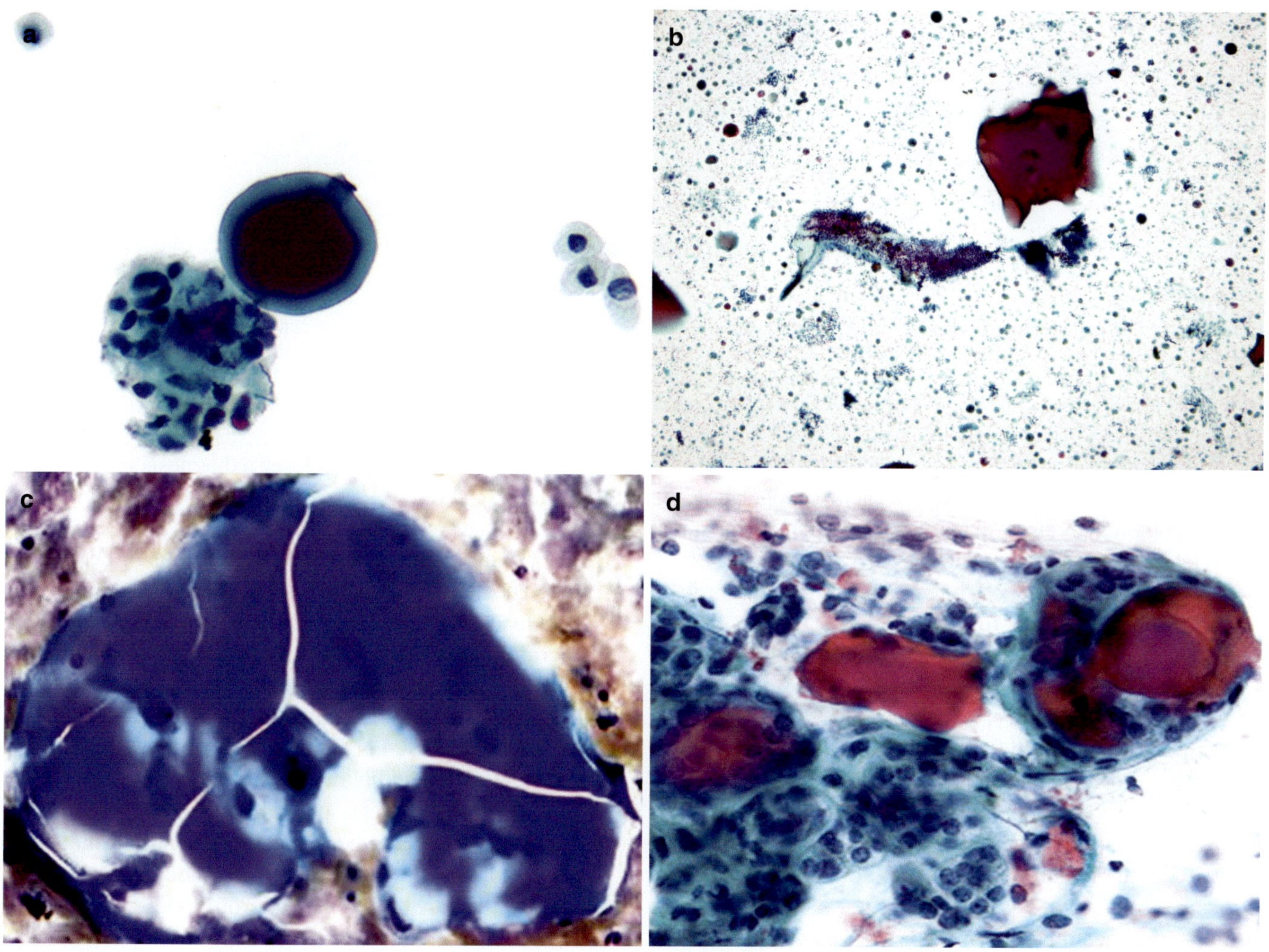

Fig. 4.6 Thick colloid in LBP and CS. (**a**, **b**) On LBP. thick colloid has a unique appearance, appearing as markedly fragmented chunks, round to oval aggregates, or dense droplets (globules), which show a dual staining pattern with a blue-staining periphery and central eosinophilia on Pap stain (**a**, Pap stain, TP; **b**, Pap stain, SP.) (**c**) On CS, this type of colloid appears as diffuse dried and cracked desert sand (DQ stain, CS). (**d**) On CS, thick colloid can appear in bigger, eosinophilic globules (Pap stain, CS)

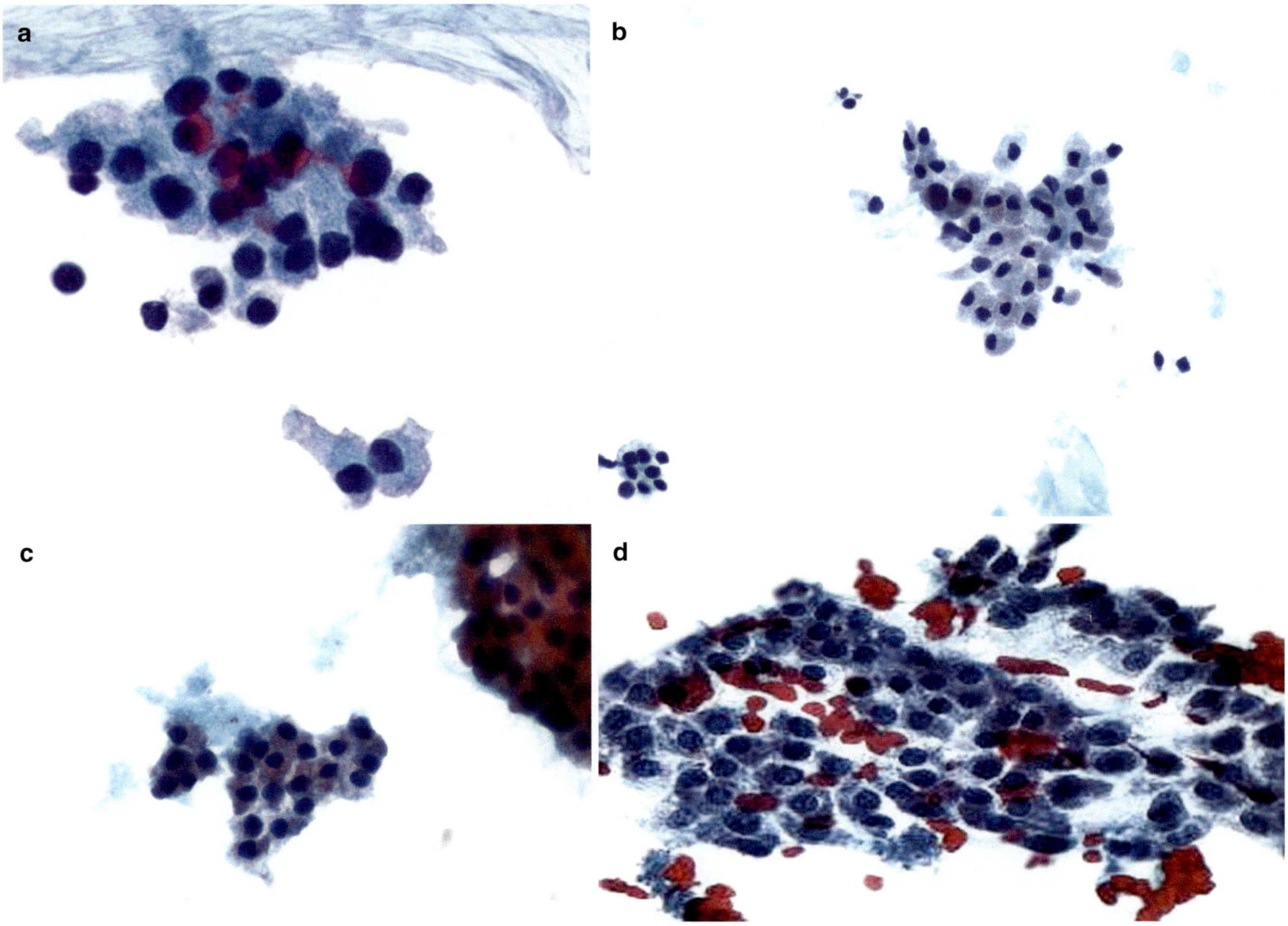

Fig. 4.7 Hürthle cell metaplasia in LBP and CS. (**a–c**) Hürthle cell metaplasia is commonly observed in MNG/BFN. In LBP, it appears similar to CS, with subtle differences. In LBP, the cells are polarized with round nuclei, granular cytoplasm, and low N:C ratio. The nuclei may appear smaller, and cytoplasm can either retain the granular quality or have a soft, lacy appearance with distinct boundaries (**a**, **b**, Pap stain, TP; **c**, Pap stain, SP). (**d**) The only difference in CS for Hürthle cell metaplasia is the larger sheet of cells (Pap stain, CS)

- Studies have demonstrated a higher incidence of thyroid cancer in patients with MNG than in the general population.
- Cytopathologists have maximum concordance for interpretation of the benign category.
- The false-negative (FN) rate of a benign diagnosis is 0–3% if noninvasive follicular thyroid neoplasm with papillary-like nuclear features (NIFTP) and microPTC are excluded.
- The main causes for FN diagnoses include errors of sampling and cytologic interpretation. Sampling errors occur with inadequate biopsy of the nodule harboring malignancy. Interpretation error may occur with poor specimen quality, such as multiple CS with air-drying artifact, thick cellular areas, and/or obscuring background blood.
- Poor specimen quality can occur when the material is not representative, scant, or poorly preserved so that neoplastic cells cannot be identified. Poor specimen quality is also implicated in false-positive (FP) diagnoses, when the cytopathologist attempts to force a diagnosis in cases with marginal material.
- FN diagnoses may also occur when focal features of classic PTC are misinterpreted as Hürthle cells or cyst-lining cells. The morphology of the latter may overlap with PTC.
- To reduce FN diagnoses, cases in which a clearly defined macrofollicular component is not identified should not be classified as benign. Whether these cases are best classified as atypical or nondiagnostic is less clear [35].
- The advent of USGFNA has decreased rates of nondiagnostic cytology and FN rates.
- False-positive diagnosis of nodular hyperplasia in LBP may occur when a hyperplastic nodule shows increased cellularity, papillary-like formation, and microfollicles. True papillae are absent and microfollicles are usually a small component.
- When the FNA yields a benign result, the NPV is >95%; when the FNA yields a malignant result, the positive predictive value (PPV) is >99%.

- The American Thyroid Association (ATA) recommends a conservative follow-up strategy for a benign cytologic diagnosis [22]

Main Differences Between LBP and CS in MNG/BFN

- As suggested by Tables 4.1 and 4.2, the morphology of MNG/BFN in LBP differs from CS in two aspects:
  - The cells in each slide are a monolayered or 3-D representative sample of the entire material collected in the vial. The residual preservative solution contains a variable amount of leftover sample.
  - The automated process causes some changes in background, architecture, and cellular morphology, the most important being the appearance of colloid, as shown on Figs. 4.5 and 4.6.
- Reduction or loss of the watery colloid makes quantitation difficult in LBP; it is more straightforward in CS. In TP, the amount of thin colloid may be diminished and therefore is difficult to quantify, requiring a closer evaluation of the architectural and cytological features.
- Cells are smaller, with pronounced shrinkage, and clusters of follicular cells are more crowded and tighter.
- Nuclear and cytoplasmic details are superior, particularly in TP, even with smaller cell size.
- Macrophages have more abundant pale cytoplasm, enlarged pale nuclei, and prominent nucleoli.
- Hürthle cells may be shrunken and more dissociated.

Partially Cystic Thyroid Nodules (PCTNs) in MNG/BFN

- Prominent cystic degeneration often occurs in MNG/BFN, comprising numerous macrophages and an adequate number of follicular cells (Fig. 4.8a).
- True epithelial cysts in the thyroid are rare.
- Thyroid cysts with an inadequate number of follicular cells should be interpreted as Nondiagnostic or Unsatisfactory (ND/Unsat), as the frequency of malignancy ranges from 5.2% to 17.6% in cystic thyroid nodules, similar to the rate for solid thyroid nodules. Some sonographic features associated with malignancy in a PCTN include microcalcifications, irregular borders, and intranodular vascularity. In the absence of worrisome US features, 2015 ATA guidelines recommend conservative management [22].
- Reparative changes of cyst-lining cells is commonly seen as a focal finding with cystic degeneration.
- Cyst-lining cells are elongated, polygonal, and cohesive, with dense or soft spindled cytoplasm, elongate to oval nuclei with grooves, powdery chromatin, and small to prominent nucleoli. The N:C ratio is low (Fig. 4.8b, c).
- Differential diagnosis of reparative changes in cyst-lining cells include cystic papillary thyroid carcinoma (PTC). Cells in cystic PTC lack spindle-cell morphology, and they show nuclear crowding and papillary microarchitecture (Fig. 4.8d).
- Immunocytochemistry for CK-19, galectin-3, HBME-1 and anti-CITED1 can be useful in distinguishing cystic PTC from benign cysts.

Thyroglossal Duct Cyst

- Thyroglossal duct cyst (TDC) is a common congenital anomaly of the thyroid gland, usually found centrally.
- Normally, the thyroglossal duct obliterates and disappears by the tenth week of gestation, but a thyroglossal remnant can remain in the form of a cyst, tract, or duct, or as ectopic thyroid within a cyst or duct.
- TDC usually presents as a painless cystic mass in the neck.
- It is treated by total thyroidectomy and surgical excision of the TDC.
- Cytologically, CS show columnar or round epithelial cells dispersed as sheets, small strips, or singly in a diffuse to granular proteinaceous background with histiocytes. Nuclei are round to oval with even chromatin. Cilia seen at the terminal end stain magenta in Diff-Quik (DQ) stain and eosinophilic Pap stain (Fig. 4.9a).
- In LBP, TDC proteinaceous material forms granular clumps and shows dispersed histiocytes and small clusters of ciliated, columnar epithelial cells. Nuclear morphology is well preserved, and the cilia stain light pink (Figs. 4.9b, c).
- The differential diagnosis of TDC includes branchial cleft cyst, lipoma, metastatic thyroid carcinoma, dermoid cyst, sebaceous cyst, and an enlarged lymph node.
- PTC can arise in a TDC, but this occurs in only 1% of all cases of TDC.

Squamous Metaplasia (SM) in Thyroid Nodules on LBP

- Squamous metaplasia (SM) is rare in thyroid nodules, but it is seen in non-neoplastic and neoplastic lesions including thyroid cysts, nodular hyperplasia, Hashimoto's thyroiditis, and PTC.
- In CS, SM shows two-dimensional sheets with a pulled-out appearance. Cells are enlarged and elongated to spindled. Nuclei are crowded, with pale to dark chromatin and

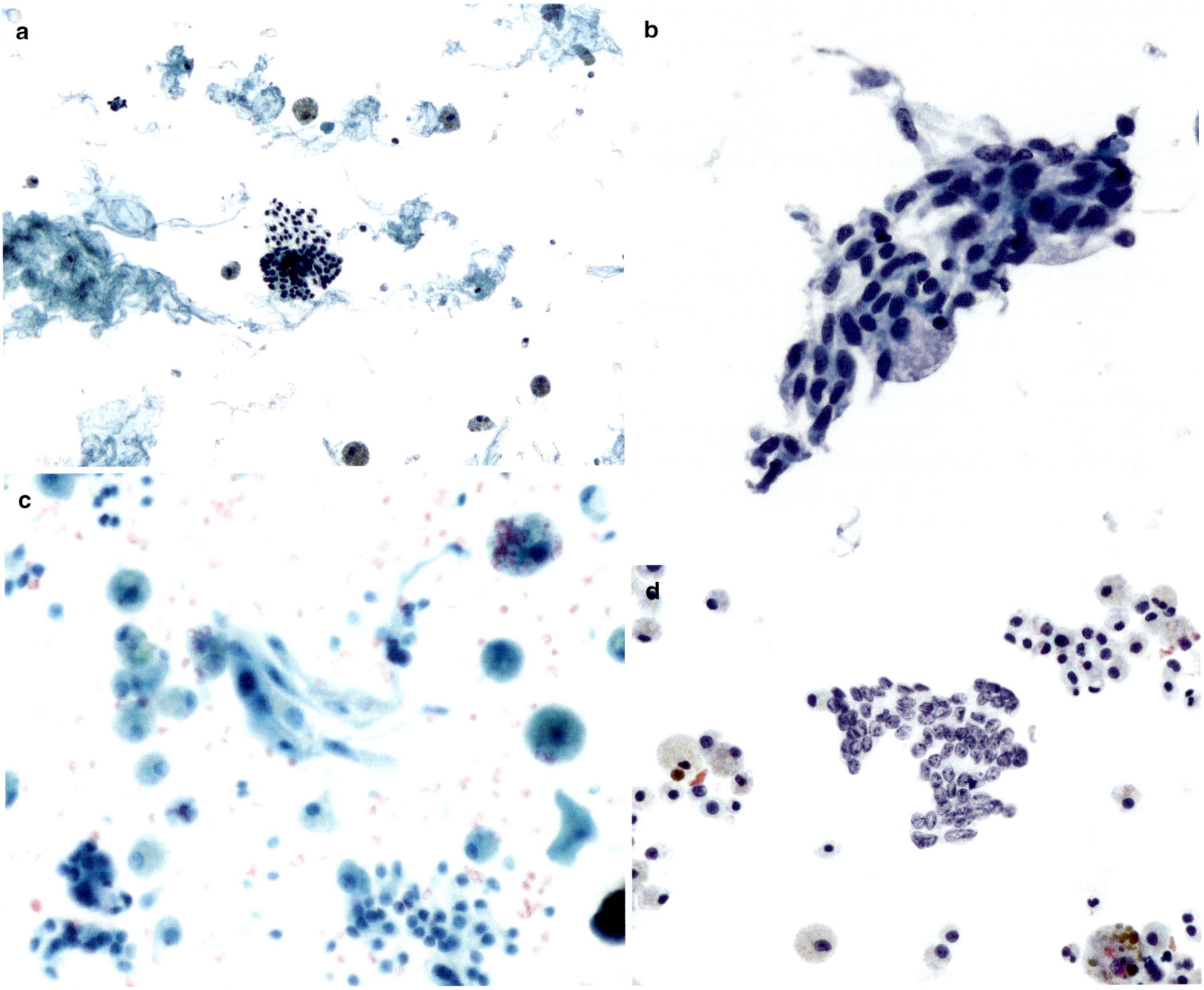

Fig. 4.8 Cystic degeneration in LBP and CS. Cystic degeneration often occurs in MNG/BFN, comprising numerous macrophages and an adequate number of follicular cells. (**a**) Cystic degeneration in a TP shows a flat sheet of uniform follicular cells in a background of abundant thin colloid and scattered hemosiderin-laden macrophages. (**b**) Reparative changes of cyst-lining cells (CLC) is commonly seen as a focal finding with cystic degeneration. CLC are elongated, polygonal, spindled, and cohesive, with slightly dense spindled cytoplasm, elongated to oval nuclei with grooves, powdery chromatin, and small to prominent nucleoli. The N:C ratio is low (**a**, **b**, Pap stain, TP). (**c**) In SP, cystic degeneration shows all features seen in TP, including sheets of uniform follicular cells and CLC in a background of abundant thin colloid and scattered hemosiderin-laden macrophages (Pap stain, SP). (**d**) Cystic papillary thyroid carcinoma (PTC) is in the differential diagnosis of CLC. Cells in cystic PTC show all nuclear features of the neoplasm, including irregularity, overlap, powdery chromatin, grooves, and pseudoinclusions. The cells lack the spindle-cell morphology of CLC. Immunocytochemistry for CK-19, galectin-3, HBME-1, and anti-CITED1 can be useful in distinguishing cystic PTC from benign CLC (Pap stain, TP)

intranuclear grooves; rarely, pseudoinclusions can be seen. Cytoplasm is dense and squamoid with distinct borders (Fig. 4.10a, b).

- In LBP, SM shows similar cells. The cells appear more cohesive and cell sheets appear tighter (Fig. 4.10c). A histologic diagnosis may show nodular hyperplasia with extensive SM (Fig. 4.10d).
- SM should be in the differential diagnosis of thyroid nodules with potentially benign cystic changes.
- Extensive SM with reactive atypia is a diagnostic dilemma in FNA. It may mimic malignancy, including PTC and squamous cell carcinoma, and lead to false-positive results.
- Surgical resection may be an appropriate approach to confirm its benign nature.

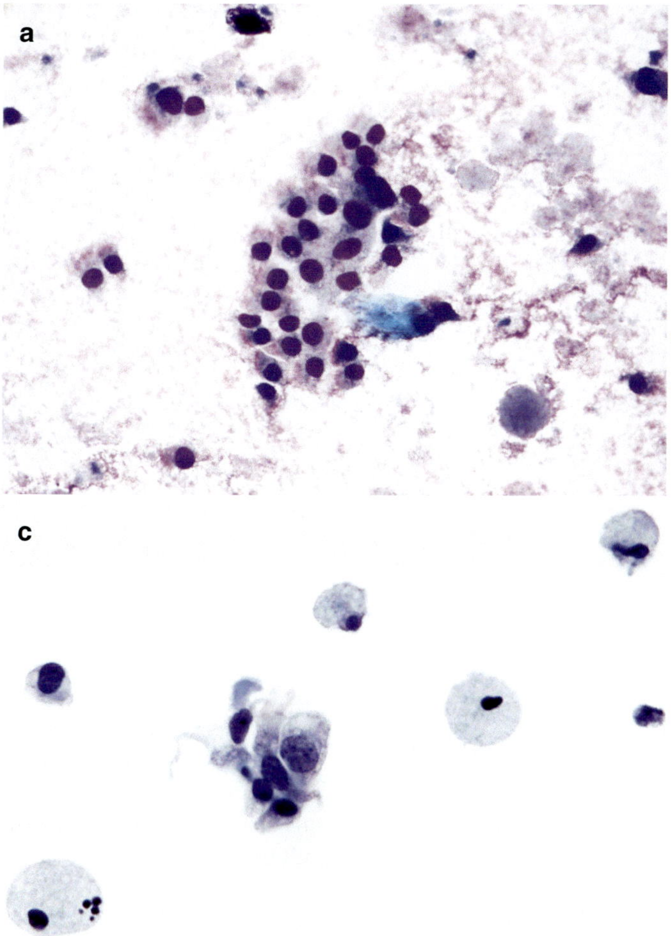

Fig. 4.9 Thyroglossal duct cyst (TDC). (**a**), CS shows small sheets and small strips of columnar to round epithelial cells in a diffuse to granular proteinaceous background with histiocytes. Nuclei are round to oval with even chromatin; magenta-staining cilia are seen at the terminal end (DQ stain, CS). (**b**, **c**) TDC in TP shows large and small granular clumps of proteinaceous material, dispersed histiocytes, and small clusters of ciliated, columnar epithelial cells. Nuclear morphology is well preserved, and cilia stain light pink (Pap stain, TP)

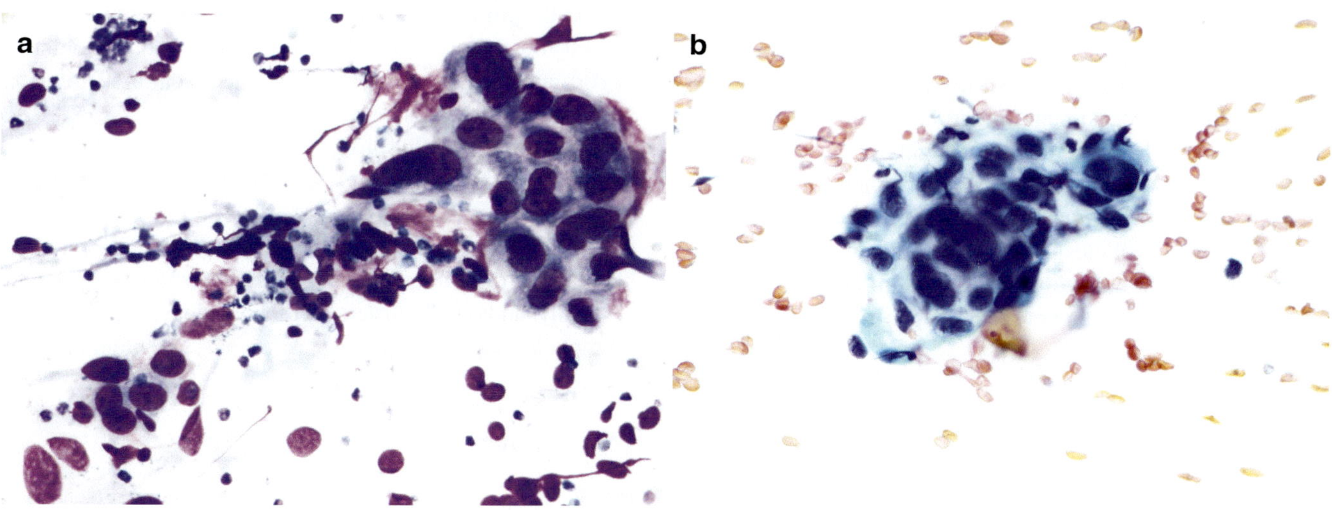

Fig. 4.10 Squamous metaplasia (SM). (**a**, **b**) In CS, SM shows two-dimensional sheets with a pulled-out appearance. Cells are enlarged, and elongated to spindled. Nuclei are enlarged with some bi-nucleation, pale to dark chromatin, and nucleoli. Intranuclear grooves occasionally can be seen, and rarely, pseudoinclusions (*not shown*). Cytoplasm is dense, squamoid, with distinct borders (**a**, DQ stain, CS; **b**, Pap stain, CS). (**c**) TP shows similar features as CS, except that the cells are in more cohesive groups with a less pulled-out 2-D appearance (Pap stain). (**d**) A histologic section of the total thyroidectomy specimen shows MNG with extensive SM. Note dilated follicles or small cysts with SM, surrounded by thyroid follicles (H&E stain)

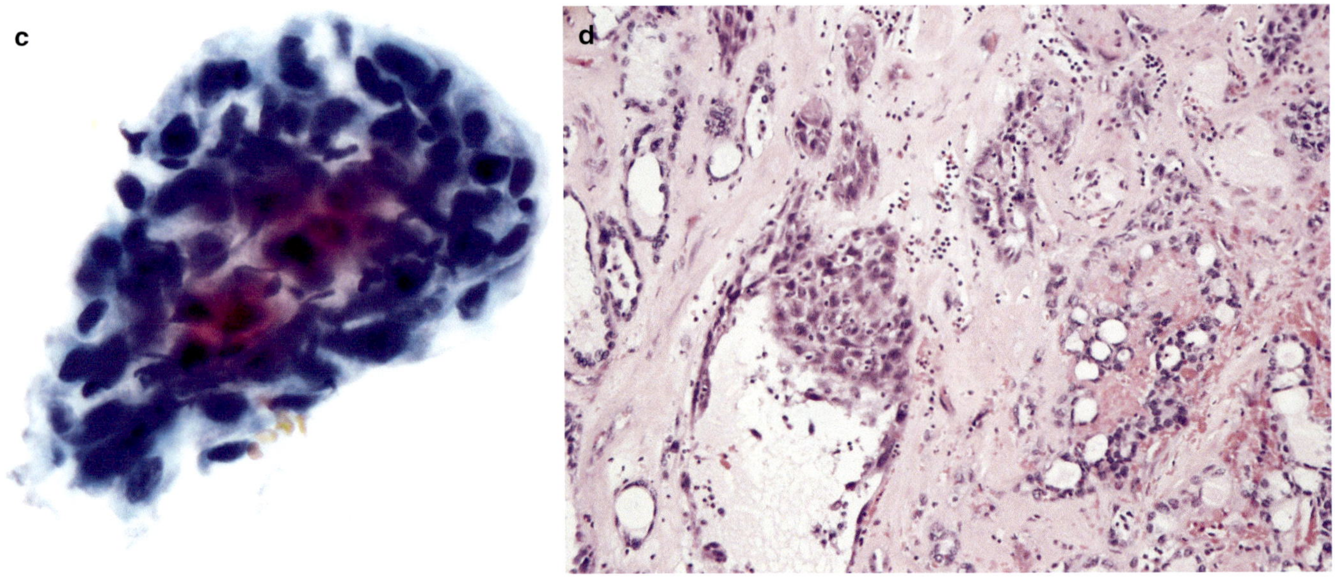

Fig. 4.10 (continued)

Hashimoto's Thyroiditis (Chronic Lymphocytic Thyroiditis)

- Hashimoto thyroiditis (HT), also known as chronic lymphocytic thyroiditis, is the most common type of lymphocytic thyroiditis.
- It is an autoimmune disease, with an incidence estimated to range from 0.3 to 1.5 cases per 1000 people.
- The disease is characterized by a cellular immune response involving T and B lymphocytic infiltration of the thyroid gland, as well as by a humoral immune response leading to the production of thyroid-specific antibodies, including antithyroid peroxidase antibodies (TPOAb).
- Grossly, the thyroid gland shows diffuse and symmetric enlargement. Occasionally it can be nodular. Cut surface is yellow-tan (Fig. 4.11a). Histologically, extensive lymphocytic infiltration with germinal center formation is seen, and some plasma cells are seen in close association with atrophic follicles lined by Hürthle cells (Fig. 4.11b). Lymphocytes are usually T-cell. Colloid is present. Giant cells and SM are also noted. HT looks similar in CS, TP, and SP.
- Diagnosis of Hürthle cell lesions is a challenge in both CS and LBP, as Hürthle cells in Hashimoto's thyroiditis, MNG/BFN, or Hürthle cell neoplasms display similar cytological appearance and may be difficult to distinguish.

Cytology of HT on LBP

- The diagnosis of HT on CS is made when increased numbers of polymorphous lymphocytes, clusters of Hürthle (oncocytic) cells, and/or thyroid follicular cells and lymphocytic infiltration of epithelial cell clusters are present in varying proportions with scanty colloid, lymphohistiocytic aggregates, lymphoid tangles, scattered plasma cells, and giant cells (Fig. 4.12a–c).
- The diagnosis of thyroiditis on TP and SP is reliable, as all characteristic findings of HT are easily identified (Figs. 4.12d–f and 4.13a–d; *see also* Fig. 3.7).
- Specimens are usually hypercellular, with both Hürthle cells and/or thyroid follicular cells and lymphocytes, noted individually and/or in clusters, lymphohistiocytic aggregates, lymphoid tangles, scattered plasma cells, and giant cells.

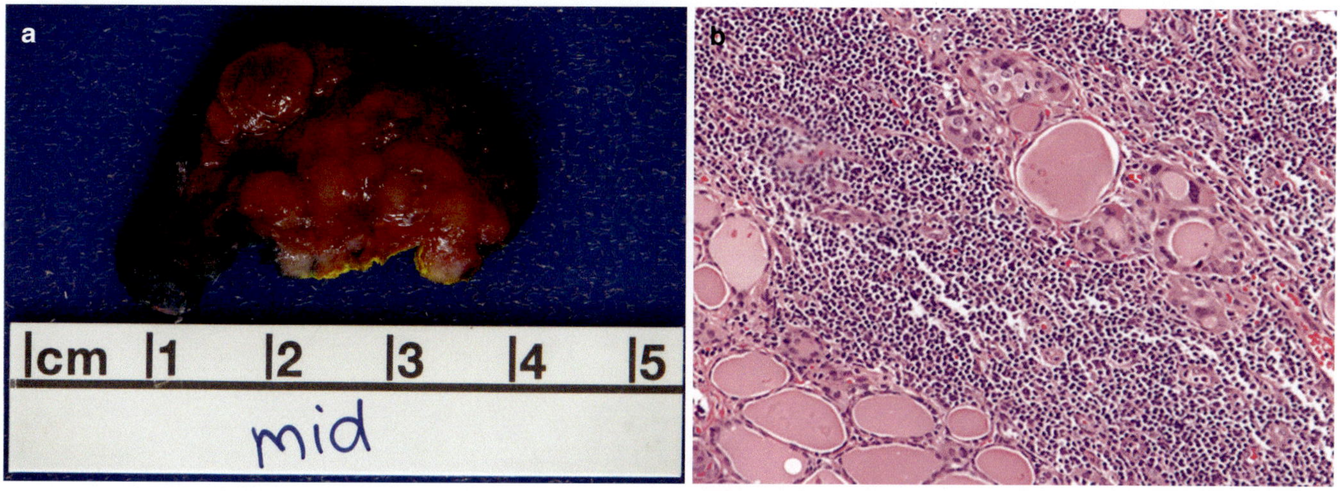

Fig. 4.11 Chronic lymphocytic thyroiditis/Hashimoto's thyroiditis (HT). (**a**) Gross specimen of a lobectomy with HT showing nodular, symmetric enlargement with a yellow-tan cut surface. (**b**) Histology shows extensive lymphocytic infiltration in close association with atrophic follicles lined by Hürthle cells. Lymphocytes are usually T cells. Colloid is present (H&E stain)

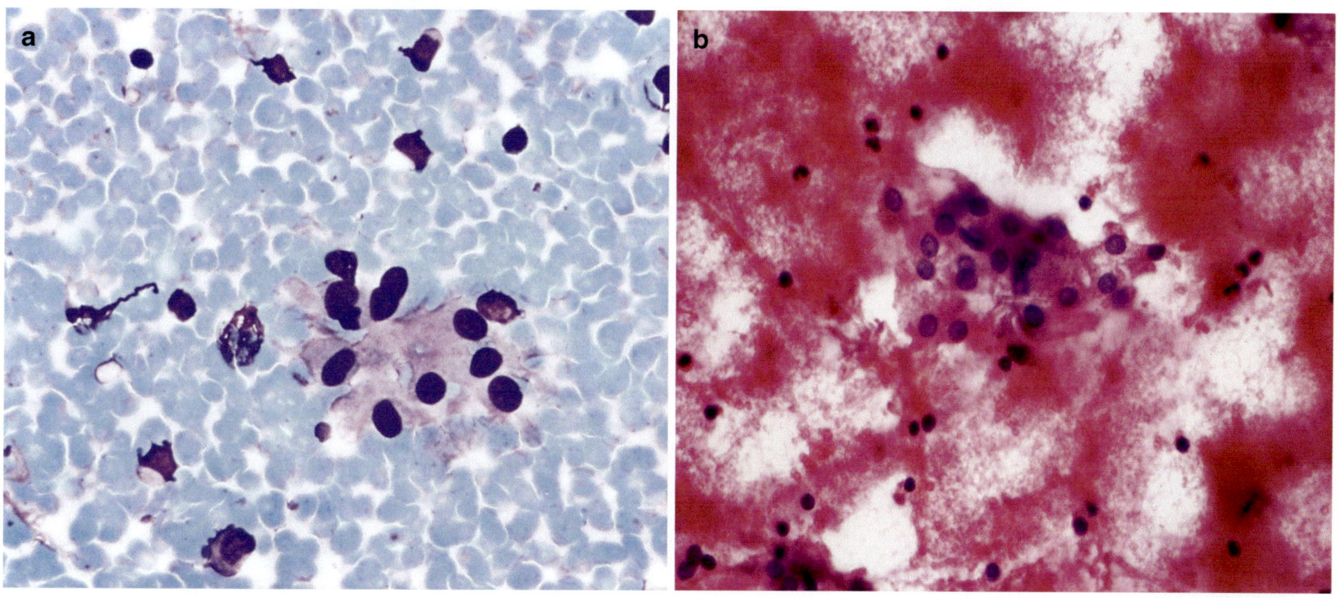

Fig. 4.12 Hashimoto's thyroiditis (HT) in CS and LBP. (**a**–**c**) Polymorphous lymphoid population, Hürthle cells, and lymphohistiocytic aggregate in HT. Note abundant blood partially obscuring cell detail in the Pap-stained CS (**a**, DQ stain CS; **b**, **c**, Pap stain CS). (**d**–**f**) TP shows a polymorphous lymphoid population, Hürthle cells, and lymphohistiocytic aggregate. Note abundant, thin tissue paper colloid, granular cytoplasm of Hürthle cells, and the crisp nuclear morphology of these cells and lymphocytes compared with the CS. Lymphohistiocytic aggregate forms a tighter cluster in TP, but the cellular morphology is similar to the CS (**d**–**f**, Pap stain TP)

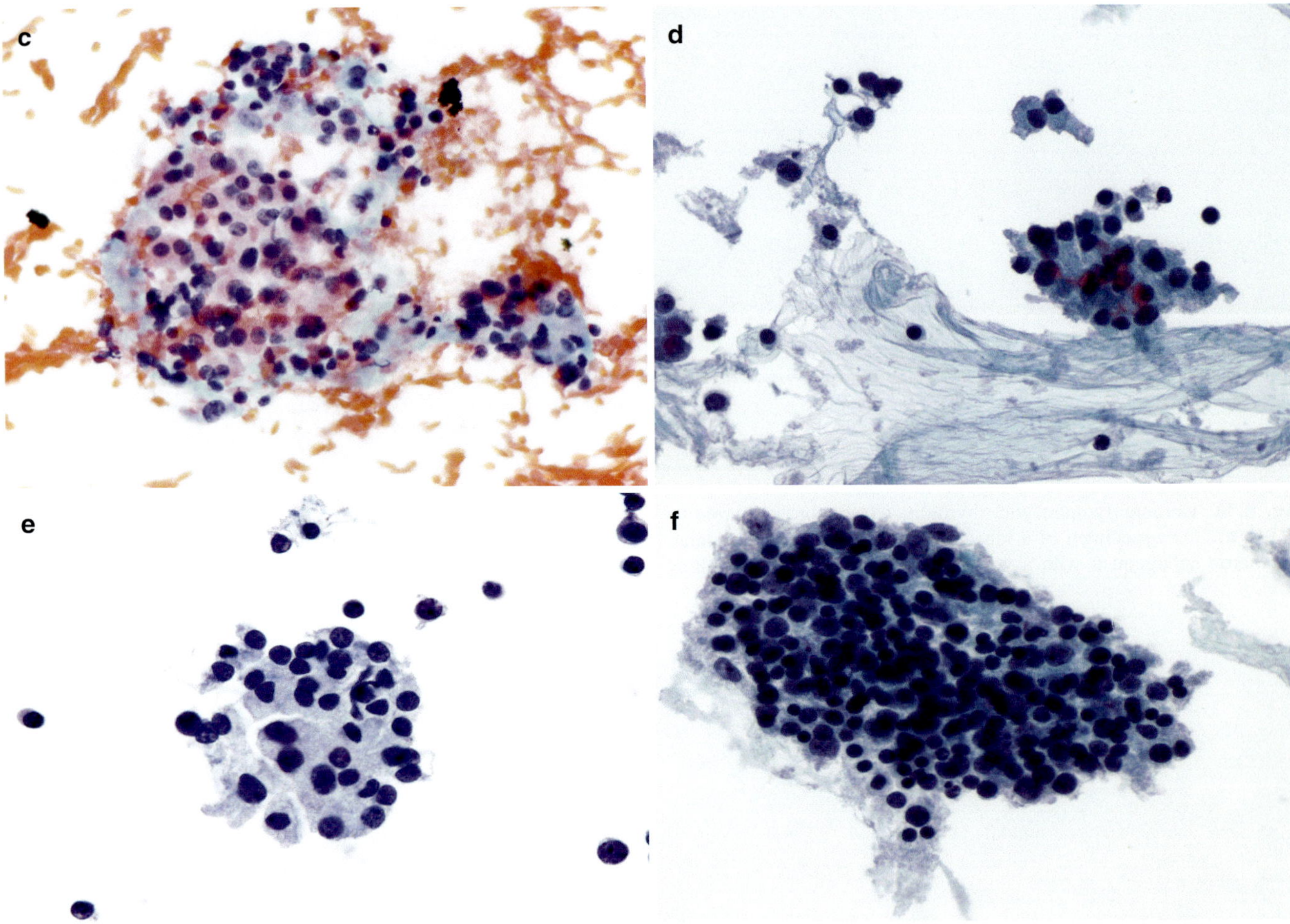

Fig. 4.12 (continued)

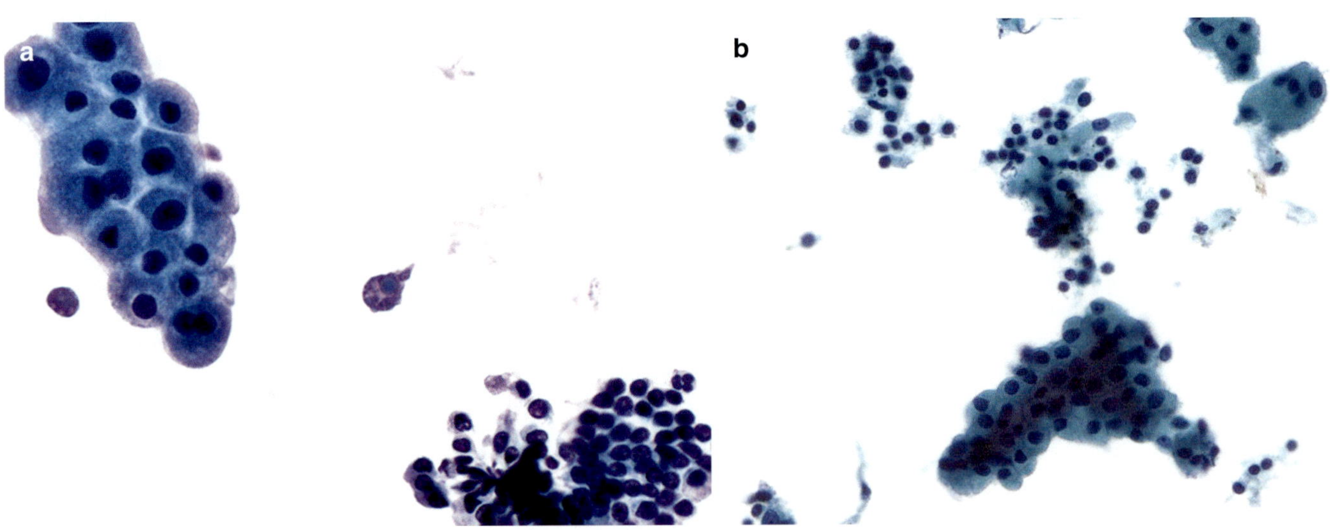

Fig. 4.13 Hashimoto's thyroiditis (HT) in TP and SP. (**a**) Characteristic cytomorphology of HT is seen on a TP slide. Lymphocytes may aggregate and clump at the periphery of the slide and mimic follicular cells (Pap stain, TP). (**b–d**) SP also shows the characteristic cytomorphology of HT. Note the distinct cytoplasmic walls of Hürthle cells and well-preserved morphology for these cells and lymphocytes. Lymphocytes are increased and appear in clusters, some adjacent to Hürthle cells. Note the somewhat 3-D appearance of cells; some lymphocytes appear on a different plane of focus (Pap stain, SP)

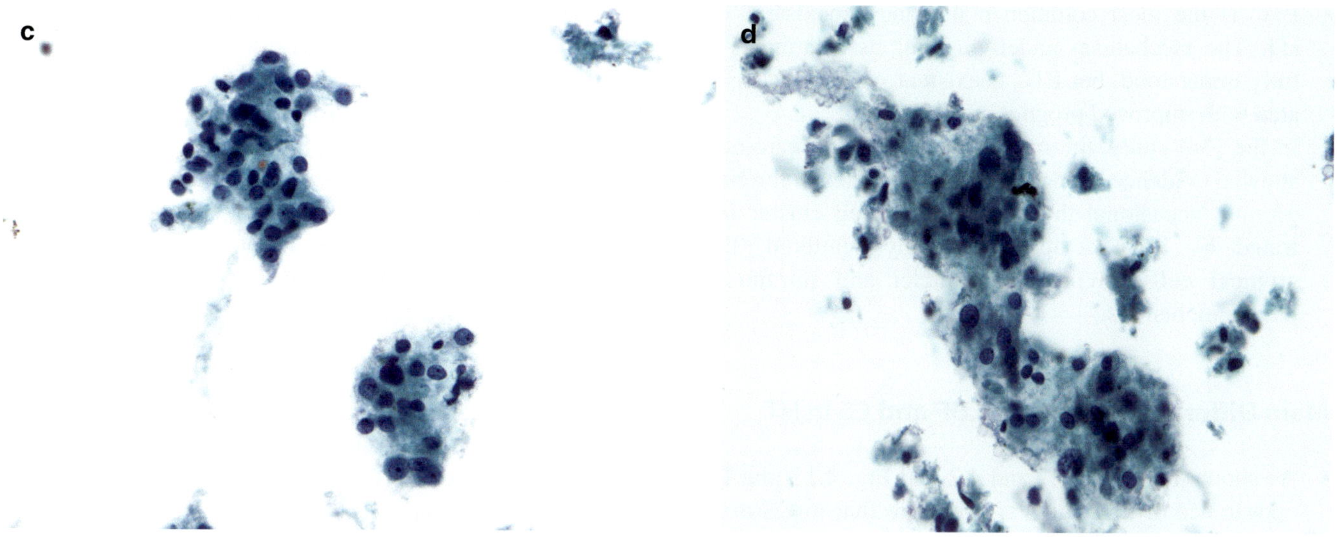

Fig. 4.13 (continued)

- The most recent TBSRTC does not require a minimum number of Hürthle cells and/or thyroid follicular cells for an adequate diagnosis of HT.
- Lymphocytes are polymorphous and dispersed as isolated cells, in clusters, and infiltrate Hürthle cells. In LBP (particularly TP), lymphocytes form clumps towards the periphery of the slide (*see* Fig. 4.13a).
- Hürthle cells are arranged in flat sheets, small clusters with infiltrating lymphocytes, or as isolated cells, showing small nuclei with or without nucleoli. The cytoplasm is well defined and granular (*see* Figs. 4.12d and 4.13a, b).
- Random cellular and nuclear atypia composed of large Hürthle cells with large nuclei and prominent nucleoli is usually present and favors a diagnosis of HT.
- Hürthle cells in HT can demonstrate atypical nuclear features, including elongation, grooves, and clearing with a less prominent HT background and can be misinterpreted as PTC.
- Plasma cells and lymphohistiocytic aggregates may be prominent and are seen in close approximation to Hürthle cell clusters.
- The appearance of HT on cytologic preparations depends on the state of the disease. In the milder early phase, LBP show follicular cell clusters infiltrated by a few lymphocytes. As the disease progresses to a more severe form, LBP show follicular cell clusters infiltrated by moderate amounts of lymphocytes. In the late phase of the disease, the background shows an increased/dense lymphocytic infiltration in various stages of transformation, with fewer Hürthle and/or follicular cells.

Salient Points for HT

- Clinical presentation is symmetric enlargement of thyroid gland.
- Diagnosis of HT is made with clinical imaging, serum thyroid peroxidase (TPO) antibody assessment, and FNA.
- Proper recognition of Hürthle cells, lymphocytes, and lymphohistiocytic aggregates virtually rules out a Hürthle cell neoplasm and prevents unnecessary surgery.
- HT may be the main cause for false-positive (FP) results on thyroid FNA. In a 2018 study by Rammeh et al. [34] of head and neck masses, all FP were reported in the thyroid group. These cases, cytologically classified suspicious for malignancy and PTC, proved to be lymphocytic thyroiditis on final histology.
- Problems in the differential diagnosis of HT may arise when there is a deviation in the proportions of the two cell components, Hürthle cells and lymphocytes. In cases of HT misdiagnosed as MNG/BFN, Hürthle cells may be present in a background of colloid with low numbers of lymphocytes. Cases of HT misdiagnosed as suspicious for PTC may show the nuclear changes described above for the cytology of HT.
- When a thyroiditis is suspected, the detection of lymphoepithelial clusters in an inflammatory background is the pivotal clue for the diagnosis in LBP.
- Neoplasia most commonly associated with HT includes PTC and non-Hodgkin's lymphoma.
- The incidence of coexisting thyroid neoplasia with HT ranges between 3% and 14%.

- PTC is the most common malignancy coexistent with HT. The mechanism underlying this association is not fully understood, but PTC coexistent with HT is associated with improved prognosis.
- In the [34] study, the only case of HT with carcinoma showed evidence of increased lymphocytes in the background, occasional thyroid follicular cell cluster infiltrated by lymphocytes, and many scattered, large atypical cells having large nuclei and intranuclear pseudoinclusions.

Main Differences Between LBP and CS in HT

- As shown in Tables 4.1 and 4.2 and Fig. 4.12, the LBP appearance of thyroiditis is similar to that in CS except that the amount of background lymphocytes in LBP can be higher than normal because of the spinning of the material before the automated process. When a thyroiditis is suspected, the detection of lympho-epithelial clusters in an inflammatory background is the pivotal clue for the diagnosis and warrants a simple follow-up for the patient.
- Lymphocytes may be more evenly dispersed, with fewer lymphohistiocytic aggregates.
- Lymphocytes may clump at the periphery of the slide (particularly in TP) and may be mistaken for follicular cells.
- Hürthle cells may be shrunken and more dissociated.

Riedel's Thyroiditis

- Riedel's thyroiditis (RT) is a rare form of chronic thyroiditis. Although the etiology is unknown, it may develop in the course of subacute thyroiditis. It may be associated with idiopathic fibrosis in other sites (retroperitoneum, lung, mediastinum, pancreas).
- Patients present with diffuse and painless enlargement of the thyroid with compressive symptoms.
- It is a fibroinflammatory process that partially destroys and replaces the thyroid parenchyma and often involves surrounding tissues.
- Grossly, the goitrous thyroid gland is hard (Fig. 4.14a). The mass may not be well defined and may involve extrathyroidal tissue, such as adjacent muscle and other structures. Cut surface is firm, yellow-tan to gray, and smooth. Histologically, spindle cells of dense fibrosis obliterate thyroid parenchyma and infiltrate adjacent skeletal muscle and other structures. Patchy perivascular and infiltrative inflammatory cells comprise lymphocytes, plasma cells, and eosinophils (Fig. 4.14b).
- On CS, FNA demonstrates moderate cellularity with fragments of fibrous tissue with bland, spindle-shaped cells, myofibroblasts, and intense inflammatory infiltrate composed of lymphocytes (Figs. 4.14c, d).
- On TP, the fibrosis forms clumps of spindle cells instead of being diffuse. Cells may be closely associated with inflammatory cells (Fig. 4.14e).
- The differential diagnosis includes a fibrous variant of HT, anaplastic carcinoma, solitary fibrous tumor, and sarcoma.
- Immunohistochemical studies (IHC) reveal a few scattered B lymphocytes (CD20 positive) and numerous scattered T lymphocytes (CD3 positive).
- RT has been claimed to be an IgG4-related disease.

Graves' Disease

- Graves' disease is an autoimmune, diffuse hyperplastic disorder that causes hyperthyroidism and is usually clinically diagnosed. It is more common in women and presents as diffuse enlargement of thyroid gland. Histologically, hyperplastic follicles with papillary infoldings without fibrovascular cores are seen. FNA is performed only when there is a dominant cold nodule that raises a suspicion for malignancy.
- On CS, Graves' disease shows a hypercellular specimen with follicular cells in large branching sheets, with thin, watery colloid in the background. The nuclei are enlarged and vesicular and may show a prominent nucleoli. Nuclear atypia may be pronounced after anti-thyroid therapies. Cytoplasm is moderate to abundant and shows small secretory vacuoles. The most distinctive feature is "flame cells" or fire-flare appearance, represented by marginal cytoplasmic vacuoles with eosinophilic frayed edges; these are best seen on DQ stain.
- In LBP, Graves' disease may be difficult to identify unless there is a clinical history. Cytology shows features similar to those in CS, including enlarged nuclei with a prominent nucleoli. Cytoplasm is moderate to abundant and shows small secretory vacuoles. The "flame cells" or fire-flare appearance, represented by marginal cytoplasmic vacuoles with frayed edges, are evident and appear different from benign follicular cells (Fig. 4.15a–c).

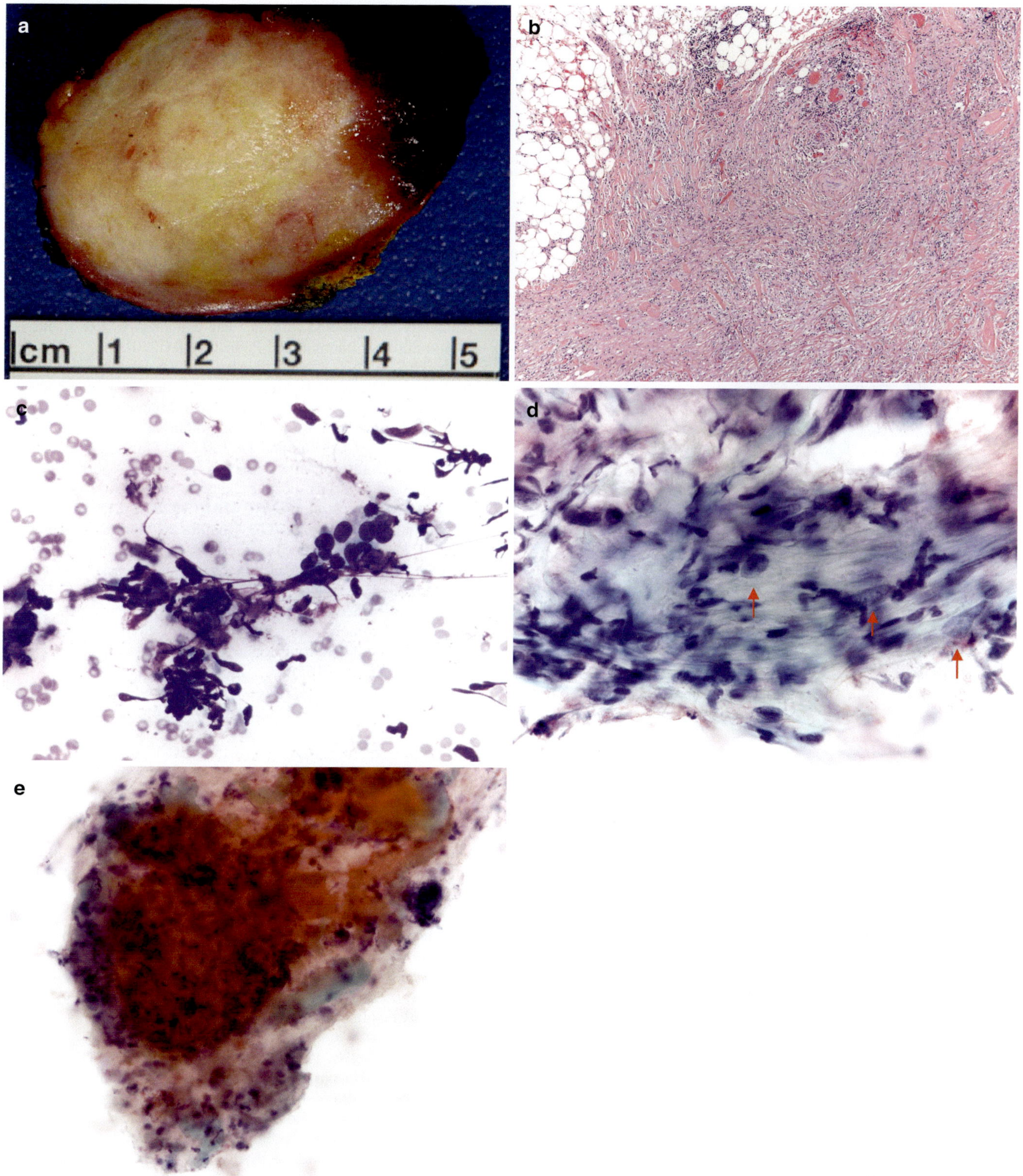

Fig. 4.14 Riedel's thyroiditis (RT). (**a**) Gross appearance of a thyroid lobe in RT appears smooth with a yellow-tan to gray cut surface. The gland was hard and firm on palpation. (**b**) Histologic section of the thyroidectomy specimen shows spindle cells of dense fibrosis with inflammatory cells obliterating thyroid parenchyma and infiltrating adjacent skeletal muscle and adipose tissue. The patchy perivascular and infiltrative inflammatory cells comprise lymphocytes, plasma cells, and eosinophils (H&E stain). (**c**, **d**) CS of RT show a moderate cellularity with loosely cohesive fragments of fibrous tissue composed of bland, spindle-shaped cells (i.e., myofibroblasts) (*arrows*). Other areas showed inflammatory infiltrate composed of lymphocytes. Note the fibrous stroma, which stains magenta in DQ (**c**) and pale green in the Pap stain (**d**). (**e**) On TP, the spindle cells of fibrosis form cohesive clumps instead of being in loosely cohesive fragments. This may occur because of the non-neoplastic nature of the lesion. Cells are closely associated with inflammatory cells (Pap stain, TP)

a
b
c

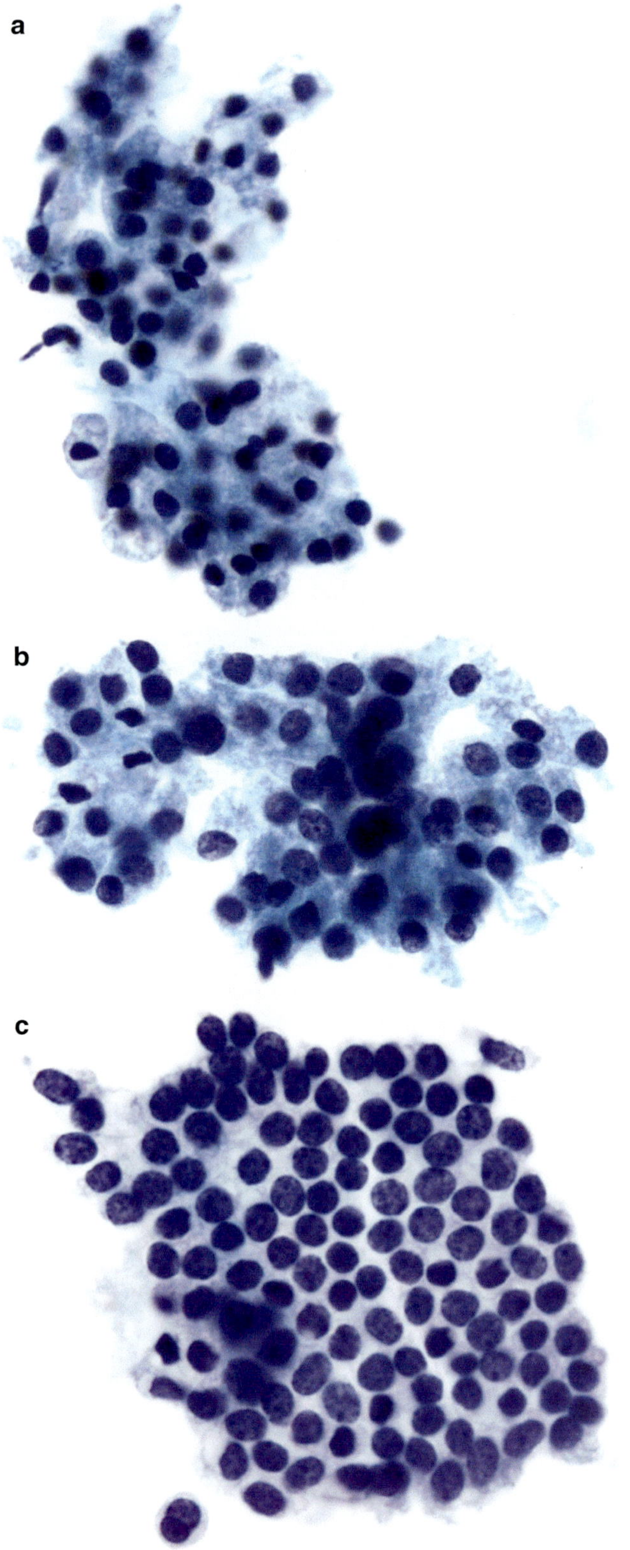

Fig. 4.15 Graves' disease. (**a**, **b**) A clinically proven case of Graves' disease shows enlarged nuclei with nucleoli. Cytoplasm is moderate to abundant and shows small secretory vacuoles. The most distinctive feature is "flame cells" or fire-flare appearance, represented by marginal cytoplasmic vacuoles with eosinophilic frayed edges; these are best seen on DQ stain. However, some peripheral cells in the two groups of follicular cells do show frayed edges. (**c**) A macrofollicle of benign follicular cells shown for comparison (**a**–**c**, Pap stain, TP)

Suggested Reading

1. Abi-Raad R, Prasad M, Baldassari R, Schofield K, Callender GG, Chhieng D, et al. The value of negative diagnosis in thyroid fine-needle aspiration: a retrospective study with histologic follow-up. Endocr Pathol. 2018;29:269–75. https://doi.org/10.1007/s12022-018-9536-5.
2. Afify AM, Liu J, Al-Khafaji BM. Cytologic artifacts and pitfalls of thyroid fine-needle aspiration using ThinPrep: a comparative retrospective review. Cancer. 2001;93:179–86.
3. Alatsakis M, Drogouti M, Tsompanidou C, Katsourakis A, Chatzis I. Invasive thyroglossal duct cyst papillary carcinoma: a case report and review of the literature. Am J Case Rep. 2018;19:757–62. https://doi.org/10.12659/AJCR.907313.
4. Ali SZ, Cibas ES. The Bethesda system for reporting thyroid cytopathology; definitions, criteria, and explanatory notes. 2nd ed. Cham: Springer International Publishing AG; 2018.
5. Alshaikh S, Harb Z, Aljufairi E, Almahari SA. Classification of thyroid fine-needle aspiration cytology into Bethesda categories: an institutional experience and review of the literature. Cytojournal. 2018;15:4. https://doi.org/10.4103/cytojournal.cytojournal_32_17.
6. Awasthi P, Goel G, Khurana U, Joshi D, Majumdar K, Kapoor N. Reproducibility of "the Bethesda system for reporting thyroid cytopathology": a retrospective analysis of 107 patients. J Cytol. 2018;35:33–6. https://doi.org/10.4103/JOC.JOC_215_16.
7. Bongiovanni M, Papadakis GE, Rouiller N, Marino L, Lamine F, Bisig B, et al. The Bethesda system for reporting thyroid cytopathology explained for practitioners: frequently asked questions. Thyroid. 2018;28:556–65. https://doi.org/10.1089/thy.2017.0685.
8. Chandanwale SS, Nair R, Gambhir A, Kaur S, Pandey A, Shetty A, et al. Cytomorphological spectrum of thyroiditis: a review of 110 cases. J Thyroid Res. 2018;2018:5246516. https://doi.org/10.1155/2018/5246516.
9. Chong Y, Ji SJ, Kang CS, Lee EJ. Can liquid-based preparation substitute for conventional smear in thyroid fine-needle aspiration? A systematic review based on meta-analysis. Endocr Connect. 2017;6:817–29. https://doi.org/10.1530/EC-17-0165.
10. Choong KC, Khiyami A, Tamarkin SW, McHenry CR. Fine-needle aspiration biopsy of thyroid nodules: is routine ultrasound-guidance necessary? Surgery. 2018;164:789–94. https://doi.org/10.1016/j.surg.2018.04.047.
11. Cibas ES, Ali SZ. The 2017 Bethesda system for reporting thyroid cytopathology. Thyroid. 2017;27:1341–6. https://doi.org/10.1089/thy.2017.0500.
12. Cipriani NA, White MG, Angelos P, Grogan RH. Large cytologically benign thyroid nodules do not have high rates of malignancy or false-negative rates and clinical observation should be considered: a meta-analysis. Thyroid. 2018. doi: https://doi.org/10.1089/thy.2018.0221. [Epub ahead of print].
13. Clark DP, Faquin WC. Thyroid cytopathology. 2nd ed. New York: Springer; 2010.
14. Cochand-Priollet B, Prat JJ, Polivka M, Thienpont L, Dahan H, Wassef M, et al. Thyroid fine needle aspiration: the morphological features on ThinPrep slide preparations. Eighty cases with histological control. Cytopathology. 2003;14:343–9.
15. Das DK, George SA, Mohammad T, John B, George SS, Behbehani AI. Papillary carcinoma in thyroglossal duct cyst: diagnosis by fine-needle aspiration cytology and immunocytochemistry. Diagn Cytopathol. 2018;46:797–800. https://doi.org/10.1002/dc.23968.
16. Duncan LD, Forrest L, Law WM Jr, Hubbard E, Stewart LE. Evaluation of thyroid fine-needle aspirations: can ThinPrep be used exclusively to appropriately triage patients having a thyroid nodule? Diagn Cytopathol. 2011;39:341–8. https://doi.org/10.1002/dc.21392.
17. Durante C, Costante G, Lucisano G, Bruno R, Meringolo D, Paciaroni A, et al. The natural history of benign thyroid nodules. JAMA. 2015;313:926–35. https://doi.org/10.1001/jama.2015.0956.

18. Fadda G, Rossi ED, Raffaelli M, Mulè A, Pontecorvi A, Miraglia A, et al. Fine-needle aspiration biopsy of thyroid lesions processed by thin-layer cytology: one-year institutional experience with histologic correlation. Thyroid. 2006;16:975–81.
19. Fischer AH, Clayton AC, Bentz JS, Wasserman PG, Henry MR, Souers RJ, et al. Performance differences between conventional smears and liquid-based preparations of thyroid fine-needle aspiration samples: analysis of 47,076 responses in the College of American Pathologists Interlaboratory Comparison Program in Non-Gynecologic Cytology. Arch Pathol Lab Med. 2013;137:26–31. https://doi.org/10.5858/arpa.2012-0009-CP.
20. Geers C, Bourgain C. Liquid-based FNAC of the thyroid: a 4-year survey with SurePath. Cancer Cytopathol. 2011;119:58–67. https://doi.org/10.1002/cncy.20125.
21. Guo HQ, Zhang ZH, Zhao H, Niu LJ, Chang Q, Pan QJ. Factors influencing the reliability of thyroid fine-needle aspiration: analysis of thyroid nodule size, guidance mode for aspiration and preparation method. Acta Cytol. 2015;59:169–74. https://doi.org/10.1159/000381412.
22. Haugen BR, Alexander EK, Bible KC, Doherty GM, Mandel SJ, Nikiforov YE, et al. 2015 American Thyroid Association management guidelines for adult patients with thyroid nodules and differentiated thyroid Cancer: the American Thyroid Association guidelines task force on thyroid nodules and differentiated thyroid Cancer. Thyroid. 2016;26:1–133. https://doi.org/10.1089/thy.2015.0020.
23. Harigopal M, Sahoo S, Recant WM, DeMay RM. Fine-needle aspiration of Riedel's disease: report of a case and review of the literature. Diagn Cytopathol. 2004;30:193–7.
24. Hoda RS. Non-gynecologic cytology on liquid-based preparations: a morphologic review of facts and artifacts. Diagn Cytopathol. 2007;35:621–34.
25. Hoda RS, VandenBussche C, Hoda SA. Diagnostic liquid-based cytology. New York: Springer; 2017.
26. Jung CK, Lee A, Jung ES, Choi YJ, Jung SL, Lee KY. Split sample comparison of a liquid-based method and conventional smears in thyroid fine needle aspiration. Acta Cytol. 2008;52:313–9.
27. Li W, Zhu Q, Jiang Y, Zhang Q, Meng Z, Sun J, et al. Partially cystic thyroid nodules in ultrasound-guided fine needle aspiration: prevalence of thyroid carcinoma and ultrasound features. Medicine (Baltimore). 2017;96:e8689. https://doi.org/10.1097/MD.0000000000008689.
28. Ljung BM. Thyroid fine-needle aspiration: smears versus liquid-based preparations. Cancer. 2008;114:144–8. https://doi.org/10.1002/cncr.23541.
29. Moon S, Chung HS, Yu JM, Yoo HJ, Park JH, Kim DS, et al. Associations between Hashimoto thyroiditis and clinical outcomes of papillary thyroid cancer: a meta-analysis of observational studies. Endocrinol Metab (Seoul). 2018;33:473–84. https://doi.org/10.3803/EnM.2018.33.4.473.
30. Nagarajan N, Schneider EB, Ali SZ, Zeiger MA, Olson MT. How do liquid-based preparations of thyroid fine-needle aspiration compare with conventional smears? An analysis of 5475 specimens. Thyroid. 2015;25:308–13. https://doi.org/10.1089/thy.2014.0394.
31. Pastorello RG, Destefani C, Pinto PH, Credidio CH, Reis RX, Rodrigues TA, et al. The impact of rapid on-site evaluation on thyroid fine-needle aspiration biopsy: a 2-year cancer center institutional experience. Cancer Cytopathol. 2018;126:846–52. https://doi.org/10.1002/cncy.22051.
32. Pellicer DL, Sadow PM, Stephen A, Faquin WC. Atypical squamous metaplasia in a benign cystic thyroid nodule mimicking high-grade carcinoma. Diagn Cytopathol. 2013;41:706–9. https://doi.org/10.1002/dc.22803.
33. Pusztaszeri MP, Krane JF, Cibas ES, Daniels G, Faquin WC. FNAB of benign thyroid nodules with papillary hyperplasia: a cytological and histological evaluation. Cancer Cytopathol. 2014;122:666–77. https://doi.org/10.1002/cncy.21441.
34. Rammeh S, Romdhane E, Sassi A, Belhajkacem L, Blel A, Ksentini M, et al. Accuracy of fine-needle aspiration cytology of head and neck masses. Diagn Cytopathol. 2018;47:394–9. https://doi.org/10.1002/dc.24120. [Epub ahead of print].
35. Renshaw AA, Gould EW. Characteristics of false-negative thyroid fine-needle aspirates. Acta Cytol. 2018;62:12–8. https://doi.org/10.1159/000481722.
36. Rossi ED, Morassi F, Santeusanio G, Zannoni GF, Fadda G. Thyroid fine needle aspiration cytology processed by ThinPrep: an additional slide decreased the number of inadequate results. Cytopathology. 2010;21:97–102. https://doi.org/10.1111/j.1365-2303.2009.00659.x.
37. Rossi ED, Raffaelli M, Zannoni GF, Pontecorvi A, Mulè A, Callà C, Lombardi CP, et al. Diagnostic efficacy of conventional as compared to liquid-based cytology in thyroid lesions: evaluation of 10,360 fine needle aspiration cytology cases. Acta Cytol. 2009;53:659–66.
38. Rossi ED, Zannoni GF, Moncelsi S, Stigliano E, Santeusanio G, Lombardi CP, et al. Application of liquid-based cytology to fine-needle aspiration biopsies of the thyroid gland. Front Endocrinol (Lausanne). 2012;3:57. https://doi.org/10.3389/fendo.2012.00057.
39. Sahin D, Yilmazbayhan D, Firat P, Hacisalihoglu UP, Kirimlioglu SH, Celenk E, et al. Comparison of conventional cytology and SurePath in split thyroid fine needle aspiration materials. Cytopathology. 2017;28:291–8. https://doi.org/10.1111/cyt.12430.
40. Sharma S, Agarwal S, Jain M, Singh GB, Andley M. Cytomorphological differences between liquid-based cytology and conventional smears in fine-needle aspirates of thyroid lesions. J Cytol. 2018;35:208–11. https://doi.org/10.4103/JOC.JOC_150_17.
41. Tripathy K, Misra A, Ghosh JK. Efficacy of liquid-based cytology versus conventional smears in FNA samples. J Cytol. 2015;32:17–20. https://doi.org/10.4103/0970-9371.155225.

Atypical Cells of Undetermined Significance/Follicular Lesion of Undetermined Significance

5

Rana S. Hoda, Rema Rao, and Theresa Scognamiglio

Introduction to Indeterminate Thyroid Nodules (ITN)

- Thyroid FNA has reduced the rate of unnecessary surgeries for benign thyroid nodules. High negative predictive value (NPV) of a benign FNA diagnosis has made it a valuable initial test for thyroid nodules.
- However, The Bethesda System for Reporting Thyroid Cytopathology (TBSRTC) classifies three of the six categories as having an indeterminate cytology on FNA, where it is not possible to specify whether a nodule is benign, neoplastic, or suspicious for malignancy:
  - Atypia of Undetermined Significance or Follicular Lesion of Undetermined Significance (AUS/FLUS)
  - Follicular Neoplasm or Suspicious for Follicular Neoplasm (FN/SFN), which includes cases of FN with Hürthle cell (oncocytic) features (FNHCT/SFNHCT)
  - Suspicious for Malignancy (SM)
- Each category is associated with a different risk of malignancy (ROM) and management options.
- Approximately 15–30% of thyroid nodules are classified as indeterminate.
- These indeterminate categories are diverse and heterogeneous, with significant interobserver and intraobserver variability due to broad overlap in their diagnostic criteria. Indeterminate cytology is also challenging for clinicians and may often lead to either unnecessary surgery or additional expensive ancillary tests.

R. S. Hoda (✉)
CBLPath, Rye Brook, NY, USA
e-mail: rhoda@cblpath.com

R. Rao · T. Scognamiglio
Department of Pathology and Laboratory Medicine, New York Presbyterian Hospital, Weill Cornell Medical College, New York, NY, USA
e-mail: rer9052@med.cornell.edu; ths9004@med.cornell.edu

- The positive predictive value (PPV) of indeterminate results is 5–48% in resected cases.
- The relatively high risk of thyroid cancer in the FN/SFN (25–40%) and SM (50–75%) categories typically warrants surgical excision of the nodule. In contrast, nodules falling in the AUS/FLUS category have a ROM of about 10–30%, which merits repeat FNA.

AUS/FLUS Definition

- TBSRTC defines AUS/FLUS specimens as those that contain cells (follicular, lymphoid, or other) with architectural and/or nuclear atypia that is not sufficient to be classified as FN/SFN, SM, or malignant, but with atypia more marked than can be ascribed confidently to benign changes.

Criteria for AUS/FLUS and Application in Liquid-Based Preparations (LBP)

- According to the second edition of TBSRTC, the types of aspirates that fall into the AUS/FLUS category are heterogeneous and apply to follicular, lymphoid, and other cells:
  - Aspirates with limited nuclear and/or architectural changes that quantitatively or qualitatively fall short of being SM or FN/SFN
  - Aspirates with artifacts (such as air-drying or excess blood) that limit optimal evaluation of the specimen. (This criterion does not apply to LBP, as specimen artifacts are few, if any.)
- Subclassification of AUS/FLUS is encouraged, to enhance communication with other pathologists and clinicians.
- Subclassification also distinguishes relevant differences in malignancy risk in this heterogeneous category, to help

R. S. Hoda et al. (eds.), *Atlas of Thyroid Cytopathology on Liquid-Based Preparations*,
https://doi.org/10.1007/978-3-030-25066-9_5

guide management. AUS/FLUS interpretation due to cytologic atypia carries a higher ROM than AUS/FLUS interpretation made for architectural atypia.

Cytology of Subcategories of AUS/FLUS and Application in LBP

- TBSRTC has described several scenarios in which AUS/FLUS diagnosis could be used. These scenarios are extremely helpful to cytopathologists in conveying their level of concern to clinicians. The sections below discuss how these scenarios appear in LBP.

Cytologic Atypia (Nuclear Atypia, AUS-N)

(a) *Focal cytologic atypia indicates the possibility of papillary thyroid carcinoma (PTC) and includes the following scenarios:*
  - Mild nuclear atypia: Follicular cells are usually in a macrofollicular arrangement (benign-appearing) with rare cells showing some, but not all, nuclear features of PTC, including mild nuclear clearing (pale chromatin), enlargement, irregular membrane, and grooves. All features seen in conventional smears (CS) are retained in LBP (Fig. 5.1a, b). LBP may show smaller macrofollicles.
  - Rare intranuclear pseudoinclusions (INPI): In LBP, INPI may appear small. If rare, they are difficult to detect and require careful screening for detection (Fig. 5.2a–c).
  - Paucicellular specimen with the above nuclear features (Fig. 5.3). In a paucicellular LBP, a second slide can be prepared to assess nuclear features.

(b) *Extensive but mild cytologic atypia:*
  - Most cells have mild nuclear enlargement and slightly pale chromatin, with occasional irregular membrane. In LBP, nuclei may appear smaller, so careful review for the other two features is important (Fig. 5.4a, b). INPI are either rare or not identified.

(c) *Atypical cyst-lining cells:*
  - Faquin et al. [11] described the cytologic features of cyst-lining cells (CLC) in benign thyroid cysts and in cystic PTC. All the features also apply to LBP, but

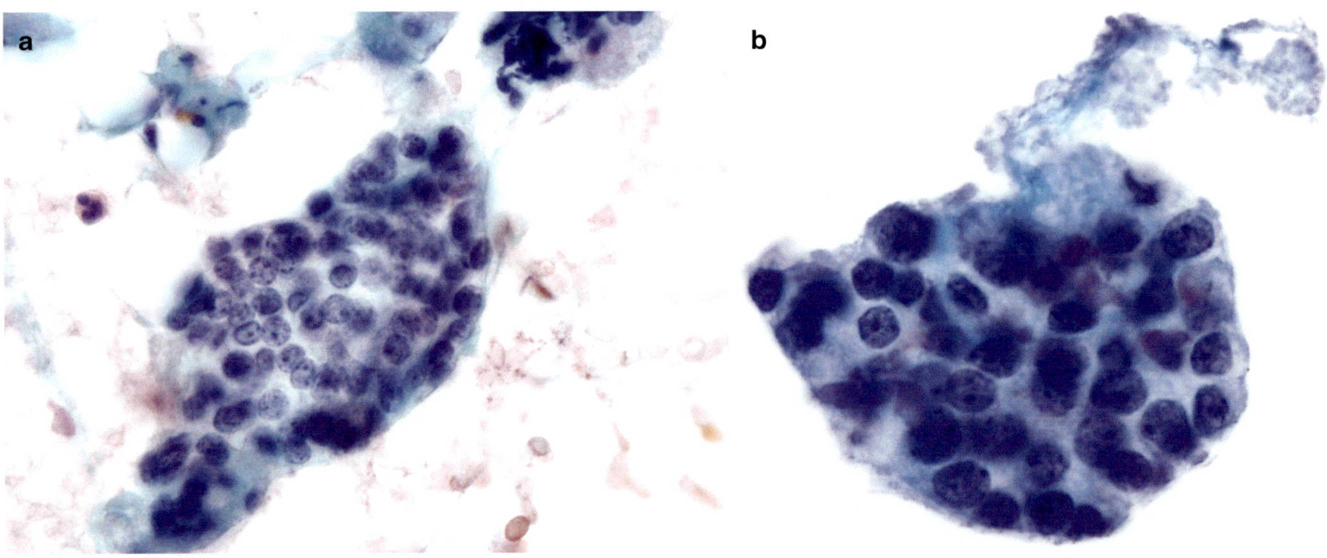

Fig. 5.1 Atypia of undetermined significance with mild nuclear atypia. (**a**) On a conventional smear (CS), follicular cells show a rare group in a macrofollicular arrangement (benign-appearing) with cells showing loss of polarity, mild nuclear clearing (pale chromatin), enlargement, irregular membrane, and grooves. Other nuclear features of papillary thyroid carcinoma (PTC), including intranuclear pseudoinclusions (INPI), nuclear overlap, and crowding, are not present. This was the only abnormal group in this case. (**b**) In the same case, a ThinPrep (TP) slide shows an atypical macrofollicular cell group. Features are similar to those seen on CS, but the nuclear morphology is crisper owing to the lack of background blood. (Compare these atypical macrofollicular structures with benign macrofollicles as shown in Chap. 4.) (**a** Pap stain, CS; **b** Pap stain, TP)

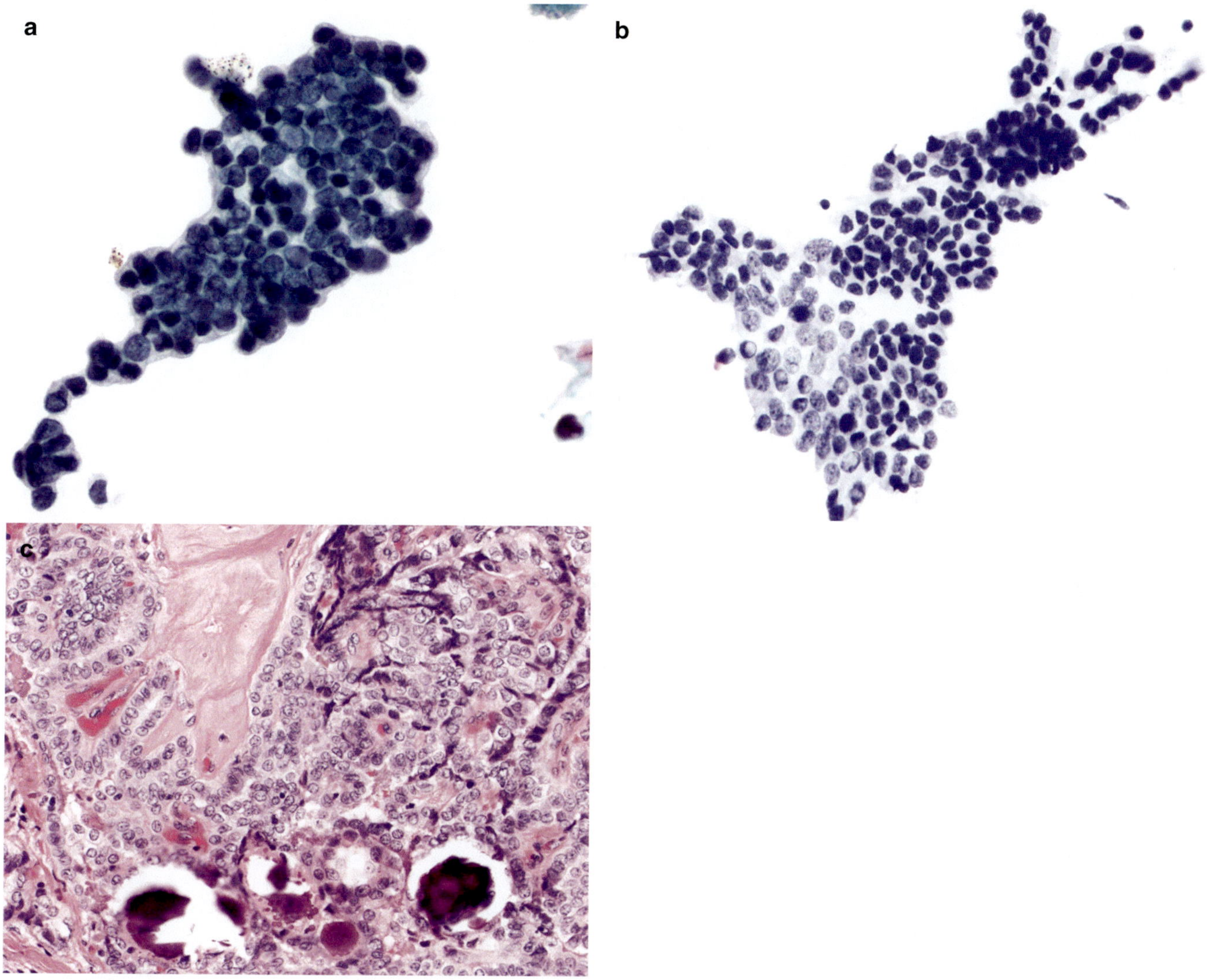

Fig. 5.2 Mild nuclear atypia with rare intranuclear pseudoinclusions (INPI). (**a**, **b**) Both these cases show rare INPI clearly visible in a single cell within the syncytial fragments. A few other nuclear features of PTC are noted, including enlargement, overlap, irregular membranes, chromatin clearing, and rare grooves. A molecular test in the case seen in **b** was abnormal and showed *BRAF* (V600E) mutation for PTC (Pap stain, TP). (**c**) Subsequent resection found PTC (H&E stain)

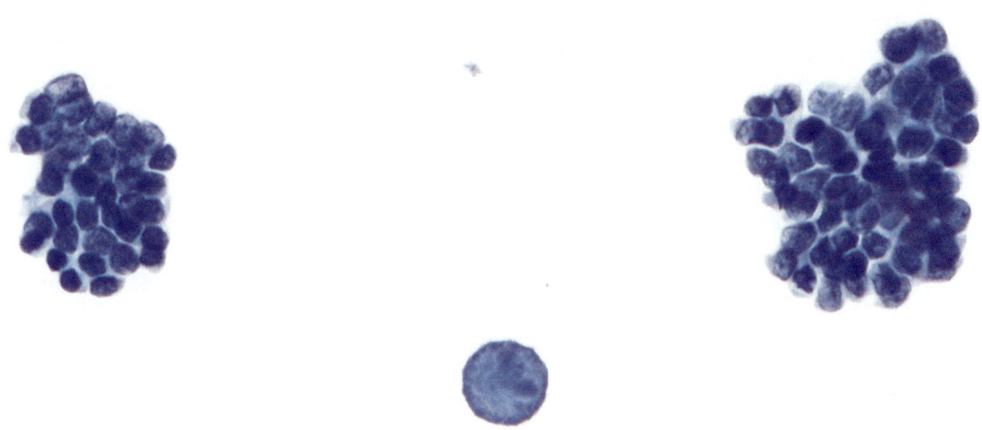

Fig. 5.3 Mild nuclear atypia in paucicellular specimen. This case shows all nuclear features of PTC except INPI (Pap stain, TP). Subsequent resection found PTC

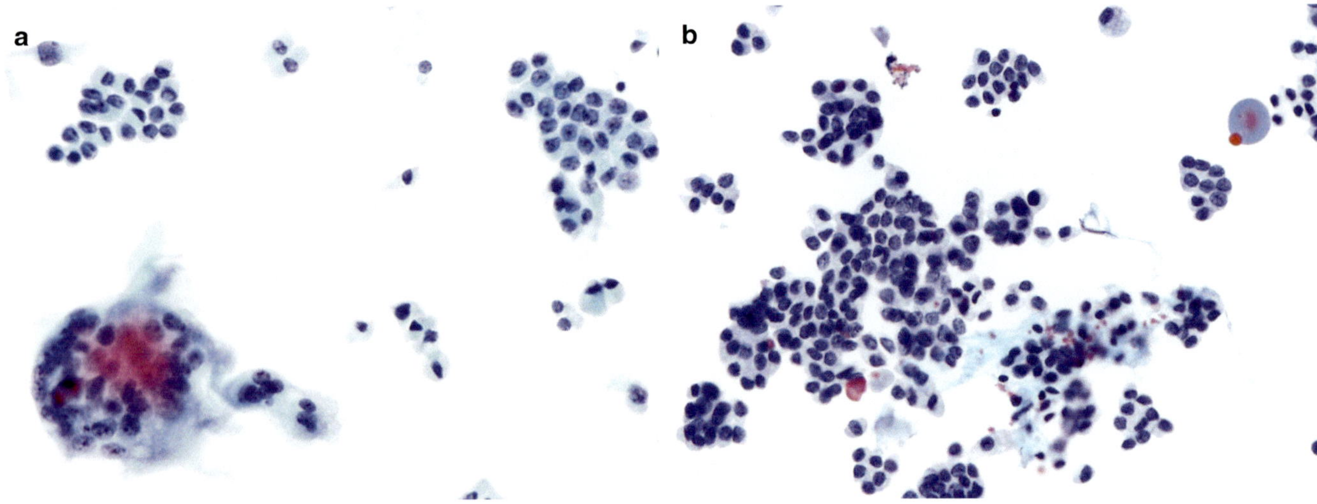

Fig. 5.4 Extensive mild nuclear atypia. (**a**, **b**) Most cells show all nuclear features of PTC except INPI. One nucleus in **a** shows a poorly formed INPI (Pap stain, TP)

subtle differences with CS will be noted, when present (*see* Chap. 4).

- Benign CLC show changes of epithelial repair, including flat two-dimensional sheets with elongated, pulled-out appearance of well-spaced cells with "windows" separating the cells. The nuclei are enlarged and pale and cytoplasm has distinct borders. Background, in an adequate sample, shows benign follicular cells, macrophages, and colloid. Cytomorphology in LBP is similar to CS, except that the CLC in SurePath™ (SP) slides show more cellular elongation (Fig. 5.5). Features seen in cystic PTC (*see below*) are lacking. In challenging cases, immunocytochemical/immunohistochemical (ICC/IHC) stains for cytokeratin (CK)-19 or galectin-3 can be performed on newly-prepared LBP slides from residual sample or on a cell block section ([27], and Chap. 14). Oertel [38] believes these cells can be diagnosed more specifically as squamous metaplasia. (*See* Chap. 4.)
- Atypical CLC (ACLC): TP shows show nuclear grooves, nucleoli, and enlargement and lacks reparative features of pulled-out appearance and elongation of cells. ACLC may also show INPI, papillary architecture, nuclear crowding, mitotic figures, and psammoma bodies. Such specimens are commonly hypocellular and pose a potential pitfall, as they cannot be reliably distinguished from a cystic PTC. In LBP, ACLC may be in small, cohesive sheets or dispersed singly. INPI may not be easily identified, and cracking of dense, inspissated colloid droplets may mimic psammoma bodies (Fig. 5.6a, b). In LBP, even benign CLC may show prominent nucleoli.
- ACLC show a similar morphology in CS (Fig. 5.6c). Cases with ACLC are either resected or tested for molecular markers. (*See* Chap. 14.) ICC/IHC staining for cytokeratin and thyroglobulin can be performed in

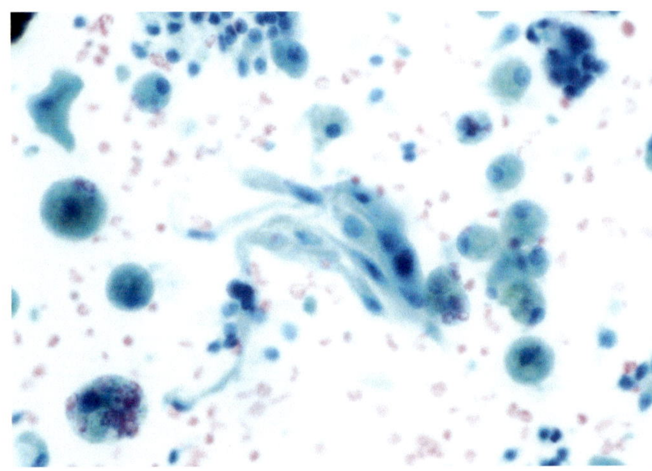

Fig. 5.5 Benign cyst-lining cells (CLC). FNA of a benign thyroid cyst showing CLC with pulled-out, spindled morphology, arranged in a small, cohesive, flat sheet. The cells display well-defined cell borders and windows similar to epithelial repair. Note benign follicular cells and hemosiderin-laden macrophages in a different plane of focus (Pap stain, SP)

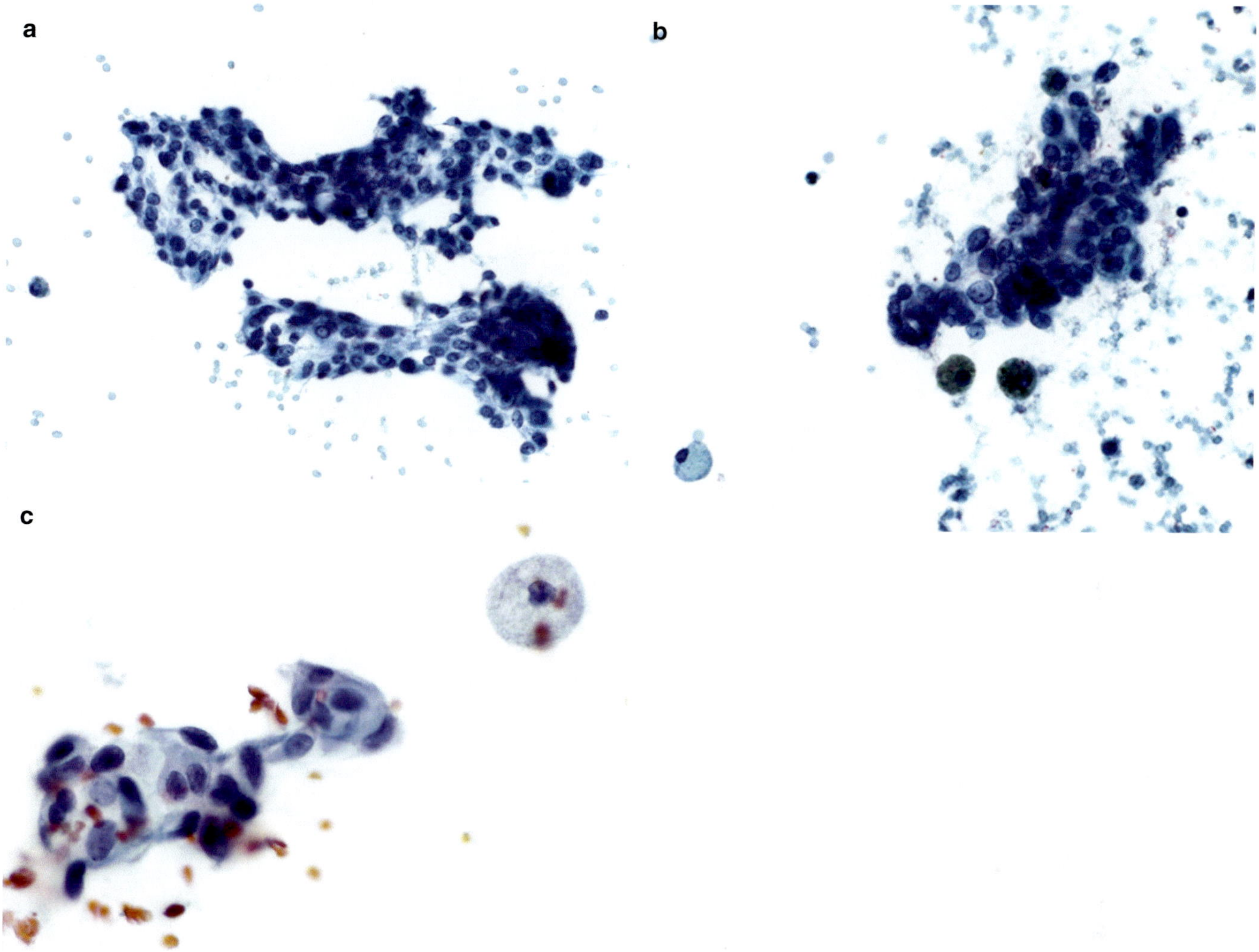

Fig. 5.6 Atypical cyst-lining cells (ACLC). (**a**, **b**) ACLC exhibit a flattened sheet of follicular cells with oval to polygonal, overcrowded nuclei displaying irregularity, grooves, and pale chromatin (Pap stain, TP). (**c**) ACLC in a loosely cohesive cluster with cells in a wrapped-around appearance. Nuclei are oval with pale chromatin and are mildly grooved (Pap stain, CS). Ultrasound had a benign solid and cystic appearance of nodular hyperplasia with no high-risk features, and a molecular test was benign

CS, cell blocks, and LBP to show that the ACLC are thyroid follicular cells.

- Cystic PTC shows nuclear enlargement, crowding and overlapping, INPI, psammoma bodies, multinucleated histiocytes, dense hypereosinophilic colloid, and papillary architecture. Cystic PTC does not display repair-like features, such as elongated or spindled cells (Fig. 5.7a–d). These features distinguish cystic PTC from ACLC of benign thyroid cysts.

(d) *Histiocytoid cells:*

- Characteristic of cystic PTC
- Histiocytoid cells are larger than histiocytes, can be single, in microfollicular arrangements or in clusters with “knobby” or “scalloped” contours. Nuclei are rounder than histiocytes, cytoplasm may be scant, harder (glassy), with distinct cell walls and may have large discrete vacuoles and lacks hemosiderin and microvacuoles. N:C ratio is high (Fig. 5.8a–d).

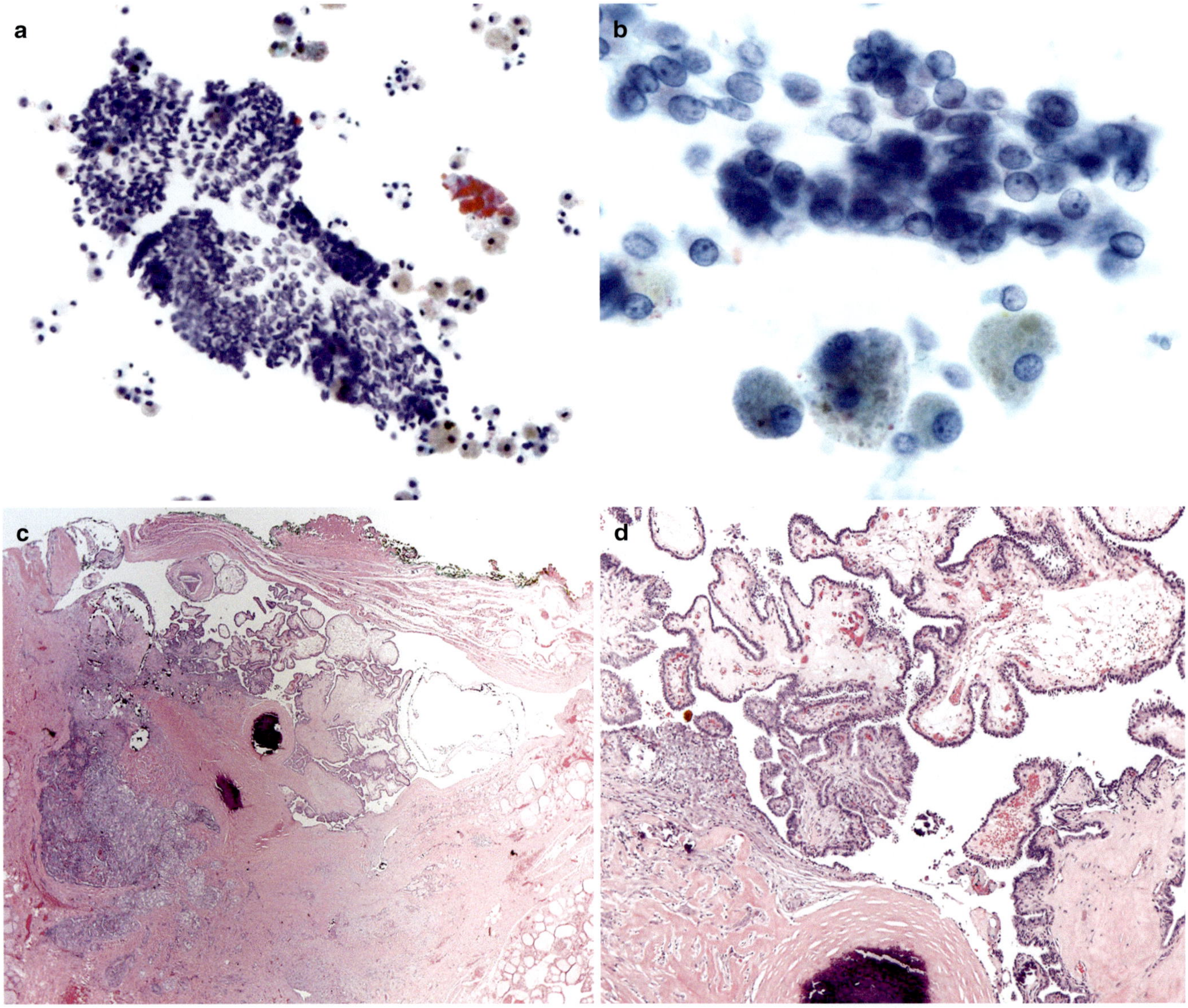

Fig. 5.7 Atypical cells of cystic PTC. (**a**) All nuclear features of PTC can be seen in this syncytial fragment in a cystic background with numerous hemosiderin-laden macrophages. Although the atypical cells of cystic PTC may be difficult to distinguish from the ACLC of benign thyroid cysts, nuclear crowding and rare INPI help distinguish cystic PTC (Pap stain, TP). (**b**) Cystic PTC in a CS displays a streaming effect, but the nuclear features of PTC are obvious (Pap stain). (**c**, **d**) Subsequent resection of cystic PTC (H&E stain)

- Rarely, cyst-lining cells have a hobnail appearance, virtually identical to the histiocytoid cells in cystic PTC, and cannot reliably be distinguished on cytology [11]. Molecular testing or surgical resection is recommended in such cases.
- Normal histiocytes are smaller, with small pale, oval, or reniform nucleus and less cytoplasm; they are negative for cytokeratin immunostain.

Architectural Atypia

(a) *Microfollicle formation:*

- Scant-cellularity specimen with follicular cells in microfollicles or crowded 3-D clusters with scant colloid. It may represent limited sampling of FN/SFN. In LBP, these structures may appear more dissociated, smaller, and tighter; nuclei are more hyperchromatic (Fig. 5.9a–f).

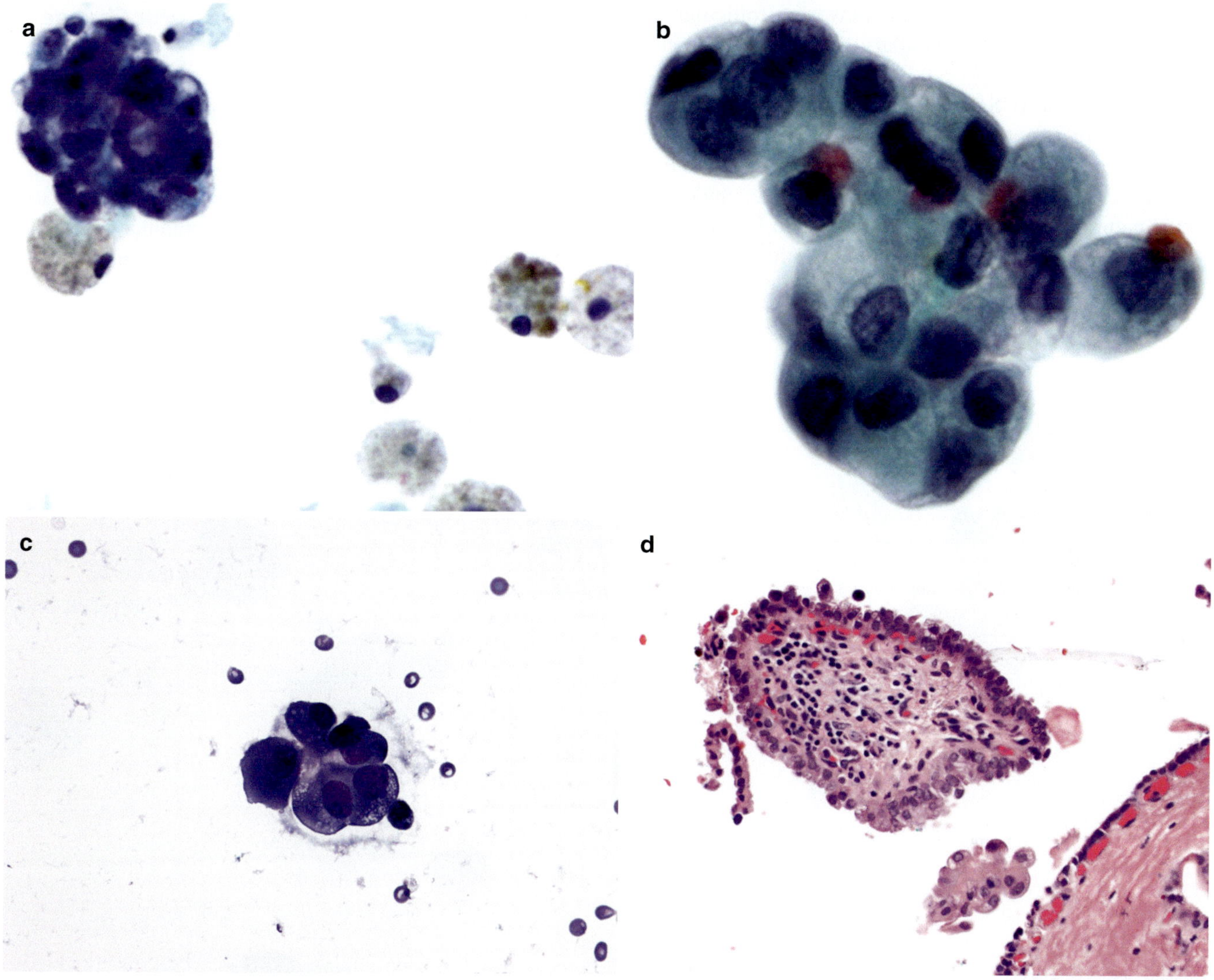

Fig. 5.8 PTC with histiocytoid cell morphology. (**a**, **b**) Two cases with histiocytoid cell morphology in cystic PTC. These nuclei are larger, round, and hyperchromatic, with grooves and small nucleoli compared with histiocytes seen in the background. In both cases, the histiocytoid cells display a clustered appearance with a "knobby" or "scalloped" contour or "hobnail" appearance. Cytoplasm is scant and finely vacuolated to hard, with distinct cell walls. The nuclear-cytoplasmic (N:C) ratio is moderately high (Pap stain, TP). (**c**) CS from the same case. Note similar morphology and hard, "glassy" cytoplasm (DQ stain, CS). A molecular test was abnormal. (**d**) Subsequent resection found an intracystic PTC. Note the knobby cluster of cells near the cyst lining (H&E stain)

(b) *Microfollicle formation and minimal nuclear atypia:*
- Markedly cellular specimen with focally prominent microfollicles with minimal nuclear atypia. In LBP, microfollicles may appear more dissociated, smaller and tighter and nuclei are more hyperchromatic.
- Parathyroid hyperplasia may also present as an AUS-F (Fig. 5.10a, b).

Cytological and Architectural Atypia

- Cytologic atypia is characterized by microfollicles and crowded 3-D configuration of follicular cells. Cytologic atypia is manifested by enlarged, overlapping nuclei with pale chromatin or clearing and grooves (Figs. 5.11a–c and 5.12a–f).

- This pattern may represent noninvasive follicular thyroid neoplasm with papillary-like nuclear features (NIFTP).
- A diagnosis of AUS/FLUS with architectural and nuclear atypia with an option of giving a differential diagnosis of the follicular variant of PTC (FVPTC) and its more indolent form, NIFTP, helps clinicians. They better understand the nature of the lesion and its associated ROM and can provide the patient optimal treatment, reducing overtreatment and morbidity.

Hürthle Cell Predominance or Oncocytic Change

(a) *Clinical setting is not suggestive of a benign lesion:*

- Scant-cellularity specimen comprising exclusively or almost exclusively of Hürthle cells with minimal colloid. It may represent limited sampling of FNHCT/SFNHCT. In LBP, cytoplasm of Hürthle cells may become less dense and lightly granular, nuclei are smaller, and nucleoli may be prominent even in benign Hürthle cells (Fig. 5.13a–d).

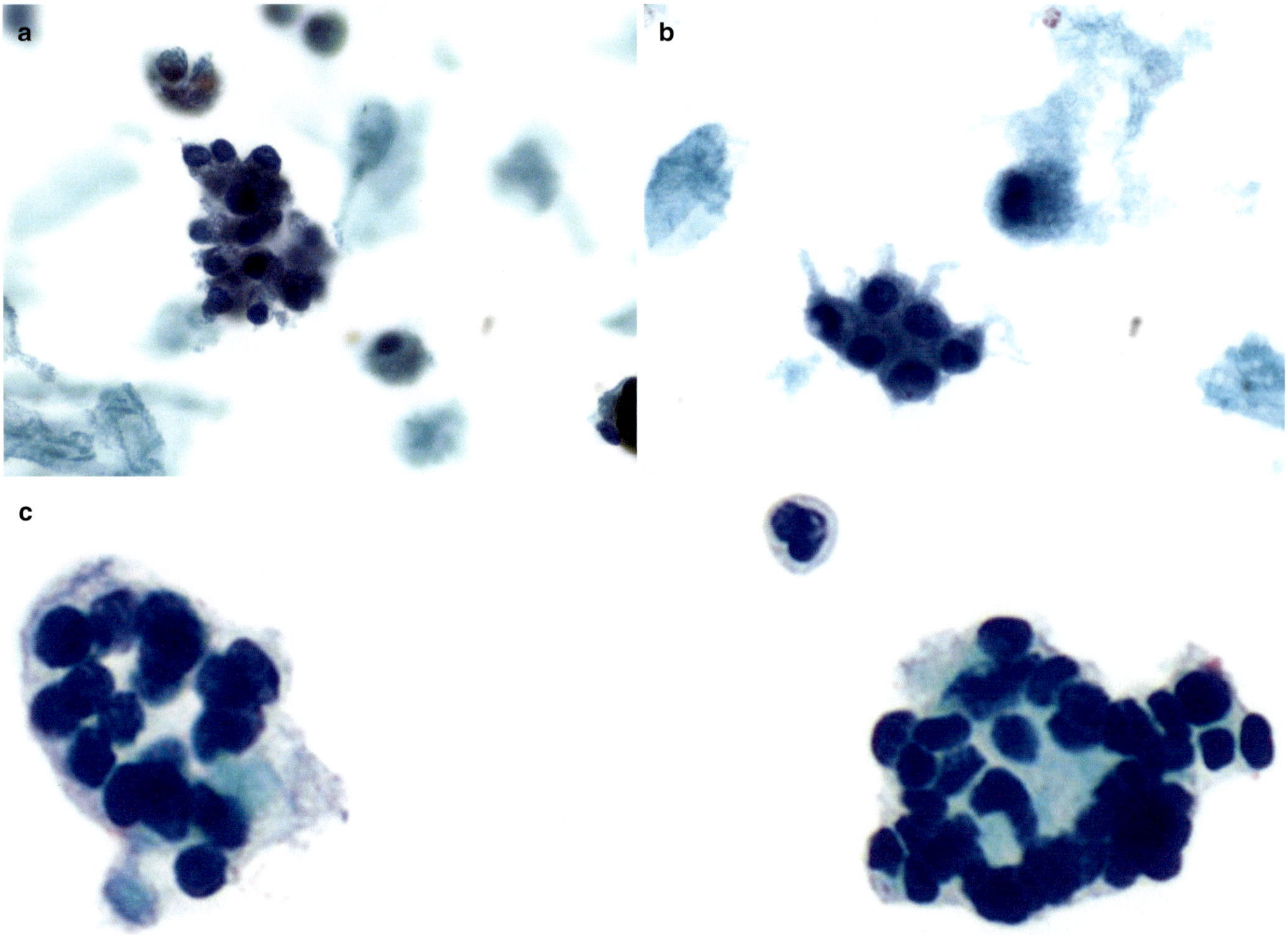

Fig. 5.9 Architectural atypia with Microfollicle Formation. (**a–c**) These three cases had scant cellularity. Follicular cells displayed smaller and tighter, crowded 3-D groups and microfollicles with nuclear overlapping and scant colloid. Note the thick, globular colloid in the first two images. These cases may represent limited sampling of FN/SFN (**a**, **b** Pap stain, SP; **c** Pap stain, TP). (**d**) Same case as above in a DQ-stained CS. Note the microfollicle formation similar to SP and TP and nuclear enlargement. (**e**, **f**) Subsequent resection showed follicular adenoma with intact capsule without capsular and vascular invasion and microfollicular pattern of arrangement (H&E stain)

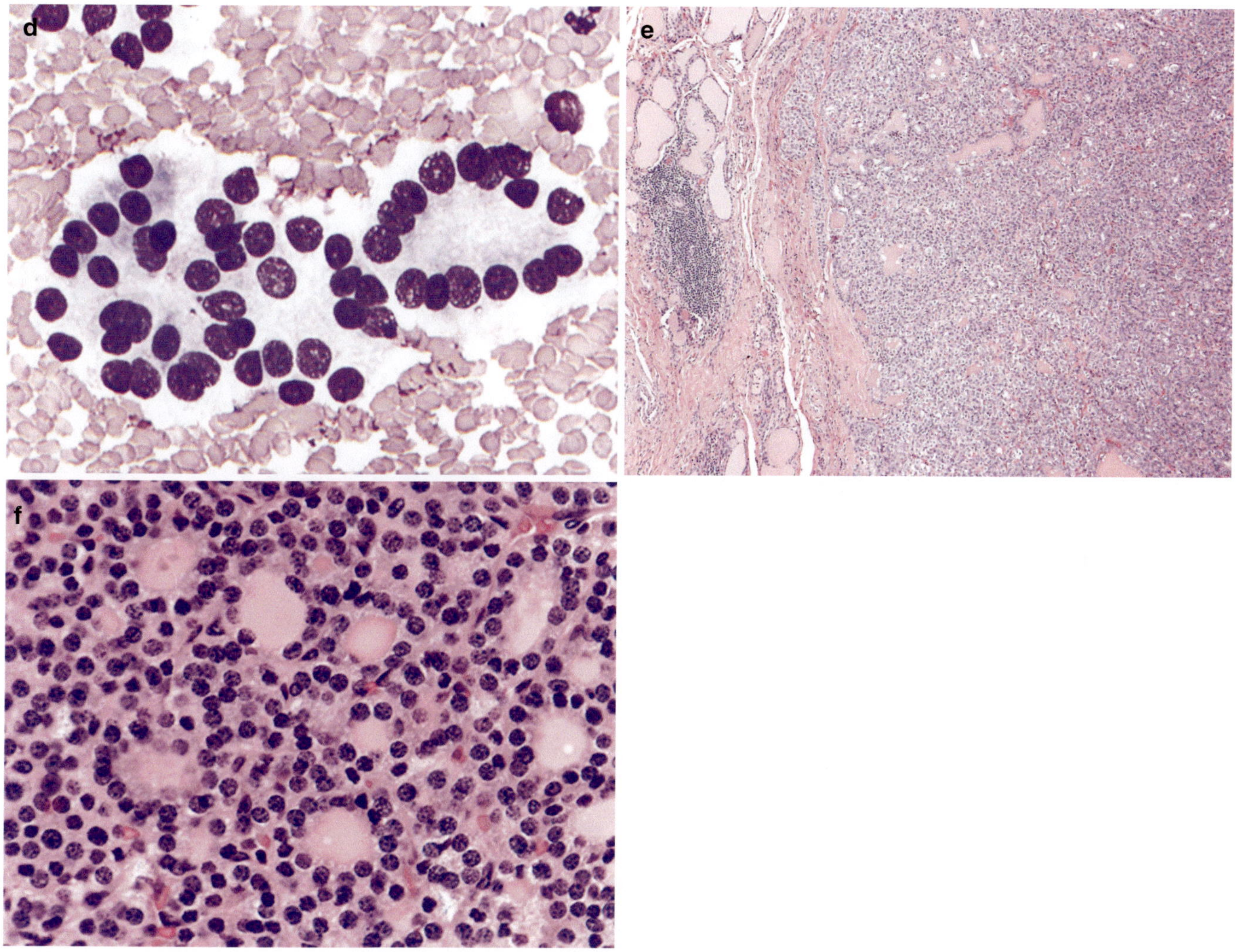

Fig. 5.9 (continued)

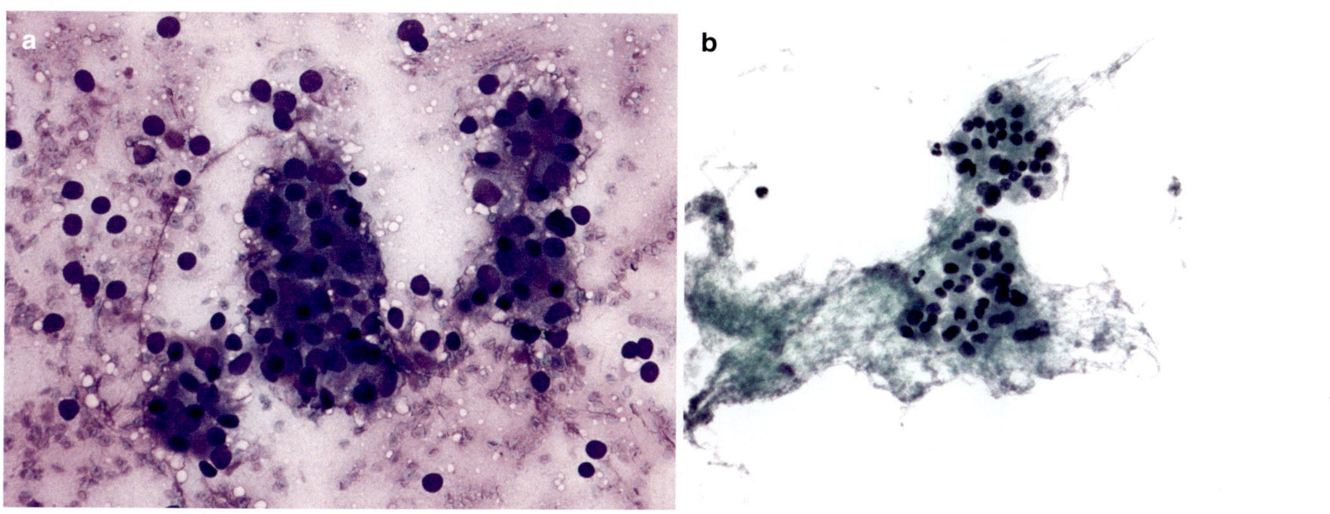

Fig. 5.10 Architectural atypia with microfollicle formation and minimal nuclear atypia. (**a**) This specimen was cellular, with focally prominent microfollicles with minimal nuclear atypia (DQ stain, CS). (**b**) TP from the same case shows microfollicles also with minimal nuclear atypia in a background of thin colloid (Pap stain). Resection showed nodular hyperplasia. (**c**) In another case, TP shows a distinct microfollicular aggregate with minimal nuclear atypia and a subtle "salt and pepper" appearance in a background of thin colloid-like material (Pap stain). Molecular testing was positive for *PTH* gene; clinically, the patient had hyperparathyroidism. FNA was performed to confirm parathyroid cells, but this information was not provided to cytopathologist. (**d**, **e**) This composite shows the resected parathyroid adenoma and the CS with cytologic features similar to the LBP (**d** H&E stain; **e** Pap stain, CS)

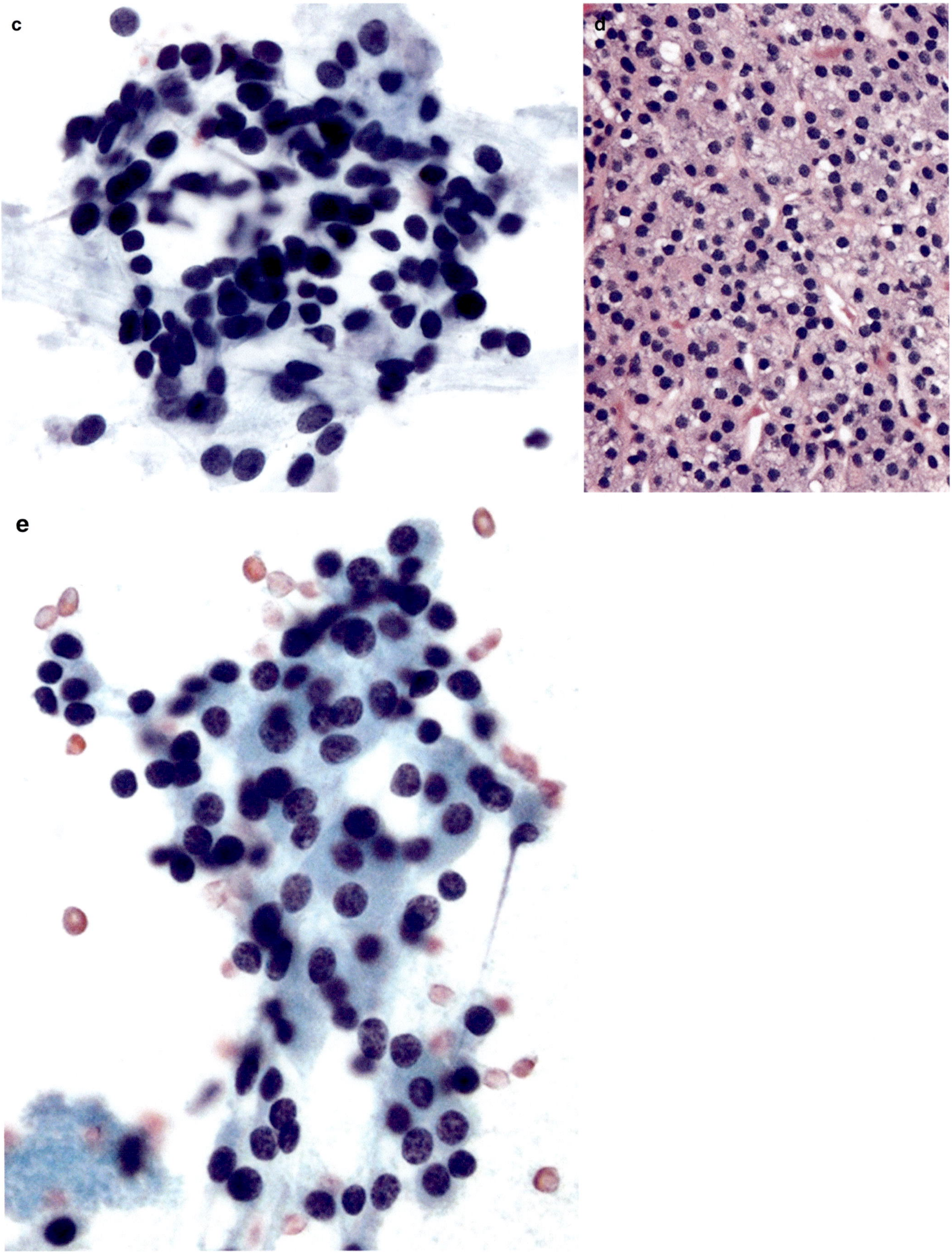

Fig. 5.10 (continued)

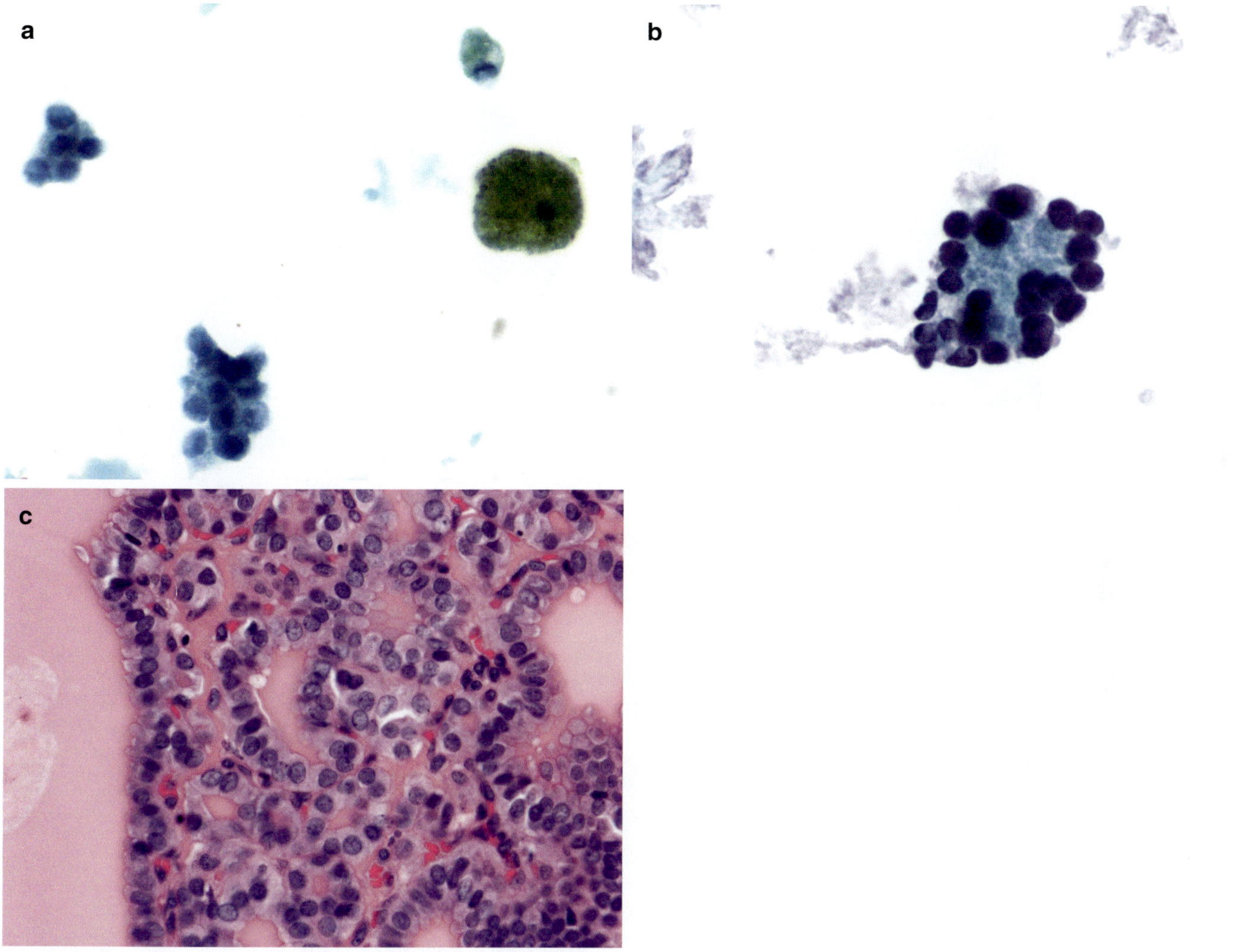

Fig. 5.11 Cytological and architectural atypia. (**a**, **b**) Architectural atypia is displayed by follicular cells in microfollicles. Cytologic atypia is manifested by enlarged, overlapping nuclei with irregularity, clearing, and grooves (**a** Pap stain, SP; **b** Pap stain, TP). Note the difference in microfollicles in SP and TP. The lumen of the microfollicle in SP was visible when the plane of focus was adjusted. (**c**) Subsequent resection showed a follicular variant of PTC (FVPTC) (H&E stain)

(b) *Clinical setting suggests a benign Hürthle cell nodule such as in Hashimoto's thyroiditis (HT) or multinodular goiter (MNG):*
- Hürthle cells in cohesive flat sheets with smaller, darker nuclei, lacking nuclear atypia and abundant colloid. In TP, some thin colloid may be lost. (*See* Chap. 4.)
- Clinical features may be of HT, but lymphocytes are lacking. Note that lymphocytes may be reduced in TP. (See benign Hürthle cell features above.)
- Hürthle cells in cohesive flat sheets with few lymphocytes; lymphocytes may be reduced in TP. In this setting, correlation with clinical and imaging findings and serum antibody assessment is advised.
- Multiple nodules with Hürthle cells may represent MNG with Hürthle cell metaplasia rather than a Hürthle cell neoplasm (Fig. 5.14a–e).

Atypia Not Otherwise Specified (AUS-NOS)

(a) *Follicular cells with pronounced nuclear enlargement and prominent nucleoli:*
- Follicular cells show nuclear enlargement and prominent nucleoli.
- This scenario lacks nuclear features of PTC.
- This subcategory is most useful when these features exist either in the absence or uncertainty about clinical history of Graves' disease, carbimazole treatment for Graves' disease, radioactive iodine or ionizing radiation to the neck, or other pharmaceutical agents (Fig. 5.15a–e).
- In LBP, prominent nucleoli alone should not be considered atypical, as this feature can also be present in benign lesions.

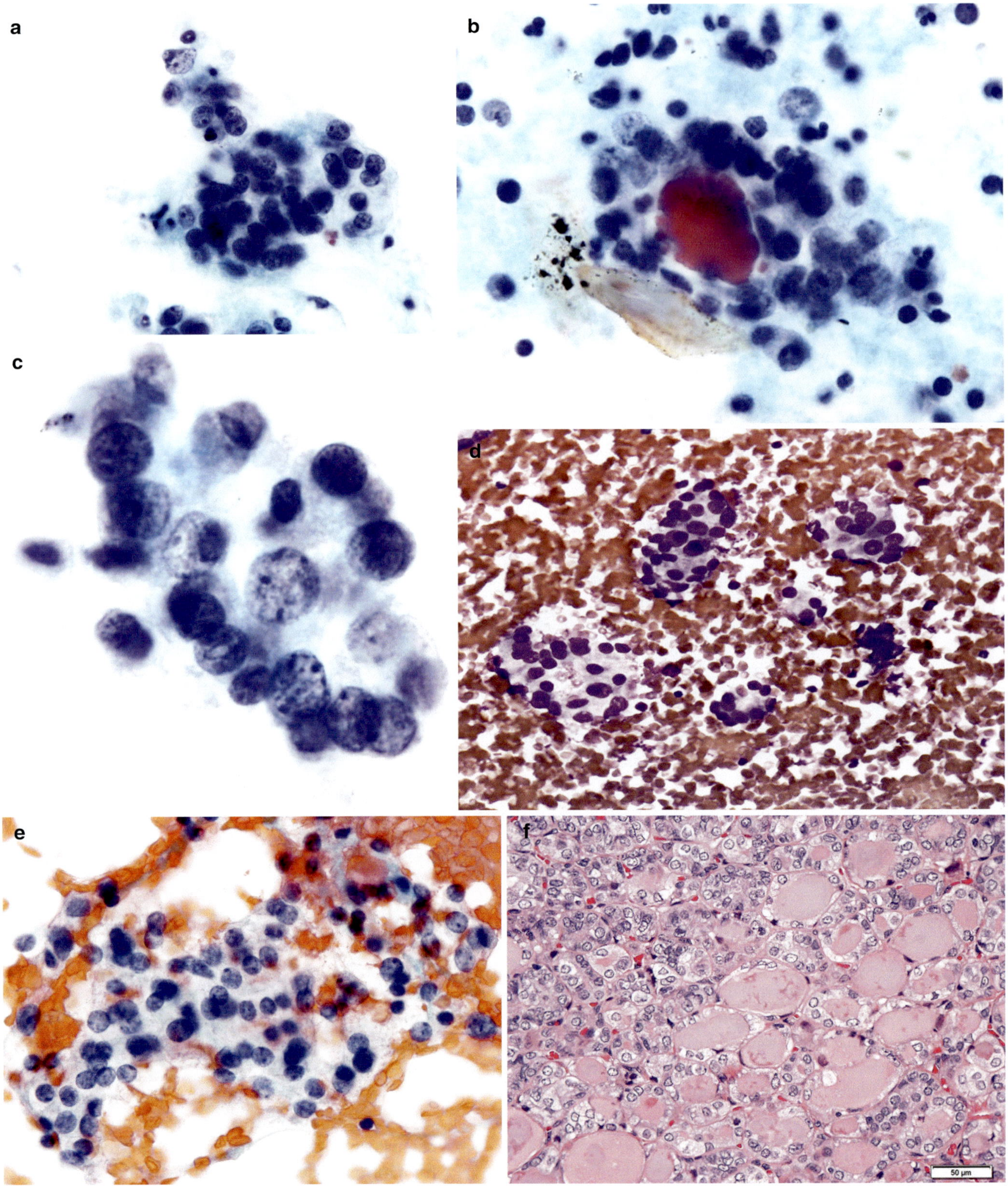

Fig. 5.12 Cytological and architectural atypia. (**a–c**) This case showed both types of atypia. Architectural atypia is displayed by follicular cells in crowded 3-D arrangements and microfollicles. Cytologic atypia is manifested by enlarged, overlapping nuclei with clearing and grooves (Pap stain, TP). (**d**) Air-dried DQ-stained CS displays microfollicular architecture. (**e**) Microfollicles and nuclear clearing and grooves are seen on Pap stain (CS). The appearance of cytology in CS is comparable to LBP, but with more abundant background blood. Molecular tests showed gene mutation. (**f**) Subsequent resection showed a noninvasive follicular thyroid neoplasm with papillary-like nuclear features (NIFTP) (H&E stain)

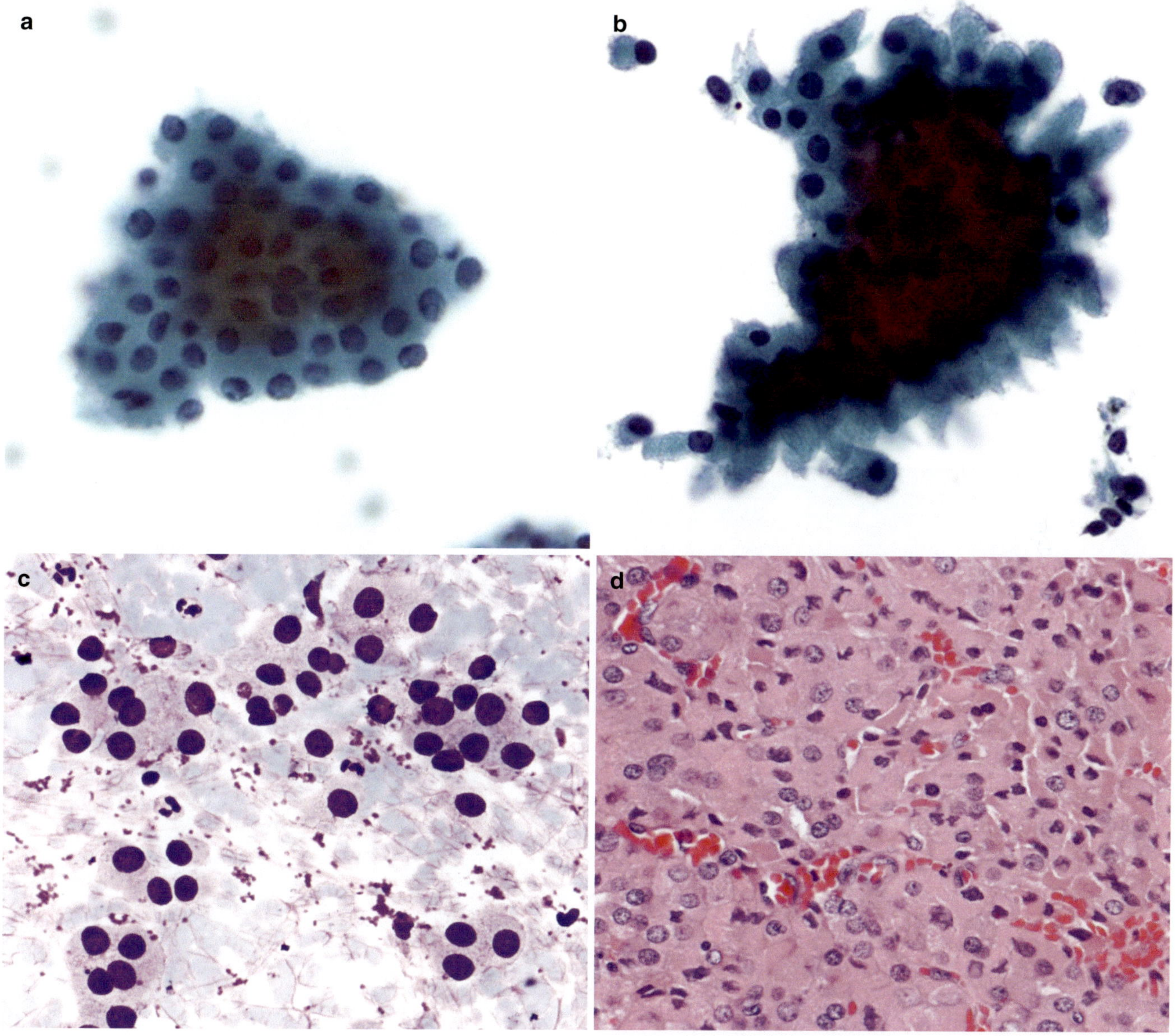

Fig. 5.13 Atypia with Hürthle cell predominance or oncocytic change. This case, processed with Pap stain and both SP (**a**) and TP (**b**), comprised exclusively of Hürthle cells with background minimal colloid. The Hürthle cells display a 3-D configuration. The nuclei are monotonous and round, with small to prominent nucleoli. Cytoplasm is moderate in amount, dense and granular, with distinct contours. Morphology is similar in both types of LBP. Such a case may represent limited sampling of FNHCT/SFNHCT. (**c**) DQ-stained CS of the same case shows less distinct cytoplasmic outlines. Note morphologic similarity with LBP. (**d**) Histologic section of Hürthle cell adenoma on lobectomy (H&E stain)

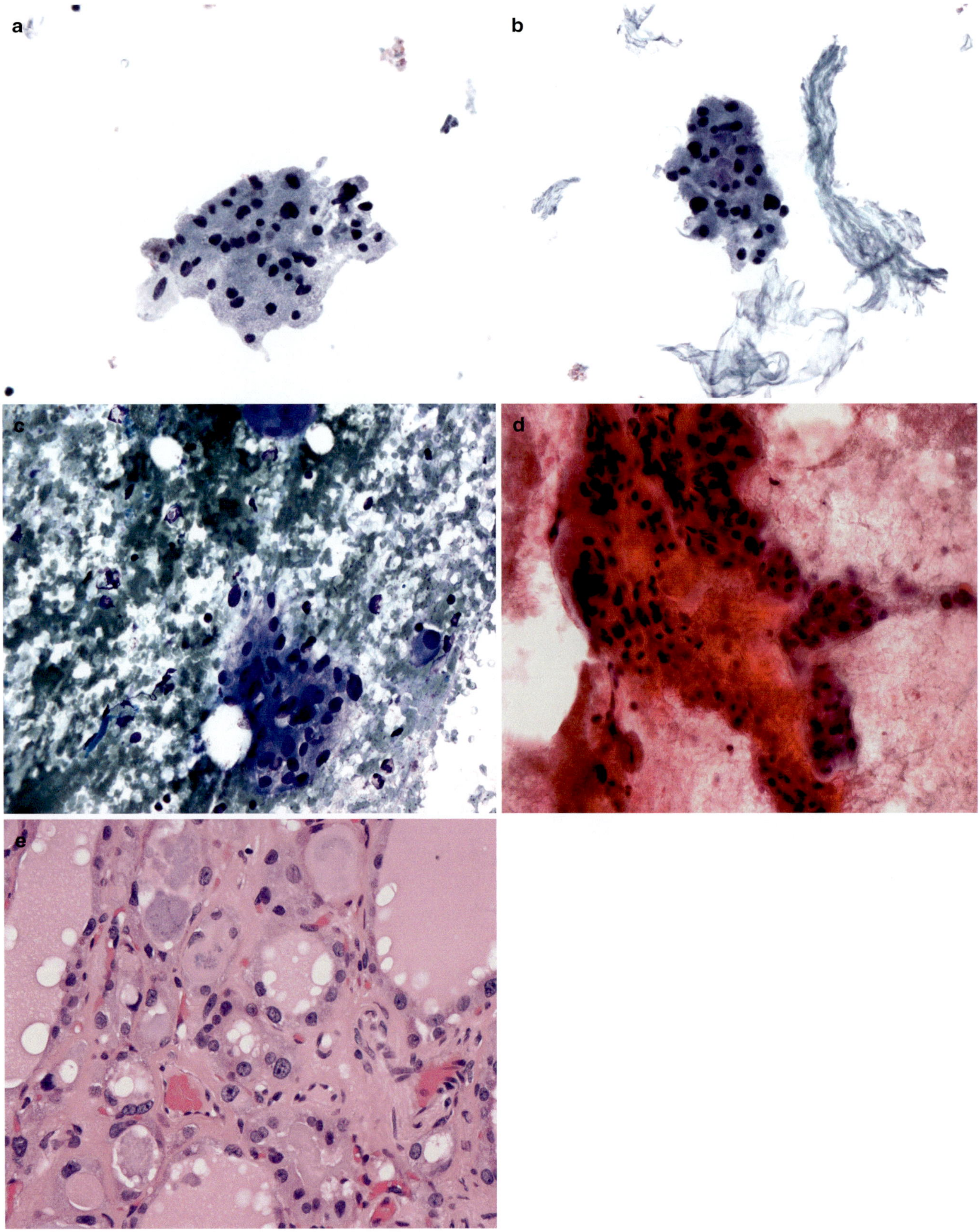

Fig. 5.14 Atypia with Hürthle cell predominance or oncocytic change. (**a**, **b**) This case presented as a multinodular goiter (MNG) and Hürthle cells. On TP and Pap stain (**a**, **b**), the Hürthle cells form flat sheets with small nuclei and abundant granular cytoplasm. Nucleoli are not present. The background shows thin colloid (Pap stain). (**c**, **d**) CS in the same case illustrate some problems associated with CS: The DQ-stained slide (**c**) is over-stained and cell morphology is barely discernible, and the Pap-stained CS (**d**) shows thick cellular clumps obscured by blood. Some macrofollicles and few Hürthle cells are also barely discernible. Lobectomy (**e** H&E stain) showed Hürthle cell metaplasia in nodular hyperplasia

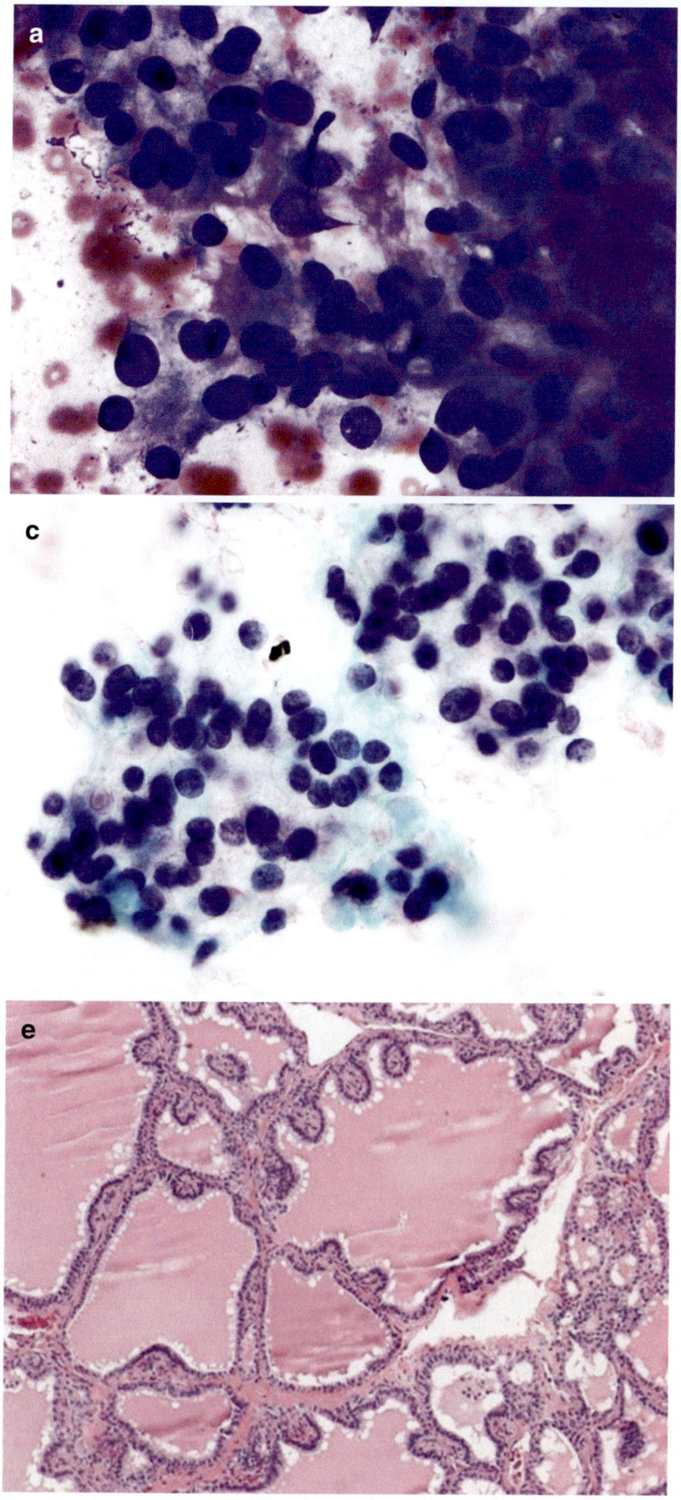

Fig. 5.15 Atypia not otherwise specified (AUS-NOS). In this patient with untreated Graves' disease, CS display large and tall follicular cells in small clusters. Nuclei are enlarged and vesicular, with abundant, finely granular cytoplasm and vacuoles of varying sizes containing deposits of colloid. In DQ stain (**a**), the marginal cytoplasmic vacuoles with colloid appear as pink-red frayed edges, hence the name "flare cells" or "flame cells." Note the edges in the Pap stain (**b**), showing the peripheral cytoplasmic vacuoles and more light-blue staining of colloid. A cytospin slide (**c**, Pap stain) shows similar morphology, as does a TP slide (**d**). The histology of Graves' disease shows scalloped colloid and tall follicular cells (**e**, H&E stain)

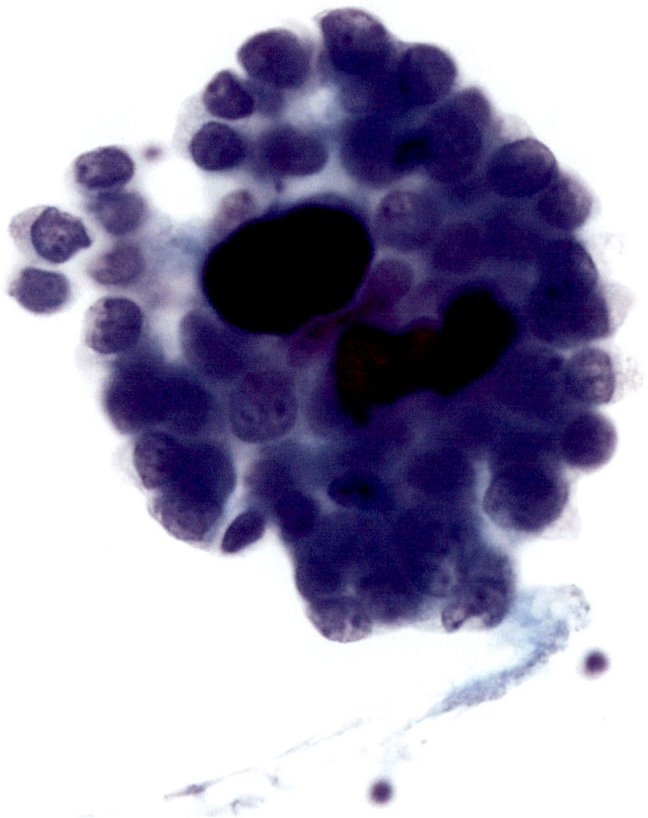

Fig. 5.16 Psammomatous calcification in the absence of nuclear features of PTC. In this case, the cells do not show all nuclear features of PTC (Pap stain, TP). Resection did show classic PTC

(b) *Psammomatous calcifications in the absence of nuclear features of PTC*
   - The specimen should be carefully screened for nuclear features of PTC. "Lamellar bodies" of inspissated colloid may be indistinguishable from true psammomatous calcifications (Fig. 5.16).
   - In LBP, small globules of thick colloid may display radial cracking and mimic psammoma bodies.

Atypical Lymphoid Cells, Rule Out Lymphoma

- There is atypia of lymphoid cells but it is not sufficient for a diagnosis of lymphoma. In LBP, morphology of atypical lymphocytes is well preserved, but they appear smaller and may clump and mimic follicular cells. Background lymphoglandular bodies may be seen as a few small, dot-like structures. In CS (particularly DQ stain), lymphoglandular bodies stain magenta and are very useful in identifying a lesion as lymphoid (Fig. 5.17a–c).
- Flow cytometry on repeat FNA can be advised if the nodule is clinically suspicious.

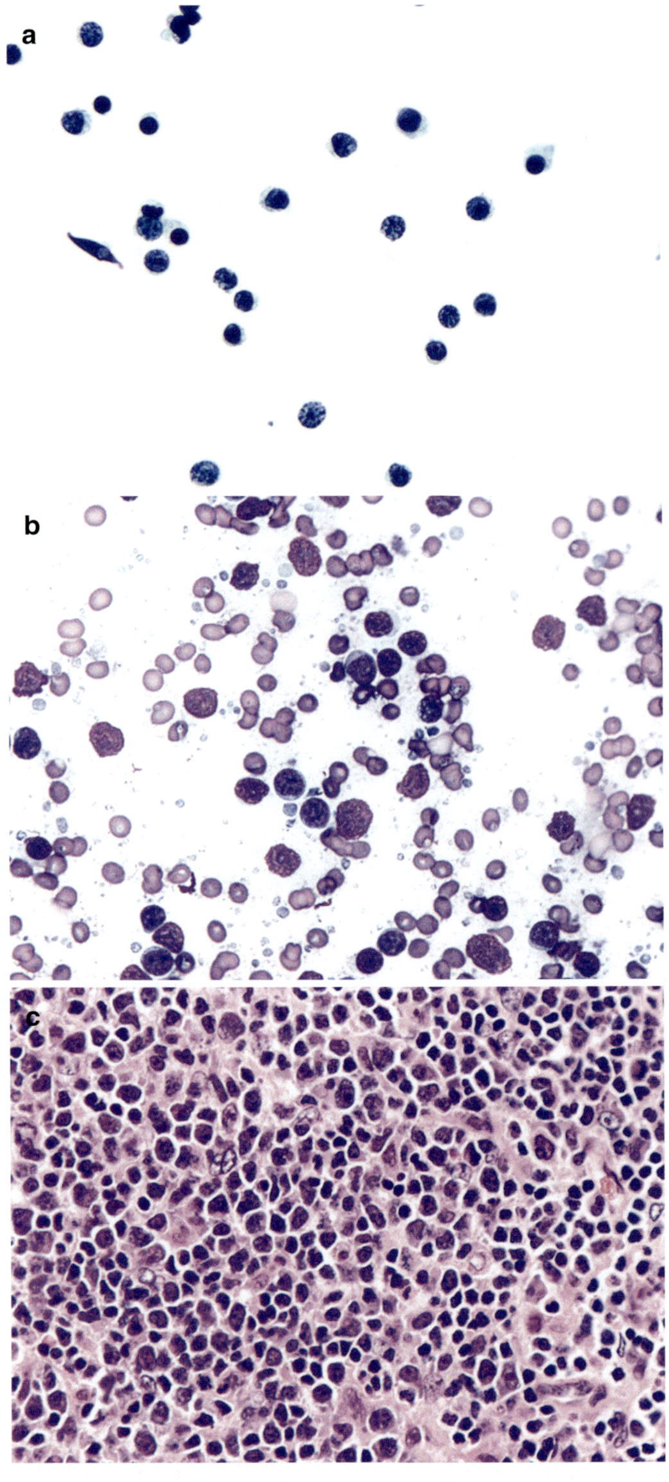

Fig. 5.17 Atypical lymphoid cells, rule out lymphoma. (**a**) Atypical lymphocytes not sufficient for a diagnosis of lymphoma. Morphology of atypical lymphocytes is well preserved. Note a bare nucleus (8 o'clock) with a tiny lymphoglandular body (Pap stain, TP). (**b**) Atypical lymphocytes with prominent lymphoglandular bodies (DQ stain, CS). Flow cytometry, performed on a repeat FNA, showed a B-cell lymphoproliferative disorder. (**c**) Histologic section from needle core biopsy showed a B-cell lymphoma (H&E stain)

Updates in TBSRTC for AUS/FLUS

- No change in terminology.
- AUS/FLUS are synonymous terms, and laboratories should only use one term.
- The category of AUS/FLUS should be used only when absolutely necessary.
- The proposed rate for this category is less than 7% of thyroid FNAs. In the literature, the range of AUS/FLUS has been reported to range from 3% to 20%.
- Intralaboratory quality assurance (QA) monitoring must be performed to prevent potential overuse.
- Reproducibility of AUS/FLUS is fair at best.

Salient Points for AUS/FLUS

- The main goal of creating a category called AUS/FLUS was to decrease unnecessary thyroid resections. Therefore, efforts have been made to identify the ROM in this category.
- The ROM in AUS/FLUS is about 10–30%.
- The malignancy rates in recently published studies using TBSRTC show a wide range of 6–48% in resected cases.
- In a systematic review and meta-analysis by Valderrabano et al. [44], the risk of cancer was 2.6 times greater in indeterminate thyroid nodules with nuclear atypia than in indeterminate thyroid nodules without nuclear atypia.
- ROM and clinical management have been updated in the new edition to reflect changes (*see* Table 2.2).
- AUS/FLUS is the most challenging category among the six diagnostic categories of TBSRTC and is interpreted as the "grey zone" by clinicians.
- Ultrasound classification of thyroid nodules is based on a standardized system for examination of the thyroid called the Thyroid Imaging Reporting and Data System (TIRADS). Ultrasound characteristics also have been shown to be helpful in stratifying the ROM in nodules with AUS/FLUS. Patients with AUS/FLUS and patients with nuclear atypia and high-risk ultrasound features according to the American Thyroid Association (ATA) (Haugen et al. 2015) are at increased risk of having a thyroid malignancy.

Role of Molecular Tests in AUS/FLUS

- The treatment approaches for TBSRTC categories II, V, and VI are well established in light of their malignancy rates, but treatments for categories III and IV, with rates of 10–30% and 25–40%, are subject to debate. Actual management may also depend on other factors besides the FNA diagnosis, such as clinical and ultrasonographic findings.
- AUS/FLUS subcategorization may have a prominent impact on the evolving landscape of molecular testing, which is fast becoming an integral part of indeterminate FNA.
- Judicious use of molecular testing in conjunction with indeterminate cytology aims to improve preoperative diagnostic accuracy. Future studies will need to validate the performance of molecular marker tests in specific cytological scenarios.
- Commercially available molecular tests such as Afirma Genomic Sequencing Classifier (GSC), ThyroSeq v3 Genomic Classifier (GC), ThyGeNEXT®, and ThyraMIR® are useful for the 15–30% of indeterminate thyroid FNAs. They may also be useful for NIFTP (*see* Chap. 14).
- Molecular tests are expensive.

Management of AUS/FLUS

- Most guidelines, including the 2015 ATA guidelines (Haugen et al.), have recommended conservative management in most instances for an initial AUS/FLUS interpretation, with either repeat ultrasound-guided FNA or molecular testing.
- A repeat FNA usually results in a more definitive diagnosis, but about 20–25% of nodules repeatedly receive a diagnosis of AUS/FLUS.

Suggested Reading

1. Absher KJ, Truong LD, Khurana KK, Ramzy I. Parathyroid cytology: avoiding diagnostic pitfalls. Head Neck. 2002;24:157–64.
2. Ali SZ, Cibas ES, editors. The Bethesda System for reporting thyroid cytopathology; definitions, criteria, and explanatory notes. 2nd ed. Cham: Springer International Publishing AG; 2018.
3. Ali SZ, Nayar R, Krane JF, Westra WH. Atlas of thyroid cytopathology with histopathologic correlations. New York: Demos Medical Publishing; 2014.
4. Baca SC, Wong KS, Strickland KC, Heller HT, Kim MI, Barletta JA, et al. Qualifiers of atypia in the cytologic diagnosis of thyroid nodules are associated with different Afirma gene expression classifier results and clinical outcomes. Cancer Cytopathol. 2017;125:313–22. https://doi.org/10.1002/cncy.21827.
5. Brandler TC, Cho M, Wei XJ, Simms A, Levine P, Hernandez O, et al. Noninvasive follicular thyroid neoplasm with papillary-like nuclear features: an interobserver study of key cytomorphological features from a large academic medical centre. Cytopathology. 2019;30:39–45. https://doi.org/10.1111/cyt.12632.
6. Cibas ES, Ali SZ. The 2017 Bethesda System for reporting thyroid cytopathology. Thyroid. 2017;27:1341–6. https://doi.org/10.1089/thy.2017.0500.
7. Cibas ES, Baloch ZW, Fellegara G, LiVolsi VA, Raab SS, Rosai J, et al. A prospective assessment defining the limitations of thyroid nodule pathologic evaluation. Ann Intern Med. 2013;159:325–32. https://doi.org/10.7326/0003-4819-159-5-201309030-00006.
8. Choong KC, Khiyami A, Tamarkin SW, McHenry CR. Fine-needle aspiration biopsy of thyroid nodules: Is routine ultrasound-guidance

necessary? Surgery. 2018;164:789–94. https://doi.org/10.1016/j.surg.2018.04.047.
9. Dincer N, Balci S, Yazgan A, Guney G, Ersoy R, Cakir B, et al. Follow-up of atypia and follicular lesions of undetermined significance in thyroid fine needle aspiration cytology. Cytopathology. 2013;24:385–90. https://doi.org/10.1111/cyt.12021.
10. Eisa N, Khan A, Akhter M, Fensterwald M, Saleem S, Fananapazir G, et al. Both ultrasound features and nuclear atypia are associated with malignancy in thyroid nodules with atypia of undetermined significance. Ann Surg Oncol. 2018;25:3913–8. https://doi.org/10.1245/s10434-018-6826-6.
11. Faquin WC, Cibas ES, Renshaw AA. "Atypical" cells in fine-needle aspiration biopsy specimens of benign thyroid cysts. Cancer. 2005;105:71–9.
12. Faquin WC, Wong LQ, Afrogheh AH, Ali SZ, Bishop JA, Bongiovanni M, et al. Impact of reclassifying noninvasive follicular variant of papillary thyroid carcinoma on the risk of malignancy in The Bethesda System for Reporting Thyroid Cytopathology. Cancer Cytopathol. 2016;124:181–7. https://doi.org/10.1002/cncy.21631.
13. Fischer AH, Clayton AC, Bentz JS, Wasserman PG, Henry MR, Souers RJ, et al. Performance differences between conventional smears and liquid-based preparations of thyroid fine-needle aspiration samples: analysis of 47,076 responses in the College of American Pathologists Interlaboratory Comparison Program in Non-Gynecologic Cytology. Arch Pathol Lab Med. 2013;137:26–31. https://doi.org/10.5858/arpa.2012-0009-CP.
14. Gan TR, Nga ME, Lum JH, Wong WM, Tan WB, Parameswaran R, et al. Thyroid cytology–nuclear versus architectural atypia within the "Atypia of undetermined significance/follicular lesion of undetermined significance" Bethesda category have significantly different rates of malignancy. Cancer Cytopathol. 2017;125:245–56. https://doi.org/10.1002/cncy.21823.
15. Geramizadeh B, Bos-Hagh S, Maleki Z. Cytomorphologic, imaging, molecular findings, and outcome in thyroid Follicular Lesion of Undetermined Significance/Atypical Cell of Undetermined Significance (AUS/FLUS): a mini-review. Acta Cytol. 2019;63:1–9. https://doi.org/10.1159/000493908.
16. Gerhard R, Boerner SL. Evaluation of indeterminate thyroid cytology by second-opinion diagnosis or repeat fine-needle aspiration: which is the best approach? Acta Cytol. 2015;59:43–50. https://doi.org/10.1159/000369332.
17. Godoi Cavalheiro B, Kober Nogueira Leite A, Luongo de Matos L, Palermo Miazaki A, Ientile JM, Kulcsar MA, Cernea CR. Malignancy rates in thyroid nodules classified as Bethesda categories III and IV: retrospective data from a tertiary center. Int J Endocrinol Metab. 2017;16:e12871. https://doi.org/10.5812/ijem.12871.
18. Haugen BR, Alexander EK, Bible KC, Doherty GM, Mandel SJ, Nikiforov YE, et al. 2015 American Thyroid Association Management Guidelines for Adult Patients with Thyroid Nodules and Differentiated Thyroid Cancer: the American Thyroid Association Guidelines Task Force on thyroid nodules and differentiated thyroid cancer. Thyroid. 2016;26:1–133. https://doi.org/10.1089/thy.2015.0020.
19. Hoda RS. Non-gynecologic cytology on liquid-based preparations: a morphologic review of facts and artifacts. Diagn Cytopathol. 2007;35:621–34.
20. Hoda RS, VandenBussche C, Hoda SA. Diagnostic liquid-based cytology. New York: Springer; 2017.
21. Hang JF, Westra WH, Zhou AG, Cooper DS, Ali SZ. The impact of noninvasive follicular thyroid neoplasm with papillary-like nuclear features on the rate of malignancy for atypia of undetermined significance subcategories. Cancer Cytopathol. 2018;126:309–16. https://doi.org/10.1002/cncy.21981.
22. Jan IS, Lee YT, Wang CM, Cheng TY, Wang CY, Chang TC, et al. The surgery and repeat aspiration outcomes of the atypia of undetermined significance/follicular lesion of undetermined significance category in The Bethesda System for Reporting Thyroid Cytopathology. Asian J Surg. 2019;42:144–7. https://doi.org/10.1016/j.asjsur.2018.02.008.
23. Jo VY, Stelow EB, Dustin SM, Hanley KZ. Malignancy risk for fine-needle aspiration of thyroid lesions according to the Bethesda System for Reporting Thyroid Cytopathology. Am J Clin Pathol. 2010;134:450–6. https://doi.org/10.1309/AJCP5N4MTHPAFXFB.
24. Jug RC, Datto MB, Jiang XS. Molecular testing for indeterminate thyroid nodules: performance of the Afirma gene expression classifier and ThyroSeq panel. Cancer Cytopathol. 2018;126:471–80. https://doi.org/10.1002/cncy.21993.
25. Jung YY, Jung S, Lee HW, Oh YL. Significance of subcategory atypia of undetermined significance/follicular lesion of undetermined significance showing both cytologic and architectural atypia in thyroid aspiration cytology. Acta Cytol. 2015;59:370–6. https://doi.org/10.1159/000441136.
26. Khalil AB, Dina R, Meeran K, Bakir AM, Naqvi S, Al Tikritti A, et al. Indeterminate thyroid nodules: a pragmatic approach. Eur Thyroid J. 2018;7:39–43. https://doi.org/10.1159/000484600.
27. Kim Y, Choi KR, Chae MJ, Shin BK, Kim HK, Kim A, et al. Stability of DNA, RNA, cytomorphology, and immunoantigenicity in residual ThinPrep specimens. APMIS. 2013;121:1064–72. https://doi.org/10.1111/apm.12082.
28. Kim SJ, Roh J, Baek JH, Hong SJ, Shong YK, Kim WB, et al. Risk of malignancy according to sub-classification of the atypia of undetermined significance or follicular lesion of undetermined significance (AUS/FLUS) category in the Bethesda System for Reporting Thyroid Cytopathology. Cytopathology. 2017;28:65–73. https://doi.org/10.1111/cyt.12352.
29. Krane JF, Cibas ES, Alexander EK, Paschke R, Eszlinger M. Molecular analysis of residual ThinPrep material from thyroid FNAs increases diagnostic sensitivity. Cancer Cytopathol. 2015;123:356–61. https://doi.org/10.1002/cncy.21546.
30. Krauss EA, Mahon M, Fede JM, Zhang L. Application of the Bethesda Classification for thyroid fine-needle aspiration: Institutional experience and meta-analysis. Arch Pathol Lab Med. 2016;140:1121–31. https://doi.org/10.5858/arpa.2015-0154-SA.
31. Lauria Pantano A, Maddaloni E, Briganti SI, Beretta Anguissola G, Perrella E, Taffon C, et al. Differences between ATA, AACE/ACE/AME and ACR TI-RADS ultrasound classifications performance in identifying cytological high-risk thyroid nodules. Eur J Endocrinol. 2018;178:595–603. https://doi.org/10.1530/EJE-18-0083.
32. Lee JH, Han K, Kim EK, Moon HJ, Yoon JH, Park VY, et al. Risk stratification of thyroid nodules with Atypia of Undetermined Significance/Follicular Lesion of Undetermined Significance (AUS/FLUS) cytology using ultrasonography patterns defined by the 2015 ATA guidelines. Ann Otol Rhinol Laryngol. 2017;126:625–33. https://doi.org/10.1177/0003489417719472.
33. Lim JXY, Nga ME, Chan DKH, Tan WB, Parameswaran R, Ngiam KY. Subclassification of Bethesda Atypical and Follicular Neoplasm categories according to nuclear and architectural atypia improves discrimination of thyroid malignancy risk. Thyroid. 2018;28:511–21. https://doi.org/10.1089/thy.2017.0274.
34. Luu MH, Fischer AH, Stockl TJ, Pisharodi L, Owens CL. Atypical follicular cells with equivocal features of papillary thyroid carcinoma is not a low-risk cytologic diagnosis. Acta Cytol. 2011;55:526–30. https://doi.org/10.1159/000333227.
35. Michael CW, Hunter B. Interpretation of fine-needle aspirates processed by the ThinPrep technique: cytologic artifacts and diagnostic pitfalls. Diagn Cytopathol. 2000;23:6–13.
36. Michael CW, McConnel J, Pecott J, Afify AM, Al-Khafaji B. Comparison of ThinPrep and TriPath PREP liquid-based

preparations in nongynecologic specimens: a pilot study. Diagn Cytopathol. 2001;25:177–84.

37. Nishino M, Wang HH. Should the thyroid AUS/FLUS category be further stratified by malignancy risk? Cancer Cytopathol. 2014;122:481–3. https://doi.org/10.1002/cncy.21412.
38. Oertel YC. “Atypical” cells in fine-needle aspiration biopsy specimens of benign thyroid cysts. Cancer. 2006;108:72; author reply 73
39. Padmanabhan V, Marshall CB, Akdas Barkan G, Ghofrani M, Laser A, Tolgay Ocal I, et al. Reproducibility of atypia of undetermined significance/follicular lesion of undetermined significance category using the Bethesda System for reporting thyroid cytology when reviewing slides from different institutions: a study of interobserver variability among cytopathologists. Diagn Cytopathol. 2017;45:399–405. https://doi.org/10.1002/dc.23681.
40. Persichetti A, Di Stasio E, Guglielmi R, Bizzarri G, Taccogna S, Misischi I, et al. Predictive value of malignancy of thyroid nodule ultrasound classification systems: a prospective study. J Clin Endocrinol Metab. 2018;103:1359–68. https://doi.org/10.1210/jc.2017-01708.
41. Steward DL, Carty SE, Sippel RS, Yang SP, Sosa JA, Sipos JA, et al. Performance of a multigene genomic classifier in thyroid nodules with indeterminate cytology: a prospective blinded multicenter study. JAMA Oncol. 2018. [Epub ahead of print]; https://doi.org/10.1001/jamaoncol.2018.4616.
42. Tripathy K, Mishra A, Singh AK, Panda PL, Mahapatra A, Lenka A. Immunocytochemistry using liquid-based cytology: a tool in hormone receptor analysis of breast cancer. J Cytol. 2018;35:260–4. https://doi.org/10.4103/JOC.JOC_23_18.
43. Tulecke MA, Wang HH. ThinPrep for cytologic evaluation of follicular thyroid lesions: correlation with histologic findings. Diagn Cytopathol. 2004;30:7–13.
44. Valderrabano P, Khazai L, Thompson ZJ, Sharpe SC, Tarasova VD, Otto KJ, et al. Cancer risk associated with nuclear atypia in cytologically indeterminate thyroid nodules: a systematic review and meta-analysis. Thyroid. 2018;28:210–9. https://doi.org/10.1089/thy.2017.0419.
45. Vivero M, Renshaw AA, Krane JF. Influence of descriptive terminology on management of atypical thyroid fine-needle aspirates. Cancer Cytopathol. 2014;122:175–81. https://doi.org/10.1002/cncy.21367.
46. Wu HH, Inman A, Cramer HM. Subclassification of “atypia of undetermined significance” in thyroid fine-needle aspirates. Diagn Cytopathol. 2014;42:23–9. https://doi.org/10.1002/dc.23052.
47. Yang J, Schnadig V, Logrono R, Wasserman PG. Fine-needle aspiration of thyroid nodules: a study of 4703 patients with histologic and clinical correlations. Cancer. 2007;111:306–15.

Follicular Neoplasm/Suspicious for Follicular Neoplasm

6

Rana S. Hoda, Rema Rao, and Theresa Scognamiglio

Introduction

- Thyroid FNA is a highly accurate modality for initial assessment of a nodule. A benign result has a negative predictive value (NPV) greater than 95%, and a malignant diagnosis has a positive predictive value (PPV) of 94–96%. But in 15% to 30% of cases, FNA renders an indeterminate diagnosis, leading to a clinical management dilemma.
- In The Bethesda System for Reporting Thyroid Cytopathology (TBSRTC), one of the indeterminate categories is Follicular Neoplasm/Suspicious for Follicular Neoplasm (FN/SFN), which carries a risk of malignancy (ROM) of 25% to 40%.
- This category also has a Hürthle cell form entitled Follicular Neoplasm Hürthle Cell (Oncocytic) Type/Suspicious for Follicular Neoplasm Hürthle Cell (Oncocytic) Type (FNHCT/SFNHCT). (See Chap. 7.)
- Follicular-patterned lesions of the thyroid can be derived from thyroid follicular cells or nonthyroid follicular cells. They can represent benign, neoplastic, or malignant entities. Benign lesions include an adenomatoid nodule; benign neoplastic lesions include follicular adenoma (FA) and parathyroid adenoma; malignant lesions include follicular carcinoma (FC), the follicular variant of papillary thyroid carcinoma (FVPTC), and its more indolent form, noninvasive follicular thyroid neoplasm with papillary-like nuclear features (NIFTP).
- Cytology cannot accurately distinguish between these entities, because of their morphologic overlap. A definitive diagnosis requires surgical resection, with histologic assessment for the presence of a capsule.
- The histologic diagnosis of FA, FC, FVPTC, and NIFTP relies on the examination of the entire capsule for the presence or absence of capsular and/or vascular invasion and certain other histologic criteria. Cytology cannot distinguish between these entities, and the accuracy of diagnosing follicular-patterned lesions in cytology will remain a "gray zone."
- The likelihood that a nodule with an FN/SFN diagnosis is neoplastic is 65–85%, and 69.7% of patients undergo surgery. The rate of malignancy is low, however; only 25–40% will have a malignant outcome on histologic examination. Papillary thyroid carcinoma (PTC) is the most common malignancy, accounting for 27–68% of cases. This wide range is due to the presence of NIFTP and FVPTC, as well as other factors [2, 18].
- Molecular markers in conjunction with cytology are recommended in this category, to better select nodules for surgery that have a high probability of malignancy.
- Because liquid-based preparations (LBP) are increasingly being used for thyroid cytology, awareness of the unique background, architecture, and nuclear features of FN/SFN is crucial to distinguish it from its mimics, and for correlation with molecular test results and histological diagnosis.

Definition of FN/SFN

- The TBSRTC defines FN/SFN as a moderately cellular or cellular aspirate composed of follicular cells, most of which are arranged in an altered architectural pattern characterized by significant cell crowding and/or microfollicle formation. Nuclear atypia is mild and includes increased nuclear size, contour irregularity, and/or chromatin clearing. True papillae and intranuclear pseudoinclusions (INPI) are absent. Some nuclear features of PTC may be present and raise the possibility of FVPTC or NIFTP.

R. S. Hoda (✉)
CBLPath, Rye Brook, NY, USA
e-mail: rhoda@cblpath.com

R. Rao · T. Scognamiglio
Department of Pathology and Laboratory Medicine, New York Presbyterian Hospital, Weill Cornell Medical College, New York, NY, USA
e-mail: rer9052@med.cornell.edu; ths9004@med.cornell.edu

R. S. Hoda et al. (eds.), *Atlas of Thyroid Cytopathology on Liquid-Based Preparations*,
https://doi.org/10.1007/978-3-030-25066-9_6

Definition of a Microfollicle

- The TBSRTC and Faquin and Clark, 2005 list the following characteristics in the definition of a microfollicle:
  - Small, flat group of 6 to 12 follicular cells arranged in a circle or wreath-like arrangement that is at least two-thirds complete.
  - Follicular cells are crowded and overlapping.
  - The lumen of the microfollicle may contain a small amount of inspissated colloid.
  - Most microfollicles are of uniform size.

Updates in TBSRTC for FN/SFN

- No change in terminology.
- The term "SFN" is preferred, because it is difficult to distinguish FN from its benign mimics on FNA cytology. Most importantly, to determine the malignant nature of follicular lesions requires histologic assessment of the capsule for capsular or vascular invasion.
- A comment can be added to the cytology report about the possibility of FVPTC or NIFTP in the presence of oval nuclei with chromatin clearing and INPI (*see* Table 6.1).

Table 6.1 Follicular thyroid lesions: diagnosis and management

Diagnosis	Ultrasound findings	Cytological features on LBP	Molecular findings	Histology	Management[a]
Hyperplastic/ adenomatoid nodule (HN)	May be solid/cystic, spongiform, isoechoic	Low to high cellularity, unremarkable follicular cells in sheets, and macrofollicles without nuclear atypia; microfollicles may be seen, cytoplasm is scant to moderate, colloid is thick and thin[b]; various degenerative changes	Genes involved in thyroid growth and hormone synthesis	Either no capsule or insufficient encapsulation with both microfollicles and some medium-sized follicles	Resection (if symptomatic) or observation
Follicular adenoma (FA)	Solitary, solid, variable echoic pattern	Low to moderate cellularity, monotonous follicular cells with minimal/no nuclear atypia, forming microfollicles, trabeculae and crowded 3-D clusters, +/− macrofollicles; scant cytoplasm; scant, dense colloid in droplets. Lacks cystic changes or nuclear atypia of PTC	*RAS* mutations	Solitary, no invasive growth pattern; surrounded by a fibrous capsule; microfollicular and macrofollicular growth pattern	Molecular test and lobectomy
Follicular carcinoma (FC)	Isoechoic to hyperechoic; thick, irregular halo; may show infiltrative features, usually macro-calcifications, solitary nodule, NS >2 cm	Low to moderate cellularity, follicular cells with minimal/no nuclear atypia in MIFC. In WIFC enlarged, pleomorphic nuclei, abnormal chromatin and/or prominent nucleoli arranged in microfollicles, trabeculae, crowded 3-D clusters, and single cells; transgressing vessels. Lacks nuclear atypia of PTC	*RAS* mutations	Large, solitary; MIFC shows capsular or vascular invasion; WIFC lacks a defined capsule and extends into the thyroid parenchyma	Molecular test; lobectomy or total thyroidectomy
FVPTC/ NIFTP	Large, hypoechoic, solid nodule; irregular margins, discontinuous halo, intranodular vascularity, microcalcifications	Microfollicles with nuclear features of PTC including nuclear enlargement, elongation, overlapping, irregularity with chromatin clearing, rare grooves, and INPI	*RAS* mutations	Nuclear features of PTC with a dominant >50% follicular growth pattern. Two subtypes: encapsulated (includes NIFTP) and infiltrative	Lobectomy or total thyroidectomy
Parathyroid adenoma (PA)	Homogeneously hypoechoic; difficult to distinguish from a thyroid follicular cell nodule	Cellular with microfollicles and cohesive clusters of cells that resemble follicular cells; nuclei are round, with coarse granular chromatin and variable atypia; cytoplasm is abundant, oncocytic. or clear; colloid is absent. Follicular and parathyroid cells cannot be cytologically distinguished; immunostains for TG and PTH help.	Parathyroid gene		

FVPTC follicular variant of papillary thyroid carcinoma, *INPI* intranuclear pseudoinclusions, *LBP* liquid-based preparations, *MIFC* minimally invasive follicular carcinoma, *NIFTP* noninvasive follicular thyroid neoplasm with papillary-like nuclear features, *NS* nodule size, *PTH* parathormone, *PTC* papillary thyroid carcinoma, *TG* thyroglobulin, *WIFC* widely invasive follicular carcinoma

[a]Actual management may depend on other factors (clinical ultrasound)

[b]See description of thick and thin colloid in LBP in Chap. 4

- Intralaboratory quality assurance (QA) monitoring and correlation with molecular test results must be performed to prevent potential overuse.
- The recommended management guidelines of the American Thyroid Association (ATA) [19] include molecular testing (*see* Chap. 14) and lobectomy.

Criteria for FN/SFN Diagnosis and Application in LBP

- The TBSRTC, as well as Clark and Faquin [10], Bommanahalli et al. [4], and Han et al. [18], have described in detail the architectural and cytological features and the differential diagnosis of follicular-patterned lesions in conventional smears (CS). These features also apply to LBP, but with some modifications, which are addressed below.
- *Cytologic criteria* in CS and the differences in LBP:
  - *Cellularity:* High in CS (Fig. 6.1a). Cellularity may be less in LBP than in CS (Fig. 6.1b, c).
  - *Colloid:* Scant and thick or absent in CS, and may form bands or big globules (Fig. 6.2a). In LBP, thick or dense colloid appears as small droplets or small globules or thick bands. The globules may become dissociated from microfollicles and appear scattered in the background (Fig. 6.2b, c). When these globules are noticed, careful screening of architecture and cells should be performed. The globules of thick colloid may crack and mimic a psammoma body (Fig. 6.2b).
- *Architecture features:* In CS, follicular cells can be arranged in microfollicular pattern, the trabecular pattern, multilayer rosettes (cellular ball clusters), branching 3-D ribbon-forming cell sheets, syncytial cellular fragments, and many isolated cells [18]. All architectural patterns are retained in LBP, with subtle alterations.

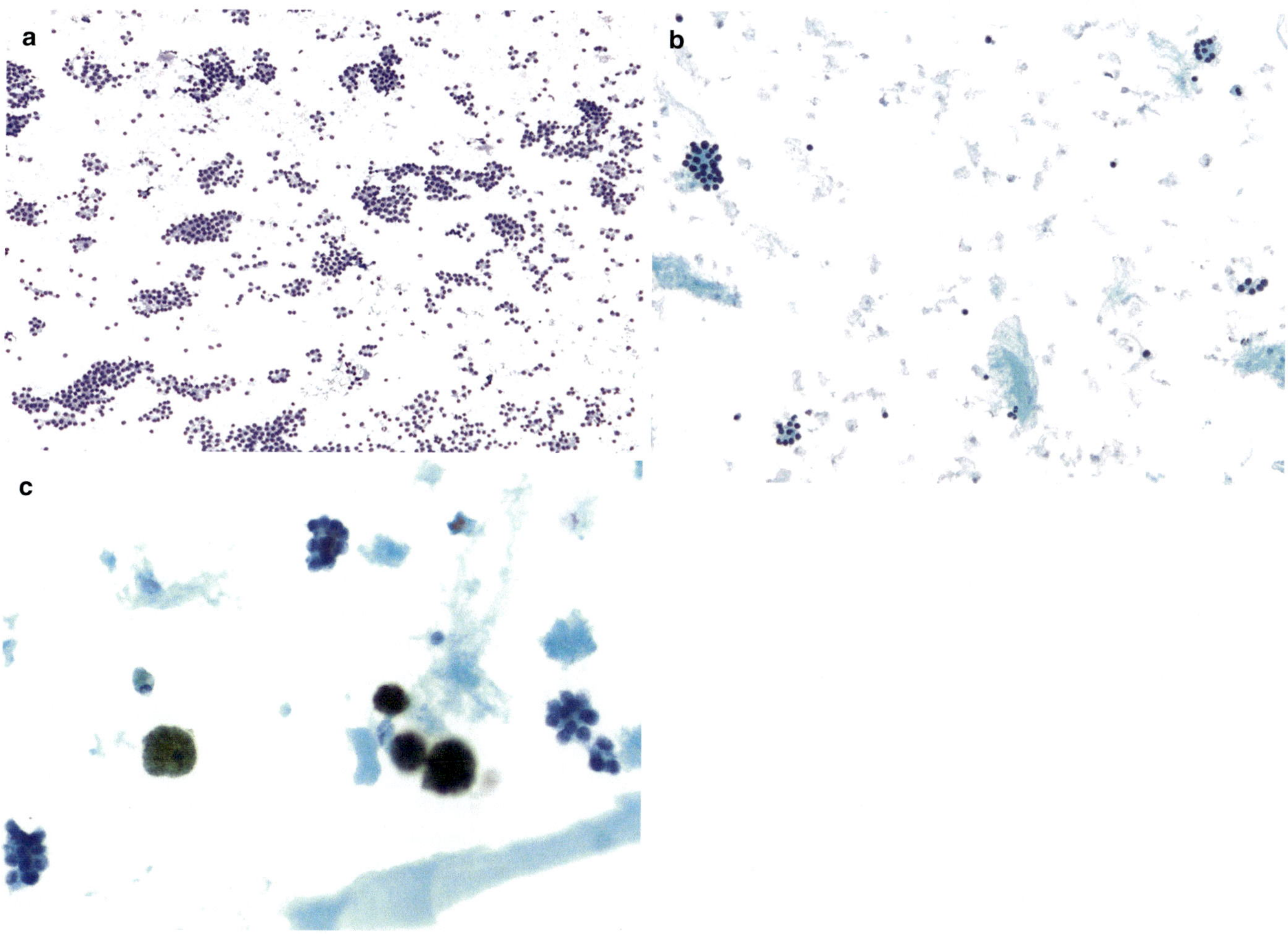

Fig. 6.1 Cellularity in FN/SFN. (**a**) Increased cellularity in Diff-Quik (DQ)–stained conventional smear (CS) in follicular adenoma (FA). (**b**, **c**) LBP with slightly less cellularity in two different cases of FA (seen in Figs. 6.10 and 6.12 respectively). Also note thick and thin colloid in both LBP. (**b** Pap stain, TP; **c** Pap stain, SP)

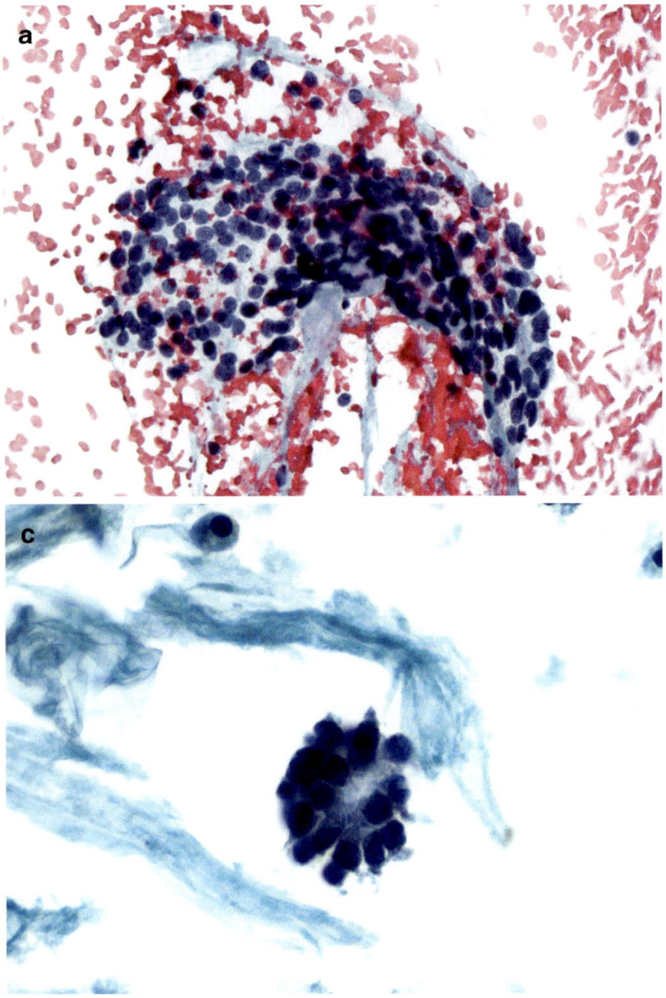

Fig. 6.2 Colloid in FN/SFN. (**a**) The CS also shows colloid as thick bands in a case of follicular variant of papillary thyroid carcinoma (FVPTC). Note the prominent nucleoli and the abundant background blood (Pap stain). (**b**) Thick globular colloid in TP from the case of noninvasive follicular thyroid neoplasm with papillary-like nuclear features (NIFTP) seen in Fig. 6.18. The globular colloid is dissociated from microfollicles and appears scattered in the background. Note the cracking of the thick globular colloid, which may mimic a psammoma body (Pap stain). (**c**) Thick colloid appears in thick bands in SurePath™ (SP) from the case of FA seen in Fig. 6.12 (Pap stain). The images below include other appearances of colloid in follicular neoplasms (FN)

- Microfollicles: In CS, microfollicles appear as a flat group of less than 15 follicular cells in a circle or wreath-like arrangement with a well-defined lumen, which sometimes contains a small amount of thick, inspissated colloid. Follicular cells are overlapping and crowded. Microfollicular pattern is seen in most cases of FN/SFN. It can also be seen in HN/adenomatoid nodule and FVPTC. So this pattern is not specific to FN/SFN. In LBP, the microfollicles may be tighter and smaller, with a preserved lumen that sometimes shows thick inspissated colloid. In ThinPrep® (TP), microfollicles may appear more isolated. In SurePath™ (SP), microfollicles appear more 3-D, with a greater depth of focus. To visualize the lumen of the microfollicle in SP requires constant focus adjustment (Fig. 6.3). It is important to understand the morphology of a macrofollicle to be able to distinguish it from a microfollicle. Macrofollicles are large, with organized and polarized cells without nuclear overlap. In LBP, macrofollicles appear as circular cell balls, whereas in CS they usually are stretched because of smearing effect (Fig. 6.4).
- Trabecular arrangement: This is also known as cellular ribbons. In CS, trabeculae are composed of crowded and overlapping follicular cells with a well-defined contour. Trabecular arrangement is mostly seen in FN/SFN. In LBP, there may be fewer trabeculae, perhaps owing to fragmentation caused by individual liquid-based processing techniques (Fig. 6.5).
- Branching 3-D ribbon-forming cell sheets: In CS, these formations appear as crowding/overlapping complex branching sheets. These can be seen in FN/

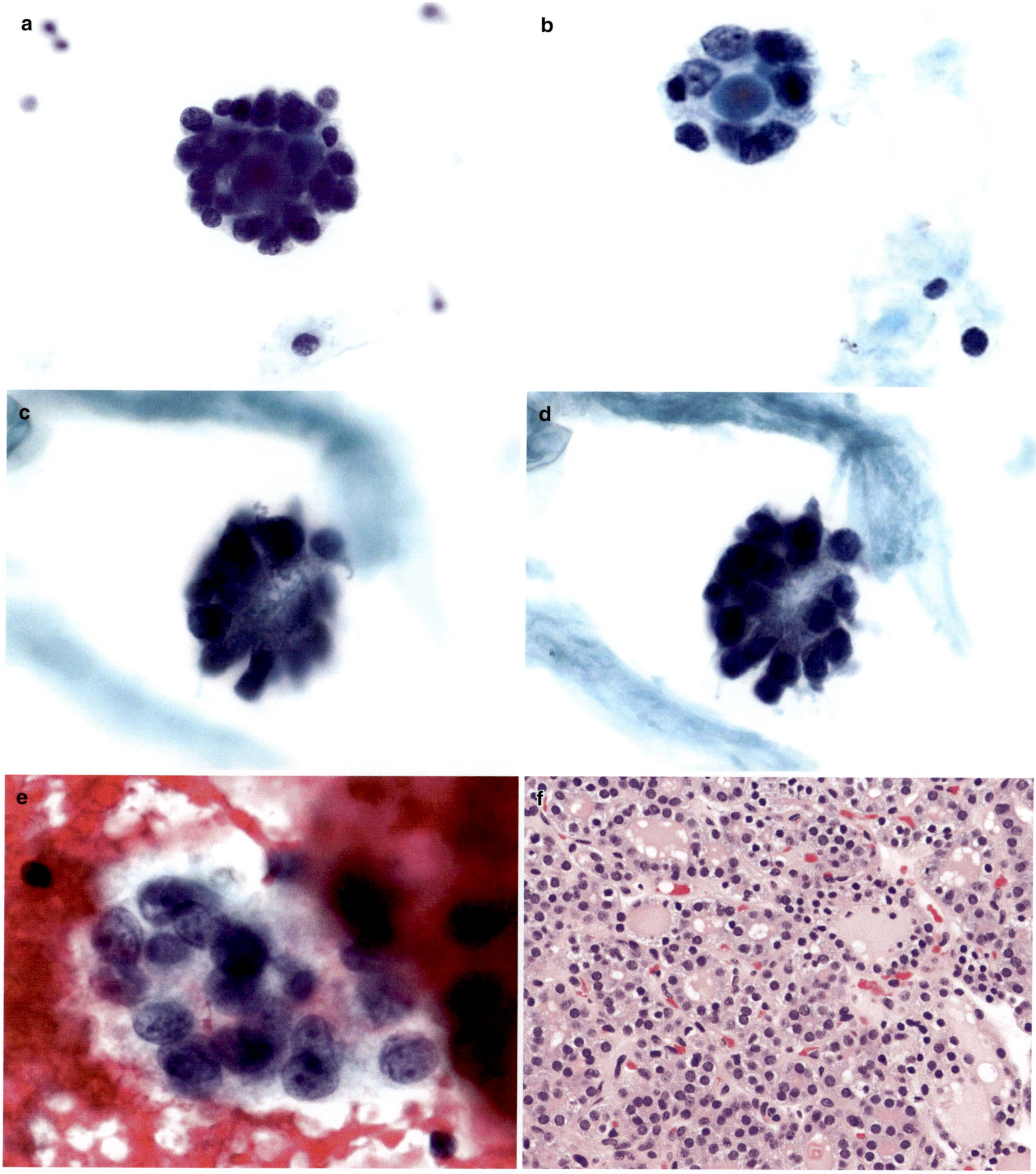

Fig. 6.3 Microfollicles in FN/SFN. (**a**) Microfollicle in a ThinPrep® (TP) slide from the case of FA in Fig. 6.10 appears as a flat group of cells, yet the three-dimensionality is retained. It comprises a tighter, wreath-like arrangement of round nuclei with overlap with dense, inspissated colloid in the lumen (Pap stain). (**b**) Another example of a microfollicle on TP (Pap stain). (**c**, **d**) Microfollicle in SP from the case of FA in Fig. 6.12; it appears more 3-D, with a greater depth of focus. The lumen of the microfollicle is visible in a different plane of focus (**c** Pap stain). (**e**) Microfollicle in CS from the case of adenomatoid nodule in Fig. 6.9 also appears as a flat group. Thick colloid is not visible in the lumen. Note the prominent nucleoli and the abundant background blood. The background is clean and devoid of blood in the two LBP. (**f**) Histologic section showing microfollicular pattern from a case of FA (H&E stain)

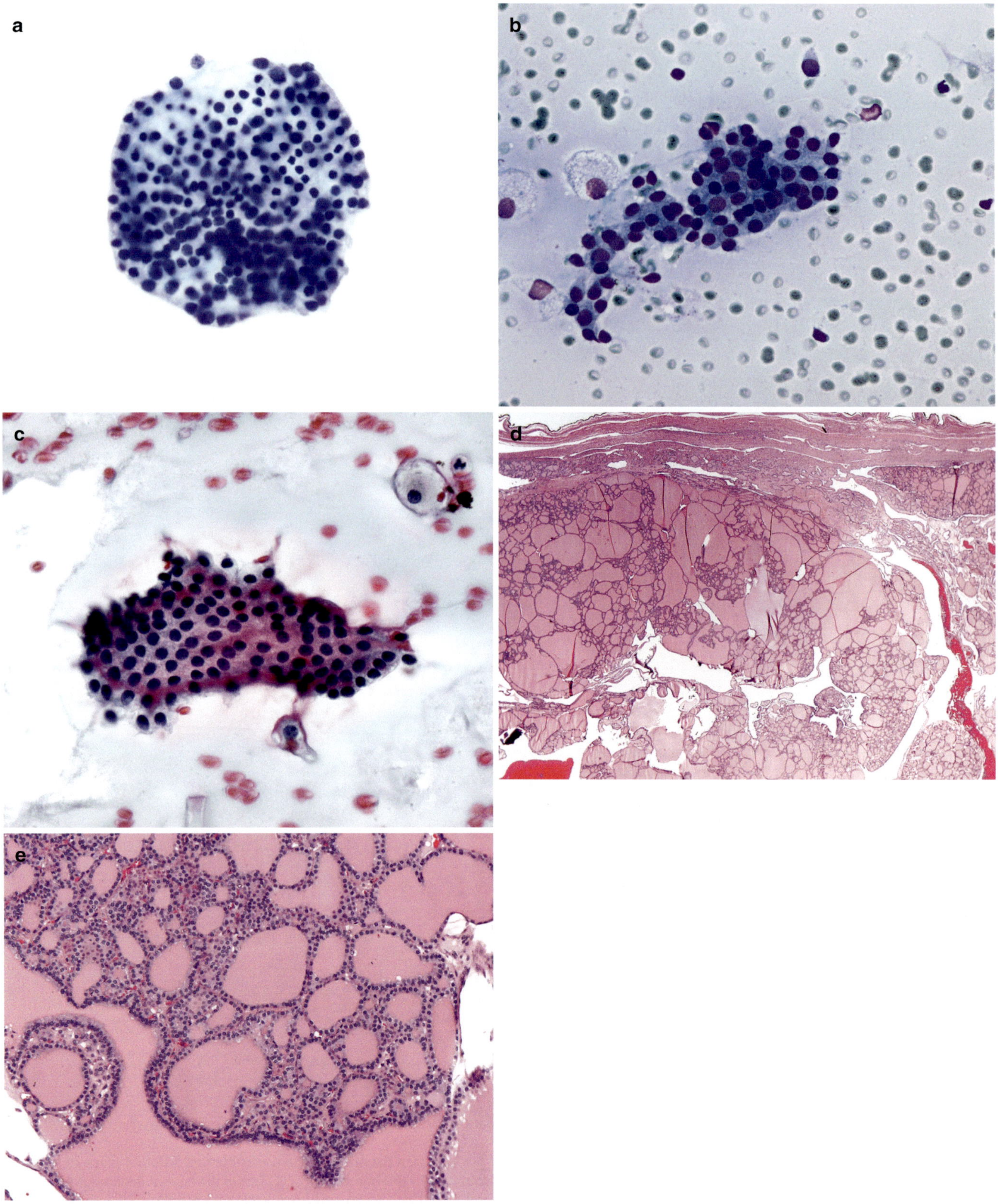

Fig. 6.4 Macrofollicular morphology in nodular hyperplasia. (**a**) Macrofollicle in TP showing a monolayered and orderly arrangement of round nuclei with granular chromatin and abundant delicate cytoplasm (Pap stain). (**b**, **c**) Macrofollicle in a CS shows a similar appearance. Note the slightly stretched-out appearance in CS (**b** DQ stain; **c** Pap stain); (**d**, **e**) Whole mount histologic section of nodular hyperplasia showing marked variation in shape and size of follicles, with large follicles showing abundant colloid. A discontinuous and thin fibrous capsule can be seen compressing the surrounding thyroid follicles. Higher magnification shows macrofollicles and microfollicles with abundant colloid relative to follicular epithelium (H&E stain)

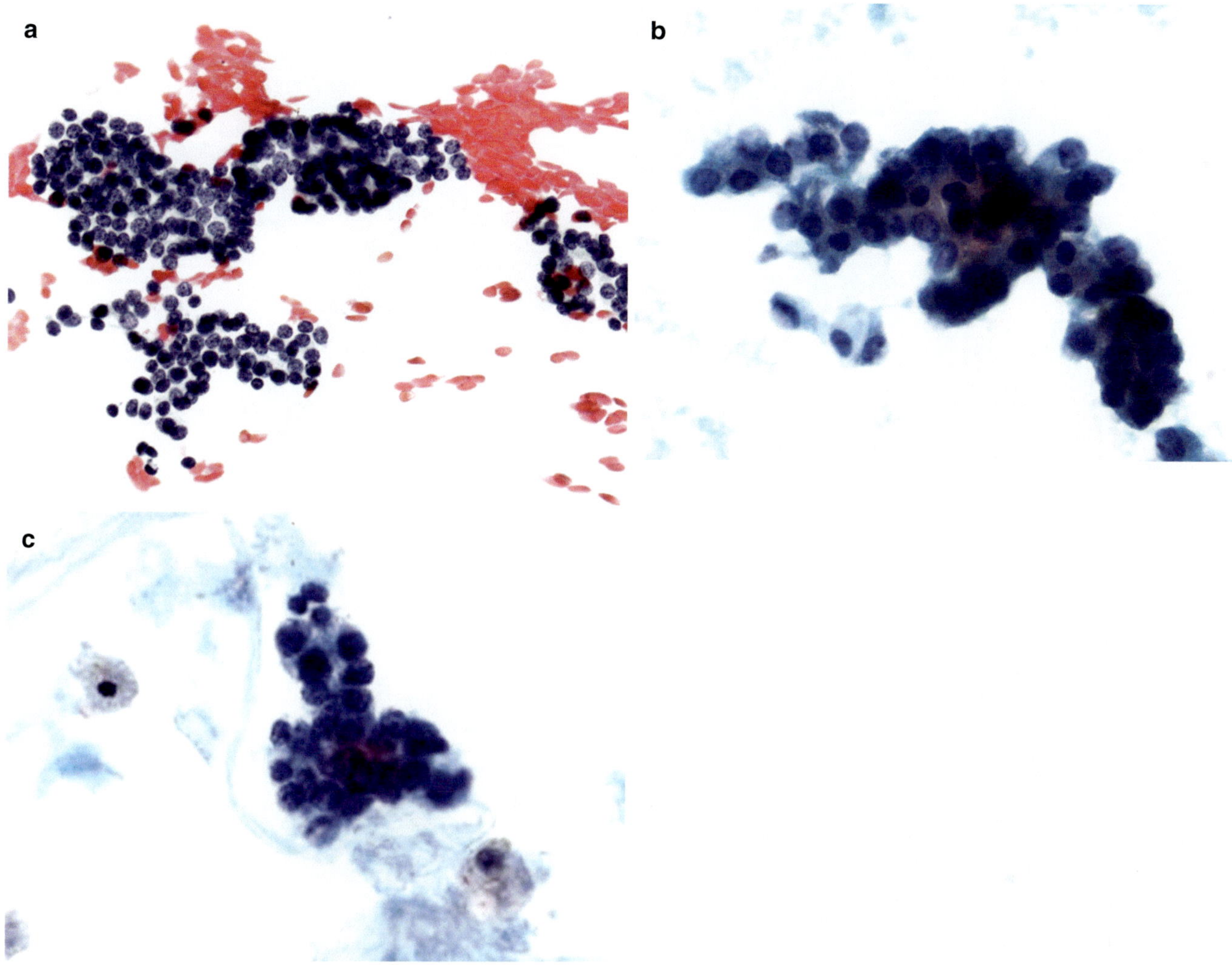

Fig. 6.5 Trabecular arrangement in FN/SFN. (**a**) In CS, trabeculae show crowding and overlapping follicular cells with a well-defined contour. (**b**) SP shows trabecular arrangement in the case of FA seen in Fig. 6.12. (**c**) TP shows trabecular arrangement in the case of NIFTP seen in Fig. 6.18. Note the crisp architectural and nuclear morphology in LBP (Pap stain)

SFN and can also be seen in FVPTC, in which they are more monolayered. In LBP, although present, there may be fewer complex branching sheets, perhaps owing to fragmentation caused by individual liquid-based processing techniques (Fig. 6.6).

- Multilayer rosettes: The well-defined lumen seen in microfollicles is not present; groups are referred to as crowded 3-D groups or microacinar arrangement or multilayered cellular ball clusters. In CS, follicular cells form variably sized groups with irregular shapes and loss of honeycomb arrangement. Unlike microfollicles, colloid is usually not associated with this pattern, so they are described as a "rosette" and are also seen in HN/adenomatoid nodules and FVPTC. In LBP, these structures appear tighter and smaller, with more crowding/overlapping of follicular cells. In TP, the rosettes appear flattened, yet all layers of cells can be appreciated. In SP, rosettes appear 3-D, and constant focusing at high magnification is required to appreciate all cells (Fig. 6.7).
- Dispersed isolated cells: CS show loosely cohesive clusters and singly dispersed follicular cells, morphologically similar to cells in groups or microfollicles. These are also more common in FN/SFN. LBP may show more dispersed single cells not only in FN/SFN but also in non-neoplastic and other neoplastic conditions (Fig. 6.8).

• *Nuclear and cytoplasmic features:* On CS, nuclei are round to ovoid with slight hyperchromasia, finely granular chromatin, overlapping, and grooves. Cytoplasm is scant. In LBP, similar nuclear features are seen. Follicular cells and nuclei appear smaller and cytoplasm is usually visible, even if scant. Note the nuclear and cytoplasmic features in the above images.

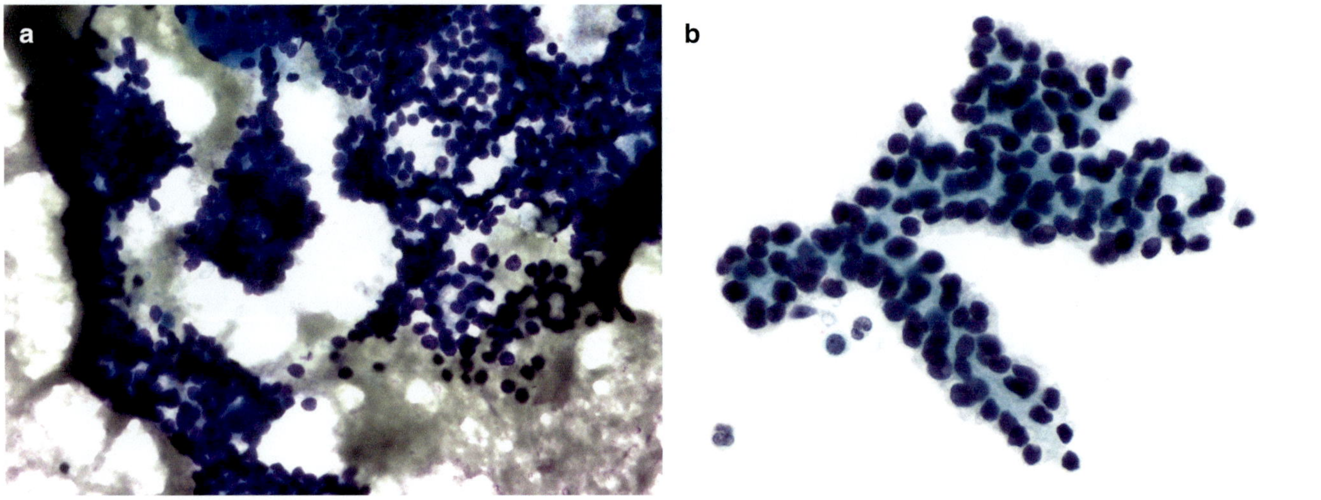

Fig. 6.6 Branching 3-D ribbon-forming cell sheets in FN/SFN. (**a**) DQ-stained CS shows monolayered crowding and overlapping complex branching sheets from the case of FVPTC shown in Fig. 6.17. (**b**) The TP from another case of FVPTC shows a well-preserved and monolayered branching ribbon-forming cell arrangement (Pap stain). This architectural feature appears monolayered in FVPTC and more 3-D in FN

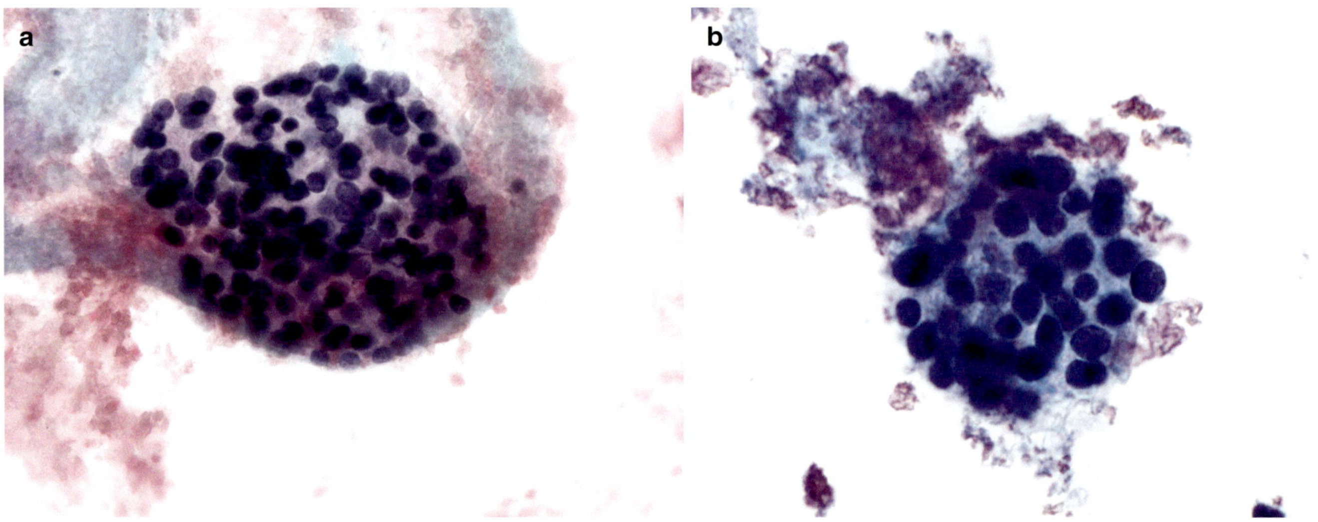

Fig. 6.7 Multilayer rosettes in FN/SFN. (**a**) CS from another case of FVPTC shows a crowded 3-D or overlapping cell group or multilayered cellular ball cluster loss of honeycomb arrangement. Compare with the benign macrofollicle in Fig. 6.4b, c. Unlike microfollicles, colloid is usually not associated with this pattern, so they are described as a "rosette." (**b**) TP from the case of follicular carcinoma (FC) in Fig. 6.15 shows a multilayered cellular ball. Note similar appearance to the CS, except that the blood clings to the tumor cells without obscuring them, instead of being diffuse as in the CS. (**a**, **b** Pap stain)

  - Nucleoli may be present. In LBP, nucleoli may be prominent even in benign lesions because of the immediate liquid fixation of the collected sample.
  - Nuclei are more uniform in FA and HN/adenomatoid nodules and show anisonucleosis in FC and FVPTC (see Figs. 6.15, 6.16, and 6.17).
  - Nuclei of HN/adenomatoid nodules are similar to those of FN/SFN except that they are evenly spaced in monolayer honeycomb sheets with no overlap.
  - Nuclei of FVPTC are slightly elongated with ground-glass or vesicular chromatin, INPI, and grooves. In LBP, nuclear changes of FVPTC may be more subtle than classic PTC, especially in NIFTP, in which the nuclei may appear smaller, with rare grooves and rare INPI.
  - Cytological atypia is not a prominent feature of follicular-patterned lesions, except for atypia of FC, when suggestive of PTC or insular carcinoma.
- In summary, the most specific criteria for FN/SFN in CS and LBP are the architectural criteria (trabecular pattern, overlapping of the branching sheets, and more isolated cells) and the nuclear criteria (round nuclei with a granular chromatin pattern).

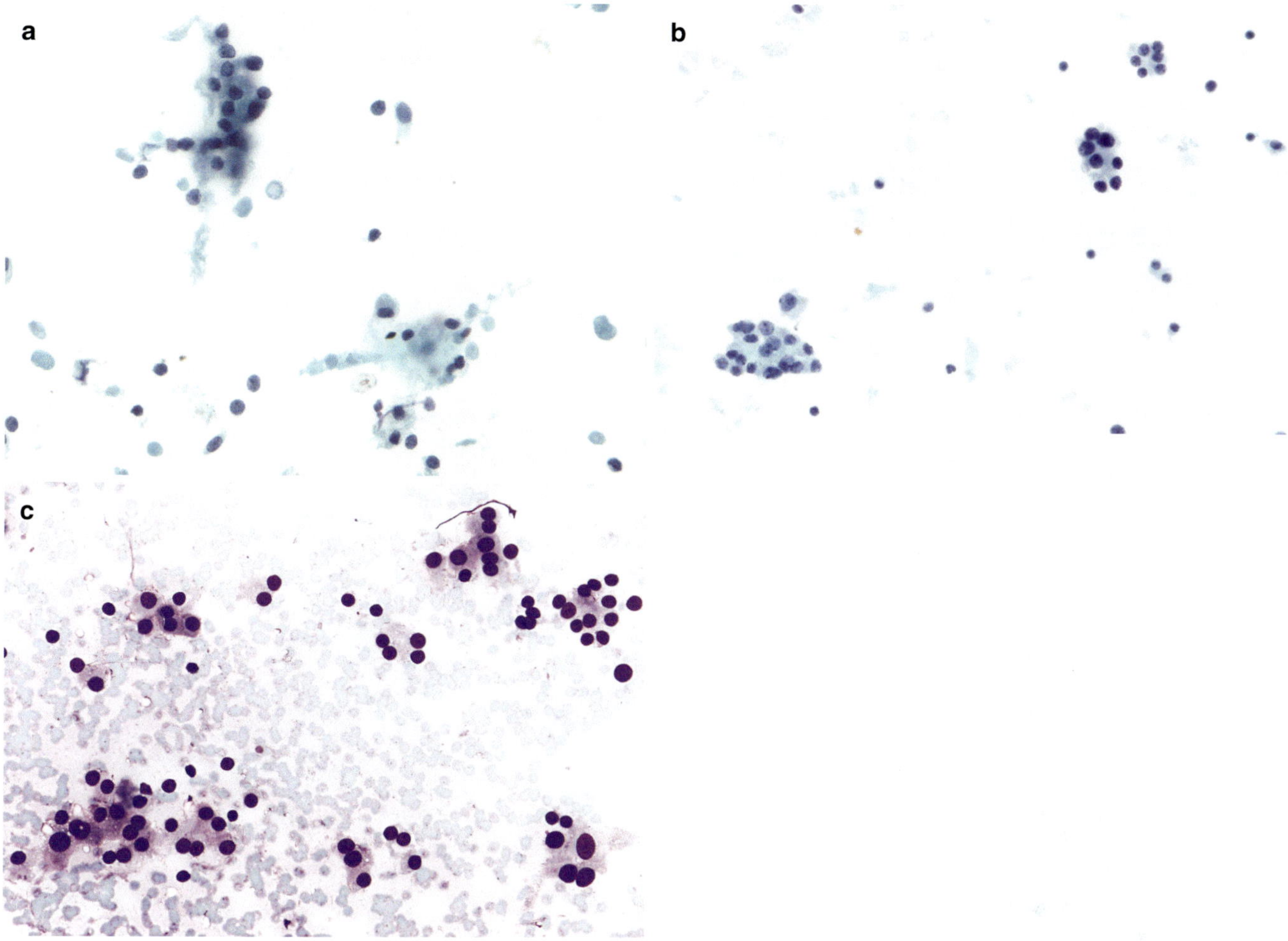

Fig. 6.8 Dispersed isolated cells in FN/SFN. (**a**, **b**) SP and TP from two different cases of FA, the latter from the case shown in Fig. 6.10. Both show loosely cohesive clusters, microfollicles, and singly dispersed follicular cells, morphologically similar to cells seen in the groups and microfollicles (Pap stain). (**c**) CS shows microfollicles and singly dispersed follicular cells from another case of FN/SFN (DQ stain). Thin colloid in DQ stain is diffuse and stains violet

Cytologic Differential Diagnosis of FN/SFN

- As shown on Table 6.1, the cytologic differential diagnosis of FN/SFN Includes hyperplastic/adenomatoid nodule, FA, FC, FVPTC, and NIFTP.

Adenomatoid Nodule

- Adenomatoid nodule is a dominant nodule in multinodular goiter.
- Histologically, adenomatoid nodule shows poor encapsulation, with a variable mixture of macrofollicles and microfollicles. Architecture and cells within the nodule are similar to surrounding thyroid parenchyma.
- Cytologically, it shows high cellularity, with uniform follicular cells in macrofollicles and microfollicles, and flat, monolayer honeycomb sheets that fold over on themselves. The nuclei are evenly spaced, round, and slightly hyperchromatic with inconspicuous nucleoli, regular nuclear contour, and coarsely-granular chromatin. Occasional larger nuclei can be seen. Colloid may be abundant, and degenerative changes of hemorrhage, fibrosis, and cyst formation and Hürthle cell metaplasia are usually present. LBP show all the above features with better-preserved cell morphology (Fig. 6.9; *see also* Figs. 4.1 and 6.4).

Follicular Adenoma

- Most patients with FA or FC present with a solid thyroid nodule while asymptomatic. Patients may also have other benign thyroid diseases.
- FA is a benign encapsulated neoplastic follicular cell proliferation.
- It is usually solitary, but rarely is multiple and solid. On imaging, the nodule is most often "cold."

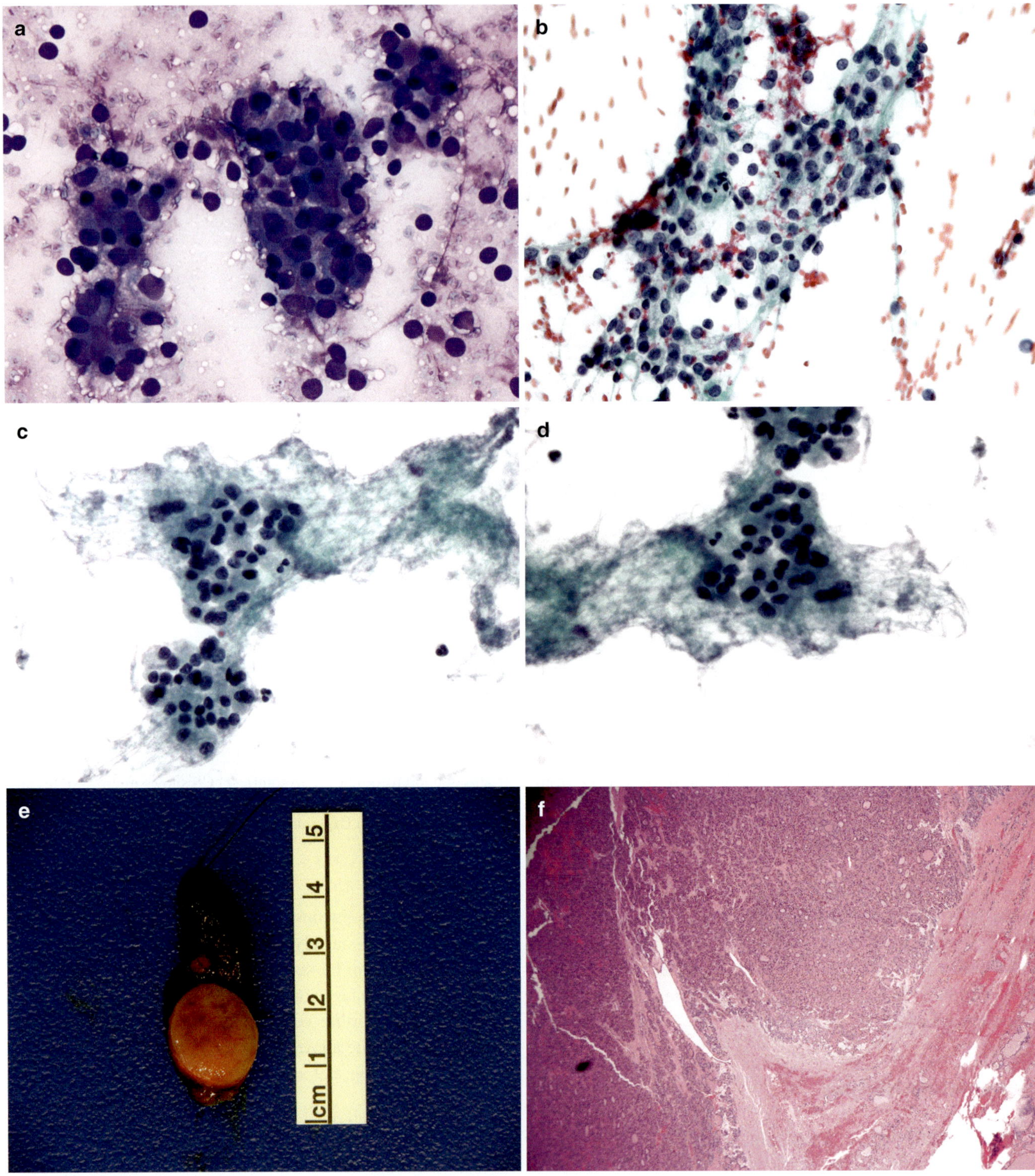

Fig. 6.9 Adenomatoid nodule. Aspirate from an adenomatoid nodule shows slightly irregularly shaped macrofollicles, few microfollicles, and few flat sheets in a background of scant, thin colloid. (**a**) Thin colloid in DQ stain (CS) is diffuse and stains violet. (**b**) In the Pap stain (CS) it appears granular and stringy. Nuclei show variable degrees of atypia with enlargement, slight overlap, hyperchromasia, small nucleoli, and occasional grooves. (**c**, **d**) The TP also shows slightly irregular macrofollicles. On higher magnification, they may appear as a conglomerate of microfollicles, but they differ from true microfollicles by the lack of overcrowding and overlapping. Nuclear features are similar to the Pap-stained CS. Note the abundant thin, tissue paper–like wrinkled, watery colloid closely associated with follicular cells (Pap stain). (**e**) Gross image of the well-defined, dominant adenomatoid nodule, which appears to be encapsulated and has a yellow-tan, shiny and bulging cut surface. (**f–h**) The nodule was partially encapsulated. Histologic section at low magnification shows surrounding fibrous tissue of varying thickness. Histologic sections of higher magnification show a microfollicular and solid growth pattern. Such cases can be misinterpreted as FA, but molecular tests would not show any abnormalities (H&E stain)

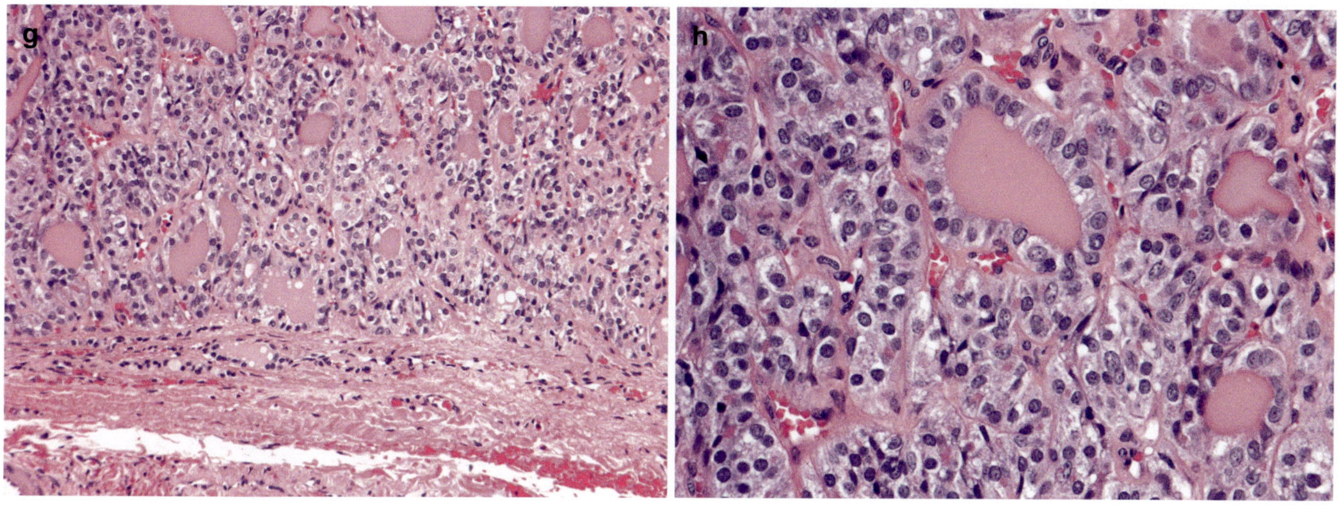

Fig. 6.9 (continued)

- Histologically, the tumor shows a predominantly microfollicular growth pattern with interspersed macrofollicles, surrounded by a fibrous capsule that compresses the surrounding thyroid parenchyma. Architecture and cells within the nodule differ from the surrounding thyroid parenchyma. Nuclear features of PTC and degenerative changes of hemorrhage, fibrosis, and cyst formation are lacking.
- Histologic subtypes include oncocytic Hürthle cell, signet-ring cell, clear cell, lipomatous, hyalinizing trabecular adenoma, and atypical FA.
- Tumor does not recur or metastasize.
- FA is treated by lobectomy.
- Cytologically, all architectural and cellular features described above are seen in LBP. Although cytology cannot distinguish FA from FC, the FA shows little or no nuclear atypia (Figs. 6.10, 6.11, and 6.12).
- Molecular alterations: Most common are *RAS* mutations; a few patients show *PAX8/PPARγ* translocations.

Adenolipoma (Lipoadenoma)

- Adenolipoma or lipoadenoma is a histologic subtype of FA.
- It is a rare benign neoplasm, encapsulated and composed of various proportions of mature adipose tissue and thyroid follicles.
- Cytologically benign follicular cells are seen with fat (Fig. 6.13).

Hyalinizing Trabecular Adenoma (HTA)

- This rare neoplasm is regarded as a histologic subtype of FA.
- Grossly, HTA is usually a single, solid, well-circumscribed or encapsulated lesion (measuring 2.5 cm or less) that presents a homogeneous and delicately lobulated yellow-tan cut surface.
- Histologically, HTA is characterized by circumscription, no invasion, a trabecular growth pattern, intratrabecular and intertrabecular hyalinization, and nuclear features of PTC, including grooves and numerous INPI.
- HTA may be difficult to distinguish from PTC in FNA cytology. Almost 60% are either diagnosed as suspicious or positive for PTC. HTA may also mimic medullary thyroid carcinoma (MTC), but immunostaining for calcitonin and chromogranin are positive in MTC.
- Cytologically, tumor cells are cohesive and radially arranged around acellular, hyaline-like stromal material. Papillary and sheet-like fragments are absent. Cells are round or fusiform (spindled) with numerous INPI and grooves. Psammoma bodies may occasionally be present (Fig. 6.14).
- The MIB-1 clone of Ki-67 immunostain shows cytoplasmic positivity, unlike the nuclear staining seen in other tumors, where it is performed to determine the proliferation index. Special requirements must be observed when using MIB-1.

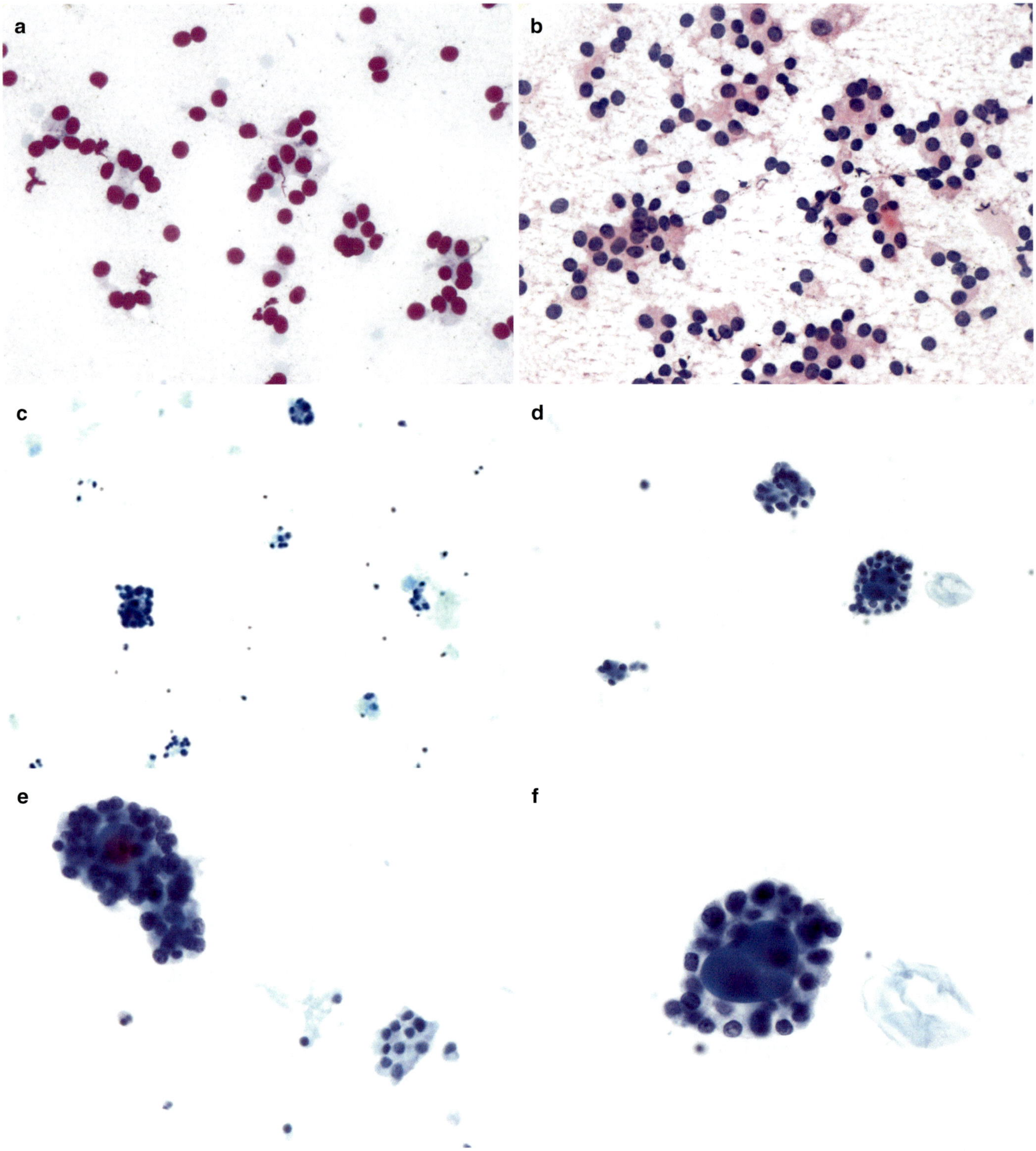

Fig. 6.10 Follicular adenoma (FA). (**a**) DQ-stained CS from fine needle aspiration (FNA) shows a cellular aspirate with follicular cells as dispersed microfollicles, and single cells that are devoid of cytoplasm or appear as naked or "bare" nuclei. Nuclei are small, round, and monomorphous with minimal or no cytological atypia. Cytoplasm is soft and ill-defined. (**b**) This is touch-imprint H&E-stained CS, which explains the high cellularity. Architectural features are similar to the DQ-stained CS. Cytologically, the nuclei show more detail, with fine chromatin with/without small nucleoli. Some microfollicles show dense eosinophilic colloid in the lumen. (**c–g**) FNA of the same case in TP (Pap stain) shows a microfollicular pattern and few single cells. Nuclear features, although better preserved, are similar to those in the H&E-stained CS. Compared with CS, the differences with TP are lower cellularity, better cellular and nuclear morphology, single cells retaining cytoplasm, well-defined cell borders, and a microfollicle lumen containing dense, inspissated colloid

g

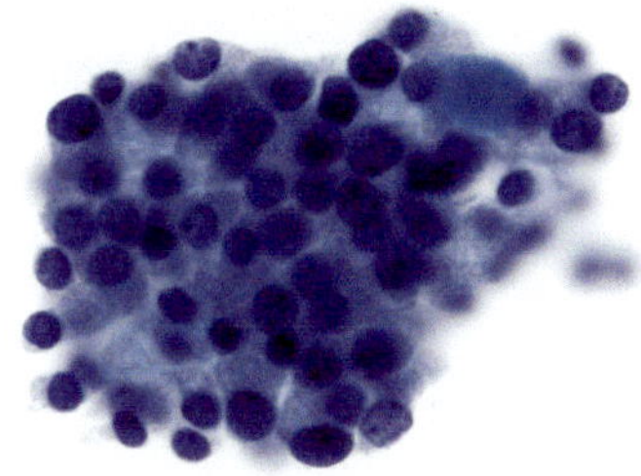

Fig. 6.10 (continued)

Follicular Carcinoma

- FC is a follicular epithelial thyroid neoplasm with capsular or vascular invasion and/or metastatic potential. It is classified as minimally invasive and widely invasive.
- It comprises 10–20% of all thyroid malignancies.
- It commonly occurs in women in the fifth or sixth decade of life, as a painless mass.
- FC differs markedly from PTC in epidemiology, ultrasound features, pathological and molecular features, and clinical behavior.
- It is usually solitary and "cold" or hypofunctioning on imaging. Most tumors are sporadic or linked to irradiation.
- Histologically, capsular and vascular invasion, invasion to thyroid parenchyma, or extrathyroidal extension (ETE) is identified. Thus, FA and FC cannot be distinguished on cytology, and the capsule must be histologically assessed. Specialized thyroid pathology textbooks list the criteria for definition and assessment of invasion.
- Cytology shows nuclear atypia (anisonucleosis), nuclear overlap, and a more 3-D appearance (Figs. 6.15 and 6.16). FA and FC cannot be distinguished on FNA cytology.
- Molecular alterations: Most common are *RAS* mutations and *PAX8/PPARγ* translocations.

Follicular Variant of PTC (FVPTC)

- This variant is the second-most-common type, after the classic variety of PTC.
- It has cytological features of classic PTC and architectural features of FC.

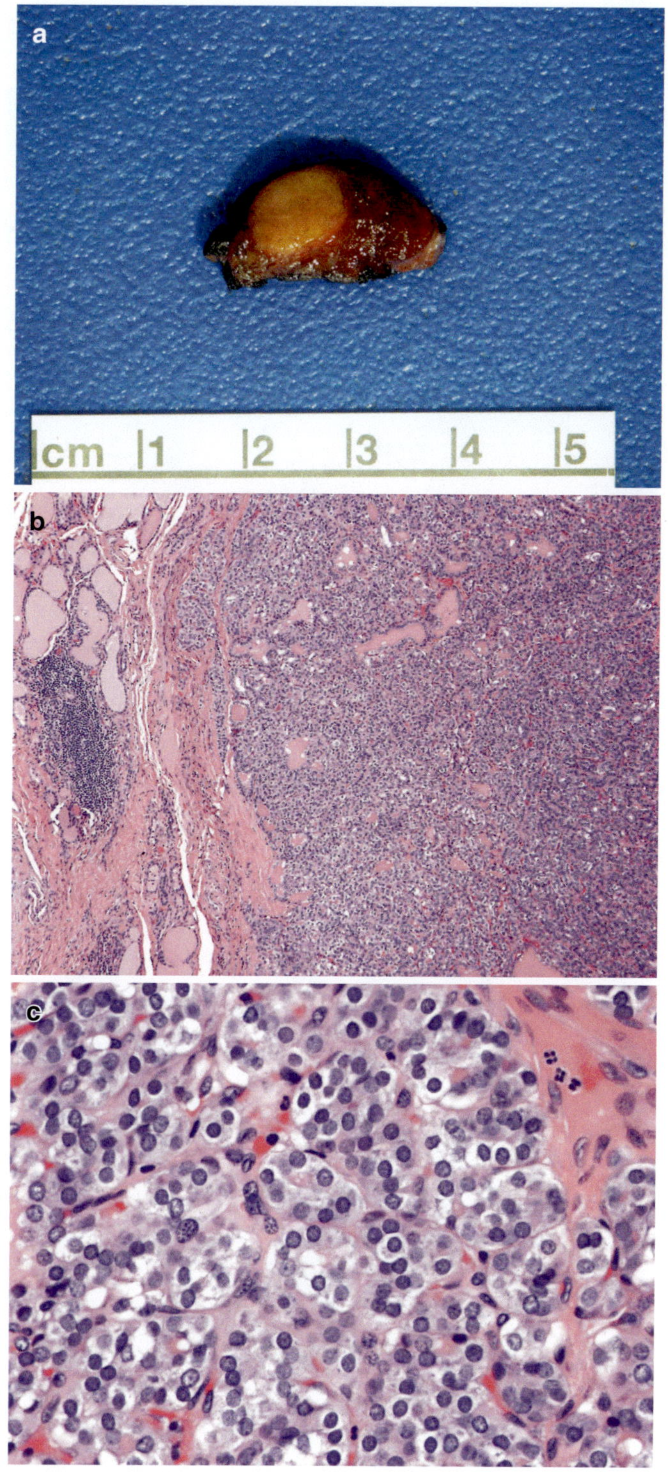

Fig. 6.11 Follicular adenoma (FA) (same case as in Fig. 6.10). (**a**) Follicular adenoma showing capsule and light tan cut surface. (**b**, **c**) This is an encapsulated tumor that is architecturally and cytologically different from the surrounding thyroid tissue. The tumor growth pattern is microfollicular; it is lined by cuboidal cells with round, uniform nuclei, few with nucleoli, and a moderate amount of amphophilic, well-defined cytoplasm (H&E stain)

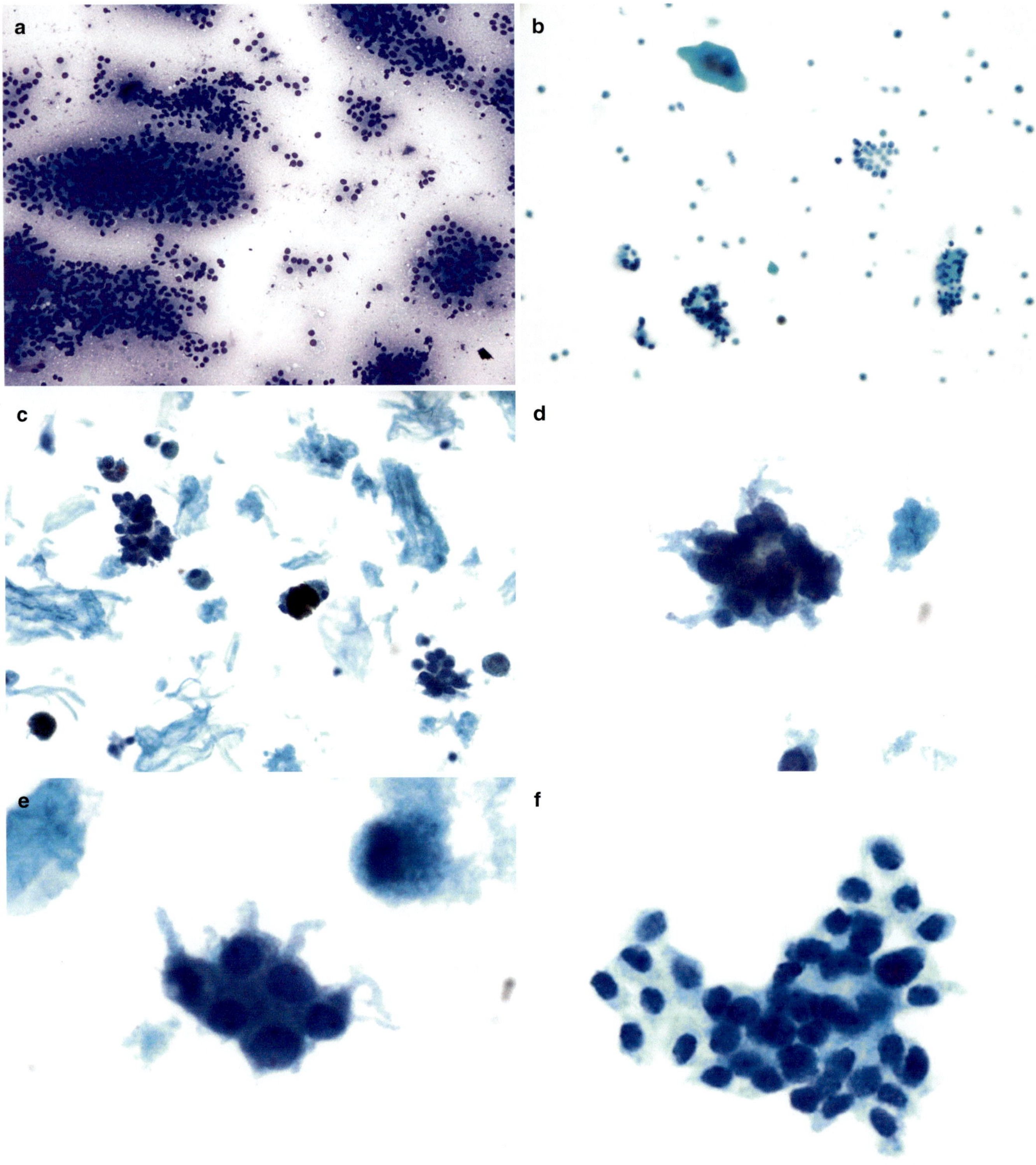

Fig. 6.12 Follicular adenoma (FA). (**a**) DQ-stained CS shows all architectural patterns seen in FA. (**b**–**f**) SP slides show moderately high cellularity (**b**), small sheets (**c**), distinct microfollicles (**d**, **e**), trabeculae (**f**), and isolated cells (**b**). Nuclei are enlarged and slightly irregular, with small nucleoli. Cytoplasm is delicate and ill-defined to well-defined. Luminal colloid is not evident, but dense clumps and bands of thick colloid can be seen (Pap stain). All features of FA in SP slides are similar to features seen on TP slides (*see* Fig. 6.10), except that the cells appear more 3-D, with a greater depth of focus and cells in different planes of focus in SP. Note out-of-focus single cells. (**g**) Gross of FA showing a solitary tumor of about 1.5 cm, with a moderately thick capsule and light brown, shiny cut surface. Minute cystic foci are noted. (**h**, **i**) Histology shows an intact fibrous capsule containing blood vessels. No invasion was identified. The tumor growth pattern is almost normofollicular, with some features of a hyperfunctioning (toxic) FA, such as the scalloping of the colloid and slight columnar morphology of cells at the bottom of the image. Some extracapsular normal thyroid is noted (H&E stain)

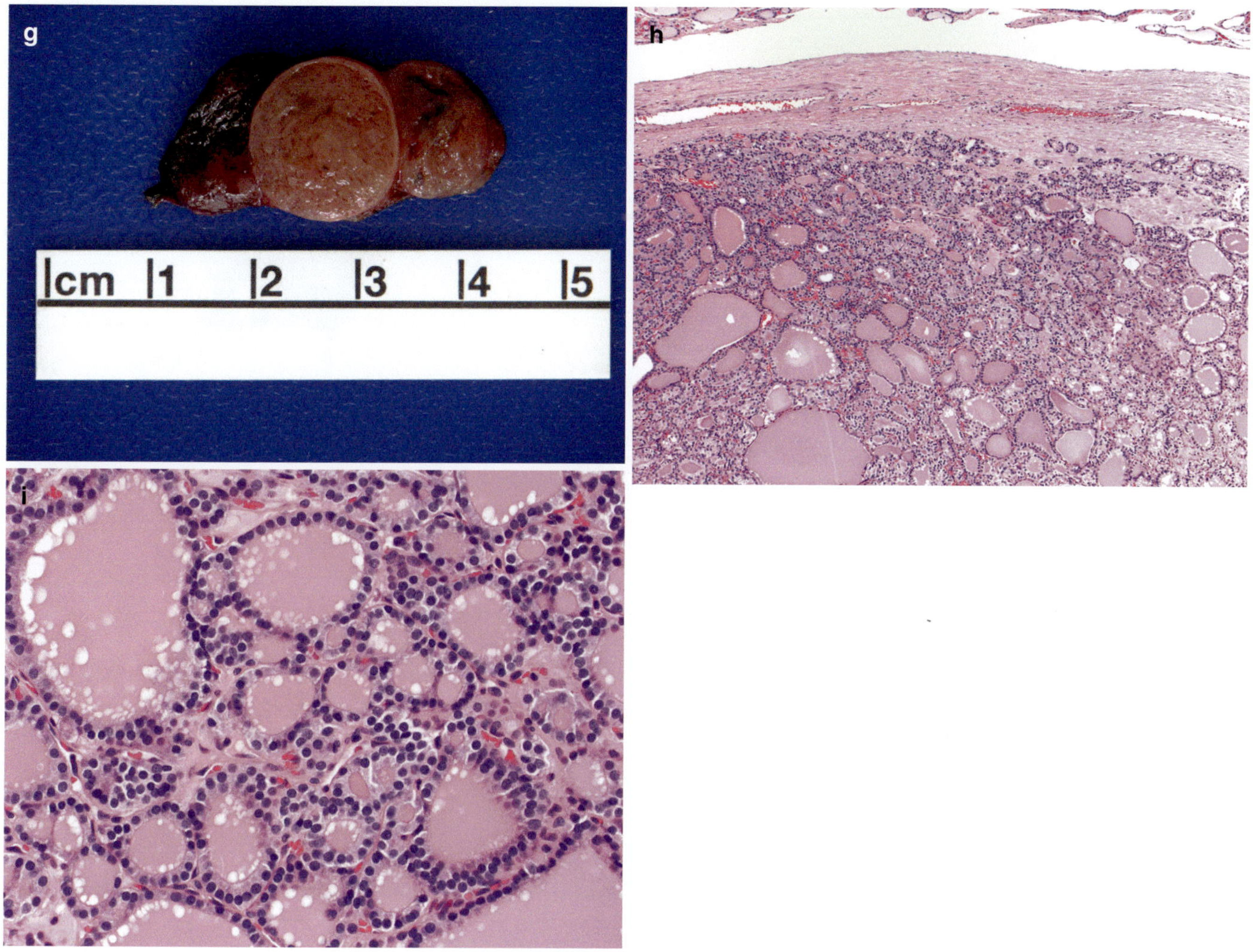

Fig. 6.12 (continued)

- For the nuclei, histologic and cytologic criteria are similar; they include nuclear enlargement, overlapping, irregularity of contour, chromatin clearing, intranuclear grooves and INPI (Fig. 6.17).
- Histologically, it is divided into two subtypes, encapsulated (eFVPTC) and infiltrative non-encapsulated (neFVPTC). The encapsulated type is split into two categories: a borderline, very low-risk tumor (NIFTP, discussed below); and a typically invasive encapsulated FVPTC. (*See* Chap. 9.)

Noninvasive Follicular Neoplasm with Papillary-like Nuclear Features (NIFTP)

- NIFTP shows nuclear atypia (anisonucleosis), nuclear overlap, and a more 3-D appearance, with a different chromatin pattern than FC (Fig. 6.18).

Parathyroid Adenoma

- There are no ultrasound features that distinguish parathyroid from thyroid.
- Parathyroid comprises three different types of cells: chief, oxyphil, and water clear cells.
- Chief cells are morphologically similar to thyroid follicular cells, and oxyphil cells are similar to Hürthle cells.
- Pathological distinction between parathyroid and thyroid can be challenging.
- Cytologically, the parathyroid samples are hypercellular, with cells arranged as disorganized two-dimensional and three-dimensional fragments. Nuclei are round, uniform, and overlapping, with stippled neuroendocrine-type chromatin, inconspicuous nucleoli, and a high nuclear-cytoplasmic (N:C) ratio. Vascular proliferation is prominent. The background shows many naked "bare" nuclei and no colloid (Fig. 6.19).

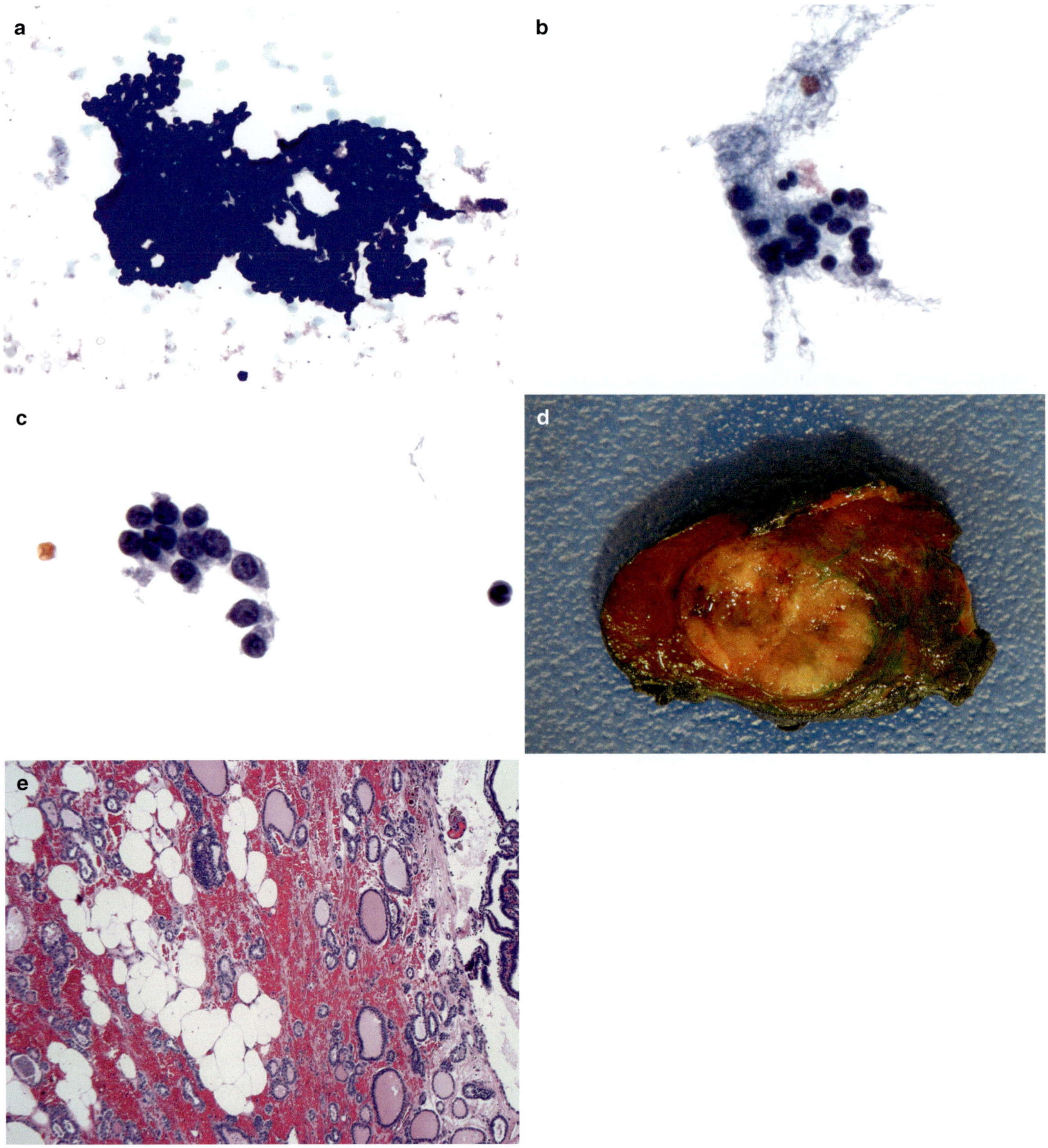

Fig. 6.13 Lipoadenoma or adenolipoma. These are rare variants of FA composed of mature adipose tissue (fat) and thyroid follicles. Fat may represent metaplastic changes. (**a**) The DQ-stained CS is overstained and shows an irregular sheet of follicular cells. No fat cells were present. (**b**, **c**) TP shows microfollicles with enlarged, slightly irregular nuclei with nucleoli. No fat cells were present (Pap stain). (**d**) Gross of adenolipoma showing a solitary nodule with a yellow and greasy cut surface and a focus of cystic change. (**e**) Histologic section shows a variable proportion of mature fat and microfollicular epithelium (H&E stain)

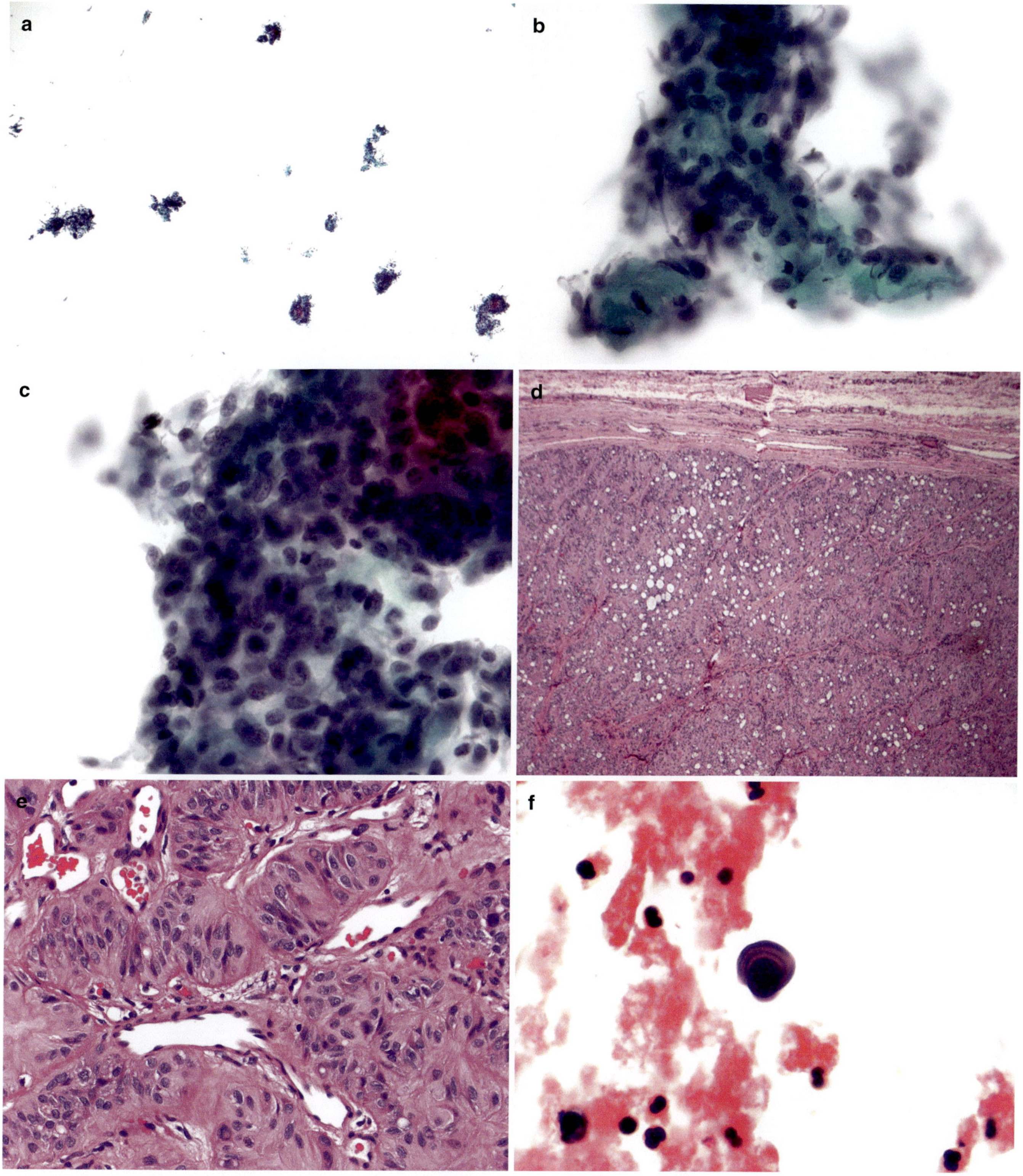

Fig. 6.14 Hyalinizing trabecular adenoma (HTA). (**a**) Low magnification shows cells organized in trabecular clusters and microfollicular structures. Hyaline material stains green-blue and is also visible. (**b**, **c**) Tumor epithelial cells are elongated and fusiform, with small nucleoli and finely granular cytoplasm associated with acellular hyaline stroma. Rare vague INPI and grooves are present, but not as frequent as they usually are in HTA (**a**–**c** Pap stain, TP); (**d**, **e**) Low magnification of the histologic section shows an encapsulated tumor with a thin capsule and trabecular architecture. High magnification shows polygonal and fusiform tumor cells arranged in trabeculae and supported by a delicate fibrovascular stroma. Nuclei are elongated, spindled, and fusiform, with scattered grooves; cytoplasm is abundant. One "yellow body" staining pink can be seen in the top of the image (H&E stain). (**f**) Cell block from another case of HTA showed one psammoma body and prompted a closer inspection of the TP slide. (**g**) The TP slide had only a few groups of cells. High magnification shows a group of elongated and fusiform cells. Intranuclear grooves and vague pseudoinclusions are seen in cells in the lower part of the image (TP, Pap stain)

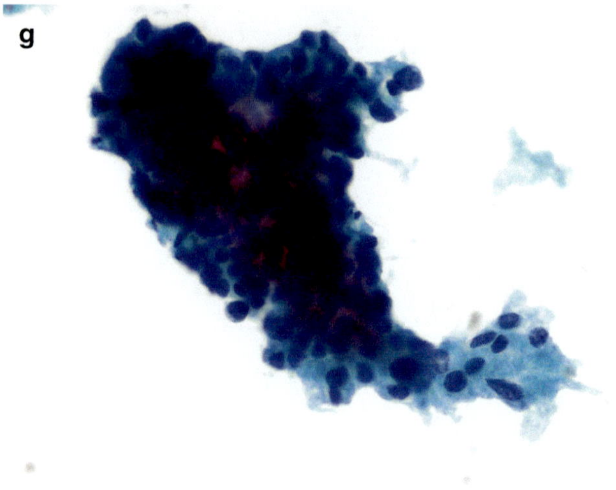

Fig. 6.14 (continued)

- Cytological features seen in follicular neoplasms, especially FC, include nuclear atypia, nucleoli, and a lower N:C ratio. Follicular cells also show cytoplasmic lipofuscin granules (*see* Fig. 6.19d).
- PTH assay or immunostaining for PTH and thyroglobulin can be of diagnostic value.
- Parathyroid lesions are usually interpreted as a follicular lesion of undetermined significance (FLUS) or FN/SFN. Subsequent molecular testing can detect the parathyroid gene and sometimes, chromogranin gene.

Cell Block Preparations from LBP Sample

- Unlike CS, a residual LBP sample can be used to process a cell block. A dedicated FNA pass is not required.

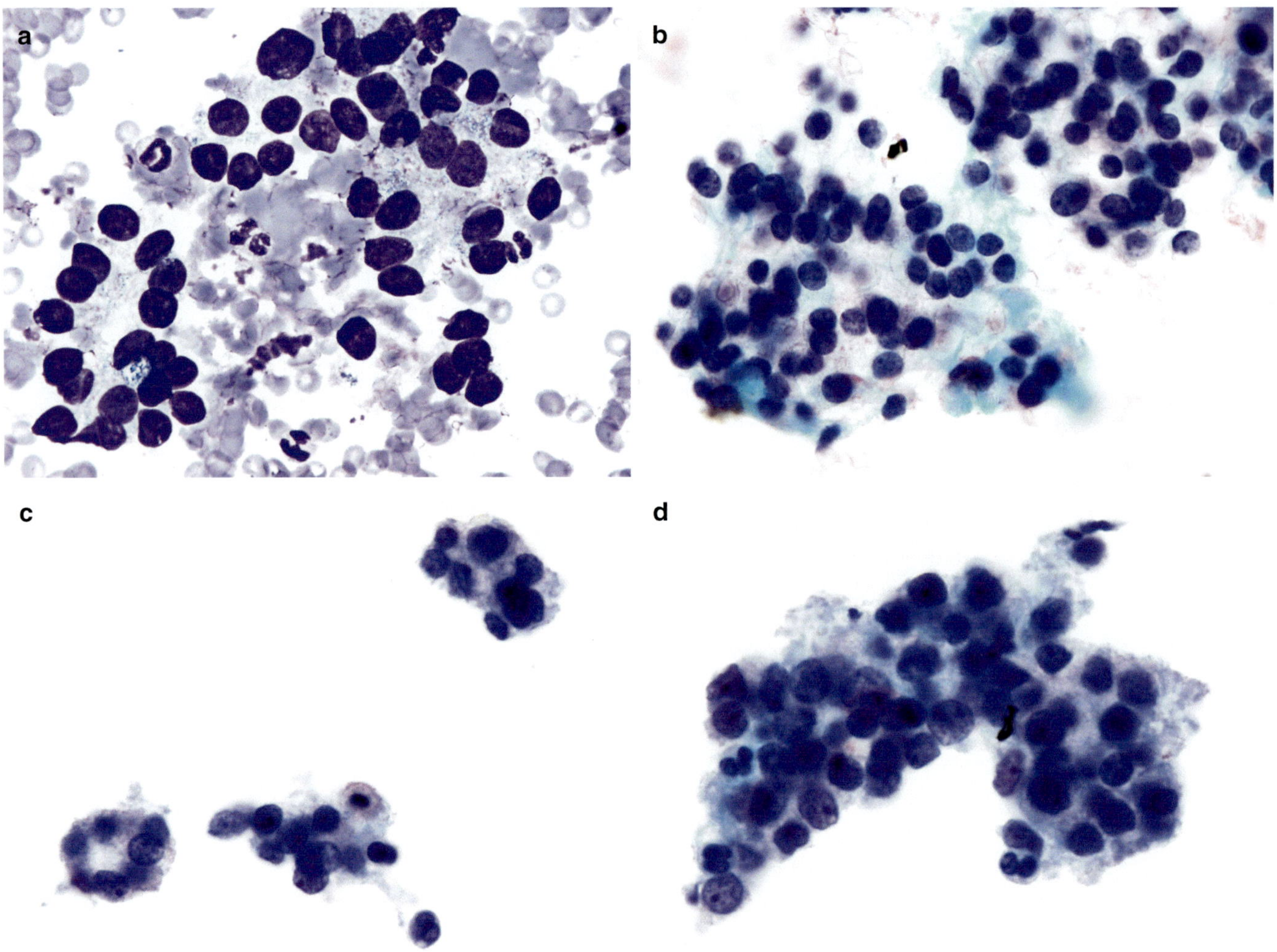

Fig. 6.15 Follicular carcinoma (FC). (**a**, **b**) Cytology of CS shows FC as microfollicles and overlapping groups of cells. Nuclei show atypia and are enlarged (compare with red blood cells), irregular, and hyperchromatic, with nucleoli (**a** DQ stain; **b** Pap stain). Scant, dense colloid is seen in the Pap-stained CS. (**c–e**) Cytological features of FC in TP. Note microfollicles and trabecular arrangement. Nuclear features are similar to those in CS, but more well-preserved. Dense colloid clings to tumor cells (Pap stain). (**f**) Cut surface of FC shows a solitary, solid tumor of about 2.5 cm, with a tan-brown surface and thick, irregular capsule. (**g**, **h**) Histology of the FC shows capsular and vascular invasion, which is a diagnostic finding. (**i**) High magnification shows a microfollicular architecture with enlarged, atypical nuclei and nucleoli (**g–i** H&E stain)

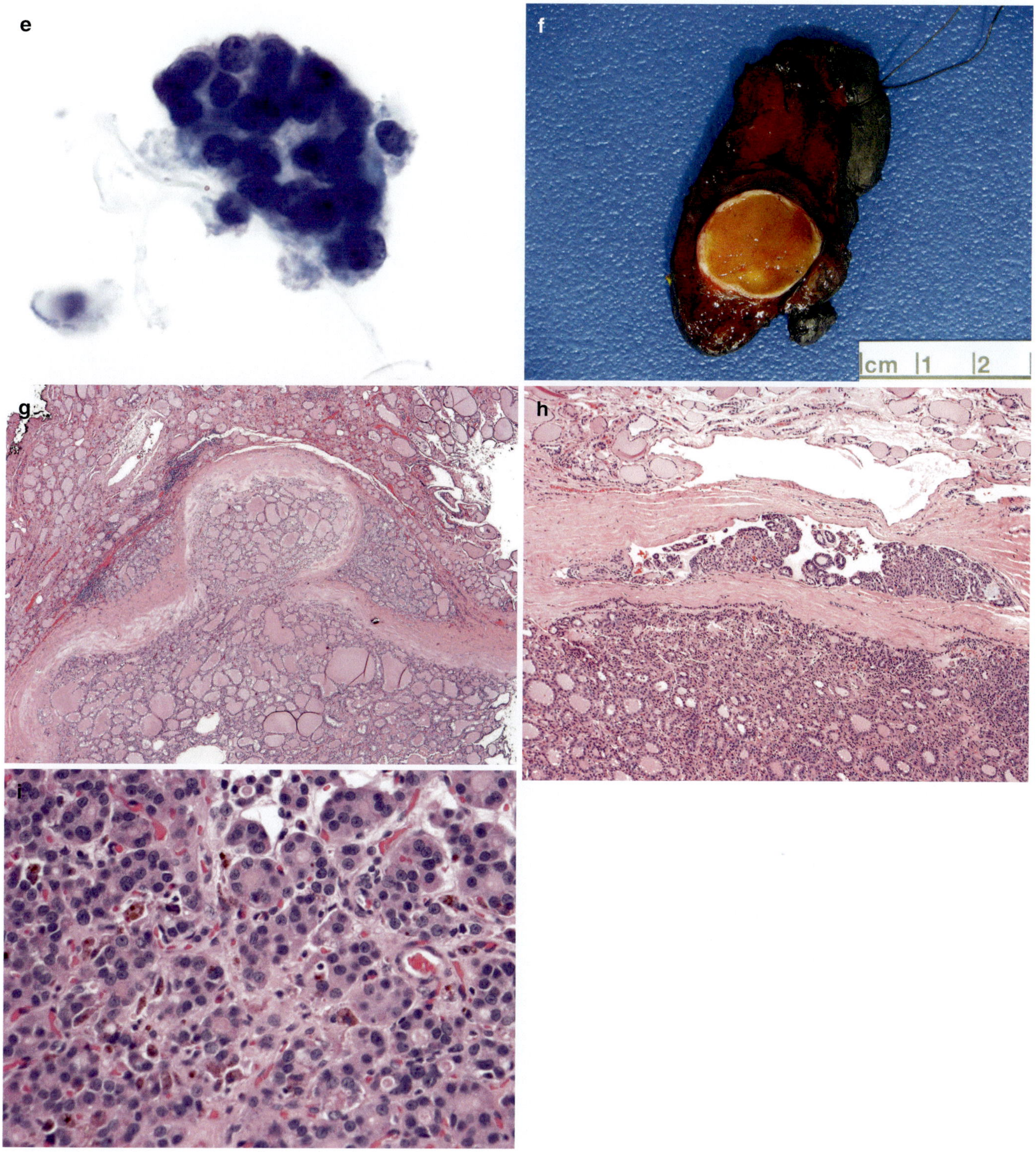

Fig. 6.15 (continued)

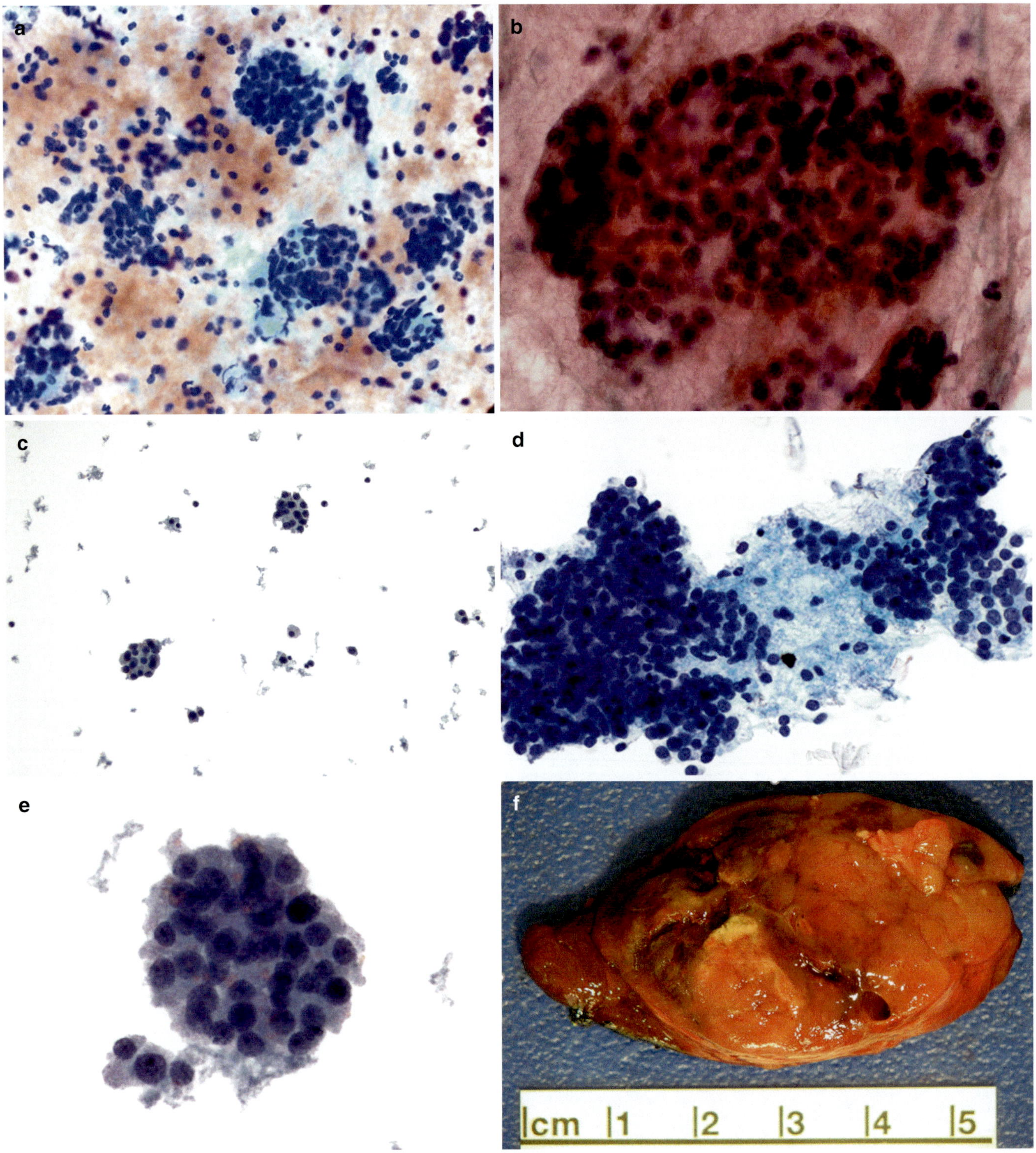

Fig. 6.16 Follicular carcinoma (FC). In another case of FC, note the similarity between CS (**a**, **b**) and TP (**c**–**e**) in architectural patterns, including microfollicles, cell balls, "rosettes," single cells, and nuclear features. The main difference is that partially obscuring blood compromises cell detail in CS. The TP shows well-preserved cells with nuclear atypia comprising enlarged, round to irregular, and hyperchromatic nuclei with nucleoli (**a** DQ stain, CS; **b** Pap stain, CS; **c**–**e** Pap stain TP). (**f**) Cut surface of the encapsulated tumor (about 4 cm); (**g**) Histologic image shows capsular invasion (H&E stain)

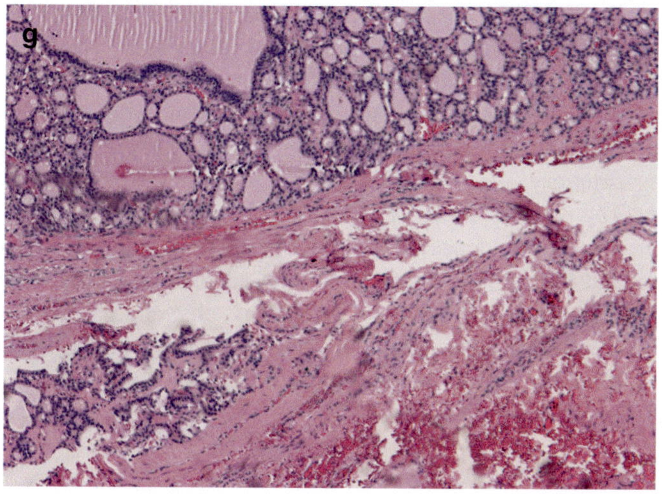

Fig. 6.16 (continued)

- Rekhtman et al. [39] described a simple and readily adoptable modification of the HistoGel method, which results in the greatest capture of cells. Using their technique, FNA collected in CytoLyt provided a significant increase in sufficiency for potential molecular and other ancillary studies.
- All cell blocks at our laboratory are being processed using this protocol, with excellent results (Fig. 6.20).

Educational Points for FN/SFN

- Histopathologic follow-up of the FN/SFN category includes benign hyperplastic/adenomatous nodule, FA, FC, FVPTC, and NIFTP.
- TBSRTC estimates the overall ROM in this category to be 25–40%. If NIFTP is not considered as carcinoma, the ROM changes to 10–40%.
- The 2015 ATA guidelines recommend molecular tests and surgical removal of the thyroid nodule because of the associated ROM.
- Subclassification based on the presence of architectural versus nuclear atypia shows significantly higher malignancy rates in FN/SFN nodules with nuclear atypia [29].
- A recent multivariate model based on several clinical, ultrasonographic, and cytological parameters concluded that calcification, nodule size, nuclear atypia, and tobacco use may predict the risk of thyroid cancer in patients with thyroid nodules diagnosed as FN/SFN on FNA [31]. In this study, 33.8% of patients had thyroid carcinoma. PTC was the most common type, seen in 66.7% of cases.
- Microfollicular patterns with nuclear atypia are associated with an ROM of 7% [25].

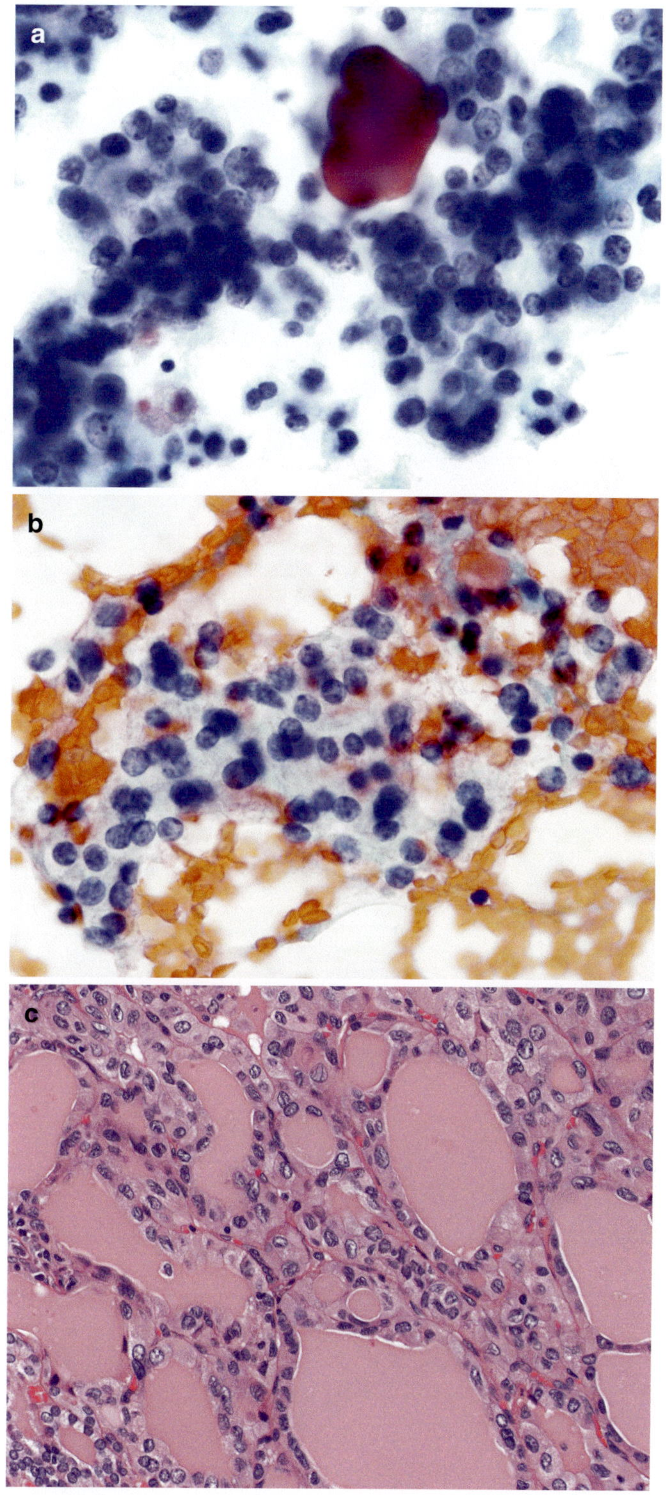

Fig. 6.17 Follicular variant of papillary thyroid carcinoma (FVPTC). (**a**) Nuclear features concerning for PTC are noted, including enlarged oval nuclei with nuclear clearing, fine (powdery) or ground-glass–appearing chromatin, and rare grooves (Pap stain, TP). (**b**) CS shows similar appearance (Pap stain). (**c**) Microscopically, the tumor shows a microfollicular architecture with clear nuclei (H&E stain)

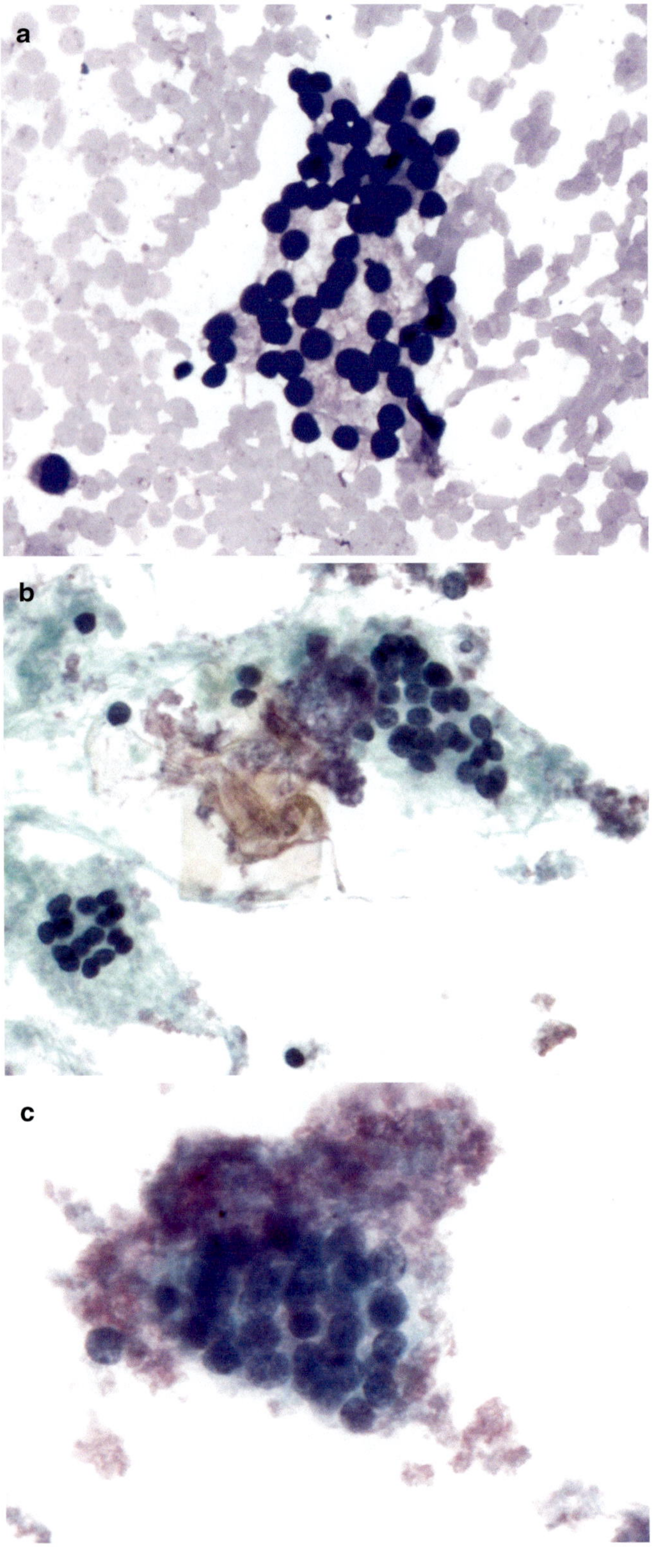

Fig. 6.18 Noninvasive follicular neoplasm with papillary-like nuclear features (NIFTP). (**a**, **b**) Note the difference of nuclear shape and chromatin between FC (Fig. 6.16) and nuclear features of NIFTP. (**c**) Tumor cells form microfollicles, which appear tighter in TP. Nuclei show mild atypia, cellular enlargement, powdery chromatin, and intranuclear grooves. The follow-up histologic examination revealed NIFTP (**a** DQ stain; **b**, **c** Pap stain, TP)

- For FN/SFN, the concordance rate between the final histological and initial cytological diagnoses on FNA ranges from 32% to 62%. Adenomatoid nodules are the main cause of poor histologic correlation with FN/SFN, the reason cytopathologists prefer "SFN" for this category.
- The diagnosis of FVPTC is most challenging because of its scant evidence of the typical nuclear features of PTC and overlapping cytological features of both benign and malignant follicular lesions. This challenge is compounded in cases with scant cellularity and subtle nuclear features of PTC within otherwise benign-appearing follicular aspirates.

Role of Molecular Tests in FN/SFN

- The treatments proposed for TBSRTC categories II, V, and VI are well established, considering their malignancy rates of 0–3%, 50–75%, and 97–99% respectively, but the best treatment options for category III (AUS/FLUS, with a 10–30% malignancy rate) and category IV (FN/SFN, 25–40%) are subject to debate about different approaches. Management of actual patients also may depend on factors in addition to the FNA diagnosis, such as clinical and ultrasonographic findings.
- The 2015 ATA guidelines recommend molecular testing in conjunction with cytopathology interpretation.
- Commercially-available molecular tests include the Afirma® Genomic Sequencing Classifier (GSC) (Veracyte, South San Francisco, CA); ThyroSeq® v3 genomic classifier (GC) (UPMC, Pittsburgh, PA); and ThyGeNEXT®/ThyraMIR® (Interpace Diagnostics, Parsippany, NJ). These are useful for the 15–30% of indeterminate thyroid FNAs and may be useful for NIFTP. (*See* Chap. 14.)
- FC and FA primarily show *RAS* point mutations (*NRAS*, *HRAS*, and less frequently *KRAS*) and *PAX8/PPARγ* rearrangements. *RAS* mutations are found in up to 40–50% of FC and 20–40% of FA; *PAX8/PPARγ* fusions are found in 30–40% of FC and 2–13% of FA [12].

Management of FN/SFN

- As per the 2015 ATA guidelines, diagnostic surgical excision (lobectomy) should be performed. Molecular testing can be performed for malignancy risk assessment in conjunction with clinical and ultrasonographic features.

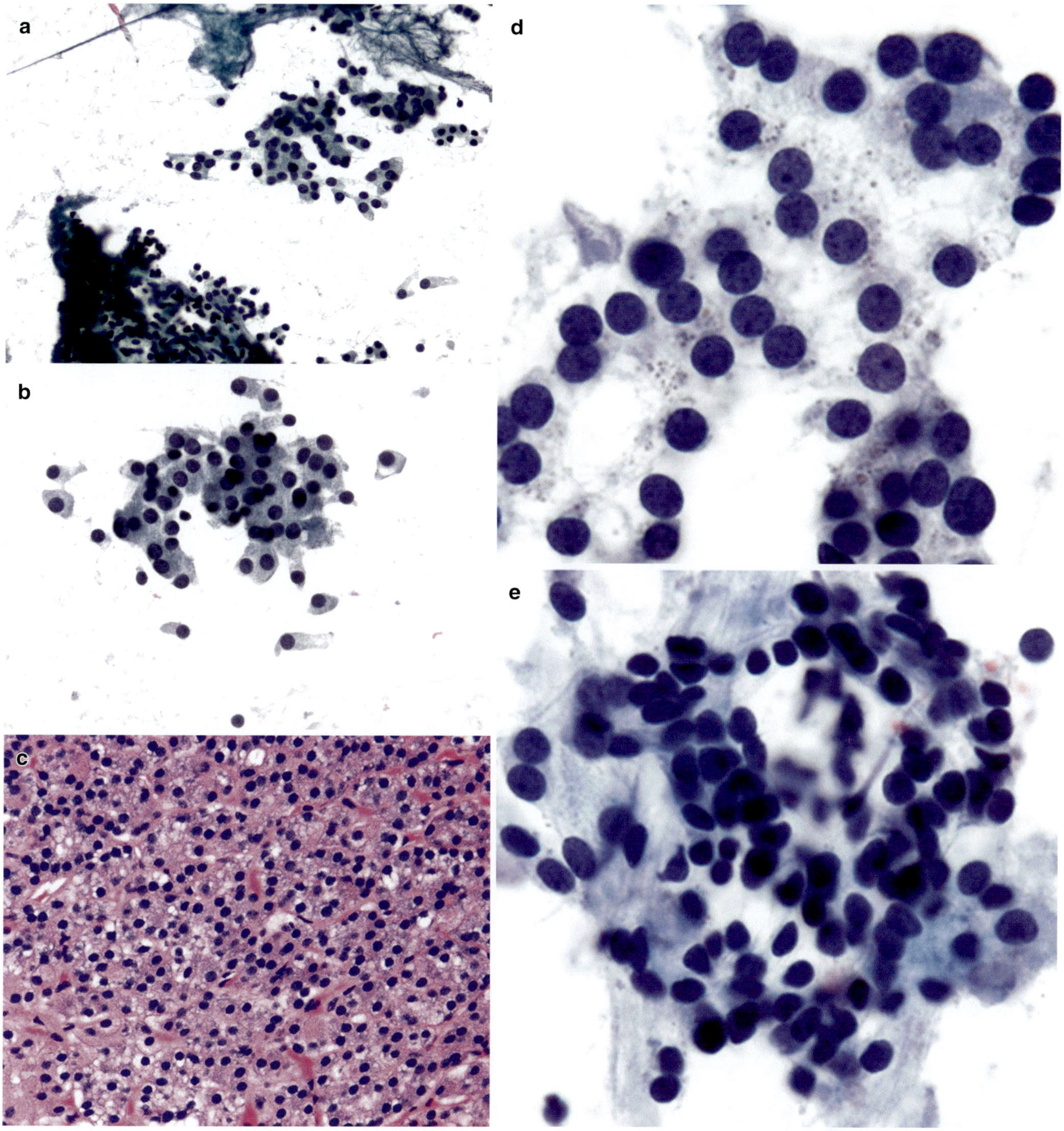

Fig. 6.19 Parathyroid adenoma. (**a**, **b**) Cellular parathyroid sample cells arranged as disorganized 2-D and 3-D fragments. Nuclei are round, monotonous, and uniform, with stippled, neuroendocrine-type chromatin, inconspicuous nucleoli, and a high nuclear-cytoplasmic (N:C) ratio. Low magnifications show vascular proliferation. The background shows single cells, some of which are "bare" nuclei, devoid of cytoplasm. Colloid is absent (Pap stain, TP). (**c**) Histology of the chief cell type of parathyroid adenoma (H&E stain). (**d**, **e**) Cytologically, parathyroid cells are difficult (if not impossible) to distinguish from thyroid follicular cells without PTH assay or immunostaining for PTH and thyroglobulin. Follicular cells show cytoplasmic lipofuscin granules, as seen on image **d** (Pap stain, TP)

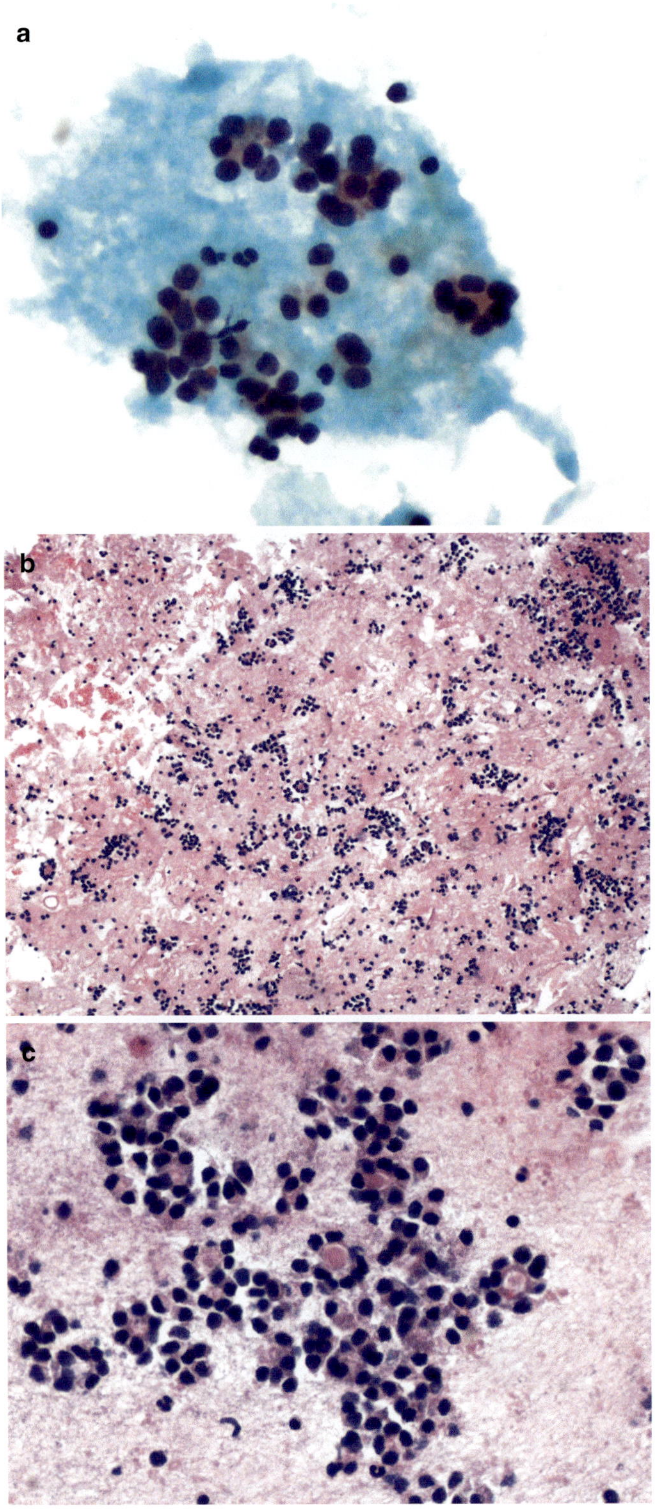

Fig. 6.20 Cell block preparation in FA. (**a**) TP from a case of FA shows microfollicles with luminal inspissated colloid (Pap stain). (**b**, **c**) Cell block section from the same case was cellular, with well-retained architecture and morphology. A cellular cell block allows for immunostaining and also can be used for molecular testing, if the specimen in the molecular vial is inadequate

Suggested Reading

1. Absher KJ, Truong LD, Khurana KK, Ramzy I. Parathyroid cytology: avoiding diagnostic pitfalls. Head Neck. 2002;24:157–64.
2. Ali SZ, Cibas ES. The Bethesda System for reporting thyroid cytopathology; definitions, criteria, and explanatory notes. 2nd ed. Cham: Springer International Publishing AG; 2018.
3. Ali SZ, Nayar R, Krane JF, Westra WH. Atlas of thyroid cytopathology with histopathologic correlations. New York: Demos Medical Publishing; 2014.
4. Bommanahalli BP, Bhat RV, Rupanarayan R. A cell pattern approach to interpretation of fine needle aspiration cytology of thyroid lesions: a cyto-histomorphological study. J Cytol. 2010;27:127–32. https://doi.org/10.4103/0970-9371.73295.
5. Brandler TC, Cho M, Wei XJ, Simms A, Levine P, Hernandez O, et al. Noninvasive follicular thyroid neoplasm with papillary-like nuclear features: an interobserver study of key cytomorphological features from a large academic medical centre. Cytopathology. 2019;30:39–45. https://doi.org/10.1111/cyt.12632.
6. Brandler TC, Liu CZ, Cho M, Zhou F, Cangiarella J, Yee-Chang M, et al. Does noninvasive follicular thyroid neoplasm with papillary-like nuclear features (NIFTP) have a unique molecular profile? Am J Clin Pathol. 2018;150:451–60. https://doi.org/10.1093/ajcp/aqy075.
7. Cibas ES, Ali SZ. The 2017 Bethesda System for reporting thyroid cytopathology. Thyroid. 2017;27:1341–6. https://doi.org/10.1089/thy.2017.0500.
8. Cibas ES, Baloch ZW, Fellegara G, LiVolsi VA, Raab SS, Rosai J, et al. A prospective assessment defining the limitations of thyroid nodule pathologic evaluation. Ann Intern Med. 2013;159:325–32. https://doi.org/10.7326/0003-4819-159-5-201309030-00006.
9. Choong KC, Khiyami A, Tamarkin SW, McHenry CR. Fine-needle aspiration biopsy of thyroid nodules: is routine ultrasound-guidance necessary? Surgery. 2018;164:789–94. https://doi.org/10.1016/j.surg.2018.04.047.
10. Clark DP, Faquin WC. Thyroid cytopathology. 2nd ed. New York: Springer; 2010.
11. Damiani D, Suciu V, Vielh P. Cytopathology of follicular cell nodules. Endocr Pathol. 2015;26:286–90. https://doi.org/10.1007/s12022-015-9386-3.
12. Daniels GH. Follicular thyroid carcinoma: a perspective. Thyroid. 2018;28:1229–42. https://doi.org/10.1089/thy.2018.0306.
13. Duncan LD, Forrest L, Law WM Jr, Hubbard E, Stewart LE. Evaluation of thyroid fine-needle aspirations: can ThinPrep be used exclusively to appropriately triage patients having a thyroid nodule? Diagn Cytopathol. 2011;39:341–8. https://doi.org/10.1002/dc.21392.
14. Faquin WC, Wong LQ, Afrogheh AH, Ali SZ, Bishop JA, Bongiovanni M, et al. Impact of reclassifying noninvasive follicular variant of papillary thyroid carcinoma on the risk of malignancy in The Bethesda System for Reporting Thyroid Cytopathology. Cancer Cytopathol. 2016;124:181–7. https://doi.org/10.1002/cncy.21631.
15. Faquin WC, Baloch ZW. Fine-needle aspiration of follicular patterned lesions of the thyroid: diagnosis, management, and follow-up according to National Cancer Institute (NCI) recommendations. Diagn Cytopathol. 2010;38:731–9. https://doi.org/10.1002/dc.21292.
16. Fischer AH, Clayton AC, Bentz JS, Wasserman PG, Henry MR, Souers RJ, et al. Performance differences between conventional smears and liquid-based preparations of thyroid fine-needle aspiration samples: analysis of 47,076 responses in the College of American Pathologists Interlaboratory Comparison Program in

non-gynecologic cytology. Arch Pathol Lab Med. 2013;137:26–31. https://doi.org/10.5858/arpa.2012-0009-CP.
17. Godoi Cavalheiro B, Kober Nogueira Leite A, Luongo de Matos L, Palermo Miazaki A, Ientile JM, Kulcsar MA, et al. Malignancy rates in thyroid nodules classified as Bethesda Categories III and IV: retrospective data from a tertiary center. Int J Endocrinol Metab. 2018;16:e12871. https://doi.org/10.5812/ijem.12871.
18. Han K, Ha HJ, Kong JS, Kim JS, Myung JK, Koh JS, et al. Cytological features that differentiate follicular neoplasm from mimicking lesions. J Pathol Transl Med. 2018;52:110–20. https://doi.org/10.4132/jptm.2018.01.17.
19. Haugen BR, Alexander EK, Bible KC, Doherty GM, Mandel SJ, Nikiforov YE, et al. 2015 American Thyroid Association Management Guidelines for adult patients with thyroid nodules and differentiated thyroid cancer: the American Thyroid Association Guidelines Task Force on thyroid nodules and differentiated thyroid cancer. Thyroid. 2016;26:1–133. https://doi.org/10.1089/thy.2015.0020.
20. Hoda RS. Non-gynecologic cytology on liquid-based preparations: a morphologic review of facts and artifacts. Diagn Cytopathol. 2007;35:621–34.
21. Hoda RS, VandenBussche C, Hoda SA. Diagnostic liquid-based cytology. New York: Springer; 2017.
22. Hang JF, Westra WH, Zhou AG, Cooper DS, Ali SZ. The impact of noninvasive follicular thyroid neoplasm with papillary-like nuclear features on the rate of malignancy for atypia of undetermined significance subcategories. Cancer Cytopathol. 2018;126:309–16. https://doi.org/10.1002/cncy.21981.
23. Jug RC, Datto MB, Jiang XS. Molecular testing for indeterminate thyroid nodules: performance of the Afirma gene expression classifier and ThyroSeq panel. Cancer Cytopathol. 2018;126:471–80. https://doi.org/10.1002/cncy.21993.
24. Kapur U, Wojcik EM. Follicular neoplasm of the thyroid: vanishing cytologic diagnosis? Diagn Cytopathol. 2007;35:525–8.
25. Kelman AS, Rathan A, Leibowitz J, Burstein DE, Haber RS. Thyroid cytology and the risk of malignancy in thyroid nodules: importance of nuclear atypia in indeterminate specimens. Thyroid. 2001;11:271–7.
26. Krauss EA, Mahon M, Fede JM, Zhang L. Application of the Bethesda Classification for thyroid fine-needle aspiration: institutional experience and meta-analysis. Arch Pathol Lab Med. 2016;140:1121–31. https://doi.org/10.5858/arpa.2015-0154-SA.
27. Kiernan CM, Solórzano CC. Bethesda category III, IV, and V thyroid nodules: can nodule size help predict malignancy? J Am Coll Surg. 2017;225:77–82. https://doi.org/10.1016/j.jamcollsurg.2017.02.002.
28. Kim HS, Yun KJ. Adenolipoma of the thyroid gland: report of a case with diagnosis by fine-needle aspiration cytology. Diagn Cytopathol. 2008;36:253–6. https://doi.org/10.1002/dc.20666.
29. Lim JXY, Nga ME, Chan DKH, Tan WB, Parameswaran R, Ngiam KY. Subclassification of Bethesda atypical and follicular neoplasm categories according to nuclear and architectural atypia improves discrimination of thyroid malignancy risk. Thyroid. 2018;28:511–21. https://doi.org/10.1089/thy.2017.0274.
30. Luu MH, Fischer AH, Stockl TJ, Pisharodi L, Owens CL. Atypical follicular cells with equivocal features of papillary thyroid carcinoma is not a low-risk cytologic diagnosis. Acta Cytol. 2011;55:526–30. https://doi.org/10.1159/000333227.
31. Macias CA, Arumugam D, Arlow RL, Eng OS, Lu SE, Javidian P, et al. A risk model to determine surgical treatment in patients with thyroid nodules with indeterminate cytology. Ann Surg Oncol. 2015;22:1527–32. https://doi.org/10.1245/s10434-014-4190-8.
32. Malheiros DC, Canberk S, Poller DN, Schmitt F. Thyroid FNAC: causes of false-positive results. Cytopathology. 2018;29:407–17. https://doi.org/10.1111/cyt.12575.
33. Manimaran D, Karthikeyan TM, Khan DM, Thulasi Raman R. Follicular variant of papillary thyroid carcinoma: cytological indicators of diagnostic value. J Clin Diagn Res. 2014;8:46–8. https://doi.org/10.7860/JCDR/2014/7477.4103.
34. Mathur A, Olson MT, Zeiger MA. Follicular lesions of the thyroid. Surg Clin North Am. 2014;94:499–513. https://doi.org/10.1016/j.suc.2014.02.005.
35. Michael CW, McConnel J, Pecott J, Afify AM, Al-Khafaji B. Comparison of ThinPrep and TriPath PREP liquid-based preparations in nongynecologic specimens: a pilot study. Diagn Cytopathol. 2001;25:177–84.
36. Nikiforov YE, Biddinger PW, Thompson LD. Diagnostic pathology and molecular genetics of the thyroid. 3rd ed. Philadelphia: Wolters Kluwer; 2020.
37. Persichetti A, Di Stasio E, Guglielmi R, Bizzarri G, Taccogna S, Misischi I, et al. Predictive value of malignancy of thyroid nodule ultrasound classification systems: a prospective study. J Clin Endocrinol Metab. 2018;103:1359–68. https://doi.org/10.1210/jc.2017-01708.
38. Pu RT, Yang J, Wasserman PG, Bhuiya T, Griffith KA, Michael CW. Does Hürthle cell lesion/neoplasm predict malignancy more than follicular lesion/neoplasm on thyroid fine-needle aspiration? Diagn Cytopathol. 2006;34:330–4.
39. Rekhtman N, Buonocore DJ, Rudomina D, Friedlander M, Dsouza C, Aggarwal G, et al. Novel modification of HistoGel-based cell block preparation method: improved sufficiency for molecular studies. Arch Pathol Lab Med. 2018;142:529–35. https://doi.org/10.5858/arpa.2017-0030-OA.
40. Schreiner AM, Yang GC. Adenomatoid nodules are the main cause for discrepant histology in 234 thyroid fine-needle aspirates reported as follicular neoplasm. Diagn Cytopathol. 2012;40:375–9. https://doi.org/10.1002/dc.21499.
41. Steward DL, Carty SE, Sippel RS, Yang SP, Sosa JA, Sipos JA, et al. Performance of a multigene genomic classifier in thyroid nodules with indeterminate cytology: prospective blinded multicenter study. JAMA Oncol. 2018. [Epub ahead of print]; https://doi.org/10.1001/jamaoncol.2018.4616.
42. Ustün H, Astarcı HM, Altunkaya C, Yılmaz S, Barın A, Ekici S, et al. Fine-needle aspiration of follicular patterned lesions of the thyroid: diagnosis, management, and follow-up according to thyroid Bethesda system. Acta Cytol. 2012;56:361–9. https://doi.org/10.1159/000338218.
43. Ustun B, Chhieng D, Van Dyke A, Carling T, Holt E, Udelsman R, Adeniran AJ. Risk stratification in follicular neoplasm: a cytological assessment using the modified Bethesda classification. Cancer Cytopathol. 2014;122:536–45. https://doi.org/10.1002/cncy.21425.

Follicular Neoplasm Hürthle Cell (Oncocytic) Type/Suspicious for Follicular Neoplasm Hürthle Cell (Oncocytic) Type

7

Rana S. Hoda, Rema Rao, and Theresa Scognamiglio

Hürthle (Oncocytic) Cells

- Hürthle cells are follicular-derived oncocytic cells originally described by Askanazy in 1898. They are also referred to as oncocytic, oxyphilic, and Askanazy cells.
- Hürthle cells are characterized as large, polygonal cells with abundant eosinophilic and granular cytoplasm, representing an abundance of mitochondria. The nuclei are enlarged and round, with a prominent nucleolus, and the cytoplasmic borders are distinct. These cells are generally larger than normal thyroid follicular cells.
- Hürthle cells can be seen in a wide range of non-neoplastic and neoplastic lesions. Thus, differentiating benign Hürthle cell (oncocytic) change from true Hürthle cell neoplasms (HCN) on fine needle aspiration (FNA) is challenging and fraught with pitfalls.
- The non-neoplastic or benign thyroid lesions that may show Hürthle cell (oncocytic) change include Hashimoto's thyroiditis (chronic lymphocytic thyroiditis [CLT]), Hürthle cell metaplasia (HCM) in multinodular goiter (MNG), and dominant adenomatous nodules.
- Neoplastic conditions of Hürthle cells include Hürthle cell adenoma (HCA), Hürthle cell carcinoma (HCC), and oncocytic variants of thyroid carcinoma such as papillary thyroid carcinoma (PTC), follicular carcinoma, and medullary thyroid carcinoma (MTC).
- WHO considers HCA and HCC as variants of follicular adenoma and follicular carcinoma. Follicular neoplasms composed predominantly of Hürthle cells (>75%) are classified as HCN.
- HCN differ from the non-Hürthle cell follicular neoplasms in cytologic appearance and have different molecular genetic profiles.

R. S. Hoda (✉)
CBLPath, Rye Brook, NY, USA
e-mail: rhoda@cblpath.com

R. Rao · T. Scognamiglio
Department of Pathology and Laboratory Medicine, New York Presbyterian Hospital, Weill Cornell Medical College, New York, NY, USA
e-mail: rer9052@med.cornell.edu; ths9004@med.cornell.edu

Clinical Significance of HCN: Impact on Risk of Malignancy

- The presence of oncocytic cells in thyroid neoplasms appears to indicate a higher risk of malignancy (ROM) and should not be overlooked on microscopic examination. However, FNA has a low sensitivity and negative predictive value (NPV) in differentiating benign from malignant HCN.
- Studies emphasize a more aggressive biological behavior and worse clinical outcome for HCC compared with non-oncocytic follicular carcinoma.
- Studies based on histological follow-up have used clinical parameters to stratify patients with an FNA diagnosis of HCN into groups with high and low risk of malignancy.
- Bronner et al. [1] found that 67–80% of Hürthle cell (oncocytic) tumors measuring at least 3.5 cm were histologically malignant.
- Giorgadze et al. [12] showed that the ROM was higher in patients at least 40 years of age and in nodules measuring at least 2 cm. Both age and size were significant. Malignant lesions were also more common in men, although the difference was not statistically significant. These authors concluded that cytological assessment combined with various clinical variables (size of the nodule, age, and sex of the patient) might be helpful in predicting malignancy.

TBSRTC Definition

- The Bethesda System for Reporting Thyroid Cytopathology (TBSRTC) defines Follicular Neoplasm Hürthle Cell (oncocytic) Type/Suspicious for Follicular

R. S. Hoda et al. (eds.), *Atlas of Thyroid Cytopathology on Liquid-Based Preparations*,
https://doi.org/10.1007/978-3-030-25066-9_7

Neoplasm Hürthle Cell (oncocytic) Type (FNHCT/SFNHCT) as a cellular aspirate that consists exclusively (or almost exclusively) of Hürthle cells.

Updates in TBSRTC for FNHCT/SFNHCT

- Both diagnostic terms, FNHCT and SFNHCT, are acceptable.
- SFNHCT is preferred over FNHCT because 16–25% of cases prove on resection to be benign Hürthle cell change rather than HCN.
- *Oncocytic* is used for Hürthle cell neoplasms.
- The implied ROM of this category is 10–40%.

Cytologic Criteria for Diagnosis of FNHCT/SFNHCT and Application in LBP

- All diagnostic criteria devised and seen in CS are evident in LBP, with subtle differences:
  - *Cellularity:* Generally high in CS. Cellularity may be less in LBP.
  - *Presentation:* Hürthle cells in CS are predominantly dispersed as isolated cells, flat sheets, loosely cohesive groups, microfollicles, papillary or syncytial tissue fragments, and crowded, irregular 3-D groups. "Bare" or naked nuclei also occur. Transgressing vessels are present. In LBP, cellular arrangements are the same, except there may be more single cells and more loosely cohesive or 3-D clusters.
  - *Hürthle cells:* Polygonal, mostly uniform or monotonous in a given tumor, but can be variable small to large cells, with well-defined cell borders. The nuclear-cytoplasmic (N:C) ratio is variable. Hürthle cells are easily recognizable in LBP, with similar features as CS.
  - *Nuclei:* Single, binucleation to multinucleation is frequent; central to eccentric location; uniform, round, smooth nuclear membrane; finely granular, evenly distributed chromatin; intranuclear grooves and pseudoinclusions (INPI) can be seen. Small and large cell dysplasias are noted. In LBP, the nucleus retains its location, shape, and nucleoli, but it may appear smaller and darker, with denser, more compact chromatin than in CS. Binucleation is present. Nuclear detail and nucleoli are more easily detected. Small and large cell dysplasia is maintained.
  - *Nucleoli:* Cherry-red macronucleoli are seen in HCN (particularly HCC). In LBP macronucleoli are retained and may appear more basophilic. LBP may also show prominent nucleoli in Hashimoto's thyroiditis. Look for lymphocytes infiltrating clusters of Hürthle cells.
  - *Cytoplasm:* Abundant, intracytoplasmic granules can be seen. The granules appear blue to gray-pink in Romanowsky-type stains and green on Papanicolaou (Pap) stain. LBP show similar features. The cytoplasm may sometimes appear frothy with microvacuoles in LBP.
  - *Background elements and colloid:* Colloid is generally scant or absent; psammoma bodies can be seen. Colloid may be apparent in LBP, though scant. Other background features are similar.
  - *Lymphoplasmacytic infiltrate and germinal center cells:* Not present. LBP shows similar feature.
  - *Histiocytes with or without hemosiderin*: Present or absent. LBP shows similar feature.
  - *Regular-type benign follicular cells:* Absent. They may be sampled from adjoining benign thyroid, particularly if FNA is performed without ultrasound guidance. LBP shows similar feature.
  - *Stroma:* Transgressing vessels, but they may not always be present. Transgressing vessels are retained and clearly evident in LBP.
- TBSRTC divides the cellular and nuclear atypia into small cell and large cell dysplasias. Both types are evident in LBP:
  - *Small cell dysplasia:* The cells have a diameter that is less than twice the nuclear diameter, often with bland cells, less abundant granular cytoplasm, and high N:C ratio.
  - *Large cell dysplasia:* The cells demonstrate at least twice the variation in the nuclear diameter, often with prominent nucleoli and irregular nuclear outlines; very large cells with abundant granular cytoplasm.
  - Some cases may show a combination of small cell and large cell dysplasia.

TBSRTC Problematic Scenarios for FNHCT/SFNHCT and Application to LBP

- All problematic scenarios outlined in the TBSRTC for CS also apply to LBP:
- *Minimum necessary criteria:* (These apply to oncocytic proliferations in patients with MNG or lymphocytic thyroiditis and distinguish FNHCT/SFNHCT from other neoplasms such as PTC, MTC, and parathyroid tumors.
  - Sparsely cellular aspirate composed entirely of Hürthle (oncocytic) cells. In LBP, cellularity may be low, as part of the specimen preparation technique. In our laboratory, such cases are interpreted as Hürthle cell nodule or AUS/FLUS with oncocytic features.

- Markedly cellular aspirate composed entirely of Hürthle (oncocytic) cells or "Hürthleoid" cells without atypia or dysplasia. This appearance of cells with non-watery colloid can be seen in LBP. Such cases in our laboratory are interpreted as Hürthle cell nodule. Subsequent molecular testing will provide helpful information for proper patient management (observation or lobectomy).
- Clearly abnormal sample with partial or minimal Hürthle (oncocytic) cell differentiation. This appearance of cells can be seen in LBP. Such cases in our laboratory are interpreted as Hürthle cell nodule or FNHCT/SFNHCT. Subsequent molecular testing will provide helpful information for proper patient management.
- Clearly abnormal sample with watery colloid. In LBP, some watery colloid is usually evident in Hürthle cell lesions.

- *Oncocytic proliferations in patients with MNG or lymphocytic thyroiditis (LT):*
  - Hürthle cell metaplasia commonly occurs in MNG. In LBP, normal follicular cells, metaplastic Hürthle cells, and colloid are seen, but metaplastic Hürthle cells predominate in some cases; in our laboratory, these are interpreted as Hürthle cell nodule. Metaplastic Hürthle cells form flat, cohesive sheets with well-defined cell borders and an organized and polarized cell arrangement with distinct cell walls. They have a low N:C and lack nuclear atypia or dysplasia. The latter feature is most important in distinguishing metaplasia from HCN.
  - In some LT cases, the lymphocytic component may be absent or less prominent. In LBP, the lymphocytic component may be reduced as part of preparation. Careful assessment of Hürthle cell morphology and finding of lymphocytes infiltrating Hürthle or follicular cell clusters and lymphohistiocytic aggregates is required to avoid pitfalls. In LT, Hürthle cells may show atypia that may mimic PTC. Correlation with serology and clinical and radiologic findings is important.
- *Distinguishing FNHCT/SFNHCT from other neoplasms:*
  - It is imperative to obtain clinical information, ultrasound findings, and results of other pertinent clinical tests.
  - Careful review of cytological features.
  - Immunohistochemistry for specific lesions, such as calcitonin or parathormone (PTH) immunostains, if MTC or parathyroid lesion are a diagnostic consideration.
  - Molecular profile will help in further characterization of the specific lesion. If MTC was a diagnostic consideration and the molecular test is positive for *RET* mutation, the patient will be treated appropriately. Similarly, *PTH* gene will be detected if the lesion is of parathyroid origin.
  - Oncocytic tumors tend to undergo ischemic necrosis, especially after FNA.

Differential Diagnosis of Hürthle Cell Lesions

- Non-neoplastic entities:
  - Hürthle cell metaplasia in MNG, adenomatoid (dominant) nodule with Hürthle cell metaplasia in MNG, and Hashimoto's thyroiditis (Table 7.1).
- Neoplastic entities:
  - HCA, HCC. It is important to note that almost all benign and malignant epithelial tumors of the thyroid and parathyroid have a Hürthle cell (oncocytic) variant, including parathyroid adenoma (PA), follicular adenoma (FA), follicular carcinoma (FC), PTC, and poorly differentiated carcinoma. Anaplastic thyroid carcinoma is an exception that does not have an oncocytic variant.

Benign Hürthle Cell Lesion Versus HCN

- Hürthle cell metaplasia in MNG (Fig. 7.1), adenomatoid (dominant) nodule in MNG with Hürthle cell metaplasia (Figs. 7.2 and 7.3) and Hashimoto's thyroiditis (Fig. 7.4) all show abundant colloid and Hürthle cells in flat 2-D sheets with honeycomb cell arrangement in CS and LBP [9].

HCN Including HCA and HCC

- HCA (Figs. 7.5 and 7.6) and HCC are relatively rare tumors of follicular cell origin.
- The true HCN category represents only 3–5% of all thyroid neoplasms, and HCC accounts for only 2–3% of all thyroid cancers.
- Similar to follicular neoplasms, invasive HCN demonstrating capsular and/or vascular invasion is defined as HCC (Figs. 7.7, 7.8, 7.9, and 7.10).
- HCC is considered as a distinct clinicopathological entity because of its genetic profile, more aggressive clinical course, and association with a higher rate of distant metastases than the other well-differentiated thyroid cancers (Fig. 7.11).
- Cytology cannot distinguish benign HCA from its malignant counterpart. HCA or HCC can only be reliably diagnosed after histological assessment of the tumor capsule and lymphovascular invasion. FNA is used as a reliable

Table 7.1 Follicular thyroid lesions, Hürthle cell (oncocytic) type: diagnosis and management

Diagnosis	Ultrasonographic findings	Cytological features on LBP	Molecular findings	Histology	Management[a]
HCM in MNG	May be solid or cystic, spongiform and isoechoic	Low to high cellularity; flat, two-dimensional sheets without nuclear atypia or dysplasia; abundant colloid	–	Unencapsulated, or insufficient encapsulation with macrofollicles and microfollicles	Observation. Resection, if symptomatic
Hashimoto thyroiditis (CLT)	Diffusely enlarged thyroid with heterogeneous echotexture	Low cellularity; >90% HC; some colloid; sheets >50%; HC with nuclear atypia of PTC; lymphocytes infiltrating follicular and Hürthle cells, plasma cells, and tingible body macrophage	–	Unencapsulated; Hürthle cells and lymphoplasmacytic infiltration; germinal center formation	Observation or conservative treatment
HCN	No specific feature predicts malignancy	Moderate to high cellularity, monotonous HC; non-macrofollicular pattern (single cells >50%, syncytia and crowded 3-D clusters); small or large cell dysplasia; smooth nuclear membrane; prominent or macronucleoli; pale blue intracytoplasmic granules; transgressing vessels; no colloid	Somatic and germline mutation in *GRIM-19*; Copy number alterations	Large, solitary, HCC capsular or vascular invasion	Lobectomy or total thyroidectomy
PTC-OV	Hypoechoic, solid; irregular, discontinuous halo, microcalcifications, intranodular vascularity	Tumor comprises HC with nuclear features of PTC, grooves, INPI, abundant colloid	*BRAFV600E* mutation, *RET/PTC* rearrangements	Encapsulated or invasive oncocytic neoplasm with nuclear features of PTC	Total thyroidectomy
MTC-OV	Usually nodule with heterogeneous echo pattern	Immunostains positive for calcitonin, negative for TG	*RET* mutation	Oncocytic neoplasm with nuclear features of MTC	Lobectomy or total thyroidectomy
Parathyroid adenoma (PA)	Homogeneously hypoechoic, difficult to distinguish from a thyroid follicular cell nodule	Cellular with microfollicles; dispersed cells resemble follicular cells; round nuclei; coarse granular chromatin; variable atypia; cytoplasm abundant oncocytic or clear, colloid absent; vascular fragments. Immunostains negative for TG, positive for PTH.	Parathyroid gene	Encapsulated; cellular; chief cells, some oxyphil cells; delicate capillary network; rim of compressed normal tissue	Lobectomy

CLT chronic lymphocytic thyroiditis, *CNAs* copy number alterations, *HC* Hürthle cells, *HCM* Hürthle cell metaplasia, *HCN* Hürthle cell neoplasm, *INPI* intranuclear pseudoinclusions, *LBP* liquid-based preparations, *MNG* multinodular goiter, *MTC-OV* medullary thyroid carcinoma, oncocytic variant, *PTC-OV* papillary thyroid carcinoma, oncocytic variant, *PTH* parathormone, *TG* thyroglobulin

[a]Actual management may depend on other factors (clinical ultrasound); also see American Thyroid Association management guidelines [13]

screening test only and classifies oncocytic tumors as indeterminate for malignancy.

- The ROM of Hürthle cell lesions reported as indeterminate on cytology is 10–40%.
- Cytological features:
  - Exclusively Hürthle cells
  - Dyshesion
  - Nuclei: small cell or large cell dysplasia where nuclei are irregular, overlapping or overcrowded, and hyperchromatic, with grooves and macronucleoli. The N:C ratio is high in small cell dysplasia and low in large cell dysplasia.
  - Transgressing vessels
  - Colloid that is absent or scant and sometimes forms basophilic structures with concentric lamellations
  - In Hashimoto's thyroiditis and MNG, Hürthle cell nuclei can show anisonucleosis and hyperchromasia but lack large nucleoli.
- Molecular tests may be helpful.
- Surgical resection (lobectomy) is the recommended management.

Cytological Criteria in the Literature for Distinguishing HCA from HCC

- There are no absolute cytological criteria (including ploidy analysis and morphometric analysis of nuclear features) or architectural criteria to distinguish between benign and malignant HCN.

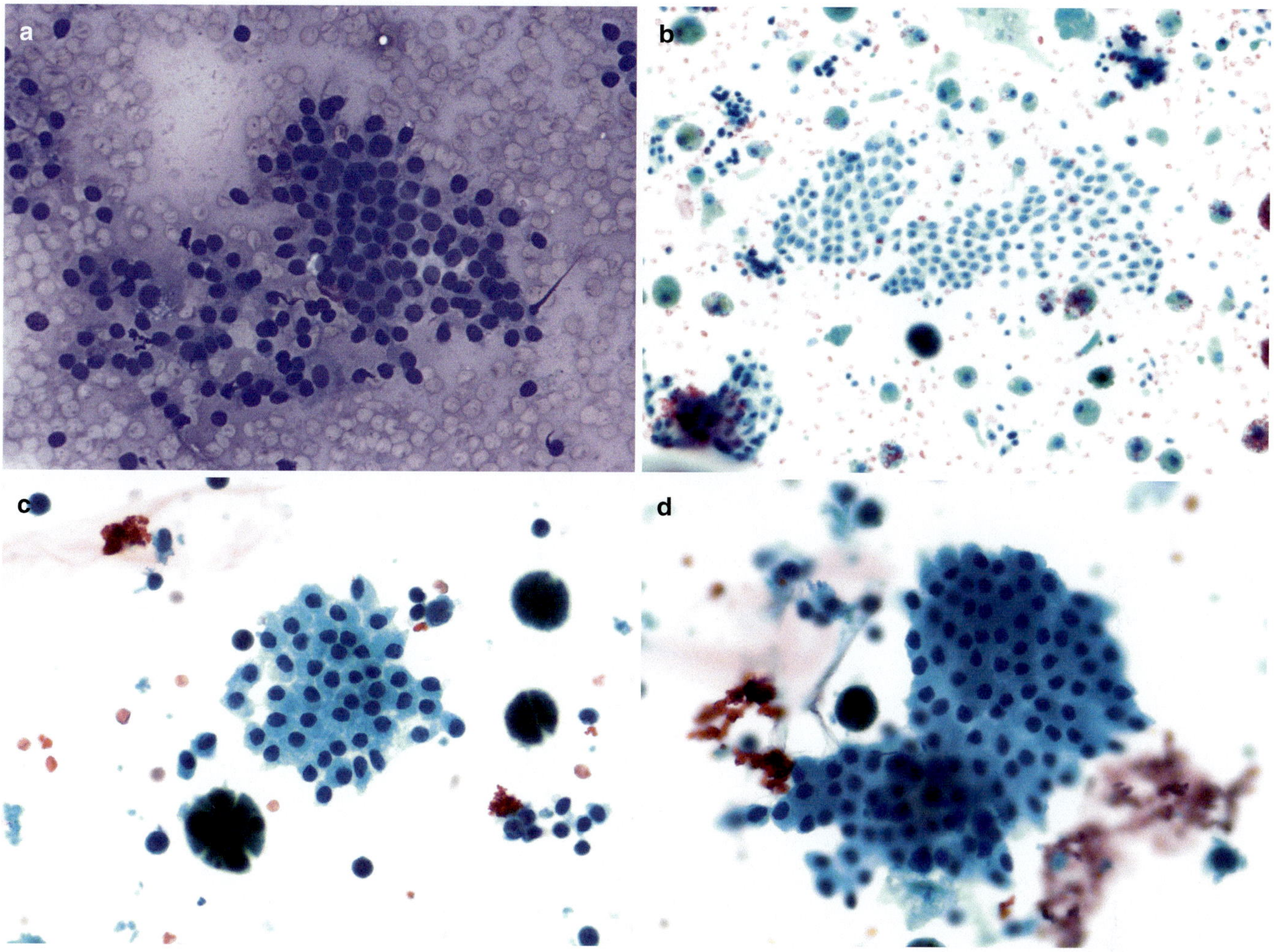

Fig. 7.1 Normal thyroid follicular cells and metaplastic Hürthle cells in a multinodular goiter (MNG). (**a**, **b**) Normal thyroid follicular cells (non-Hürthle cells) are smaller than Hürthle cells and have a different cell shape, with smaller nuclei. Compare the size of normal thyroid follicular cells with red blood cells (RBCs). (**a** DQ stain, CS; **b** Pap stain, SurePath™ [SP]). (**c**, **d**) Hürthle cell metaplasia in MNG. Hürthle cells form flat, cohesive sheets with organized and polarized cell arrangement, well-defined cell borders, and a low nuclear-cytoplasmic (N:C) ratio; they lack nuclear atypia or dysplasia. The latter feature is most important in distinguishing metaplasia from Hürthle cell neoplasms (HCN). Hürthle cells are large and polygonal, with enlarged round to oval nuclei, small nucleoli, and abundant dense and granular cytoplasm with distinct cytoplasmic borders. Compare the size of metaplastic Hürthle cells with RBCs. (**c** Pap stain, ThinPrep® [TP]; **d** Pap stain, SP). Hürthle cells appear similar in both liquid-based preparations (LBP), but in SP, the cells appear in different planes of focus

- 10–25% of HCA are aneuploid, but aneuploidy predicts a more aggressive clinical behavior in histologically proven HCC.
- Elliot et al. [11] performed a morphologic study to distinguish benign Hürthle cell lesions from HCN. The authors found that 6 of 14 cytologic features were statistically significant in predicting HCN:
  - Non-macrofollicular architecture
  - Absence of background colloid
  - Absence of chronic inflammation
  - Presence of transgressing vessels
  - >90% Hürthle cells
  - >10% single Hürthle cells
- They also found that the first four features, when present in combination, are highly predictive of HCN.
- Other published features of HCN include predominantly Hürthle cells, monotonous population, marked dyshesion, the presence of microfollicles, nuclear crowding, small cell and large cell dysplasia, and intracytoplasmic vacuoles. All these features are clearly applicable to LBP.
- Renshaw et al. [25] focused on features seen more commonly in HCC rather than HCN. These include predominantly Hürthle cells, scant colloid, and one of the following: small cell dysplasia, large cell dysplasia, crowding or syncytia, and dyshesion (numerous single cells and barely cohesive cells). All HCC in the study

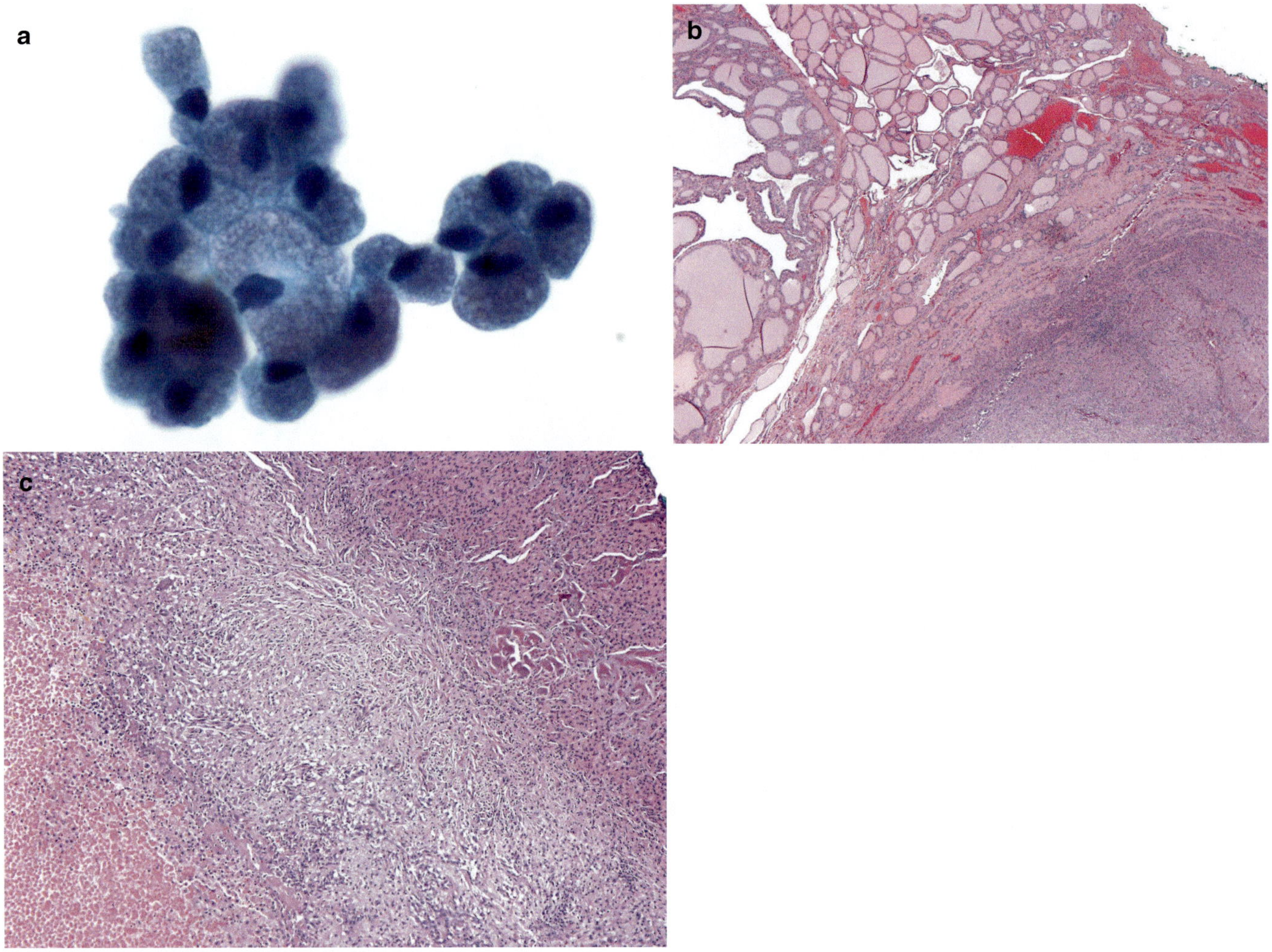

Fig. 7.2 Hürthle cell metaplasia in an adenomatoid nodule (SP). This nodule presented as a dominant solid, 1.5-cm nodule in MNG. Cytology was interpreted as a Hürthle cell nodule/lesion. A lobectomy revealed nodular hyperplasia with a dominant 1.5-cm oncocytic nodule. (**a**) SP shows Hürthle cells arranged in a cluster with small nuclei and no apparent nucleoli (Pap stain). (**b**, **c**) Histologic sections show the oncocytic nodule with no capsule and surrounding hyperplastic features. Note the infarcted focus in image (**c**) which resulted from a prior FNA of the nodule (H&E stain)

could be identified using these criteria, but 63% of HCA and 25% of non-neoplastic Hürthle-cell lesions could not be reliably classified as benign using these criteria.

- Díaz del Arco and Fernández Aceñero [9] concluded that the absence of colloid, high cellularity, >25% of isolated Hürthle cells, the presence of 3-D groups, transgressing vessels, nuclear irregularity, prominent nucleoli or macronucleoli, coarse chromatin, hyperchromatism, pleomorphism, and diffuse large cell dysplasia were features significantly associated with malignancy.
- To heighten awareness about cytological diagnosis of HCN, cytological criteria should be assessed in conjunction with the clinical parameters and correlated with molecular and subsequent histological findings.

Parathyroid Adenoma

- There are no ultrasound features that distinguish parathyroid from thyroid. Thus, pathological distinction between parathyroid and thyroid can be challenging.
- Parathyroid comprises three different types of cells: chief, oxyphil, and water clear cells.
- Chief cells are morphologically similar to thyroid follicular cells, and oxyphil cells are similar to Hürthle cells.
- Cytologically, the parathyroid samples are hypercellular, with cells arranged as disorganized 2-D and 3-D fragments. Nuclei are round, uniform, and overlapping, with stippled "salt-and-pepper" neuroendocrine-type chromatin, inconspicuous nucleoli, and a high N:C ratio. Vascular

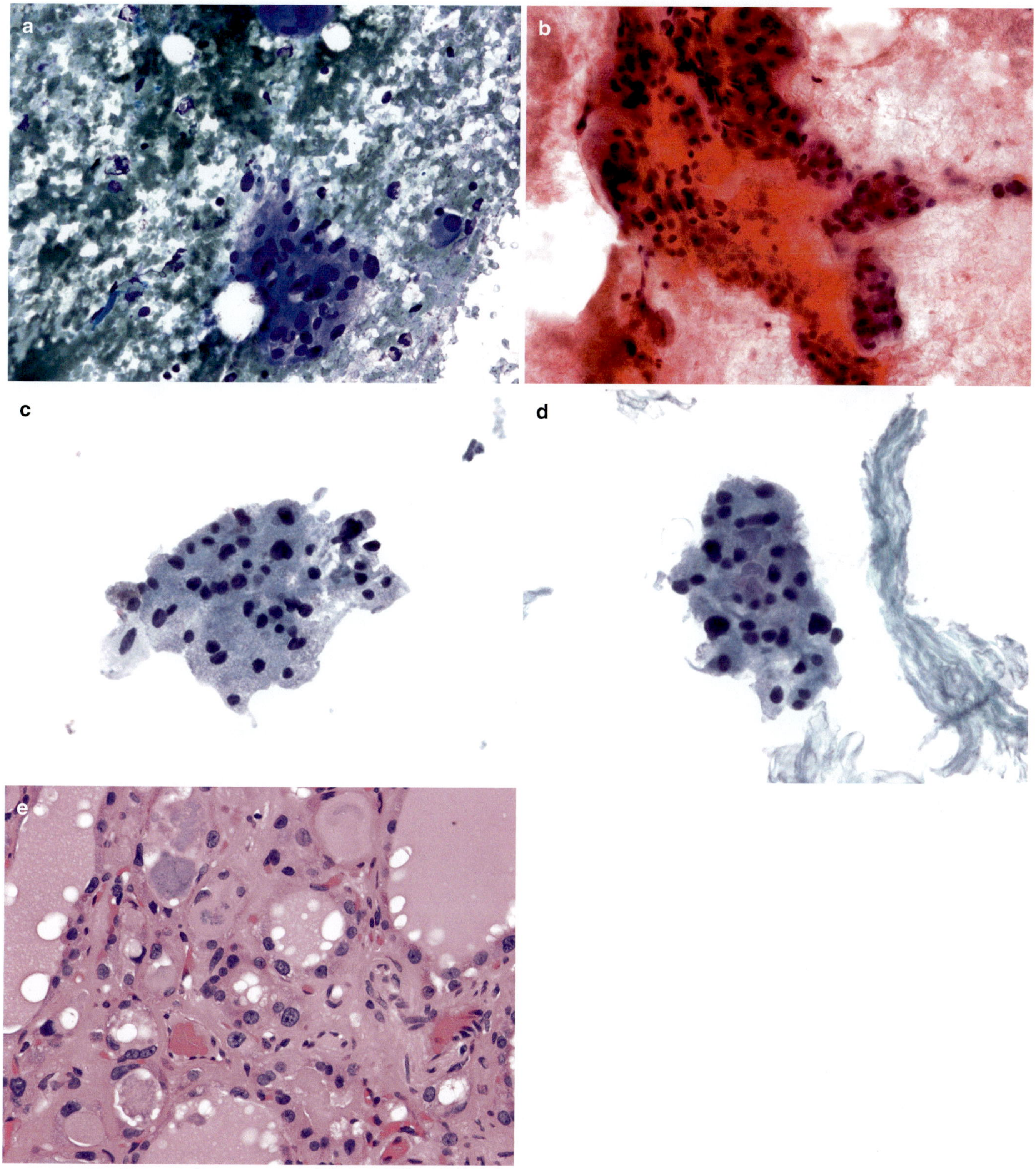

Fig. 7.3 Hürthle cell metaplasia in an adenomatoid nodule (TP). This nodule presented as a stable, predominantly solid, 1.2-cm nodule with punctate internal echogenic foci. Cytology was interpreted as a Hürthle cell nodule/lesion. A lobectomy revealed nodular hyperplasia with a dominant 1.2-cm oncocytic nodule. (**a, b**) Conventional smears (CS) show variably sized Hürthle cell nuclei with nucleoli. Note the abundant blood in the Pap-stained slide (**a** DQ stain; **b** Pap stain). (**c, d**) TP from the same case, with well-preserved morphology and granular oncocytic cytoplasm (Pap stain). (**e**) Histologic section shows the adenomatoid nodule with oncocytic features (H&E stain)

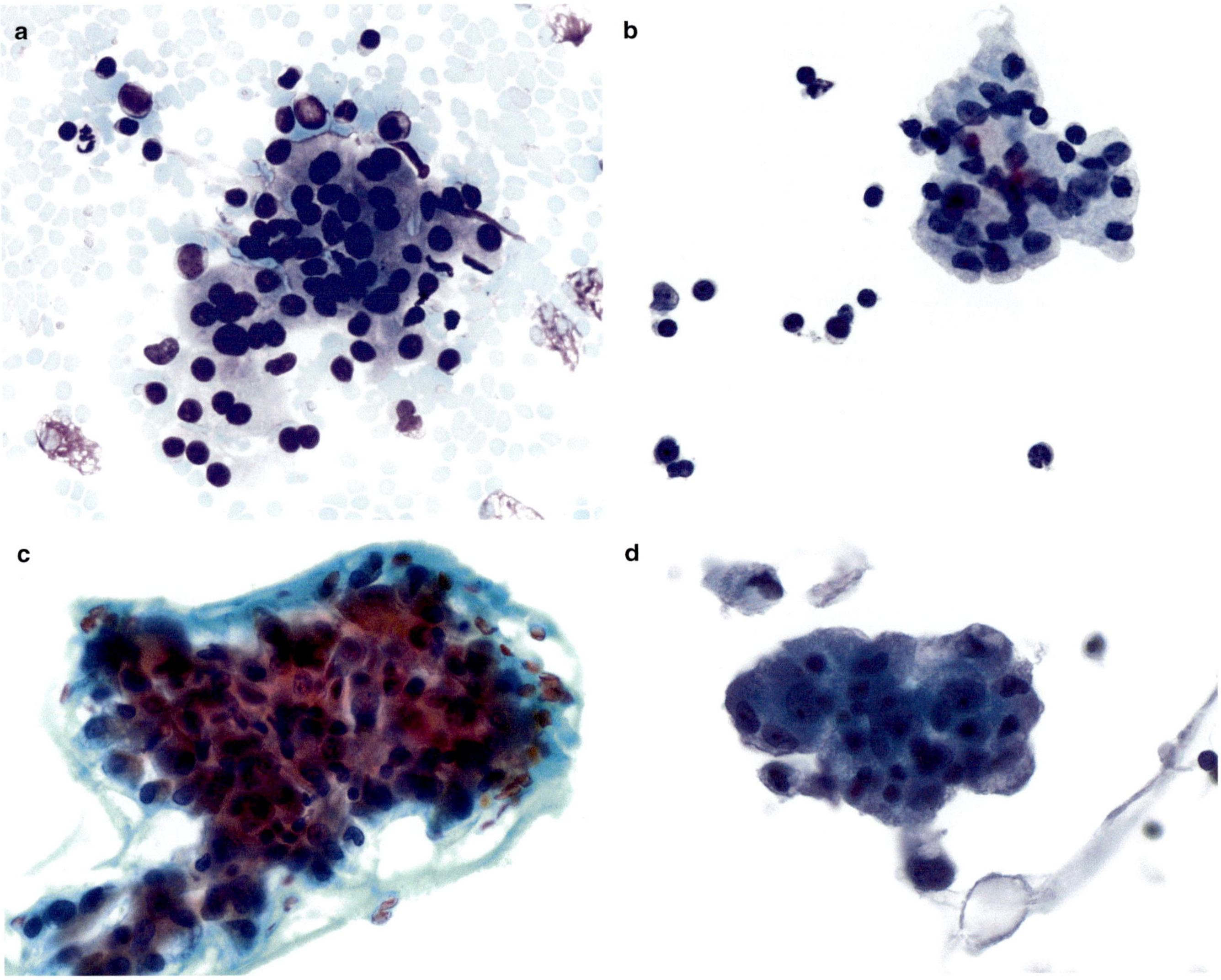
Fig. 7.4 Chronic lymphocytic (Hashimoto's) thyroiditis (CLT). (a) CS showing an aggregate of Hürthle cells with lymphohistiocytic cells close to the group (DQ stain). (b) In the same case, TP shows Hürthle cells with lymphoid cells and histiocytes in close association (Pap stain). (c) A lymphohistiocytic aggregate in Hashimoto's thyroiditis (CLT) in a CS (Pap stain). (d) A lymphohistiocytic aggregate in Hashimoto's thyroiditis (CLT) in TP (Pap stain). Note the similarity in cytomorphology

proliferation is prominent. The background shows many naked "bare" nuclei and no colloid.

- Parathyroid cells may be distinguished cytologically as follicular cells in a FN/SFN, showing nuclear atypia and nucleoli. Follicular cells also show cytoplasmic lipofuscin granules.
- PTH assay or immunostaining for PTH and thyroglobulin can be of diagnostic value and can be used for confirmation.
- Clinical correlation with PTH assay performed from the aspirated sample can also be confirmatory of parathyroid cells.
- Parathyroid lesions are usually interpreted as a follicular lesion of undetermined significance (FLUS) or FN/SFN. Subsequent molecular testing can help in further characterization. If the lesion is a parathyroid lesion, the test may detect parathyroid gene.

Follicular Carcinoma, Oncocytic Type

- The lesion comprises >75% oncocytic cells. Diagnostic criteria are the same as for conventional follicular carcinoma (Fig. 7.12). For comparison, Fig. 7.13 shows a case of follicular adenoma with oncocytic features.

Papillary Thyroid Carcinoma, Oncocytic Type

- The oncocytic variant of PTC (PTC-OV) is composed of oncocytic cells with abundant granular and eosinophilic cytoplasm and classic nuclear features of PTC, including enlarged, elongated, crowded, and overlapping nuclei showing irregularity, small nucleoli, chromatin clearing, prominent grooves, and INPI. The

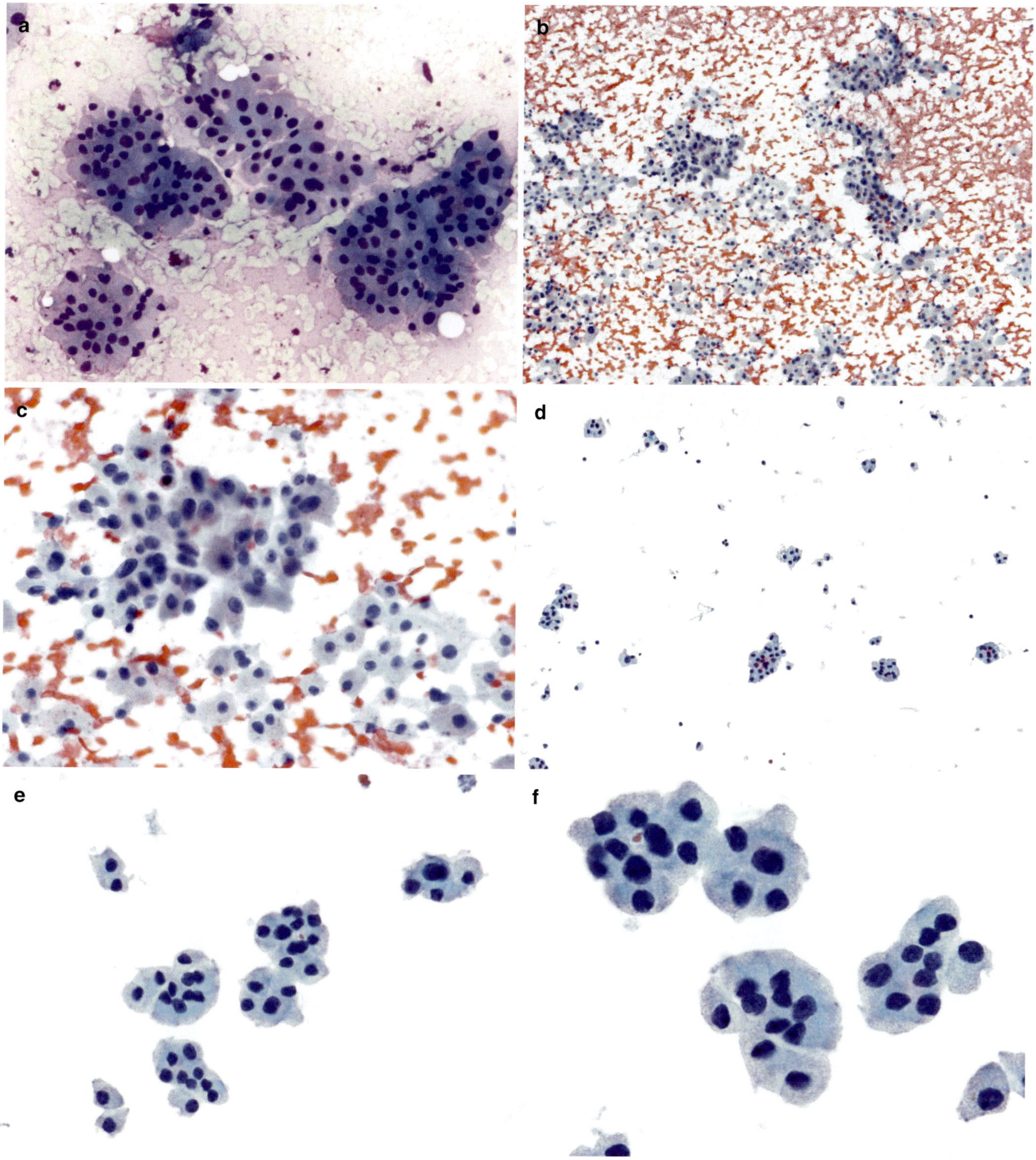

Fig. 7.5 Histologically proven Hürthle cell adenoma (HCA). (**a–c**) On CS, HCA shows high cellularity with dense cytoplasm, small to prominent nucleoli, and a relatively low N:C ratio. The lesion was diagnosed as SFNHCT (**a** DQ stain; **b**, **c** Pap stain). (**d–f**) When the same case was processed as TP, all cytologic features of CS are retained. Although the cytoplasm appears dense, the cytoplasmic granularity is more apparent in LBP (Pap stain). (**g**) Gross image of HCA showing a well-circumscribed and encapsulated 1.5-cm tumor. (**h**, **i**) Histologic sections of HCA. Note the thin capsule (H&E stain)

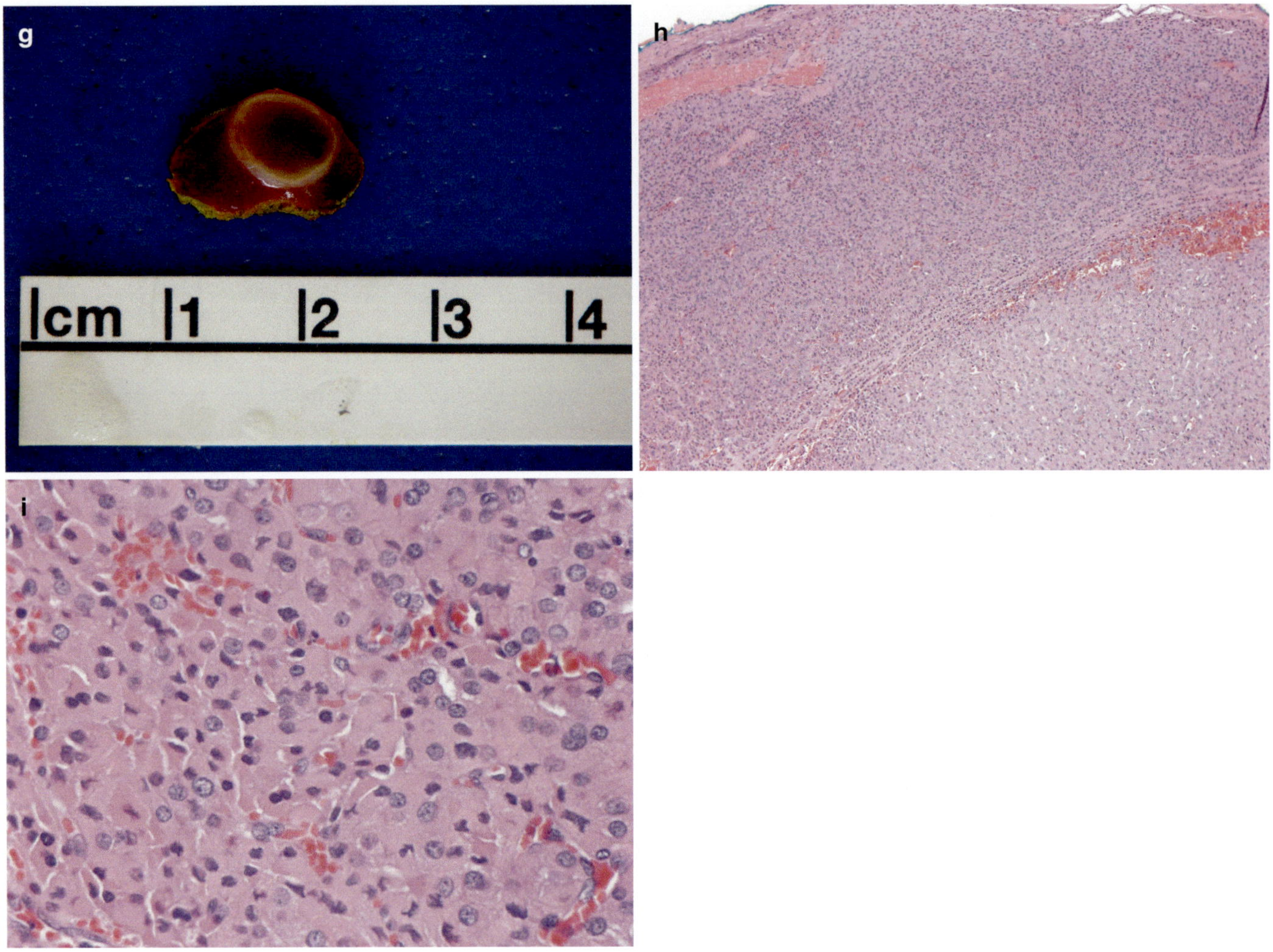

Fig. 7.5 (continued)

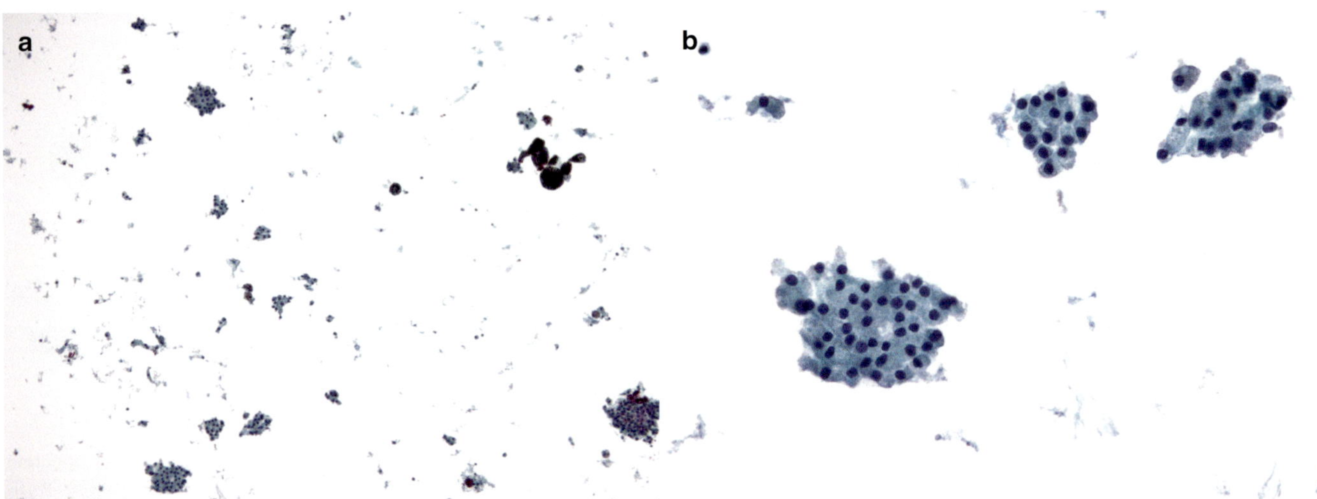

Fig. 7.6 Cytologic diagnostic criteria for FNHCT/SFNHCT in LBP. (**a–c**) Another case of HCA showing high cellularity, with cells dispersed singly, flat sheets, and clusters. Nucleoli are present and the N:C ratio is relatively low compared with the case of HCA above. Colloid is absent (Pap stain, TP). (**d**) Cluster of neoplastic Hürthle cells with transgressing vessels (Pap stain, TP). Note cytoplasmic granularity and eosinophilia

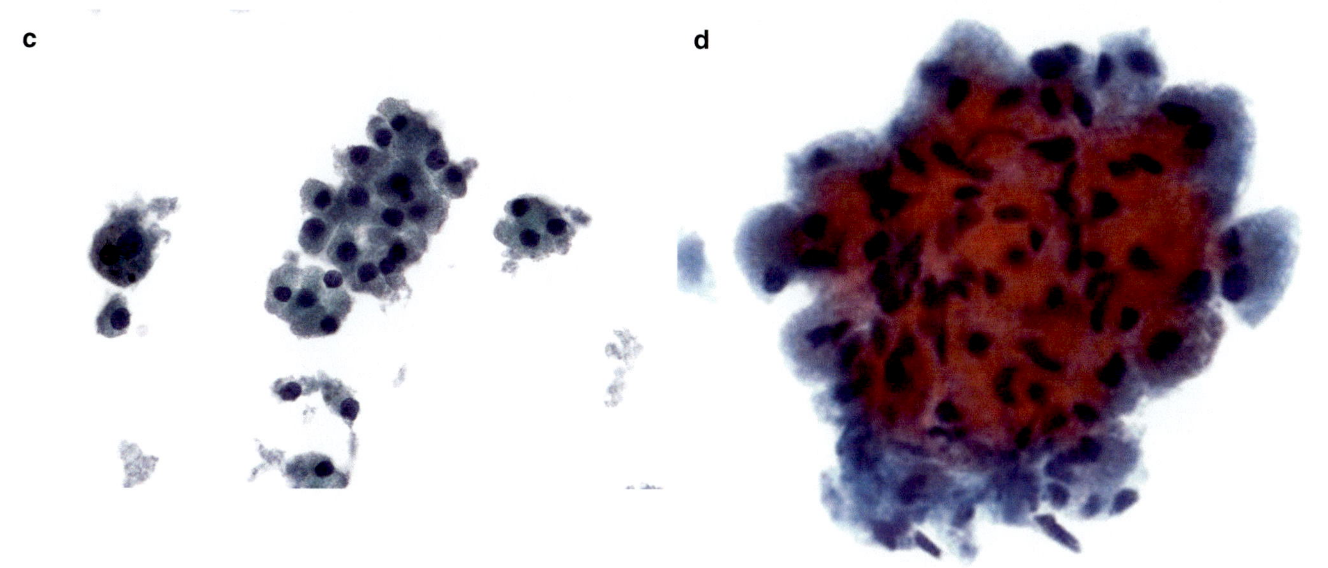

Fig. 7.6 (continued)

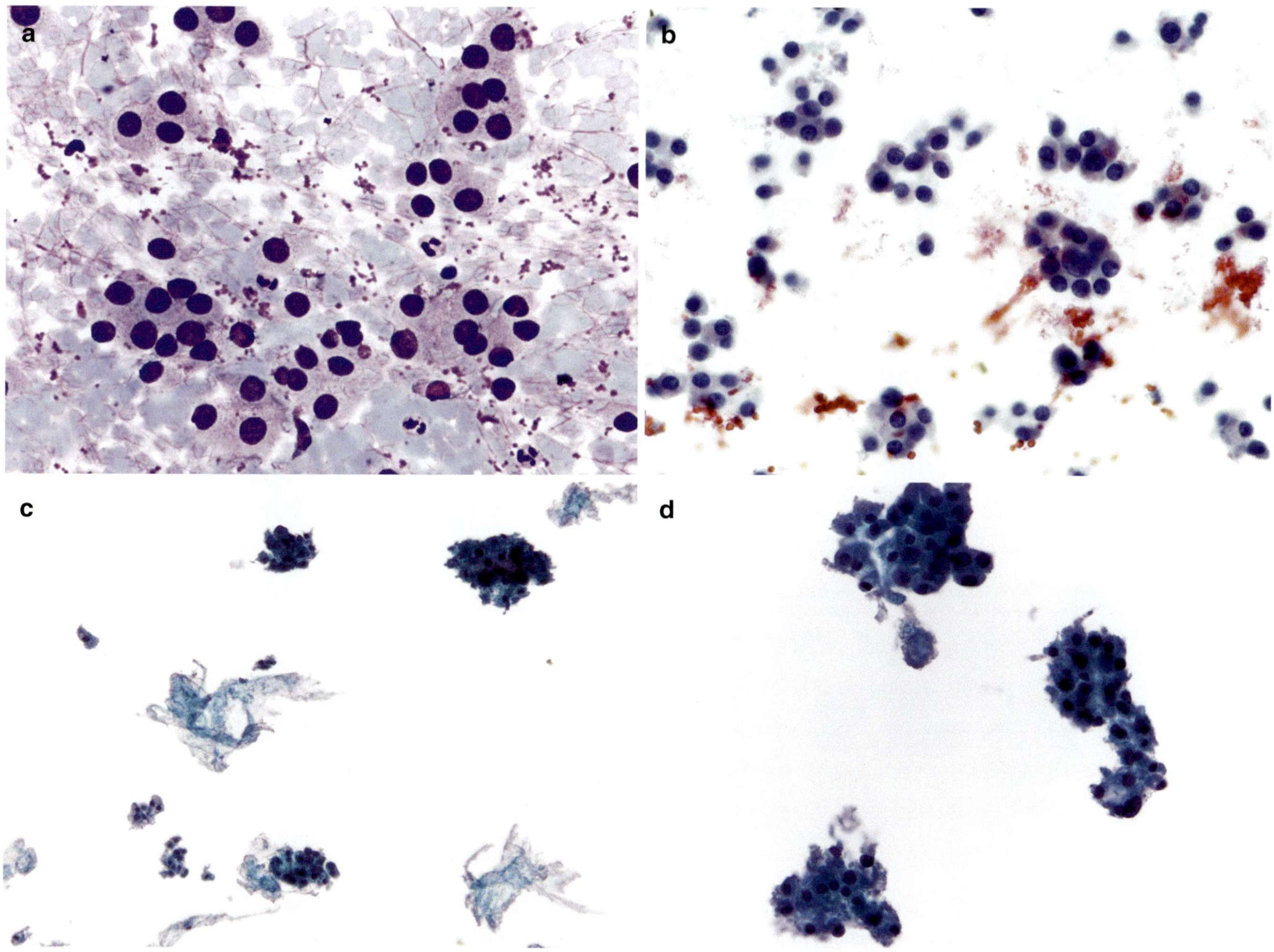

Fig. 7.7 FNHCT/SFNHCT with small cell dysplasia. (**a**, **b**) CS shows small cells with less abundant cytoplasm, eosinophilic granules, and high N:C ratio. Nuclei are enlarged, central to eccentrically placed, and have prominent nucleoli. (**a** DQ; **b** Pap stain). (**c**–**e**) Small cell dysplasia in TP showing similar cytology as CS. Some thin colloid is evident (Pap stain). (**f**) Histologic section from Hürthle cell carcinoma (HCC) (H&E stain)

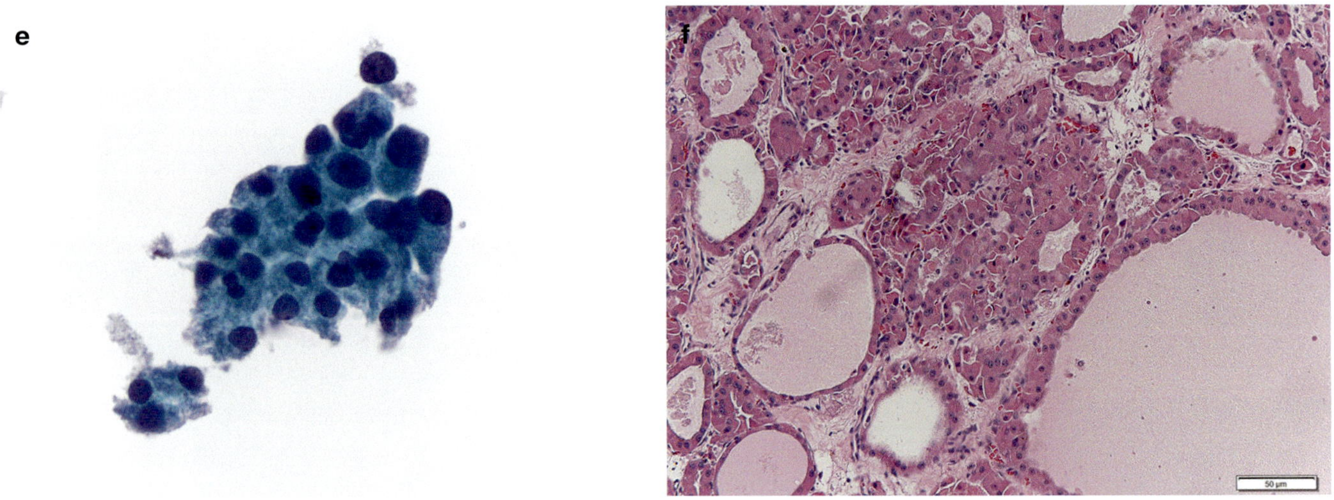

Fig. 7.7 (continued)

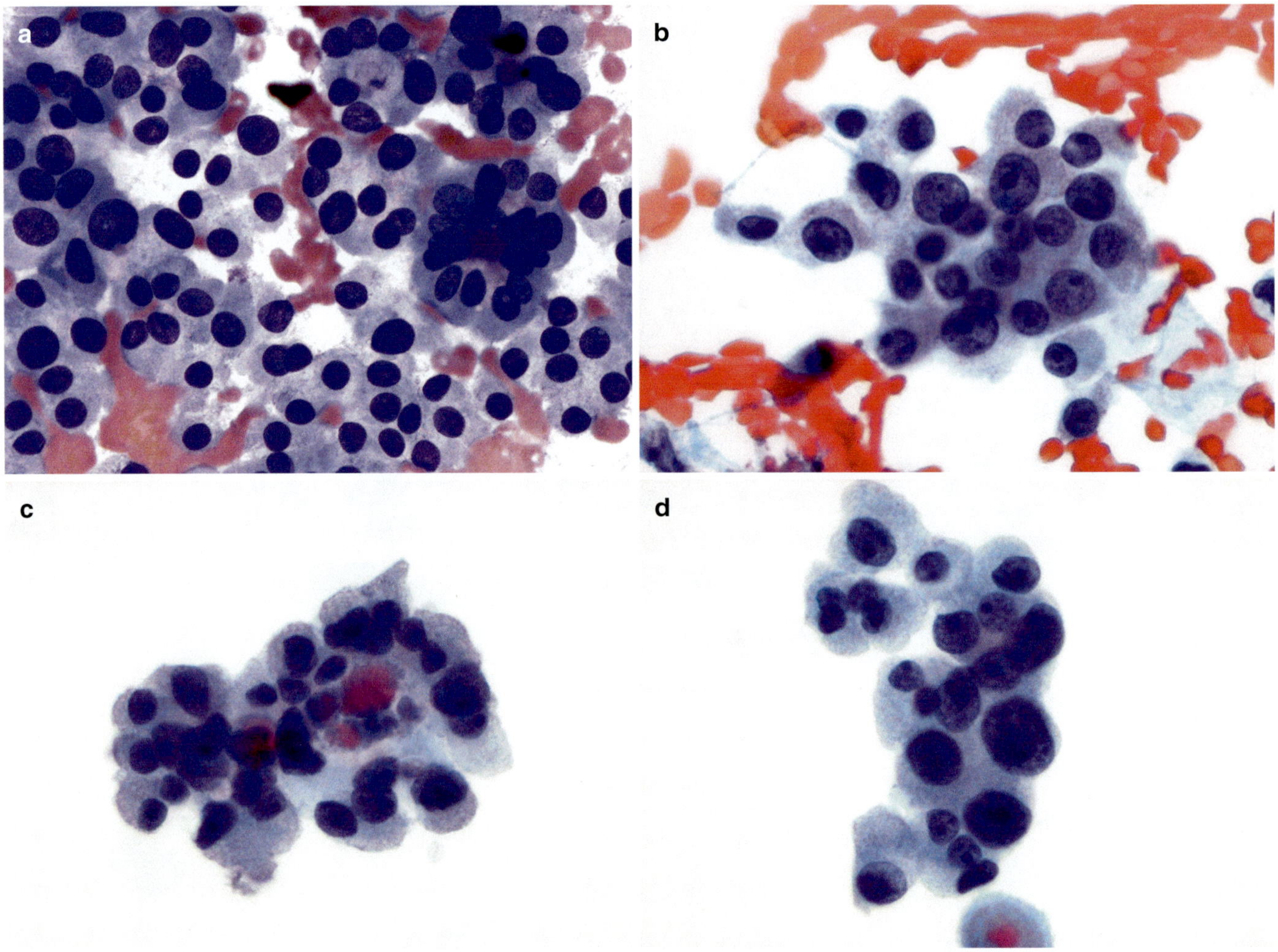

Fig. 7.8 FNHCT/SFNHCT with large cell dysplasia. (**a**, **b**) CS shows loosely cohesive and cohesive large cells with abundant granular cytoplasm and macronucleoli (**a** DQ; **b** Pap stain). (**c**, **d**) In TP, the same case shows similar features (Pap stain). A subsequent molecular test showed CNAs. (**e**) Gross specimen of Hürthle cell carcinoma. *Lower left* shows normal thyroid. (**f**, **g**) Resected HCC showing capsular invasion; high magnification shows cytology similar to the CS and TP (H&E stain)

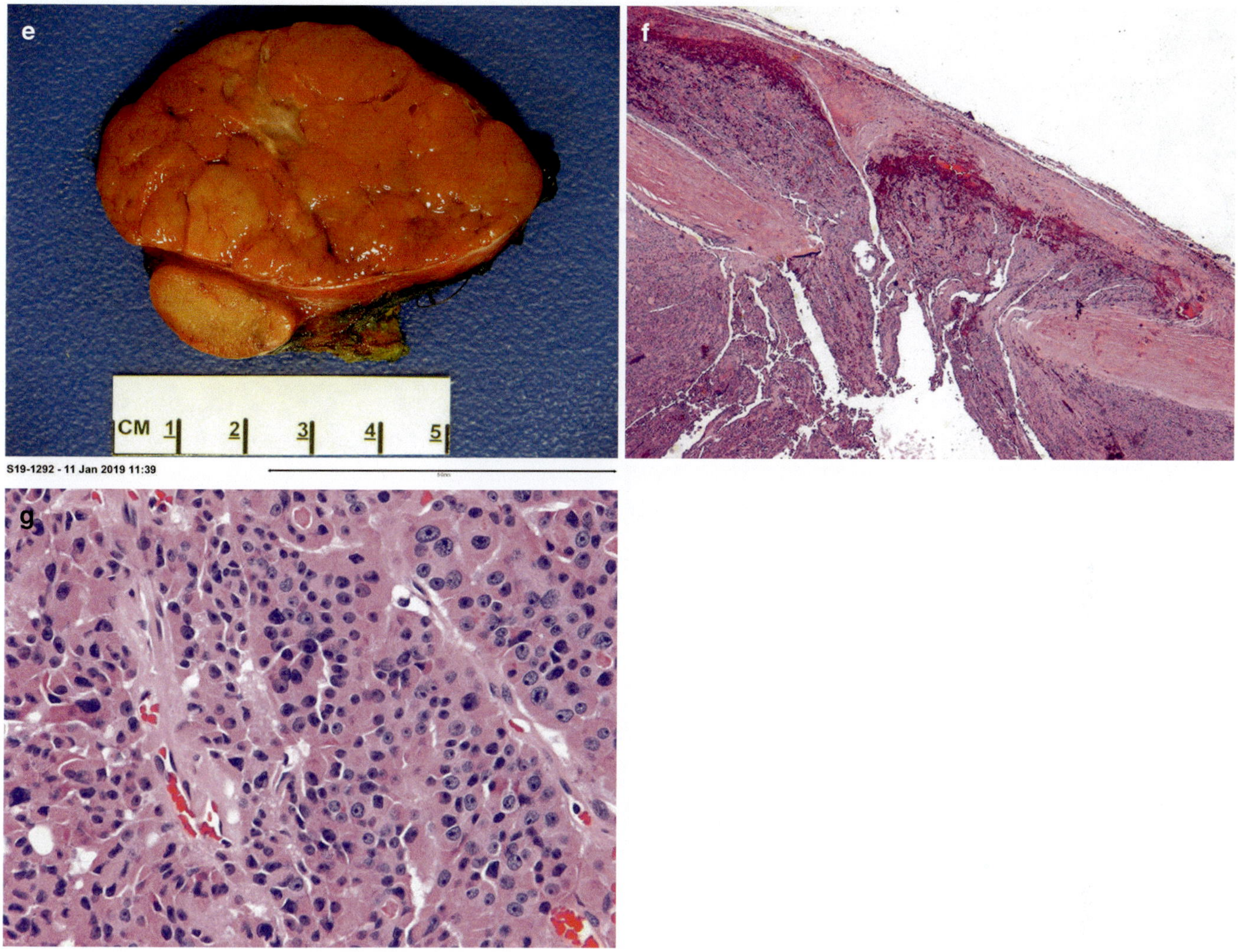

Fig. 7.8 (continued)

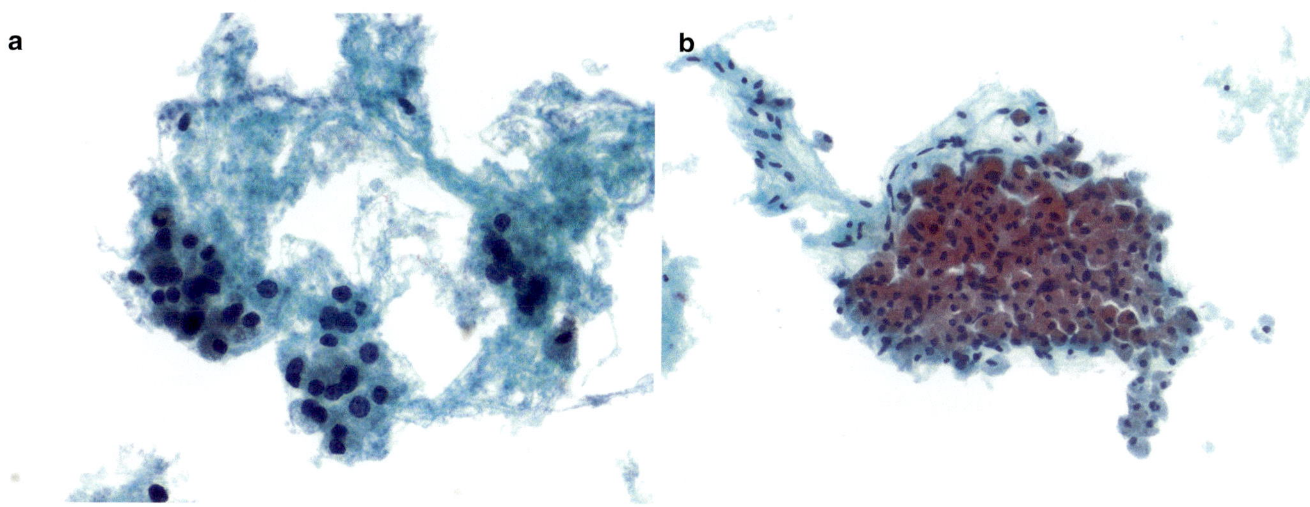

Fig. 7.9 FNHCT/SFNHCT with vascular proliferation. (**a**, **b**) On TP, this HCA shows a loosely-cohesive group of tumor cells and another fragment with vascular endothelial cells surrounding and transgressing the cell group (Pap stain). (**c**–**e**) Cell block made from residual TP vial showing HCA (H&E stain). Note abundant material with Hürthle cells in microfollicles and intact vascular fragments in the cell block, similar to the vascular fragment seen in the TP. The cell block was processed utilizing the technique published by Rekhtman et al. [24]

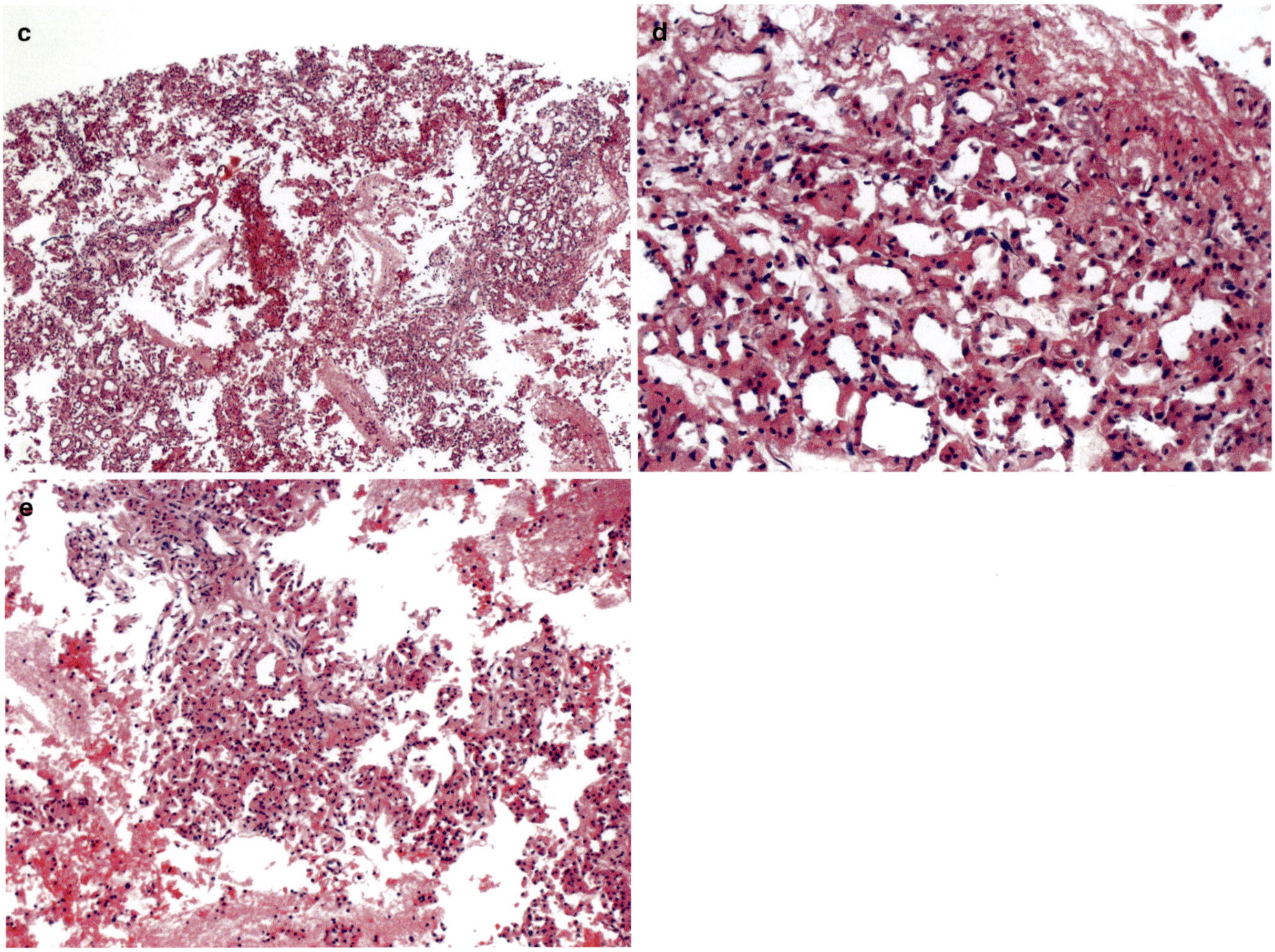

Fig. 7.9 (continued)

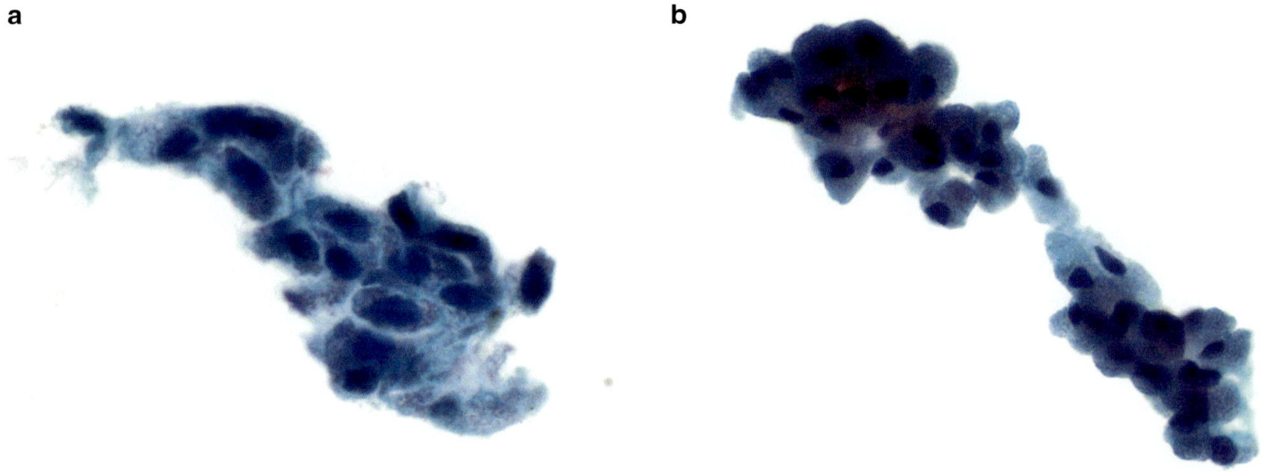

Fig. 7.10 FNHCT/SFNHCT on SP. (**a–d**) Mix of small and large cell dysplasia of tumor cells with granular cytoplasm, relatively high N:C ratio, and small to large nuclei with nucleoli. Note eosinophilic cytoplasmic granules in image **a**. (Pap stain, SP)

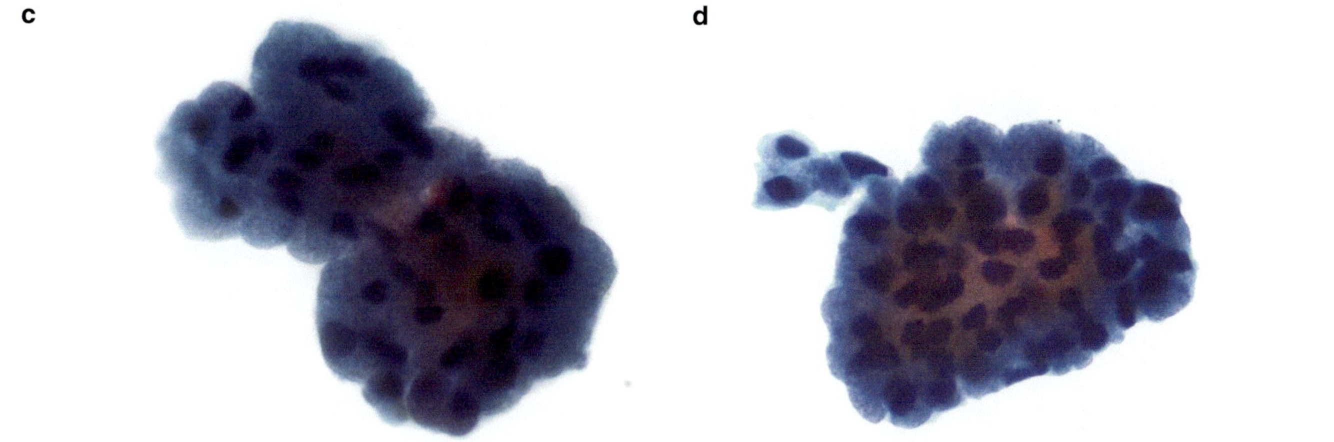

Fig. 7.10 (continued)

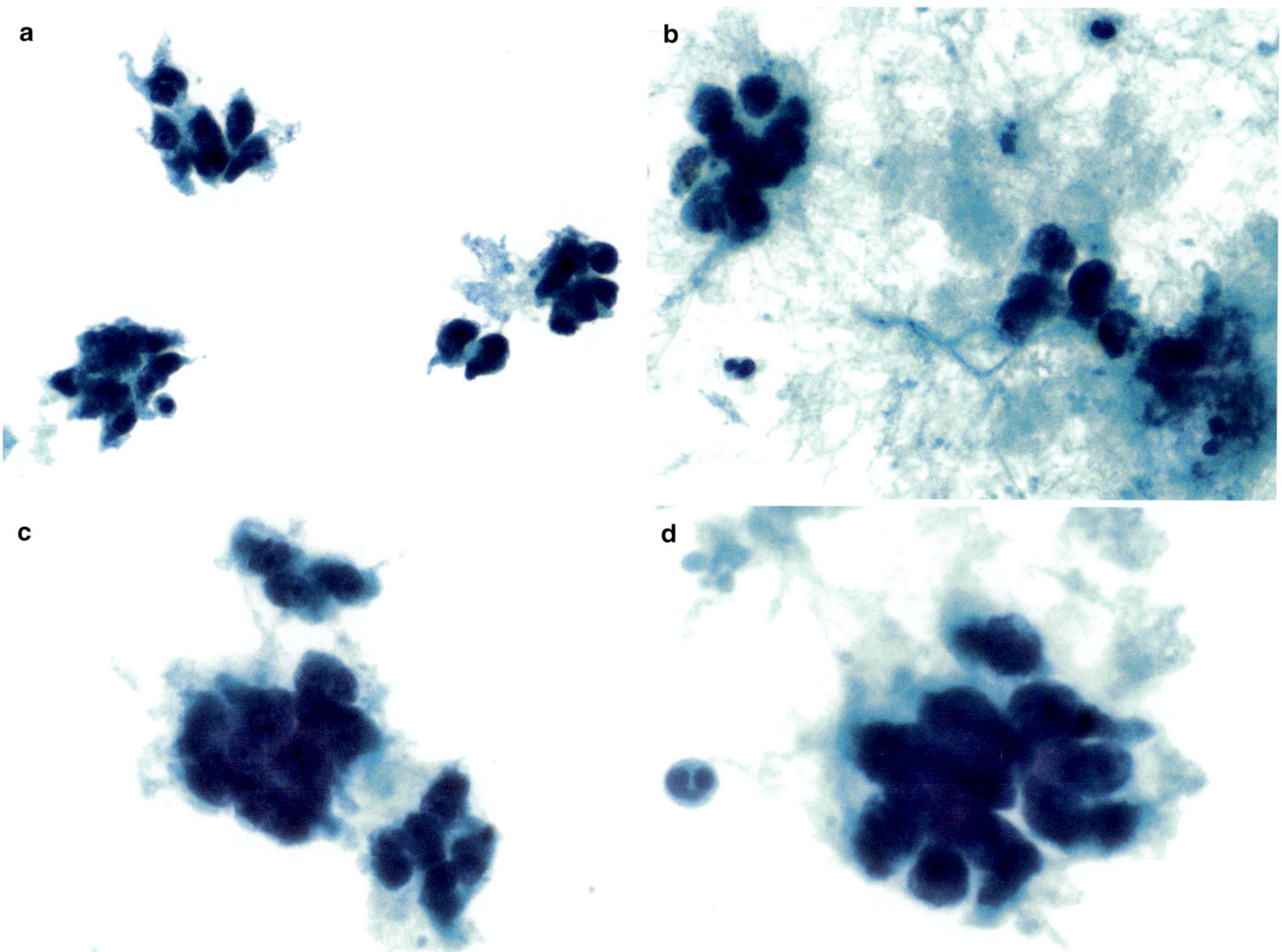

Fig. 7.11 Hürthle cell carcinoma (HCC) first diagnosed as metastasis to hip bone. The thyroid HCC was discovered after the patient first presented with metastasis to the hip bone. (**a–d**) Oncocytic tumor cells with high N:C ratio, enlarged hyperchromatic nuclei with prominent nucleoli, and cytoplasm with eosinophilic granules (Pap stain, SP); (**e–g**) Cell block (CB) section from the hip FNA shows an oncocytic tumor. Immunohistochemistry was positive for thyroglobulin and showed cytoplasmic staining; *PAX8* was positive with nuclear staining (**e** H&E stain, CB); **f** thyroglobulin immunostain; **g** *PAX8* immunostain). (**h**) Histologic section of HCC from the needle core biopsy of hip metastasis (H&E stain). Thyroid FNA was later performed on a solitary 2.5-cm nodule and was diagnosed as HCC, after review of the prior hip metastasis. The tumor was not resected

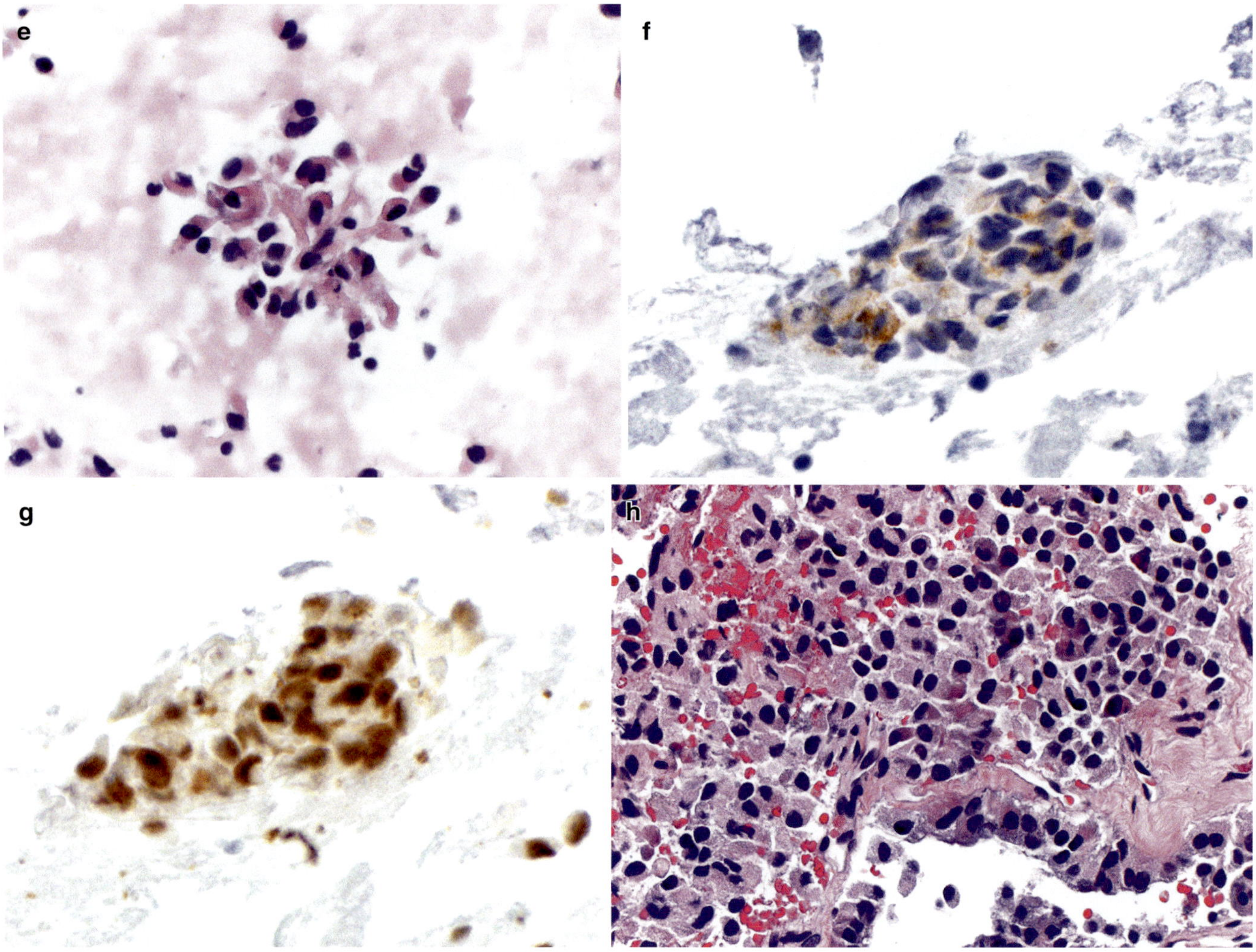

Fig. 7.11 (continued)

follicular variant of PTC may show a microfollicular architecture with similar nuclear features, but fewer INPI (Fig. 7.14).
- PTC-OV is rare, with a reported incidence of 1–11%.
- The pure form of PTC-OV is very rare and must be differentiated from the HCN and tall cell variant (TCV) of PTC, both of which also have abundant eosinophilic cytoplasm. The latter is also characterized by cells that are two to three times as tall as they are wide. PTC-OV can be distinguished from HCN based on nuclear features.
- It is debatable whether PTC-OV confers a more aggressive clinical course and increased risk of recurrence when compared with classic PTC.
- Management and follow-up of patients should be based on American Thyroid Association guidelines [13].

Medullary Thyroid Carcinoma, Oncocytic Type

- Medullary thyroid carcinoma (MTC), the most common tumor to be distinguished from HCN, is covered in detail in Chap. 10.
- Both tumors are characterized by a single-cell monomorphous pattern, round plasmacytoid nuclei that may be single or binucleated to multinucleated, and oncocytic cytoplasm. MTC can be cytologically distinguished from HCN by the presence of a double population of variable plasmacytoid and spindle cells, coarsely granular neuroendocrine-type chromatin, and lack of prominent nucleoli.
- Immunocytochemistry can be performed to avoid diagnostic pitfalls. For MTC, negativity for thyroglobulin of the neoplastic parafollicular C-cells and positivity for calcitonin should be confirmed.

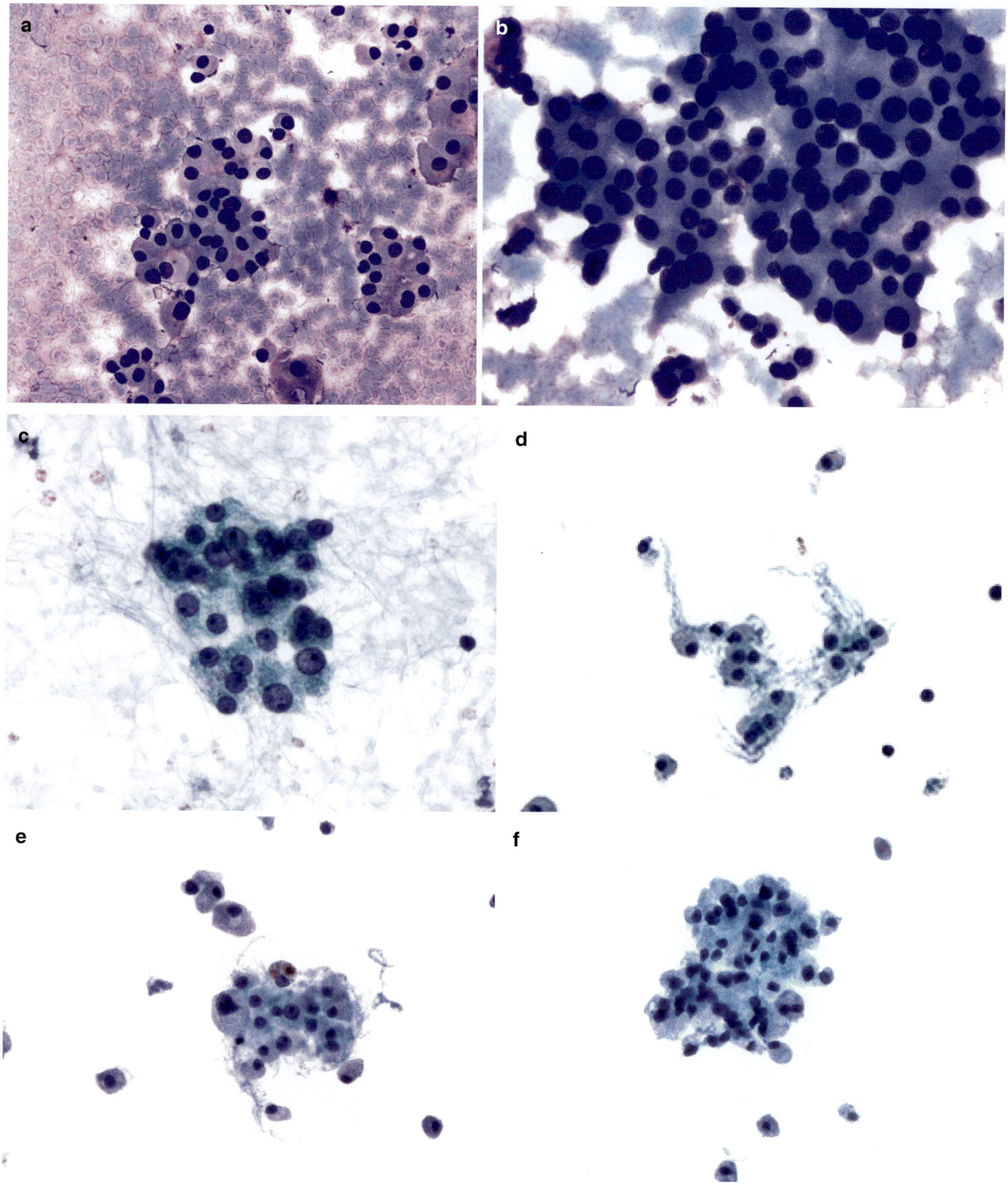

Fig. 7.12 Follicular carcinoma, oncocytic variant (FC-OV). This case was diagnosed on FNA as FNHCT/SFNHCT with large cell dysplasia. (**a–c**) CS displays enlarged, round to oval nuclei, and macronucleoli. Cytoplasm appears denser on the DQ stain and more granular on the Pap stain (**a**, **b** DQ stain; **c** Pap stain). (**d–f**) The same case processed as TP showed similar cytoplasmic and nuclear morphology. Note monomorphous nuclei, cytoplasmic granules staining pale green, rare histiocytes with hemosiderin, and some thin colloid clinging to tumor cells (Pap stain). (**g**) Histologic section of FC-OV from the resection specimen (H&E stain). After comparison with the case of HCC shown in Fig. 7.8, it becomes evident that these two tumors cannot be distinguished cytologically. Molecular testing may be helpful, as the two tumors have different genetic profiles. For example, the *PAX8/PPARγ* rearrangement seen in 26–53% of FC is rare in HCC ([6]; Máximo et al. 2016)

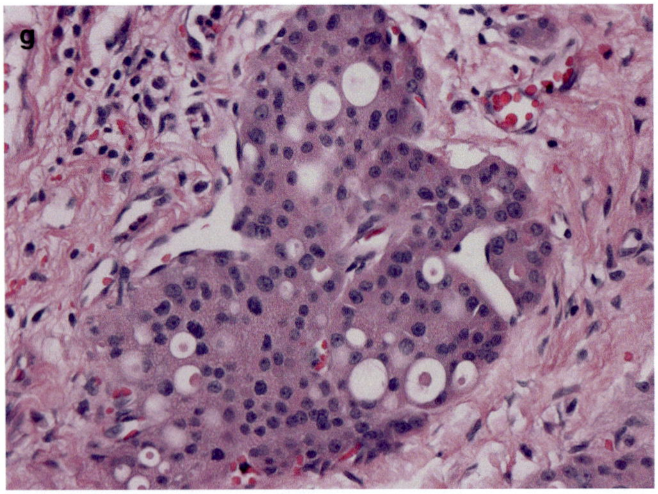

Fig. 7.12 (continued)

- Immunocytochemistry works well on LBP owing to the more visible neoplastic cells and clean background. A small amount of monoclonal antibody is required for LBP.

Metastatic Carcinoma Mimicking Thyroid Hürthle Cell Neoplasm

- Usually, there is a clinical history of a non-thyroid malignancy.
- Metastatic tumors of breast, kidney, or melanoma, among other oncocytic tumors, may mimic primary thyroid HCN (*see* Chap. 11).
- Immunocytochemistry can be performed on LBP for confirmation of primary *versus* metastatic tumor.

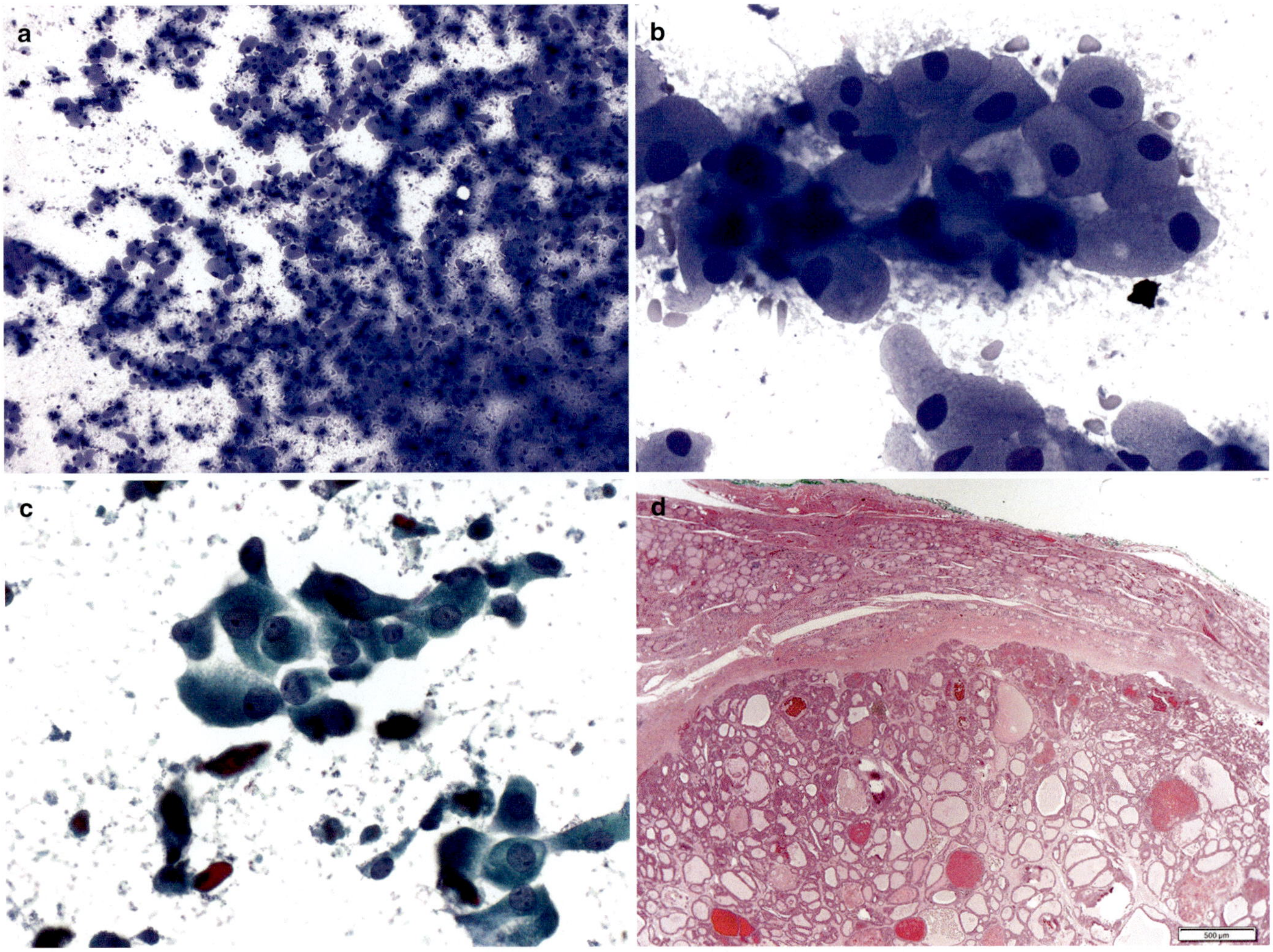

Fig. 7.13 Follicular adenoma, oncocytic variant (FA-OV). This case of HCA was also diagnosed on FNA as FNHCT/SFNHCT. (**a**, **b**) DQ-stained CS shows a cellular aspirate with singly dispersed, large polygonal cells with abundant dense cytoplasm, distinct cell borders, small round to oval nuclei, and a low N:C ratio. (**c**) A Pap-stained Cytospin™ slide shows similar morphology with small nucleoli and thin granular colloid in the background. (**d**) Histologic section of FA-OV. Note the intact capsule and compressed, benign thyroid parenchyma (H&E stain). After comparison with the case of HCC shown in Fig. 7.8 and FC-OV in Fig. 7.12, it becomes evident that distinguishing Hürthle cell tumors on cytology is challenging. Molecular testing may be helpful in detecting the genetic profile

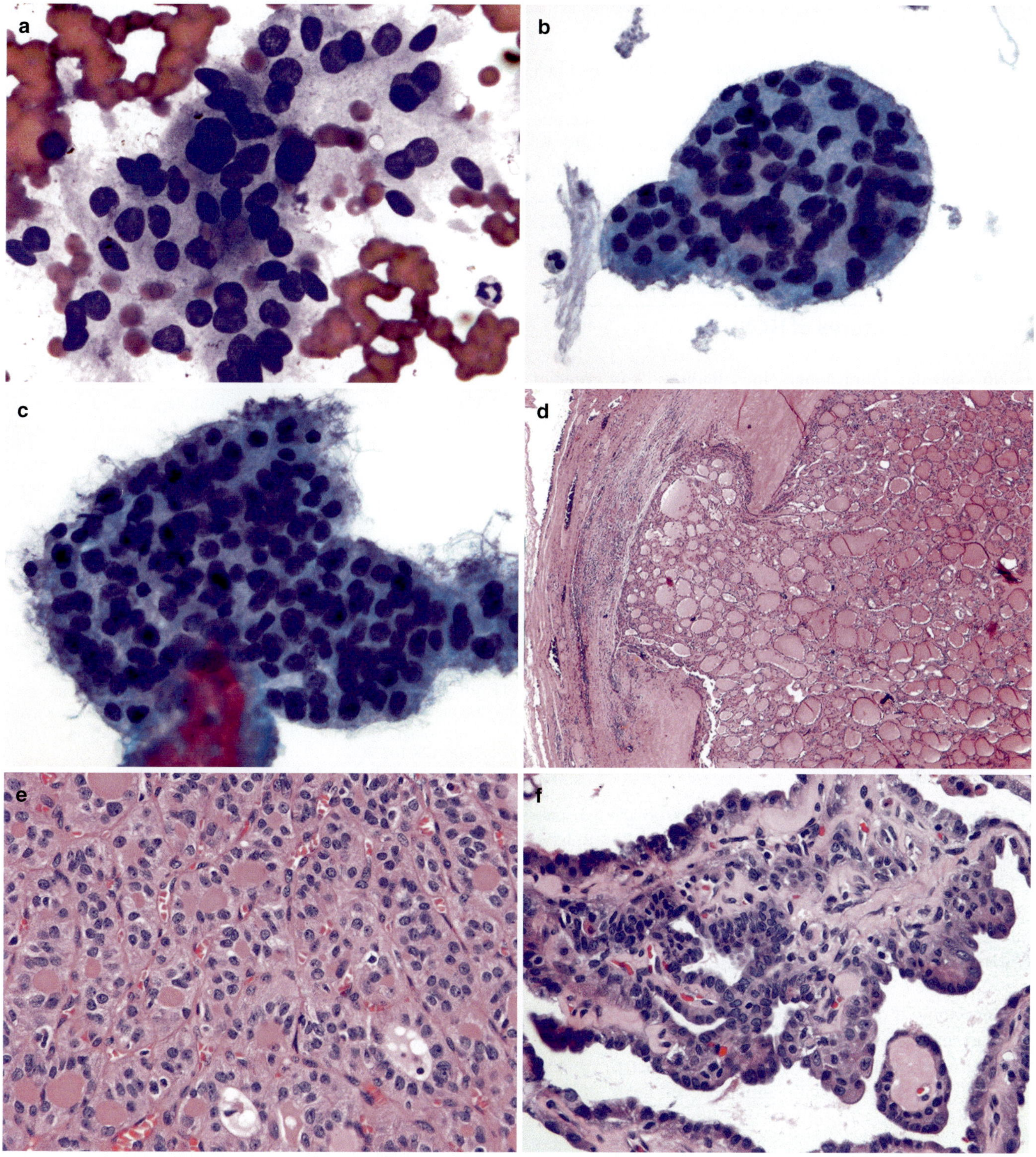

Fig. 7.14 Papillary thyroid carcinoma, follicular variant (FVPTC) with Hürthle cell features. (**a**) DQ-stained CS shows a microfollicular fragment of tumor cells with enlarged round to oval nuclei, nucleoli, nuclear overlap, and occasional intranuclear grooves (*left side*). Intranuclear pseudoinclusions (INPI) were rare. (**b, c**) The Pap-stained TP shows similar cytological features. One vague INPI can be seen at the 12 o'clock position in image **b**. Architecturally, a microfollicular arrangement and syncytial pattern are evident. (**d, e**) Histologic section from the FVPTC with Hürthle cell features showing capsular invasion. A rare INPI can be seen in the high magnification in the middle of the field (H&E stain). (**f**) Histologic section of metastatic PTC with Hürthle cell features in one positive cervical lymph node (H&E stain)

Salient Points for FNHCT/SFNHCT

- The diagnostic accuracy of detecting HCNs by FNA cytology of thyroid nodules is in the range of 85–90%.
- Salient cytological criteria for diagnosis of a HCN include overall high cellularity comprising predominantly of Hürthle (oncocytic) cells that are dispersed mostly in a single-cell pattern, large cell and small cell dysplasia, prominent nucleoli, transgressing vessels, absent colloid, and lack of background chronic inflammation.

Ultrasound Features of HCN

- No specific ultrasonographic findings can predict malignancy.

Molecular/Genetic alterations in HCN: The Role of Molecular Tests

- HCA:
  - *RET/PTC* and *PAX8/PPARγ* gene rearrangements
  - *RAS* mutations are less common than in follicular adenoma (FA); they are seen in about 30% of cases.
  - Monosomies are more frequent than polysomies.
  - Somatic and germline mutation in *GRIM-19*
- HCC:

  Most important is:

- Copy Number Alterations (CNAs). ThyroSeq® v3, performed on the FNA, includes CNAs and is found to have greater positive predictive value (PPV) for identifying HCC.

Management of FNHCT/SFNHCT

- Lobectomy if cytology indicates HCN, as per ATA 2015 management guidelines (Haugen et al. 2015)
- Molecular finding of CNAs with ThyroSeq® v3 may make a more convincing argument in favor of total thyroidectomy.
- HCC often has less radioiodine avidity, and patients may benefit from a more complete thyroidectomy.

Suggested Reading

1. Bronner MP, Clevenger CV, Edmonds PR, Lowell DM, McFarland MM, LiVolsi VA. Flow cytometric analysis of DNA content in Hürthle cell adenomas and carcinomas of the thyroid. Am J Clin Pathol. 1988;89:764–9.
2. Canberk S, Griffin AC, Goyal A, Wang H, Montone K, Livolsi V, et al. Oncocytic follicular nodules of the thyroid with or without chronic lymphocytic thyroiditis: an institutional experience. Cytojournal. 2013;10:2. https://doi.org/10.4103/1742-6413.106686.
3. Carpi A, Rossi G, Mechanick JI, Nicolini A, Camici M, Russo MA, et al. Large needle aspiration biopsy histology for preoperative selection of Hürthle cell thyroid nodules. Histopathology. 2011;59:892–6. https://doi.org/10.1111/j.1365-2559.2011.04014.x.
4. Carr AA, Yen TWF, Ortiz DI, Hunt BC, Fareau G, Massey BL, et al. Patients with oncocytic variant papillary thyroid carcinoma have a similar prognosis to matched classical papillary thyroid carcinoma controls. Thyroid. 2018;28:1462–7. https://doi.org/10.1089/thy.2017.0603.
5. Ali SZ, Cibas ES. The Bethesda System for reporting thyroid cytopathology; definitions, criteria, and explanatory notes. 2nd ed. Cham: Springer International Publishing AG; 2018.
6. Cibas ES, Ali SZ. The 2017 Bethesda System for reporting thyroid cytopathology. Thyroid. 2017;27:1341–6. https://doi.org/10.1089/thy.2017.0500.
7. Clark DP, Faquin WC. Thyroid cytopathology. 2nd ed. New York: Springer; 2010.
8. Cochand-Priollet B, Prat JJ, Polivka M, Thienpont L, Dahan H, Wassef M, et al. Thyroid fine needle aspiration: the morphological features on ThinPrep slide preparations. Eighty cases with histological control. Cytopathology. 2003;14:343–9.
9. Díaz Del Arco C, Fernández Aceñero MJ. Preoperative diagnosis of neoplastic or malignant Hürthle cell lesions: a chimera? Acta Cytol. 2018;62:193–203. https://doi.org/10.1159/000488441.
10. Duncan LD, Forrest L, Law WM Jr, Hubbard E, Stewart LE. Evaluation of thyroid fine-needle aspirations: can ThinPrep be used exclusively to appropriately triage patients having a thyroid nodule? Diagn Cytopathol. 2011;39:341–8. https://doi.org/10.1002/dc.21392.
11. Elliott DD, Pitman MB, Bloom L, Faquin WC. Fine-needle aspiration biopsy of Hürthle cell lesions of the thyroid gland: a cytomorphologic study of 139 cases with statistical analysis. Cancer. 2006;108:102–9.
12. Giorgadze T, Rossi ED, Fadda G, Gupta PK, Livolsi VA, Baloch Z. Does the fine-needle aspiration diagnosis of "Hürthle-cell neoplasm/follicular neoplasm with oncocytic features" denote increased risk of malignancy? Diagn Cytopathol. 2004;31:307–12.
13. Haugen BR, Alexander EK, Bible KC, Doherty GM, Mandel SJ, Nikiforov YE, et al. 2015 American Thyroid Association Management Guidelines for adult patients with thyroid nodules and differentiated thyroid cancer: the American Thyroid Association Guidelines Task Force on thyroid nodules and differentiated thyroid cancer. Thyroid. 2016;26:1–133. https://doi.org/10.1089/thy.2015.0020.
14. Hoda RS. Non-gynecologic cytology on liquid-based preparations: a morphologic review of facts and artifacts. Diagn Cytopathol. 2007;35:621–34.
15. Hoda RS, VandenBussche C, Hoda SA. Diagnostic liquid-based cytology. New York: Springer; 2017.
16. Jung CK, Lee A, Jung ES, Choi YJ, Jung SL, Lee KY. Split sample comparison of a liquid-based method and conventional smears in thyroid fine needle aspiration. Acta Cytol. 2008;52:313–9.
17. Kasper KA, Stewart J 3rd, Das K. Fine-needle aspiration cytology of thyroid nodules with Hürthle cells: cytomorphologic predictors for neoplasms, improving diagnostic accuracy and overcoming pitfalls. Acta Cytol. 2014;58:145–52. https://doi.org/10.1159/000358264.
18. Lloyd R, Osamura R, Klöppel G, Rosai J. WHO classification of tumours of endocrine organs. Lyon: International Agency for Research on Cancer; 2017.
19. Malle D, Valeri RM, Pazaitou-Panajiotou K, Kiziridou A, Vainas I, Destouni C. Use of a thin-layer technique in thyroid fine needle aspiration. Acta Cytol. 2006;50:23–7.

20. Máximo V, Lima J, Prazeres H, Soares P, Sobrinho-Simões M. The biology and the genetics of Hürthle cell tumors of the thyroid. Endocr Relat Cancer. 2012;19:R131–47. https://doi.org/10.1530/ERC-11-0354.
21. Mete O, Asa SL. Oncocytes, oxyphils, Hürthle, and Askanazy cells: morphological and molecular features of oncocytic thyroid nodules. Endocr Pathol. 2010;21:16–24. https://doi.org/10.1007/s12022-009-9102-2.
22. Nikiforov YE, Biddinger PW, Thompson LDR. Diagnostic pathology and molecular genetics of the thyroid: a comprehensive guide for practicing thyroid pathology. 3rd ed. Philadelphia: Wolters Kluwer/Lippincott Williams & Wilkins; 2019.
23. Pearlstein S, Lahouti AH, Opher E, Nikiforov YE, Kuriloff DB. Thyroseq V3 molecular profiling for tailoring the surgical management of Hürthle cell neoplasms. Case Rep Endocrinol. 2018;2018:9329035. https://doi.org/10.1155/2018/9329035.
24. Rekhtman N, Buonocore DJ, Rudomina D, Friedlander M, Dsouza C, Aggarwal G, et al. Novel modification of HistoGel-based cell block preparation method: improved sufficiency for molecular studies. Arch Pathol Lab Med. 2018;142:529–35. https://doi.org/10.5858/arpa.2017-0030-OA.
25. Renshaw AA. Hürthle cell carcinoma is a better gold standard than Hürthle cell neoplasm for fine-needle aspiration of the thyroid: defining more consistent and specific cytologic criteria. Cancer. 2002;96:261–6.
26. Rossi ED, Martini M, Straccia P, Raffaelli M, Pennacchia I, Marrucci E, et al. The cytologic category of oncocytic (Hürthle) cell neoplasm mostly includes low-risk lesions at histology: an institutional experience. Eur J Endocrinol. 2013;169:649–55. https://doi.org/10.1530/EJE-13-0431.
27. Rossi ED, Zannoni GF, Moncelsi S, Stigliano E, Santeusanio G, Lombardi CP, et al. Application of liquid-based cytology to fine-needle aspiration biopsies of the thyroid gland. Front Endocrinol (Lausanne). 2012;3:57. https://doi.org/10.3389/fendo.2012.00057.
28. Sobrinho-Simões M, Máximo V, Castro IV, Fonseca E, Soares P, Garcia-Rostan G, et al. Hürthle (oncocytic) cell tumors of thyroid: etiopathogenesis, diagnosis and clinical significance. Int J Surg Pathol. 2005;13:29–35.
29. Tuzun D, Ersoy R, Yazgan AK, Kiyak G, Yalcin S, Cakir B. Cytomorphologic features and ultrasonographic characteristics of thyroid nodules with Hürthle cells. Ann Diagn Pathol. 2015;19:175–9. https://doi.org/10.1016/j.anndiagpath.2015.03.002.

8 Suspicious for Malignancy

Rana S. Hoda, Rema Rao, and Theresa Scognamiglio

Introduction

- The majority of thyroid nodules are benign, but a small percentage, about 10–15%, are malignant. According to The Bethesda System for Reporting Thyroid Cytopathology (TBSRTC), 3% of all thyroid fine needle aspiration (FNA) specimens are classified as Suspicious for Malignancy (SM).
- Ultrasound (US) and cytopathology are the two initial modalities in the assessment of the thyroid nodule.
- FNA of the thyroid is the most important test to determine whether a thyroid nodule that is suspicious on US is benign or malignant. A review by Jackson [11] reported sensitivity of 89–98% and specificity of 92%.
- Molecular tests can be performed in suspicious thyroid nodules to assist in the preoperative clinical decision making, for selection of the most appropriate surgical management.
- Diagnosis of "Suspicious for Malignancy (SM)" is included in the indeterminate category of TBSRTC. Other entities in this category include Atypia of Undetermined Significance or Follicular Lesion of Undetermined Significance (AUS/FLUS, Chap. 5), Follicular Neoplasm or Suspicious for a Follicular Neoplasm (FN/SFN, Chap. 6), and Follicular Neoplasms of Hürthle Cell Type (FNHCT/SFNHCT, Chap. 7).
- The category of SM is used mainly for cases with features that are not quantitatively or qualitatively sufficient to make a definitive diagnosis of malignancy.
- SM is applied mainly to cases that are suspicious for papillary thyroid carcinoma (PTC), which have subtle nuclear and architectural changes of PTC such as enlarged, irregular nuclei with grooves and fine, pale chromatin with clearing. Intranuclear pseudoinclusions (INPI) are scarce or absent, and papillary structures with fibrovascular cores and psammoma bodies are absent.
- Other cases in the SM category include those with features suggestive of medullary thyroid carcinoma (MTC), lymphoma, or malignancy not otherwise specified (NOS).
- Cases diagnosed cytologically as SM can be triaged to molecular testing for more diagnostic information.
- Management is usually a conservative resection, such as a lobectomy. A more extensive surgical procedure may be undertaken if molecular tests show a high-risk mutation such as *BRAF*V600E, seen in PTC.
- If lymphoma is suspected, repeat FNA is recommended for flow cytometry, and needle core biopsy to determine the type of lymphoma, in order to select the proper management.

TBSRTC Definition of Suspicious for Malignancy (SM)

- TBSRTC defines "Suspicious for Malignancy (SM)" to be used when cytologic features (most often of PTC) raise a strong suspicion of malignancy but the findings are not sufficient for a conclusive diagnosis. Cases suspicious for a follicular or Hürthle cell neoplasm are excluded from this category. Cases diagnosed as SM are more likely to be malignant.

R. S. Hoda (✉)
CBLPath, Rye Brook, NY, USA
e-mail: rhoda@cblpath.com

R. Rao · T. Scognamiglio
Department of Pathology and Laboratory Medicine, New York Presbyterian Hospital, Weill Cornell Medical College, New York, NY, USA
e-mail: rer9052@med.cornell.edu; ths9004@med.cornell.edu

R. S. Hoda et al. (eds.), *Atlas of Thyroid Cytopathology on Liquid-Based Preparations*,
https://doi.org/10.1007/978-3-030-25066-9_8

Updates in TBSRTC for SM

- SM has an implied risk of malignancy (ROM) of 45–60% if noninvasive follicular thyroid neoplasm with papillary-like nuclear features (NIFTP) is not considered as cancer; if it is, the ROM is 50–75%.
- The positive predictive value (PPV) of an SM diagnosis is 70%.
- Because the risk of malignancy in the SM category is high, the distinction between SM and the "Malignant" category may not be of much clinical significance. Most patients are managed by total thyroidectomy. Preoperative molecular testing may be helpful in identifying high-risk mutations.

Differential Diagnosis of SM

- Table 8.1 lists the of SM:
  - PTC

Table 8.1 Suspicious for malignancy category: differential diagnosis on liquid-based preparations (LBP)

Diagnosis	Cytological features on LBP	Distinguishing features for differential diagnosis	Molecular findings	Management
A. Suspicious for PTC (classic)	Review the 4 TBSRTC-described patterns for this category. Most nuclear features of PTC are present, with few INPI. Papillary structures and psammoma bodies are absent.		*BRAF*V600E mutation, *RET/PTC* 1 and 3 gene rearrangement	Lobectomy/total thyroidectomy[a]
1. DDX: Hashimoto thyroiditis (CLT)	Follicular/Hürthle cells with lymphocytes, plasma cells, and lymphohistiocytic aggregates. PTC-like nuclear atypia (including focal enlargement, grooves, and chromatin clearing) may be seen.	Focal nuclear changes of PTC; prominence of nucleoli. Serum antibodies against thyroid-specific antigens.	Molecular findings of PTC are absent.	Observation or treated by thyroid hormone replacement
2. DDX: Hyperplastic nodule	Smaller, darker nuclei; prominent nucleoli; grooves; rare INPI. Papillary structures are few, short, with fewer ramifications, and are mixed with benign macrofollicles and microfollicles, brown pigment in cytoplasm, background of a cyst (abundant watery colloid & macrophages).	History of Graves' disease; smaller, darker nuclei; prominent nucleoli, no other atypia, cytologic variation, abundant thin colloid	Molecular findings of PTC are absent.	
3. DDX: Hyalinizing trabecular adenoma (HTA)	Usually many nuclear features of PTC, including grooves and many INPI. Trabecular pattern and intracellular hyaline material is present.	Cytoplasmic staining with MIB-1 immunostain, unlike typical nuclear staining	*RET/PTC1* gene rearrangement	Lobectomy
B. Suspicious for cystic PTC	Hypocellular specimen with blood, foamy and hemosiderin-laden macrophages, epithelial cells with nuclear features of PTC, atypical histiocytoid cell clusters with abundant dense or vacuolated cytoplasm and scalloped borders, epithelioid giant cells with dense cytoplasm and rare psammoma bodies		Mutations present	Lobectomy/total thyroidectomy[a]
1. DDX: Normal cyst- lining cells	Reparative, stretched-out/streaming 2-D cohesive sheets of spindled or polygonal polarized cells with distinct borders, mildly enlarged pale nuclei with smooth contours, grooves, moderate to dense granular cytoplasm, associated hemosiderin-laden macrophages and benign follicular cells	Patchy changes, elongated or spindled nuclei, large nucleoli, associated benign follicular cells	Molecular findings of PTC are absent.	Observation
C. Suspicious for MTC	Low cellularity or poorly preserved specimen with mostly singly dispersed, small spindled cells with spindled or oval eccentric nuclei. Background amyloid may be present. Immunostain positive for calcitonin and chromogranin, negative for thyroglobulin.		*RET* mutation	Total thyroidectomy and cervical lymph node dissection, if proven
Suspicious for lymphoma	Low cellularity or poorly preserved specimen with mostly singly dispersed small, round cells with irregular round, central or eccentric nuclei, small nucleoli. Background lymphoglandular bodies may be present. Immunostain positive for LCA and negative for thyroglobulin.		Mutations of thyroid neoplasia absent	Flow cytometry, incisional biopsy for typing and pertinent treatment

CLT chronic lymphocytic thyroiditis, *DDX* differential diagnosis, *PTC* papillary thyroid carcinoma

[a]Usual management is lobectomy, but total thyroidectomy may be performed if molecular test shows a high-risk mutation such as *BRAF*V600E

- MTC
- Lymphoma
- Metastatic malignancy
- Other malignant tumors, NOS

Cytologic Features of PTC

- High cellularity with cells arranged in syncytial fragments, cellular swirls, papillary fragments
- Nuclear features of enlargement, intranuclear pseudoinclusions, grooves, molding, nucleoli, and chromatin pallor and clearing.
- Liquid-based preparations (LBP) easily display all the architectural and nuclear features of PTC.

TBSRTC Criteria for Diagnosis of SM and Application in LBP

Suspicious for PTC

- TBSRTC has put forth four cytological patterns, A–D, for cases suspicious for PTC.
- These patterns were described on conventional smears but are applicable to LBP.
  - *Pattern A (Patchy nuclear changes of PTC)*: Specimens are of moderate or high cellularity with cells arranged in macrofollicles and display patchy nuclear changes of PTC including, enlargement, pallor, grooves, membrane irregularity, molding, and few or no INPI. Papillary structures and psammoma bodies are not present (Figs. 8.1a–e, 8.2a–c, and 8.3).
  - *Pattern B (Incomplete nuclear changes of PTC)*: Specimens are of moderate or high cellularity with generalized but incomplete nuclear changes of PTC, including mild to moderate enlargement, mild pallor, grooves, and few or no INPI. Nuclear membrane irregularity and molding, papillary structures, and psammoma bodies are not present (Figs. 8.4a–h and 8.5a–d).
  - *Pattern C (Sparse cellularity with nuclear changes of PTC)*: Specimens show many nuclear changes of PTC, but the specimen is of sparse cellularity (Figs. 8.6a, b and 8.7).
  - *Pattern D (Cystic degeneration)*: Cases show cystic degeneration with hemosiderin-laden macrophages, some nuclear features of PTC, few or absent INPI, occasional atypical "histiocytoid" cells, and no papillary structures or psammoma bodies (Figs. 8.8a–d and 8.9a, b).

Suspicious for MTC

- Specimens are sparsely or moderately cellular; they quantitatively or qualitatively fall short of a definitive diagnosis of MTC:
  - Singly dispersed, small to medium-sized monomorphic cells with eccentric round to oval nuclei and a high nuclear-cytoplasmic (N:C) ratio. Cellular and nuclear morphology may be poorly preserved.
  - Because the specimens have low cellularity, there may not be enough sample for ancillary immunocytochemical or immunohistochemical (ICC/IHC) studies.
  - If LBP are used, an attempt can be made to process additional LBP slides for immunocytochemistry (ICC), but only if the laboratory has validated ICC on LBP as per the guidelines of the College of American Pathologists (CAP) [13].
- All diagnostic criteria seen in conventional smears (CS) are evident in LBP with subtle differences (Figs. 8.10, 8.11, and 8.12).

Suspicious for Lymphoma

- Specimens are sparsely or moderately cellular; they quantitatively or qualitatively fall short of a definitive diagnosis of lymphoma:
  - Singly dispersed, small to medium-sized, monomorphic, atypical lymphoid cells with round to irregular

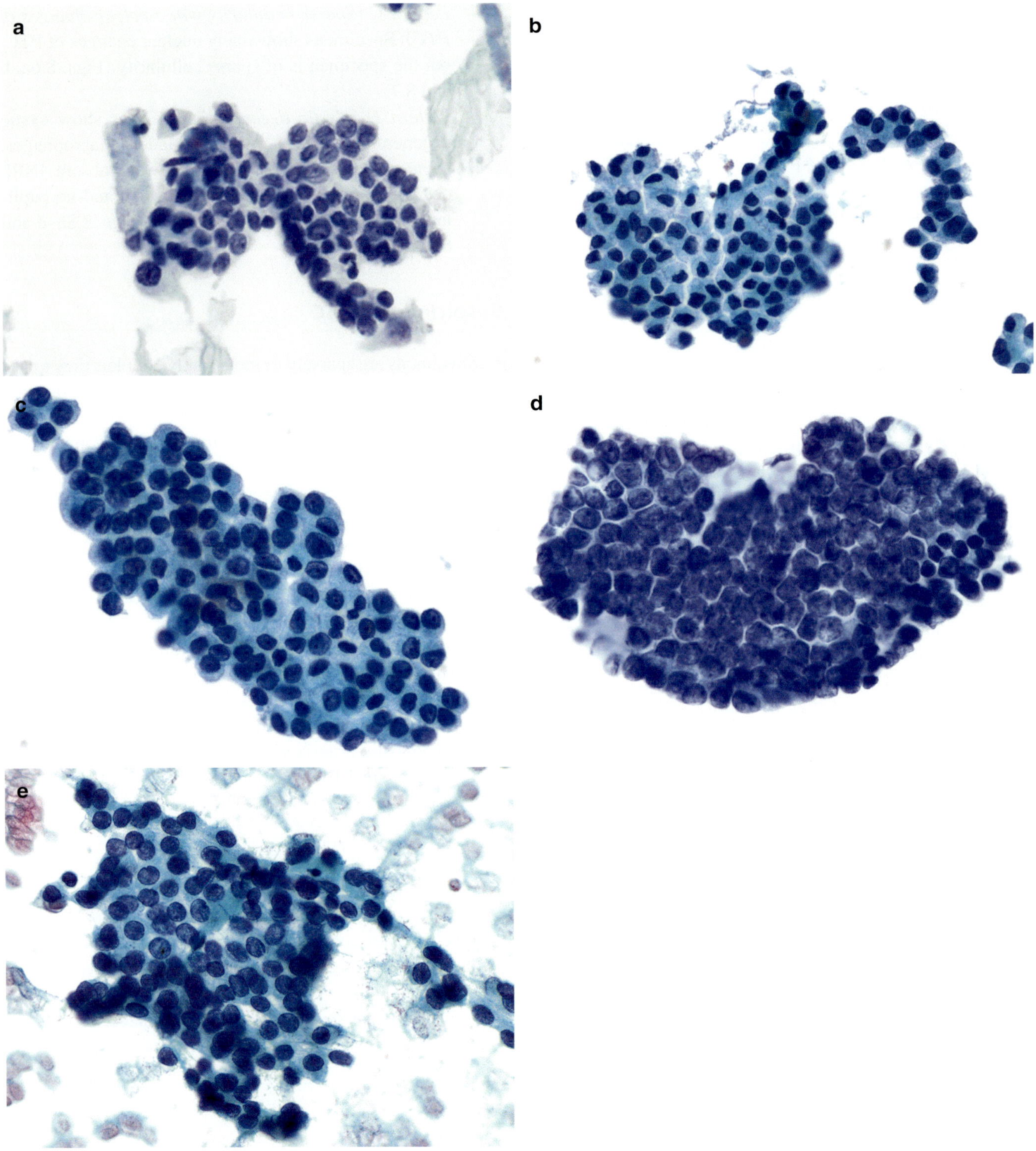

Fig. 8.1 Suspicious for papillary thyroid carcinoma (PTC): patchy nuclear changes of PTC in ThinPrep® (TP) (TBSRTC Pattern A). In all these four separate cases, nuclear features of PTC were patchy and intermixed with benign follicular cells. All were submitted for molecular testing, which showed *BRAF*V600E mutations. Subsequent total thyroidectomy found classic PTC. (**a**) This irregular sheet shows all nuclear features of PTC (except intranuclear pseudoinclusions [INPI]), including enlargement, membrane irregularity, grooves, chromatin clearing, "powdery chromatin," and small nucleoli. (**b**) This sheet shows all nuclear features of PTC, including one well-formed INPI. (**c**) This sheet shows all nuclear features of PTC, with a suggestion of INPI in the center of the field. (**d**) This sheet shows all nuclear features of PTC, including nuclear molding. One poorly-formed INPI is noted at the 11 o'clock position. (**a**–**d** Pap stain, TP) **e**, Conventional smear (CS) preparation (Pap stain) from the case seen in **a**. Note similar cytology

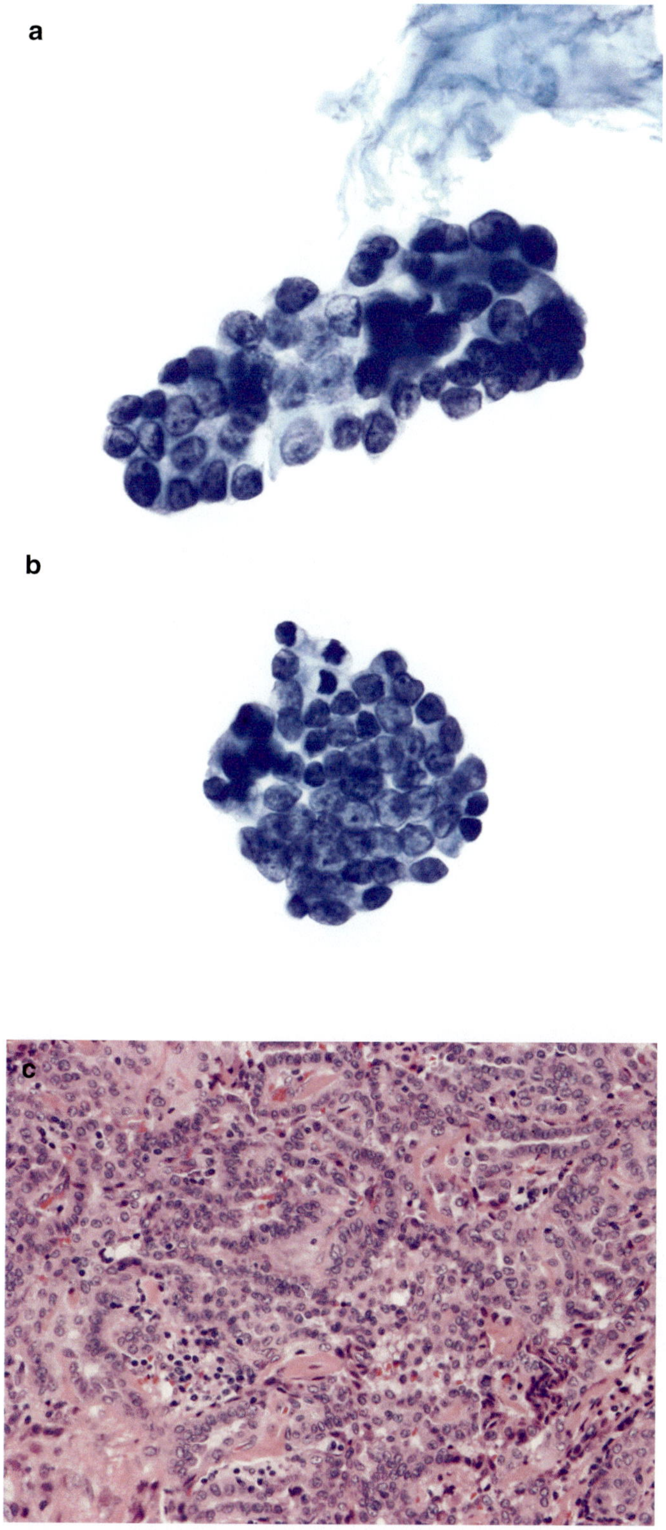

Fig. 8.2 Suspicious for PTC: patchy nuclear changes of PTC in ThinPrep® (TBSRTC Pattern A). (**a**, **b**) This nodule showed patchy nuclear features of PTC including enlargement, molding, membrane irregularity, grooves, chromatin clearing, "powdery chromatin," and small nucleoli. No INPI were noted (Pap stain, TP). (**c**) Histologic section shows classic PTC (H&E stain)

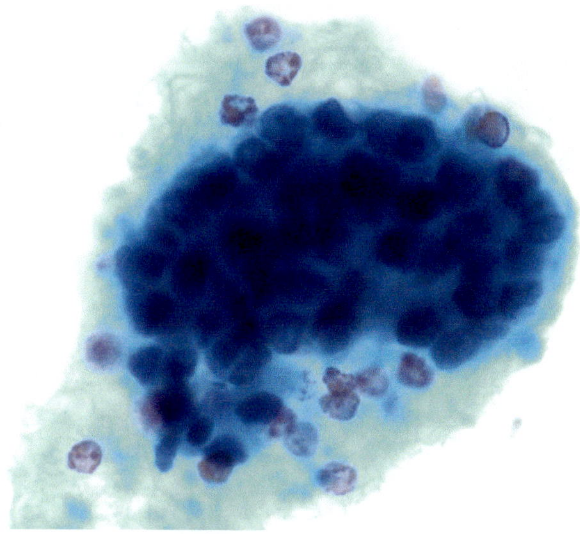

Fig. 8.3 Suspicious for PTC: patchy nuclear changes of PTC in SurePath™ (SP) (TBSRTC Pattern A). This macrofollicular sheet shows all nuclear features of PTC except INPI, including enlargement, molding, membrane irregularity, grooves, chromatin clearing, "powdery chromatin," and small nucleoli. Note the more three-dimensional (3-D) appearance in SP (Pap stain)

nuclei, nucleoli, and a high N:C ratio. Cellular and nuclear morphology may be poorly preserved.
  - Rarely, lymphocytes in a case of lymphocytic thyroiditis may be deemed atypical.
  - Since the specimens have low cellularity, there may not be enough sample for ancillary ICC/IHC studies.
  - If LBP are used, an attempt can be made to process additional LBP slides for ICC, but only if the laboratory has validated ICC on LBP as per CAP guidelines [13].
  - Repeat FNA to collect a sample for flow cytometry can be recommended.
- All diagnostic criteria seen in CS are evident in LBP with subtle differences (Figs. 8.13a–e and 8.14a–c).

Suspicious for Metastatic Malignancy

- Tumors of breast, kidney, melanoma, and lymphoma may metastasize to the thyroid and may mimic primary thyroid malignancy. (*See* Chap. 11.)
- Metastatic tumor can be suspected if cytological features and ICC/IHC do not corroborate a thyroid tumor.
- Usually, there is a clinical history of a nonthyroid malignancy.
- Review of the prior primary and pertinent ICC/IHC can be performed on additional LBP for confirmation of primary versus metastatic tumor.

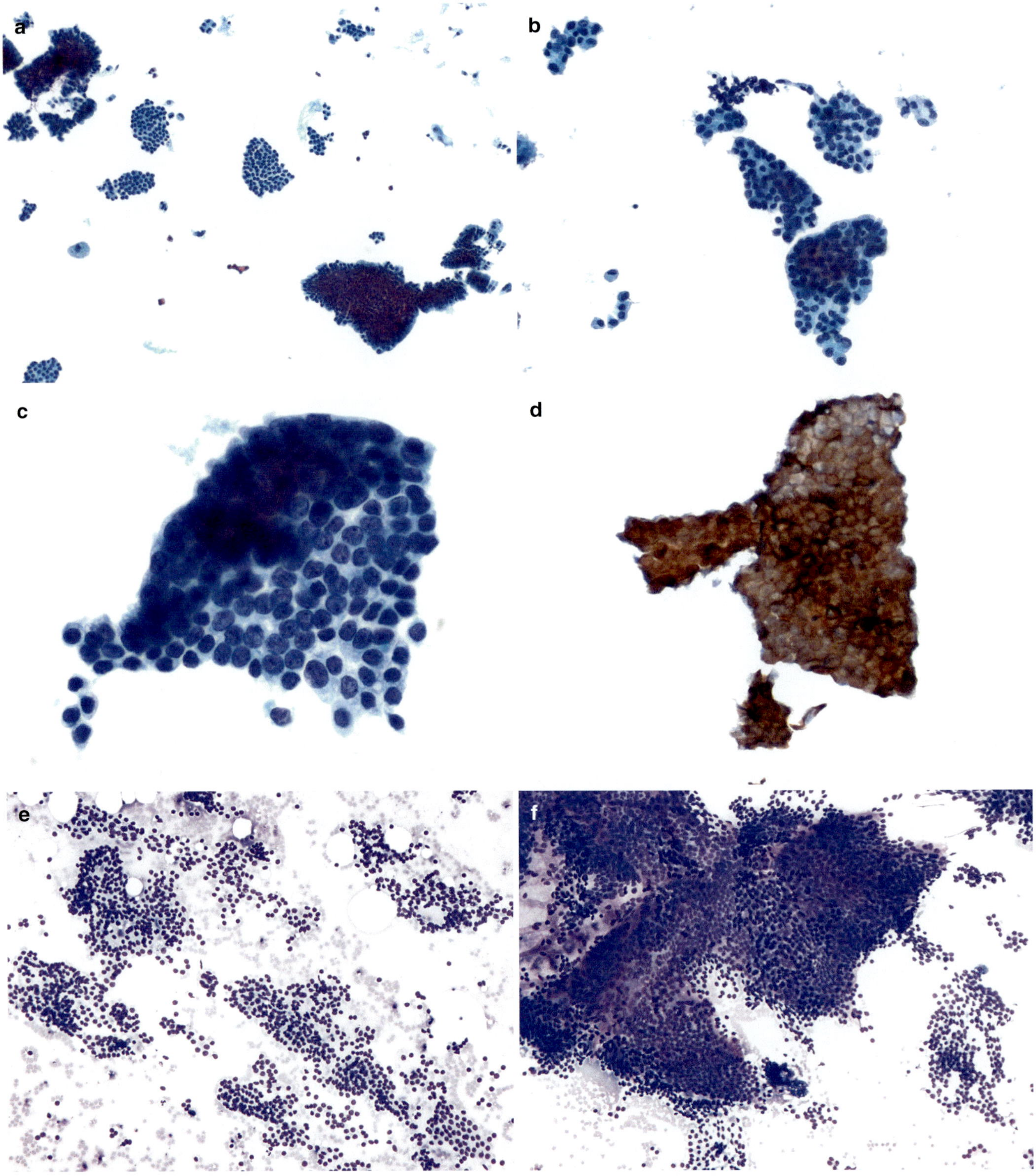

Fig. 8.4 Suspicious for PTC: incomplete nuclear changes of PTC in ThinPrep® (TBSRTC Pattern B). (**a–c**) The specimen was cellular and showed syncytia, papillae, and single cells with mild to moderate PTC-like atypia. Nuclear features included enlargement, grooves, chromatin clearing, "powdery chromatin," and small nucleoli. Membrane irregularity was mild and no INPI were noted (Pap stain, TP). (**d**) Immunostain for CK19 was strongly positive, and a diagnosis of suspicious for PTC was rendered (TP). (**e–g**) Diff-Quik (DQ) stain of CS on the same case show morphologic similarity. (**h**) Histologic section shows classic PTC (H&E stain)

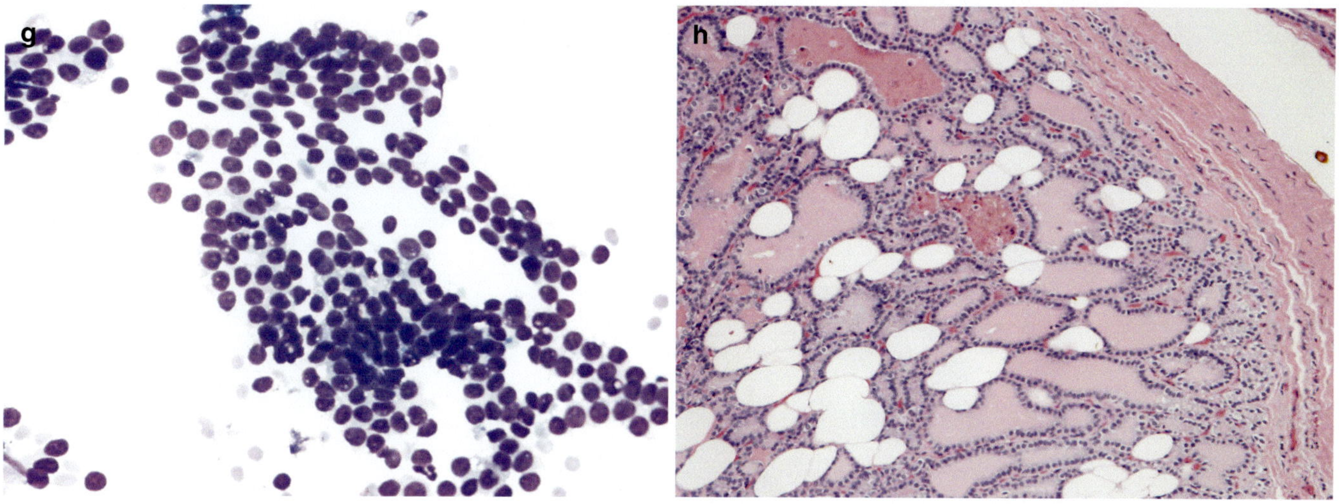

Fig. 8.4 (continued)

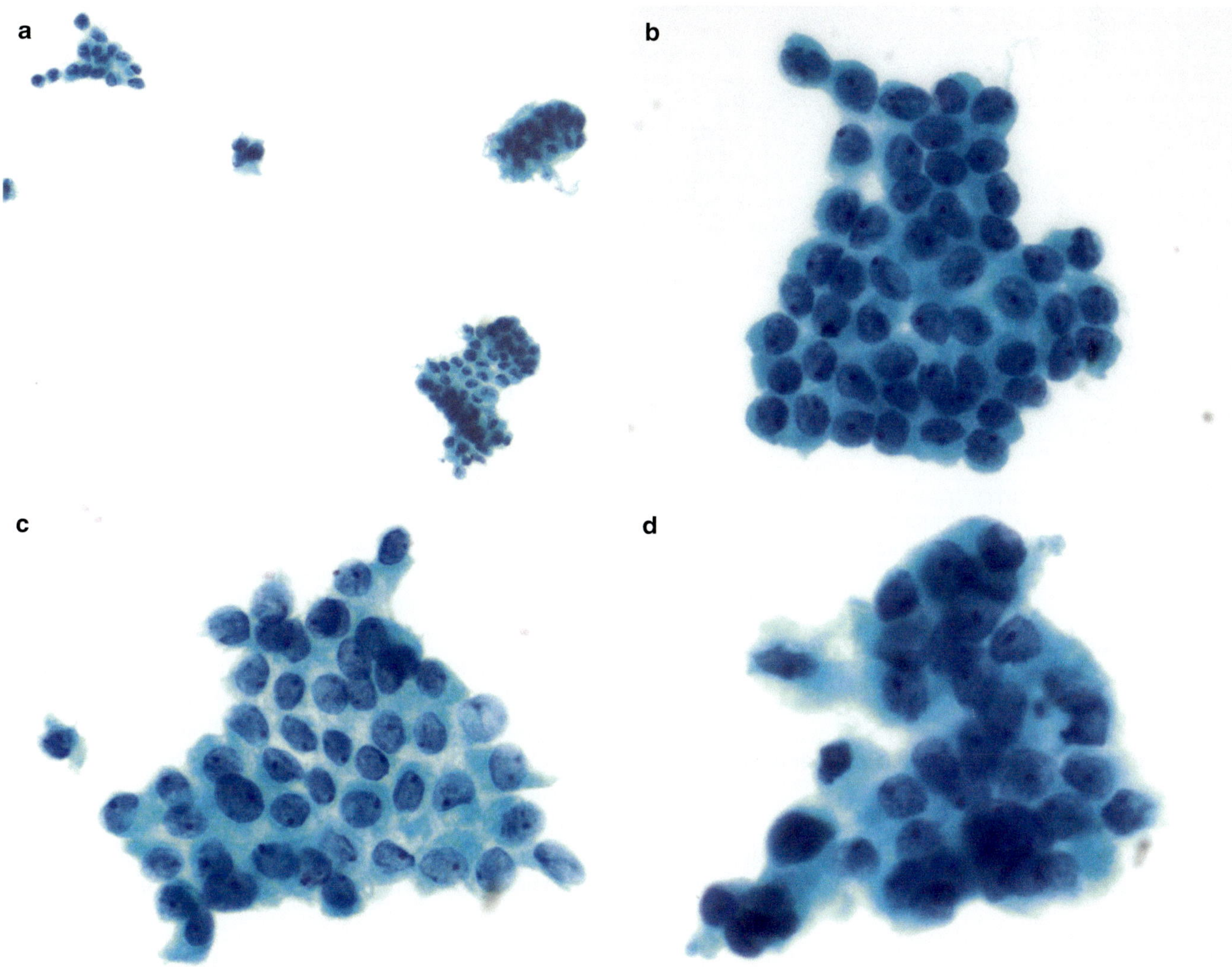

Fig. 8.5 Suspicious for PTC: incomplete nuclear changes of PTC in SurePath™ (TBSRTC Pattern B). (**a–d**) Specimen was moderately cellular and showed syncytia, papillae, and few single cells with mild to moderate PTC-like atypia. Nuclear features included enlargement, focal molding, grooves, chromatin clearing, "powdery chromatin," and small nucleoli. Membrane irregularity was mild and no INPI were noted (Pap stain, SP)

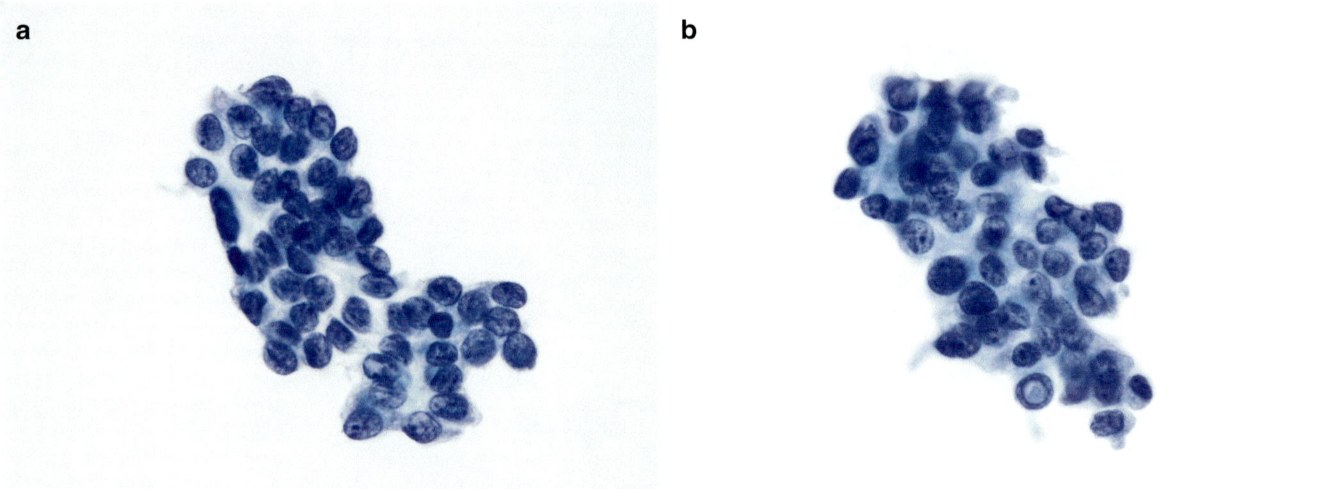

Fig. 8.6 Suspicious for PTC: sparse cellularity with most nuclear changes of PTC in ThinPrep® (TBSRTC Pattern C). (**a**, **b**) This specimen was sparsely cellular but displayed all nuclear features of PTC (Pap stain, TP)

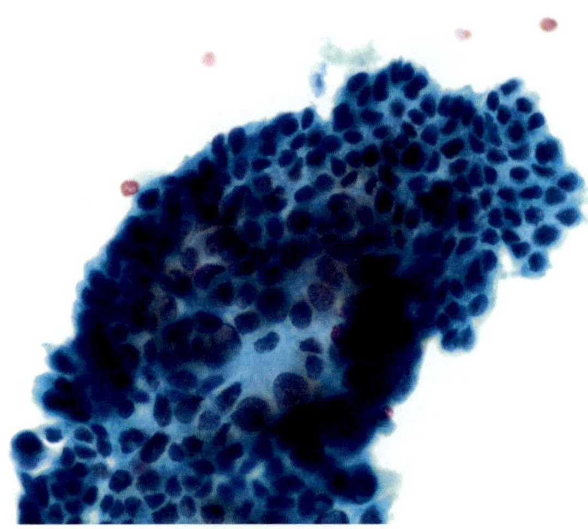

Fig. 8.7 Suspicious for PTC: sparse cellularity with most nuclear changes of PTC in SurePath™ (TBSRTC Pattern C). This specimen was sparsely cellular but displayed all nuclear features of PTC (Pap stain, SP)

- All diagnostic criteria seen in CS are evident in LBP with subtle differences.

Suspicious for Malignancy, Not Otherwise Specified (SM-NOS)

- SM-NOS is a category reserved for anaplastic or undifferentiated thyroid carcinoma or other tumors that cannot be categorized further because of an inability to perform immunostaining and/or molecular testing (Fig. 8.15a–f).

Salient Points for SM

- Yang et al. [20] studied the causes of cyto-histologic correlations and discrepancies. The overall discrepancy rate between cytology and histology was 15.3%. The most frequent cause of false-negative cytologic diagnoses was sample inadequacy. Cases of PTC that were false-negative were of inadequate or borderline cellularity. The new TBSRTC patterns for cases suspicious for PTC may help reduce the false-negative rate. The diagnosis of a benign thyroid lesion should be made only on adequate samples, but the presence of atypical cells or cellular patterns always should be addressed regardless of cellularity.
- In the same study, Yang et al. also indicated that cystic PTC is a cause for false-negative cytology diagnosis because of scant abnormal cells in a cystic background. The presence of clusters of epithelial cells with dense, squamous-like cytoplasm, enlarged nuclei containing multiple vacuoles (histiocytoid cells), a necrotic background, and papillary structures should suggest cystic PTC, especially in patients with lymph node metastasis.
- In the study by Yang et al. [20], the follicular variant of PTC (FVPTC) accounted for almost 68% of the malignancies that were diagnosed as a follicular neoplasm (FN)

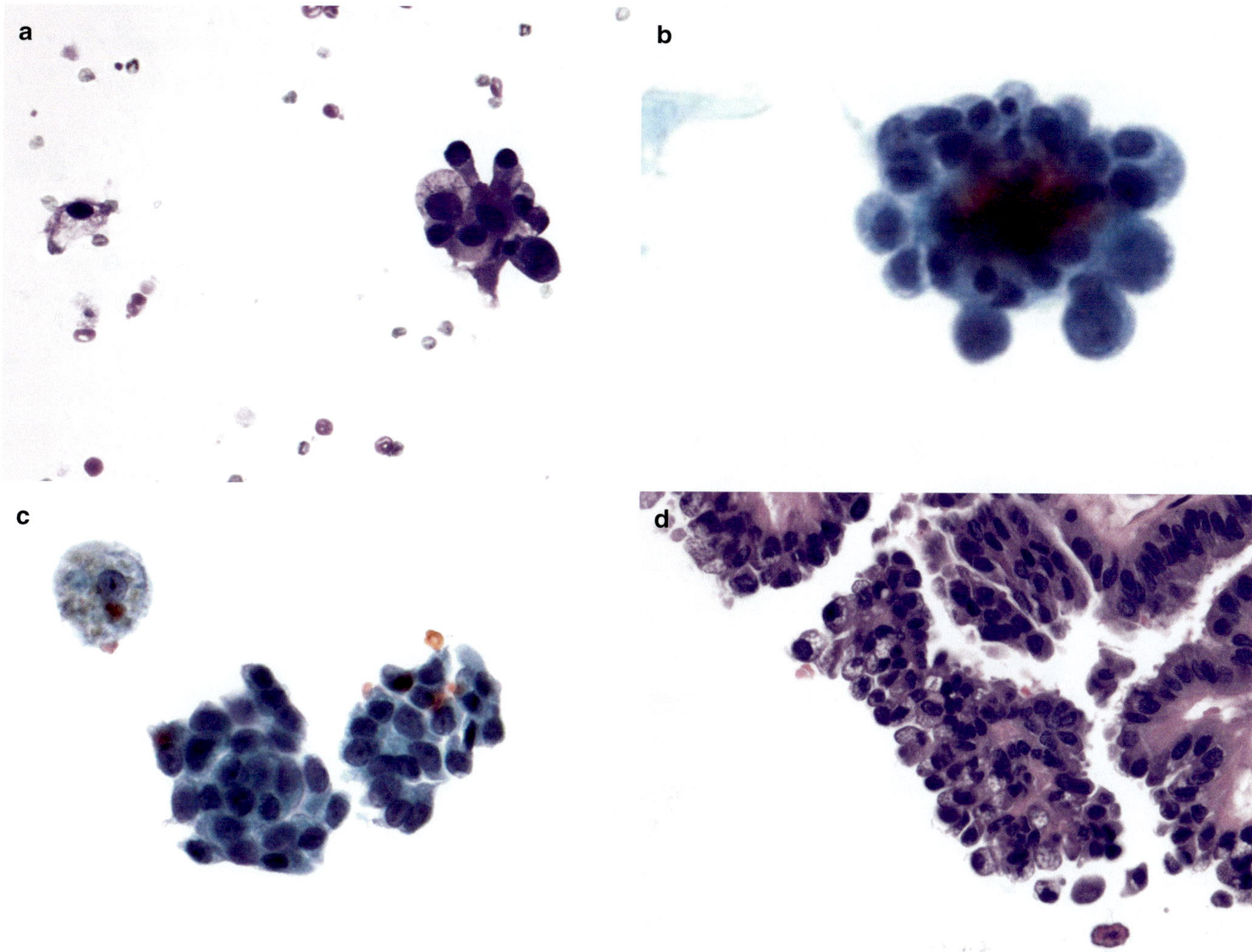

Fig. 8.8 Suspicious for PTC: changes of cystic degeneration in ThinPrep® (TBSRTC Pattern D). (**a**) DQ-stained CS shows a cystic background with hemosiderin-laden macrophage and a cluster of atypical "histiocytoid" cells with enlarged nuclei with occasional grooves and nucleoli and vacuolated cytoplasm. (**b**) In the same case, TP shows similar cytological features. Note the "histiocytoid" cell cluster with enlarged round nuclei, nucleoli, occasional grooves, and denser cytoplasm. (**c**) Less scalloped (histiocytoid) group with a macrophage in the background. Note well-preserved nuclear features suspicious for PTC (**b, c** Pap stain). (**d**) Histologic section shows intracystic PTC (H&E stain)

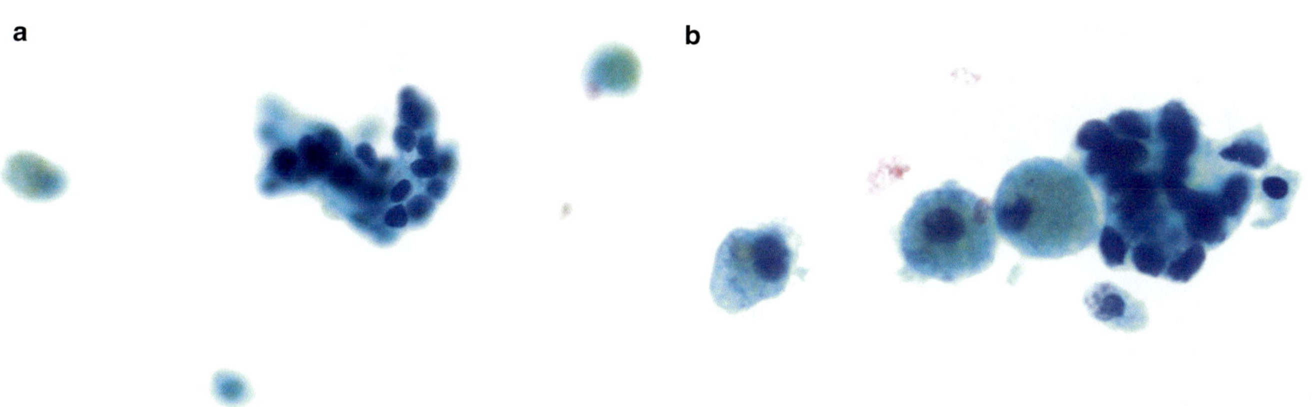

Fig. 8.9 Suspicious for PTC: changes of cystic degeneration in SurePath™ (TBSRTC Pattern D). (**a, b**) Pap-stained SP shows a cystic background with hemosiderin-laden macrophage and clusters of atypical cells with "histiocytoid cell-like" morphology. Nuclei were enlarged, with occasional grooves and nucleoli and vacuolated cytoplasm. Although the case has a more 3-D appearance, the nuclear changes of PTC as outlined above are evident (Pap stain)

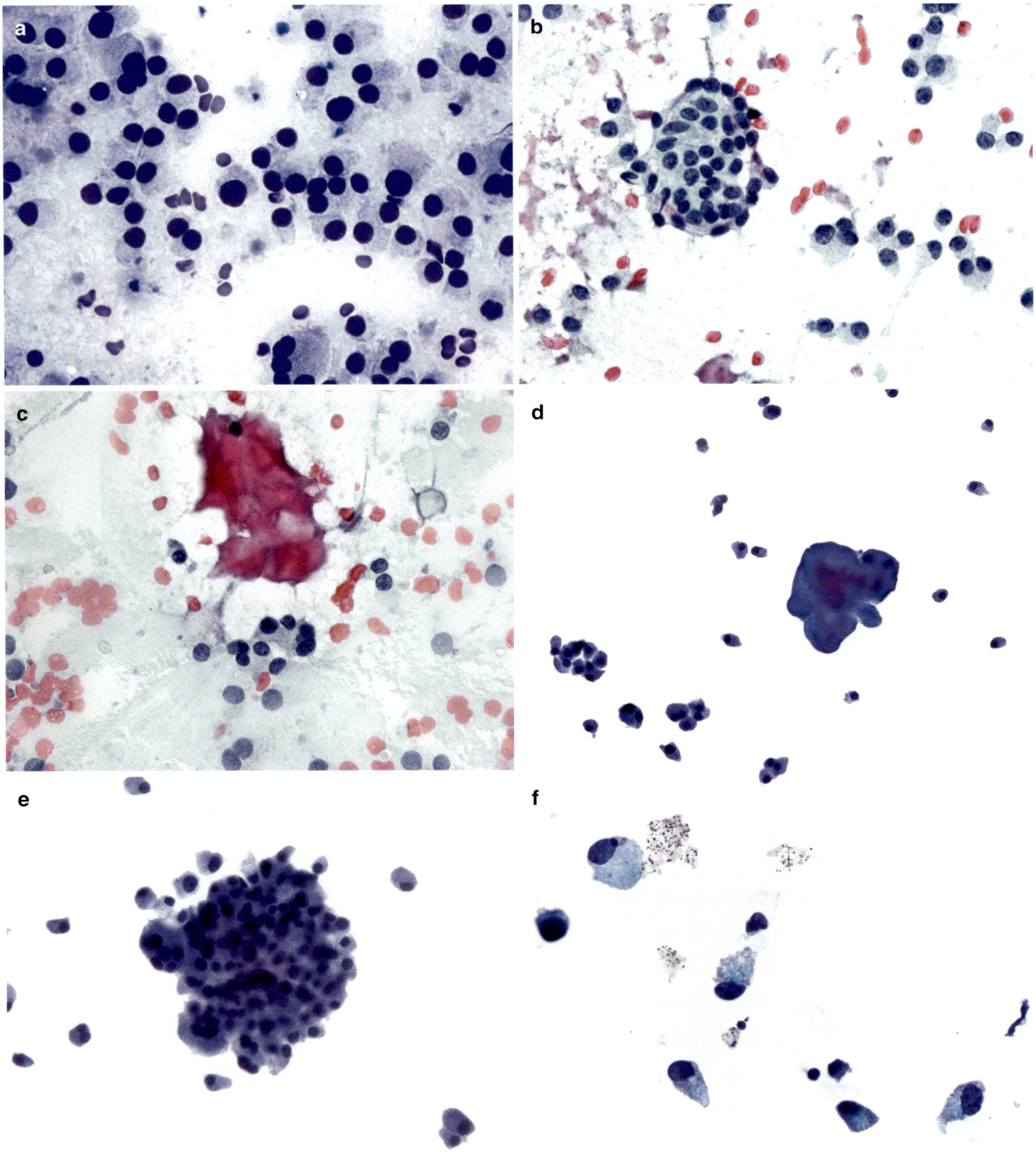

Fig. 8.10 Suspicious for medullary thyroid carcinoma (MTC) in ThinPrep®. (**a–c**) The foci shown in these CS were the only diagnostic cells. The smears show large, singly dispersed cells and a cluster of plasmacytoid cells (compare size with RBCs). Nuclei appear round and uniform with occasional nucleoli, which are more apparent in the Pap-stained CS (**b**, **c**). Almost all cells have retained their cytoplasm. Note the eosinophilic, acellular, amorphous thick colloid-like or amyloid-like material (**a** DQ stain, CS; **b**, **c** Pap stain, CS). (**d–g**) Pap-stained TP of the same case shows similar morphology. Note the more basophilic, acellular, amorphous thick colloid-like or amyloid-like material in **d**. The singly dispersed plasmacytoid cells were more prominent towards the periphery of the slide. Molecular test showed *RET* mutation. **h** The lobectomy showed a 2-cm firm tumor. (**i**) The tumor was histologically diagnosed as MTC (H&E stain)

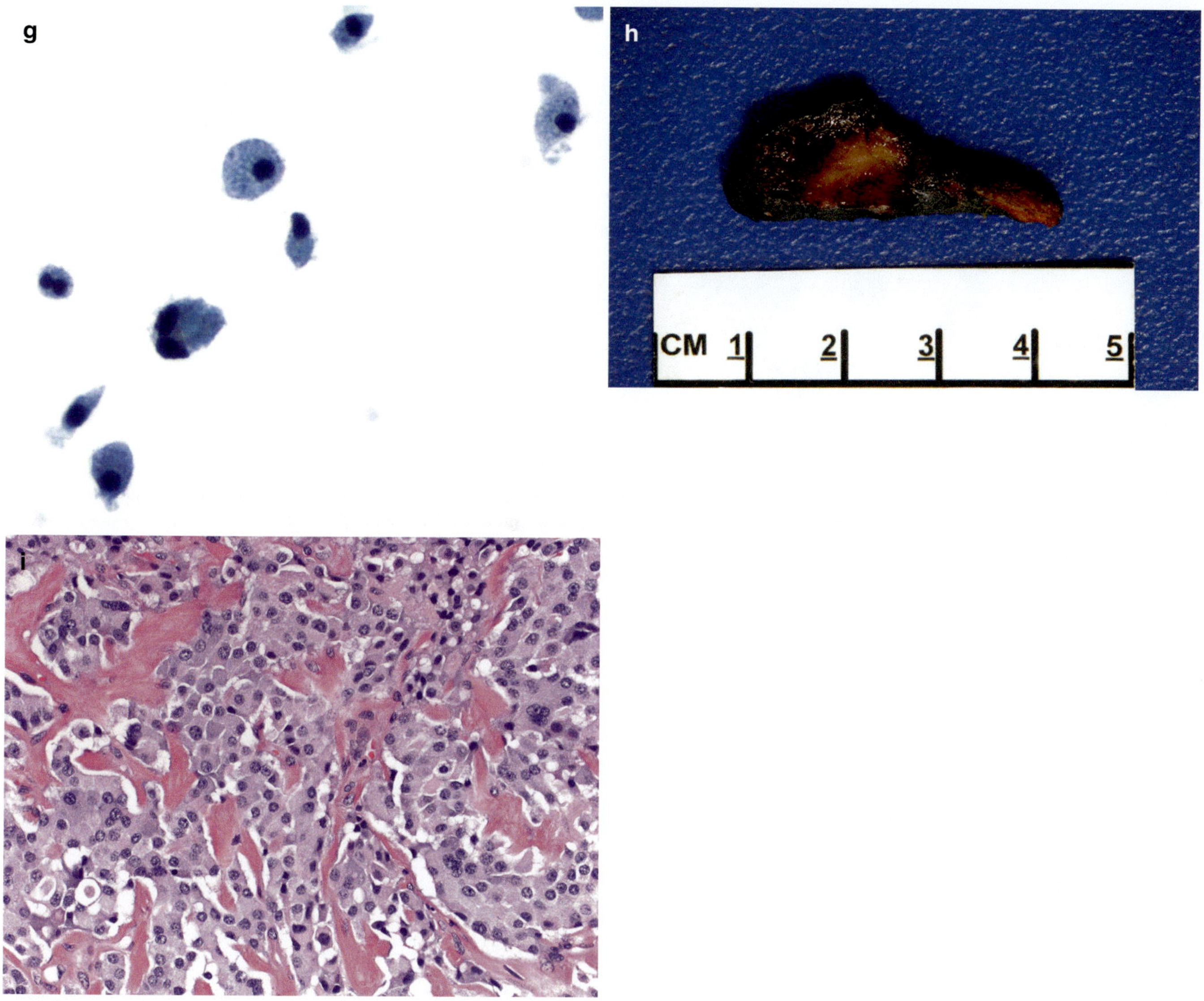

Fig. 8.10 (continued)

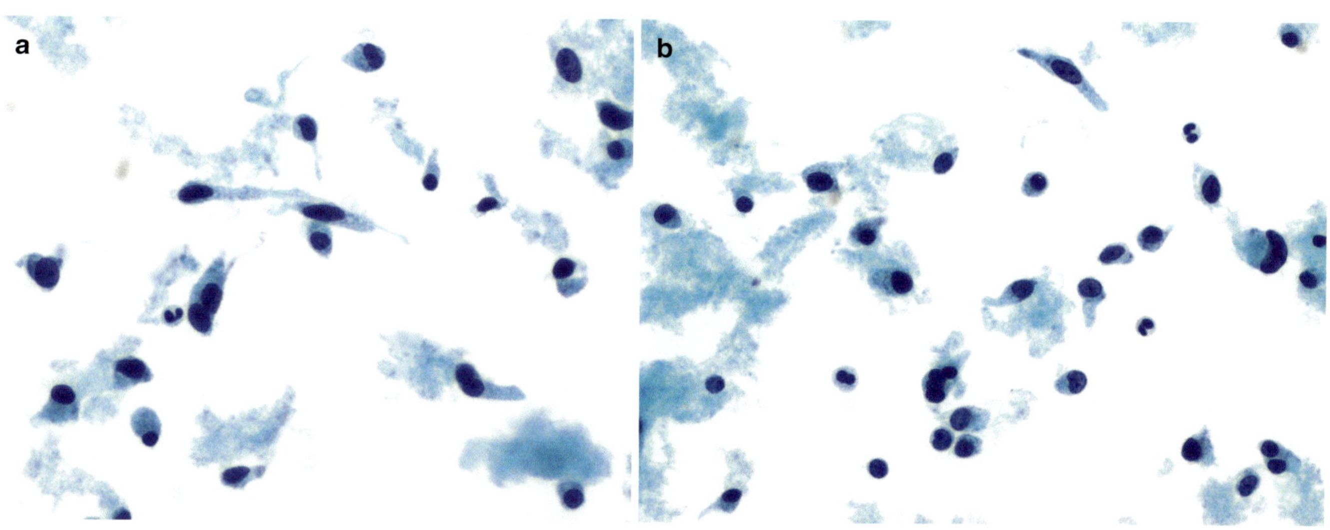

Fig. 8.11 Suspicious for MTC in ThinPrep®. (**a**, **b**) Another case suspicious for MTC processed with TP showed a sparsely cellular sample with singly -dispersed, spindled cells with spindled to round nuclei, small nucleoli, and occasional binucleation (Pap stain)

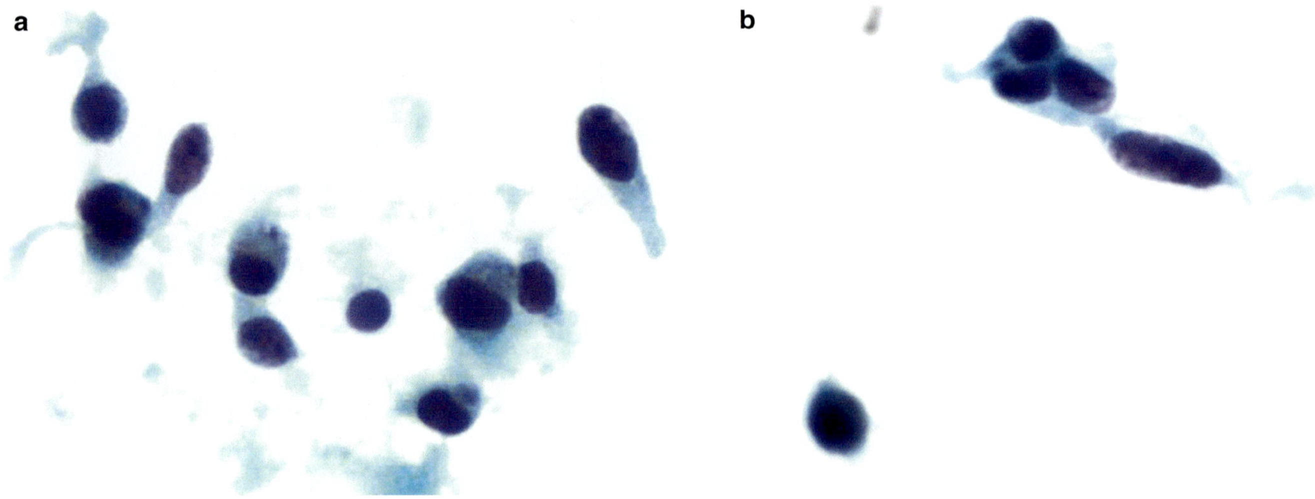

Fig. 8.12 Suspicious for MTC in SurePath™. (**a**, **b**) A case suspicious for MTC processed with SP showed a sparsely cellular sample with poorly preserved, enlarged, singly dispersed spindled cells with spindled to round nuclei, small nucleoli, and occasional binucleation (Pap stain)

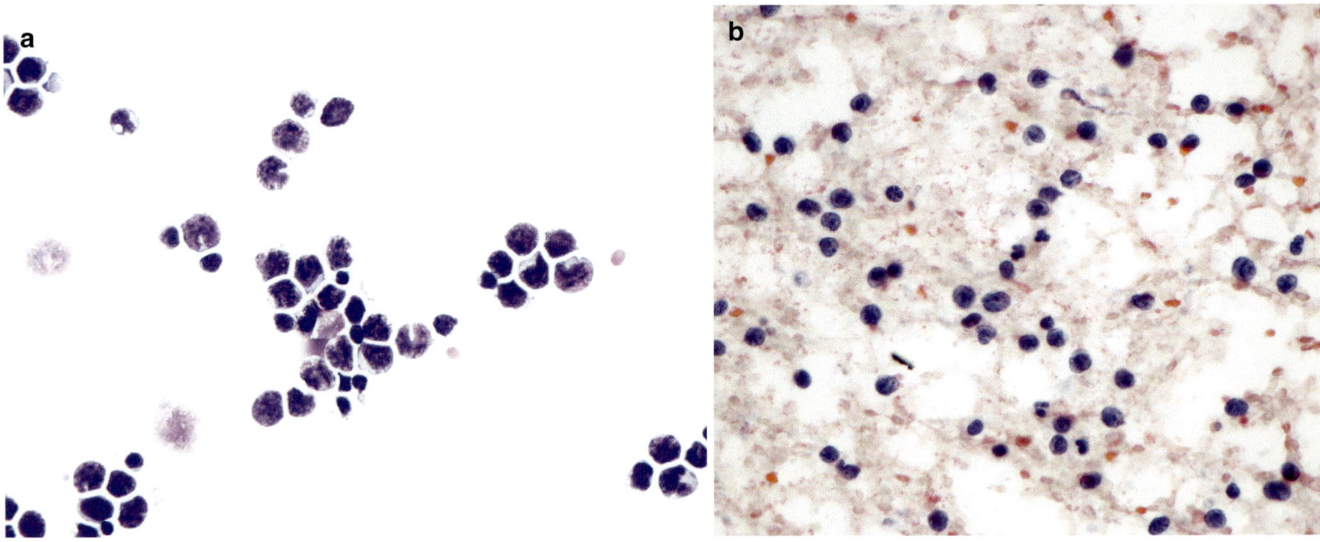

Fig. 8.13 Suspicious for lymphoma. (**a**, **b**) CS show a relatively monomorphic population of enlarged, atypical lymphoid cells (**a** DQ stain; **b** Pap stain). (**c**, **d**) The same case in TP shows predominantly large, atypical lymphoid cells with cleaved, irregular nuclei and few nucleoli. Note a few lymphoglandular bodies in the background. This case is suspicious for lymphoma (**c**, **d** Pap stain, TP). Repeat FNA for flow cytometry was performed and was interpreted as CD10-positive B-cell lymphoproliferative disorder with kappa light chain restriction, compatible with follicular lymphoma. (**e**) Needle core biopsy of the thyroid showed follicular lymphoma (H&E stain)

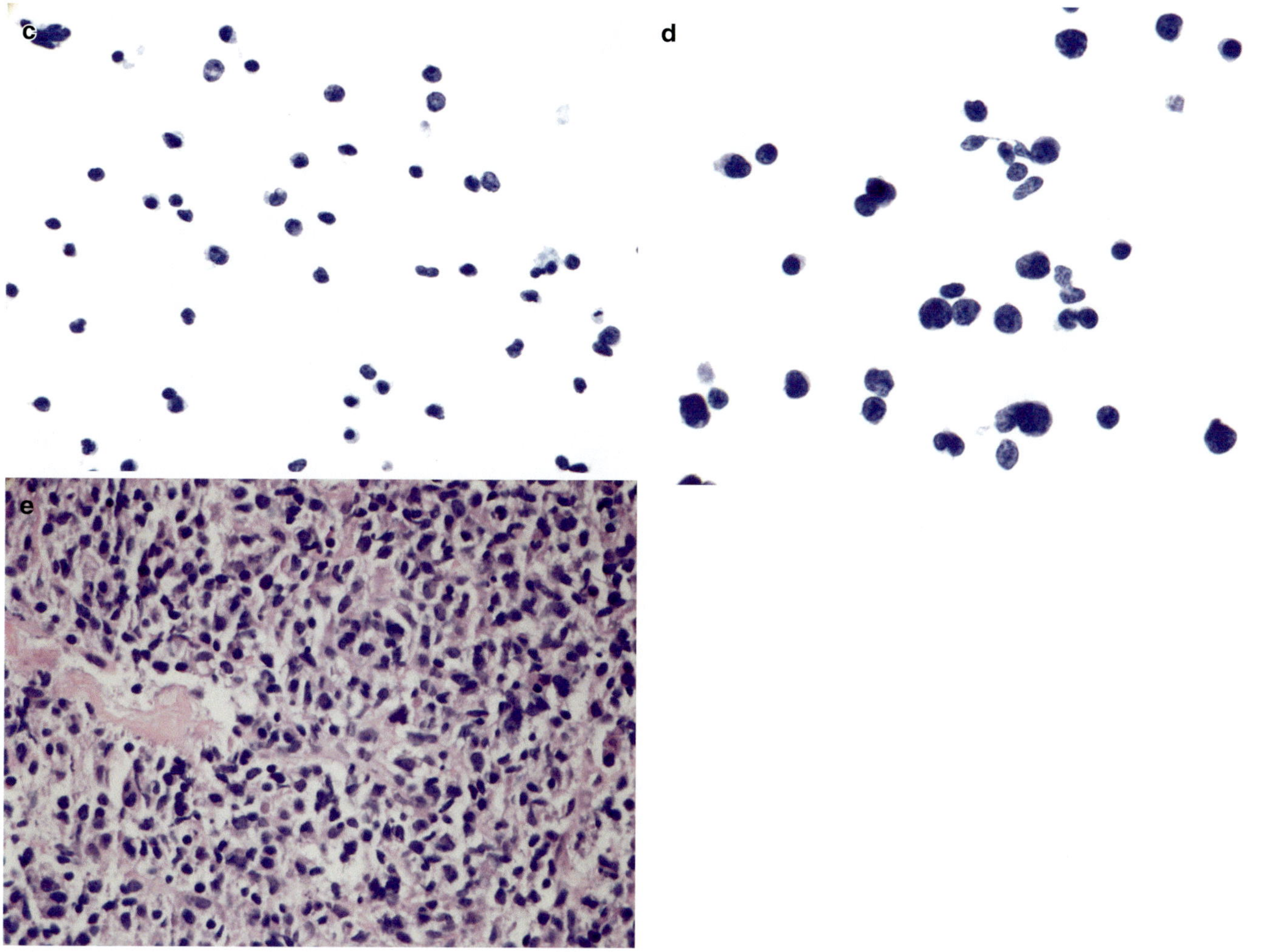

Fig. 8.13 (continued)

on FNA. An effort should be made to distinguish between FN and FVPTC, mainly by looking for nuclear features of PTC, which will be present in FVPTC. The distinction is important, as the management is lobectomy for FN but total thyroidectomy for FVPTC.

- In a study by Luu et al. [14], an SM diagnosis predicted cancer 67.9% of the time in the ThinPrep® (TP) group and 78.6% of the time in the CS group.

Ultrasound (US) Features of SM

- General high-risk US features include a solitary, solid, and hypoechoic nodule with microcalcifications, a taller-than-wide shape, irregular margins, increased intranodular vascularity, the absence of a "halo," and evidence of local invasion.
- In addition to high-risk US features, high-risk clinical parameters should also be considered before treatment options are selected:
  - Family medical history (genetic background), including family history of thyroid cancer
  - Age <20 or >70 years
  - Irradiation of the neck and head area (particularly in childhood)
  - Male gender
  - Rapid growth of nodule during follow-up
  - Nodule larger than 4 cm
  - Compression symptoms of hoarseness, dysphagia, and pain caused by a large tumor
  - Fixation of the nodule to surrounding tissue
  - Ipsilateral cervical lymphadenopathy
- Most clinical thyroid societies recommend that FNA should be performed on all thyroid nodules 1 cm or larger.

The Role of Molecular Tests

- SM is included in the indeterminate category.

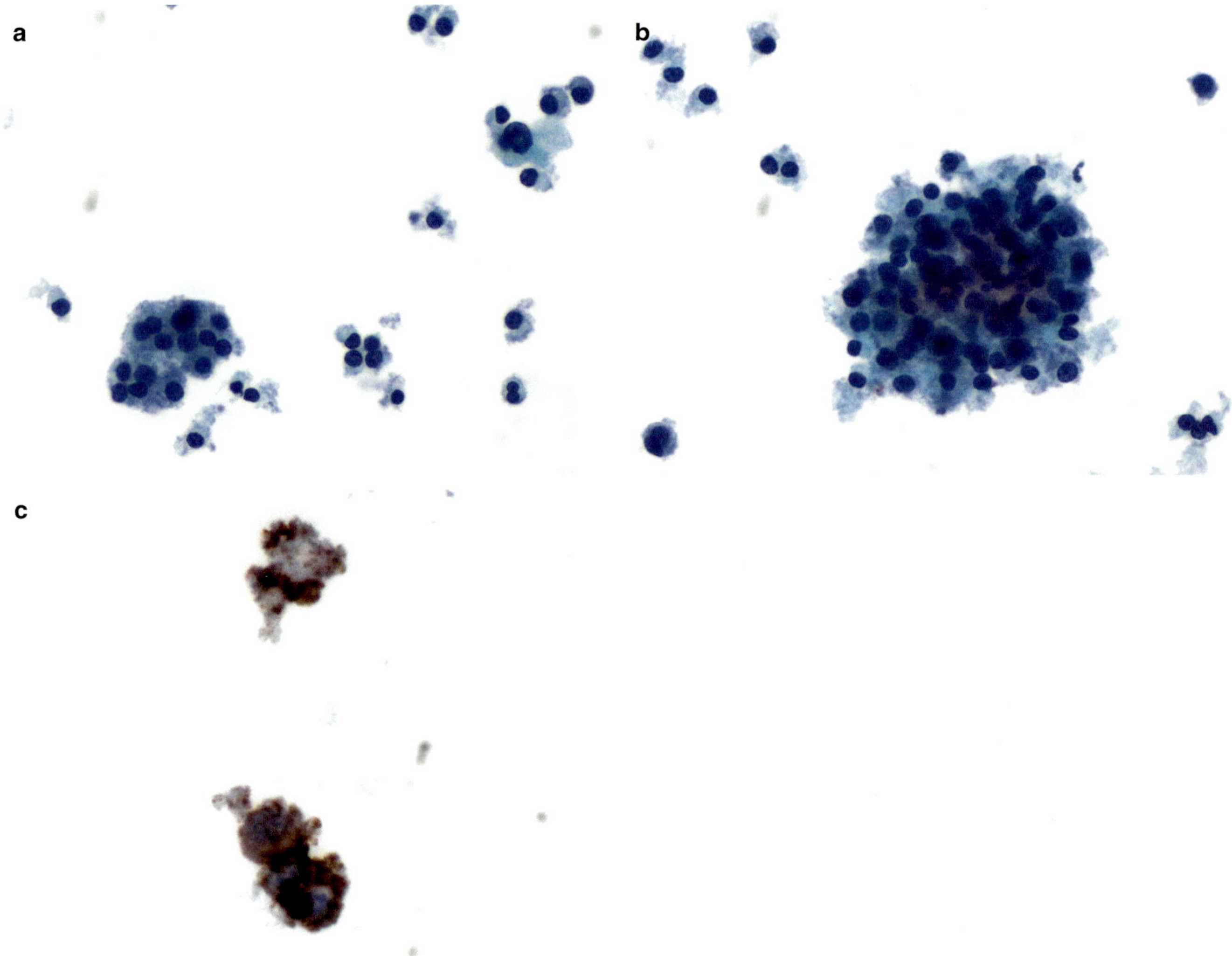

Fig. 8.14 Suspicious for lymphoma. (**a**, **b**) In this case suspicious for lymphoma, clinical information was that the patient had Waldenström macroglobulinemia. TP showed atypical cells that appeared to have a lymphoplasmacytic cell morphology (Pap stain). (**c**) Immunostain for CD38 was positive. Repeat FNA for flow cytometry showed lymphoplasmacytic lymphoma

- Many clinicians now request molecular analysis for this diagnosis, and many insurance companies will reimburse for the test.
- Specific types of genetic alterations may lead to a more definitive preoperative diagnosis. (*See* Table 8.1.)

Management of SM

- Management of patients with an SM diagnosis is complex and is influenced by many factors.
- Guidelines of the American Thyroid Association (ATA) recommend molecular testing for the SM category after review of clinical and radiological information. Molecular testing is recommended if the nodule and cytology are suspicious for PTC. Final management depends on patient preference after surgical consultation.
- Molecular testing will also be helpful if MTC is suspected.
- If lymphoma is suspected, flow cytometry and an incisional biopsy are recommended.
- Metastatic tumors are treated accordingly.

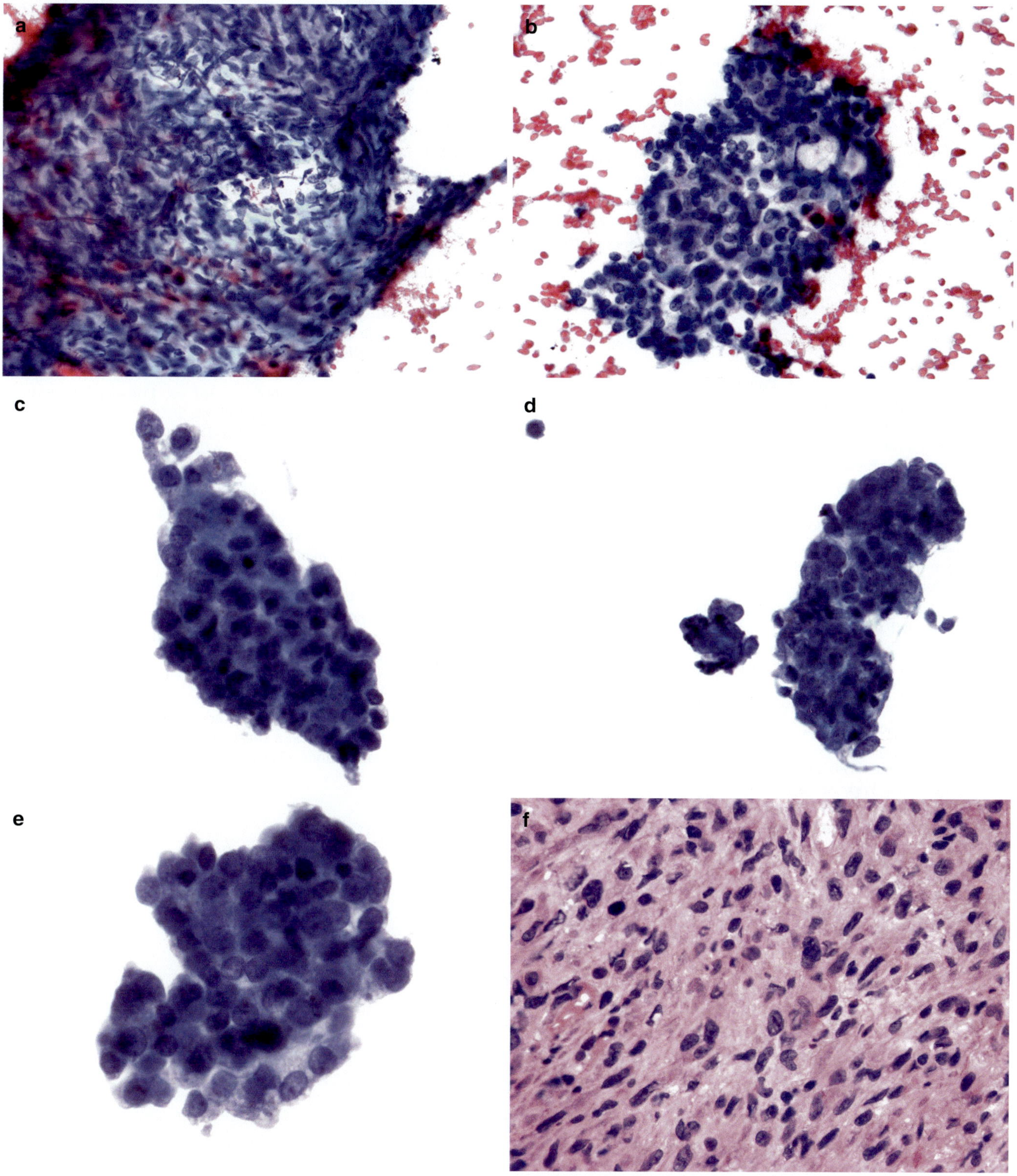

Fig. 8.15 Suspicious for malignancy, not otherwise specified (NOS). (**a**, **b**) The CS showed sheets and clusters of cohesive cells with spindled to oval, enlarged nuclei with stippled, clumped chromatin and small nucleoli. Nuclear features of PTC were not present (Pap stain). (**c**–**e**) TP shows cohesive clusters of cells with more overlapping and crowding and better nuclear morphology than seen in CS. Note the clean background in TP (Pap stain). (**f**) Histologic section from the lobectomy showed a spindle-cell tumor that was positive only for vimentin (H&E stain)

References

1. Adamczewski Z, Lewiński A. Proposed algorithm for management of patients with thyroid nodules/focal lesions, based on ultrasound (US) and fine-needle aspiration biopsy (FNAB); our own experience. Thyroid Res. 2013;6:6. https://doi.org/10.1186/1756-6614-6-6.
2. Ali SZ, Cibas ES. The Bethesda system for reporting thyroid cytopathology; definitions, criteria, and explanatory notes. 2nd ed. Cham: Springer International Publishing AG; 2018.
3. Azar N, Lance C, Nakamoto D, Michael C, Wasman J. Ultrasonographic thyroid findings suspicious for malignancy. Diagn Cytopathol. 2013;41:1107–14. https://doi.org/10.1002/dc.23058.
4. Cibas ES, Ali SZ. The 2017 Bethesda system for reporting thyroid cytopathology. Thyroid. 2017;27:1341–6. https://doi.org/10.1089/thy.2017.0500.
5. Clark DP, Faquin WC. Thyroid cytopathology. 2nd ed. New York: Springer; 2010.
6. Cochand-Priollet B, Prat JJ, Polivka M, Thienpont L, Dahan H, Wassef M, et al. Thyroid fine needle aspiration: the morphological features on ThinPrep slide preparations. Eighty cases with histological control. Cytopathology. 2003;14:343–9.
7. Duncan LD, Forrest L, Law WM Jr, Hubbard E, Stewart LE. Evaluation of thyroid fine-needle aspirations: can ThinPrep be used exclusively to appropriately triage patients having a thyroid nodule? Diagn Cytopathol. 2011;39:341–8. https://doi.org/10.1002/dc.21392.
8. Haugen BR, Alexander EK, Bible KC, Doherty GM, Mandel SJ, Nikiforov YE, et al. 2015 American Thyroid Association Management Guidelines for adult patients with thyroid nodules and differentiated thyroid cancer: the American Thyroid Association Guidelines Task Force on thyroid nodules and differentiated thyroid cancer. Thyroid 2016;26:1–133. https://doi.org/10.1089/thy.2015.0020. Review.
9. Hoda RS. Non-gynecologic cytology on liquid-based preparations: a morphologic review of facts and artifacts. Diagn Cytopathol. 2007;35:621–34.
10. Hoda RS, VandenBussche C, Hoda SA. Diagnostic liquid-based cytology. New York: Springer; 2017.
11. Jackson BS. Controversy regarding when clinically suspicious thyroid nodules should be subjected to surgery: review of current guidelines. Medicine (Baltimore). 2018;97:e13634. https://doi.org/10.1097/MD.0000000000013634.
12. Jung CK, Lee A, Jung ES, Choi YJ, Jung SL, Lee KY. Split sample comparison of a liquid-based method and conventional smears in thyroid fine needle aspiration. Acta Cytol. 2008;52:313–9.
13. Lin F, Chen Z. Standardization of diagnostic immunohistochemistry: literature review and Geisinger experience. Arch Pathol Lab Med. 2014;138:1564–77. https://doi.org/10.5858/arpa.2014-0074-RA.
14. Luu MH, Fischer AH, Pisharodi L, Owens CL. Improved preoperative definitive diagnosis of papillary thyroid carcinoma in FNAs prepared with both ThinPrep and conventional smears compared with FNAs prepared with ThinPrep alone. Cancer Cytopathol. 2011;119:68–73. https://doi.org/10.1002/cncy.20124.
15. Malle D, Valeri RM, Pazaitou-Panajiotou K, Kiziridou A, Vainas I, Destouni C. Use of a thin-layer technique in thyroid fine needle aspiration. Acta Cytol. 2006;50:23–7.
16. Nikiforov YE, Biddinger PW, Thompson LDR. Diagnostic pathology and molecular genetics of the thyroid: a comprehensive guide for practicing thyroid pathology. 3rd ed. Philadelphia: Wolters Kluwer/Lippincott Williams & Wilkins; 2019.
17. Pusztaszeri MP, Krane JF, Cibas ES, Daniels G, Faquin WC. FNAB of benign thyroid nodules with papillary hyperplasia: a cytological and histological evaluation. Cancer Cytopathol. 2014;122:666–77. https://doi.org/10.1002/cncy.21441.
18. Rekhtman N, Buonocore DJ, Rudomina D, Friedlander M, Dsouza C, Aggarwal G, et al. Novel modification of HistoGel-based cell block preparation method: improved sufficiency for molecular studies. Arch Pathol Lab Med. 2018;142:529–35. https://doi.org/10.5858/arpa.2017-0030-OA.
19. Rossi ED, Zannoni GF, Moncelsi S, Stigliano E, Santeusanio G, Lombardi CP, et al. Application of liquid-based cytology to fine-needle aspiration biopsies of the thyroid gland. Front Endocrinol (Lausanne). 2012;3:57. https://doi.org/10.3389/fendo.2012.00057.
20. Yang J, Schnadig V, Logrono R, Wasserman PG. Fine-needle aspiration of thyroid nodules: a study of 4703 patients with histologic and clinical correlations. Cancer. 2007;111:306–15.

Positive for Malignancy: Papillary Thyroid Carcinoma and Its Variants

9

Rana S. Hoda, Rema Rao, and Theresa Scognamiglio

Classic Papillary Thyroid Carcinoma (PTC)

- Approximately 5% (2–16%) of all thyroid fine needle aspiration (FNA) results are malignant.
- PTC is the most common form of thyroid cancer, comprising 83% of all diagnosed thyroid cancers.
- Diagnostic accuracy of cytology for PTC is high; when a diagnosis of PTC is rendered, 94–96% prove to be PTC on resection.
- It occurs in all age groups, including children, and peaks in the 3rd and 4th decade. The male-to-female ratio is 1:4.
- The incidence of thyroid carcinoma has almost tripled. The most common type is classic PTC (c-PTC), but the follicular variant of PTC (FVPTC) and noninvasive follicular thyroid neoplasm with papillary-like nuclear features (NIFTP) are also being diagnosed with increasing frequency.
- Risk factors for PTC include exposure to radiation during childhood, ionizing radiation to the neck, and genetic susceptibility.
- PTC usually presents as a thyroid nodule (which may be incidental); sometimes lymph node metastasis is the initial presentation.
- PTC spreads via lymphatics to regional lymph nodes and less commonly to the lungs.
- Overall, the long-term prognosis for patients with c-PTC is excellent. Variants such as the tall cell variant, columnar cell variant, and diffuse sclerosing PTC have a more aggressive behavior, with higher rates of metastases, recurrence, and possibly mortality.

R. S. Hoda (✉)
CBLPath, Rye Brook, NY, USA
e-mail: rhoda@cblpath.com

R. Rao · T. Scognamiglio
Department of Pathology and Laboratory Medicine, New York Presbyterian Hospital, Weill Cornell Medical College, New York, NY, USA

Pathologic Features of Classic PTC (c-PTC)

- Grossly, c-PTC appears as an ill-defined nodule with irregular borders. It is commonly multifocal. The cut surface is variable; the tumor usually lacks a capsule, can be solid or friable with some cystic areas or can show evidence of papillary structures, is tan-brown in color with whitish foci of fibrosis, and may show gross calcifications (Figs. 9.1a and 9.6i).
- Histologically, c-PTC shows an infiltrative tumor comprising papillary architecture with a component of neoplastic follicles, classic nuclear features (as described below), psammoma bodies, and fibrosis (Figs. 9.1b–d and 9.6j, k).

TBSRTC Definition of c-PTC

- The Bethesda System for Reporting Thyroid Cytopathology (TBSRTC) defines c-PTC as a malignant neoplasm of follicular epithelial cells with a papillary architecture and a constellation of characteristic nuclear features.

Cytologic Criteria of c-PTC

Architectural Criteria

- Papillary architecture (Fig. 9.2).

Nuclear Criteria (Figs. 9.3, 9.4, 9.5, and 9.6)

- Enlargement and/or elongation
- Irregularities in size, shape, and membrane
- Pale and dispersed, "powdery" or fine chromatin
- Crowding (nuclear molding) and overlapping
- Grooves

R. S. Hoda et al. (eds.), *Atlas of Thyroid Cytopathology on Liquid-Based Preparations*,
https://doi.org/10.1007/978-3-030-25066-9_9

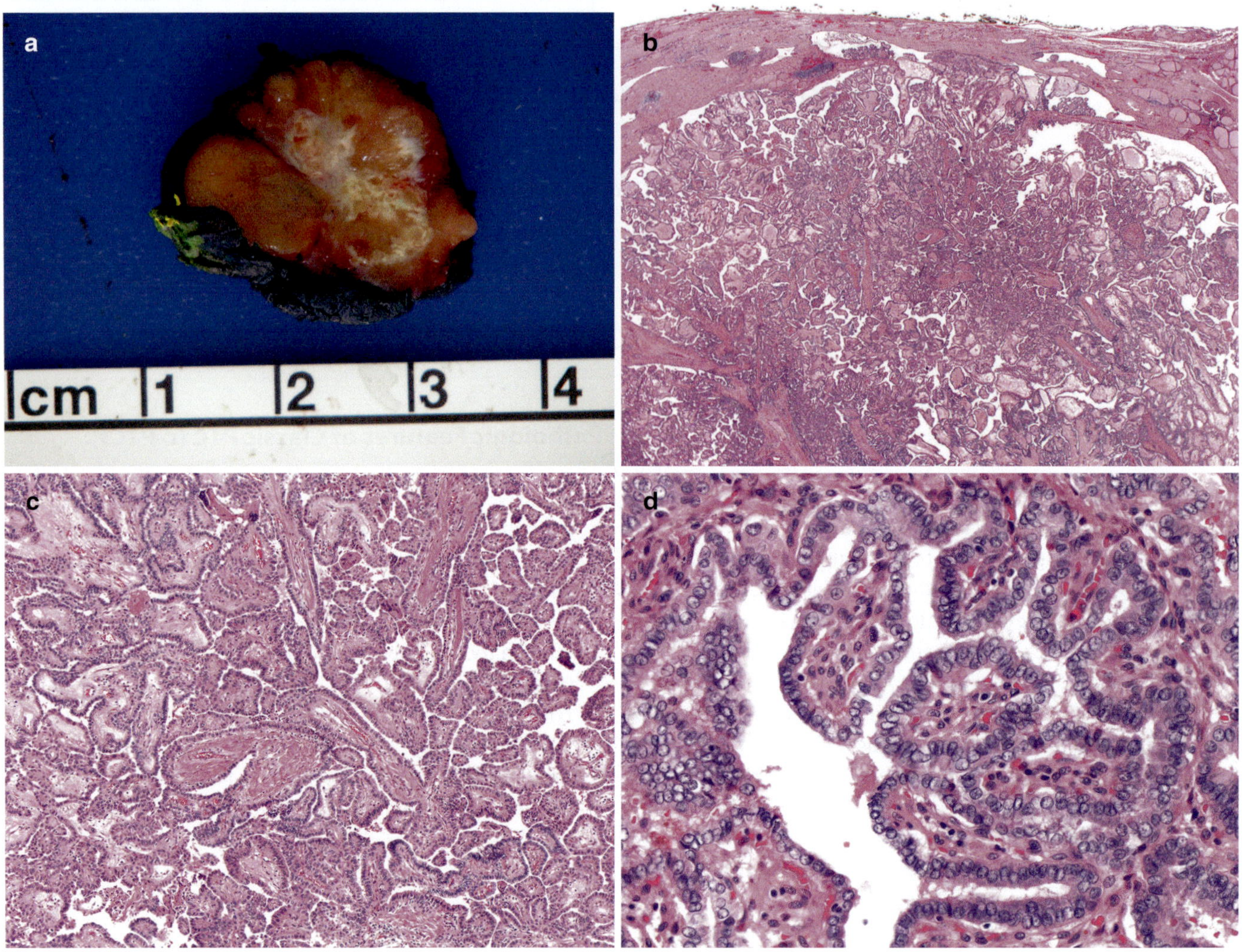

Fig. 9.1 Classic papillary thyroid carcinoma (c-PTC): Pathologic features. (**a**) The solitary tumor is about 2.5 cm and shows a discrete but ill-defined mass. The cut surface is tan-brown with whitish areas representing intramural fibrosis. (**b**) Low magnification of a histologic section of the tumor shows an infiltrative tumor comprising papillary architecture with a component of neoplastic follicles. (**c**) The tumor is composed predominantly of well-formed papillae. Scattered multinucleated giant cells can be seen. (**d**) The nuclei are enlarged and elongated and demonstrate overlapping. Chromatin clearing (Orphan Annie nuclei) is appreciated, as well as nuclear irregularity and grooves. Intranuclear pseudoinclusions (INPI), which represent invaginations of the cytoplasm into the nucleus, are also present (**b–d**, H&E stain)

- Cytoplasmic invagination into the nucleus (intranuclear pseudoinclusions [INPI])
- Small, peripherally located nucleoli

Psammoma Bodies

- Less frequently seen on FNA than in histology (Fig. 9.7)
- When psammoma bodies are associated with nuclear features of PTC, the positive predictive value (PPV) is 100%.

Other Features of c-PTC

- Architectural features of papillae, monolayered syncytial fragments, and cellular swirls (*see* Figs. 9.3, 9.4, 9.5, and 9.6).
- Cellular features of "hobnail" cells, Hürthle cells, and squamoid metaplasia (Fig. 9.8).
- Background features of a variable amount of thick, ropy or "bubble-gum" colloid and multinucleated giant cells (Fig. 9.9).

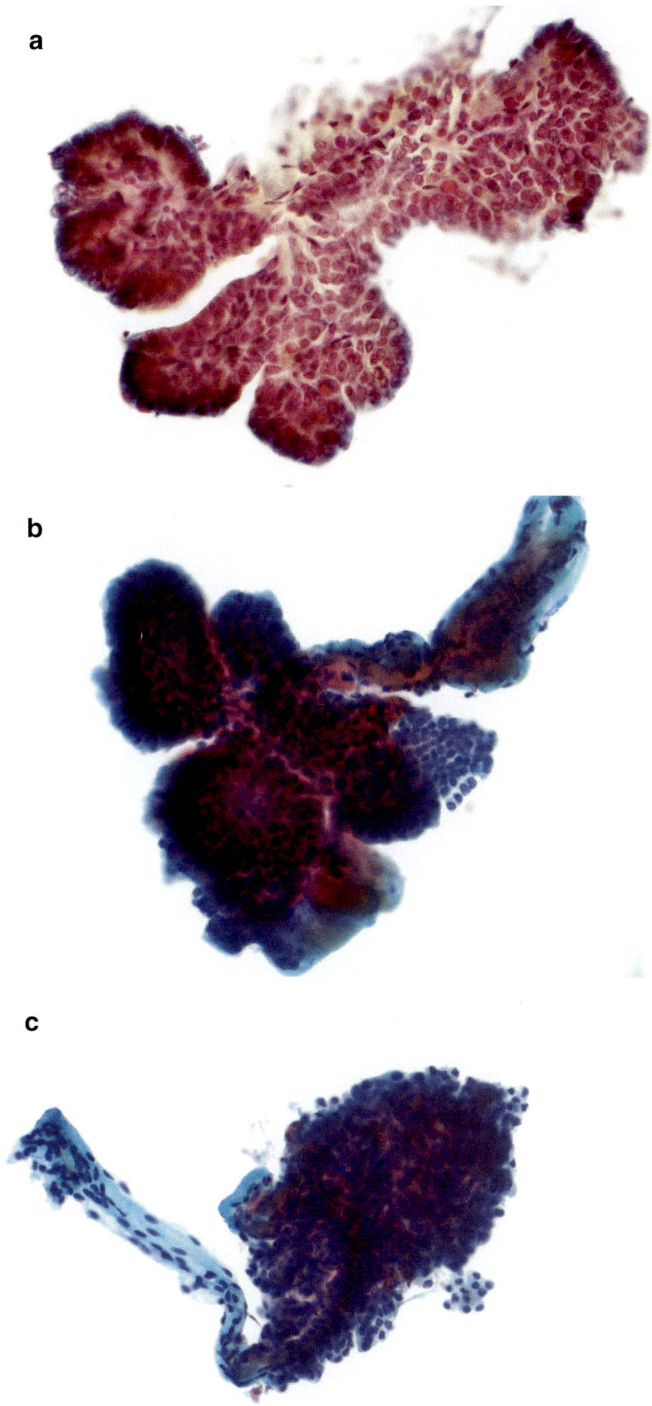

Fig. 9.2 Cytologic features of c-PTC: Papillary structures on conventional smears (CS) and ThinPrep® (TP). (**a**) Intact papillary structure with fibrovascular core seen on CS (Pap stain). (**b**) Intact papillary structure with fibrovascular core, seen on TP (Pap stain). In liquid-based preparations (LBP), such intact branching papillary architecture is rare. (**c**) The papillary structure shown is the form usually seen in LBP (TP, Pap stain)

TBSRTC Modification in the Definition of PTC

- The definition of PTC was modified with the reclassification of NIFTP as a neoplasm rather than malignancy. To avoid false positives due to NIFTP, TBSRTC suggests limiting use of the "malignant" category to cases with "classic" features of PTC (papillary fragments with fibrovascular cores, psammoma bodies, and INPI). The modified definition conforms to the histological criteria of c-PTC and may help improve cyto-histological correlations.
- TBSRTC emphasizes that a small number of malignant cytologic interpretations will be followed by a histologic NIFTP diagnosis, and thus an optional note may be used when the diagnosis "malignant: PTC" is rendered: "Note: A small proportion of cases (~3–4%) diagnosed as malignant, PTC, may prove to be NIFTP on histopathologic examination."
- TBSRTC also recommends that follicular-patterned tumors with some nuclear features of PTC but lacking true papillary structures, INPI, and psammoma bodies may represent NIFTP and should be designated either as a follicular neoplasm or suspicious for a follicular neoplasm (FN/SFN) or as suspicious for malignancy.
- Cases that do not show unequivocal features of PTC are best characterized as suspicious for PTC or atypia of undetermined significance (AUS), depending on the quantity and quality of cellular material. In such cases, molecular testing will prove helpful in further patient management.

Cytomorphologic Differences Between LBP and CS

- Morphologic differences between liquid-based preparations (LBP) and conventional smears (CS), as seen in many of the figures, are predominantly due to immediate liquid fixation, lack of the smearing effect, and automated processing techniques of LBP, as detailed in Chap. 1.
- In LBP, architecturally, there is fragmentation of large papillary fragments, more 3-D cell clusters, and more single cells as a result of the homogenizing step of LBP.
- All nuclear features of PTC are retained in LBP, but nuclear size is smaller; nucleoli are more prominent, appear eosinophilic, and may be associated with a perinuclear "halo"; nuclear membrane irregularity and nuclear grooves become more obvious; INPI are small or less evident; cytoplasm is scantier; and the nuclear-cytoplasmic (N:C) ratio is higher. These differences from CS are due to immediate liquid fixation and lack of the smearing effect.

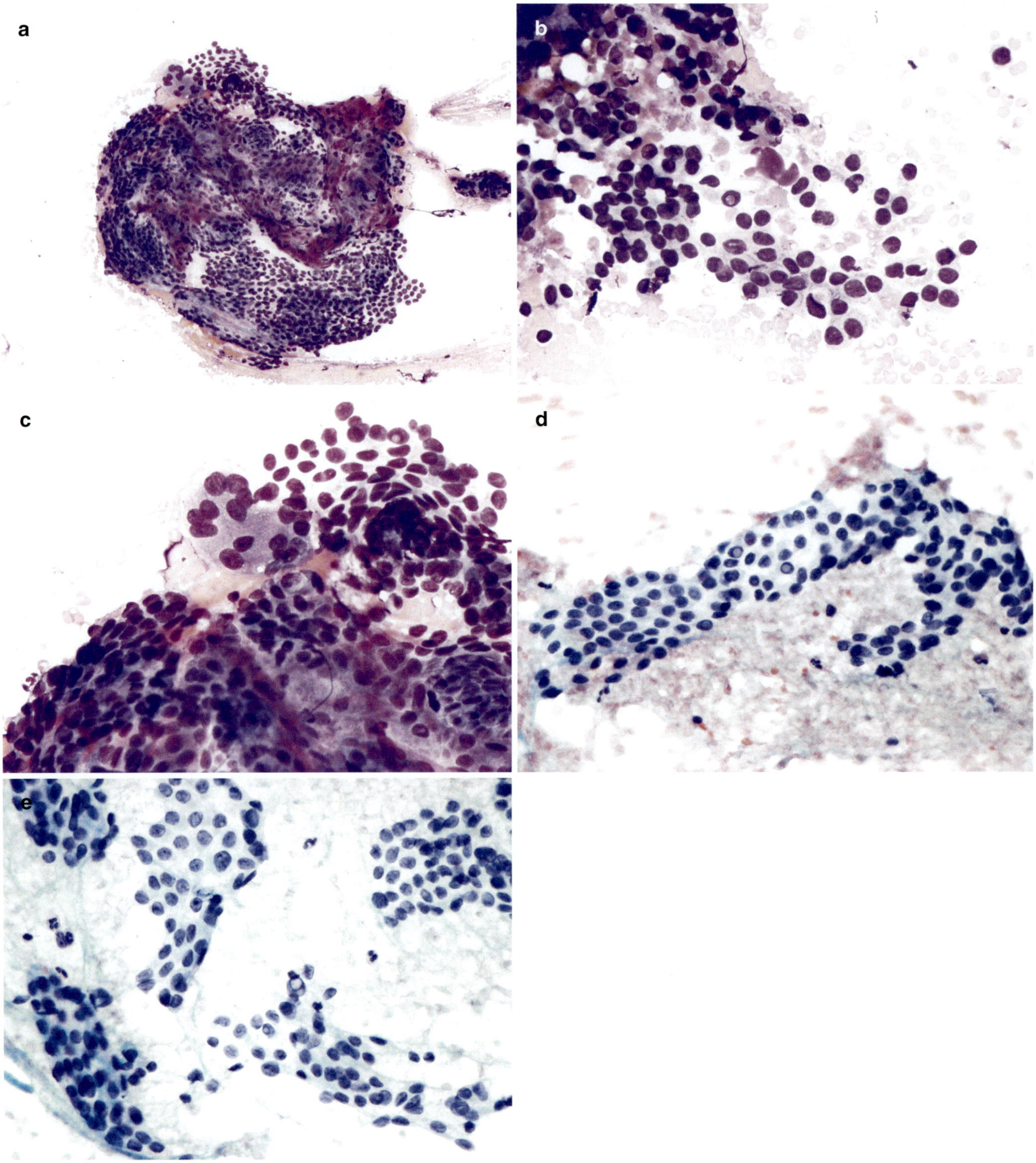

Fig. 9.3 Cytologic features of c-PTC on CS. (**a**) Diff-Quik (DQ)–stained CS of c-PTC showing a monolayered sheet of tumor cells with cellular swirling. Fibrosis is indicated by magenta bands interspersed within the sheet of cells. (**b**, **c**) Higher magnification shows elongated nuclei with intranuclear grooves and INPI. A lightly stained DQ slide can display nuclear features and background elements. (**d**, **e**) Pap-stained CS shows similar cellular morphology

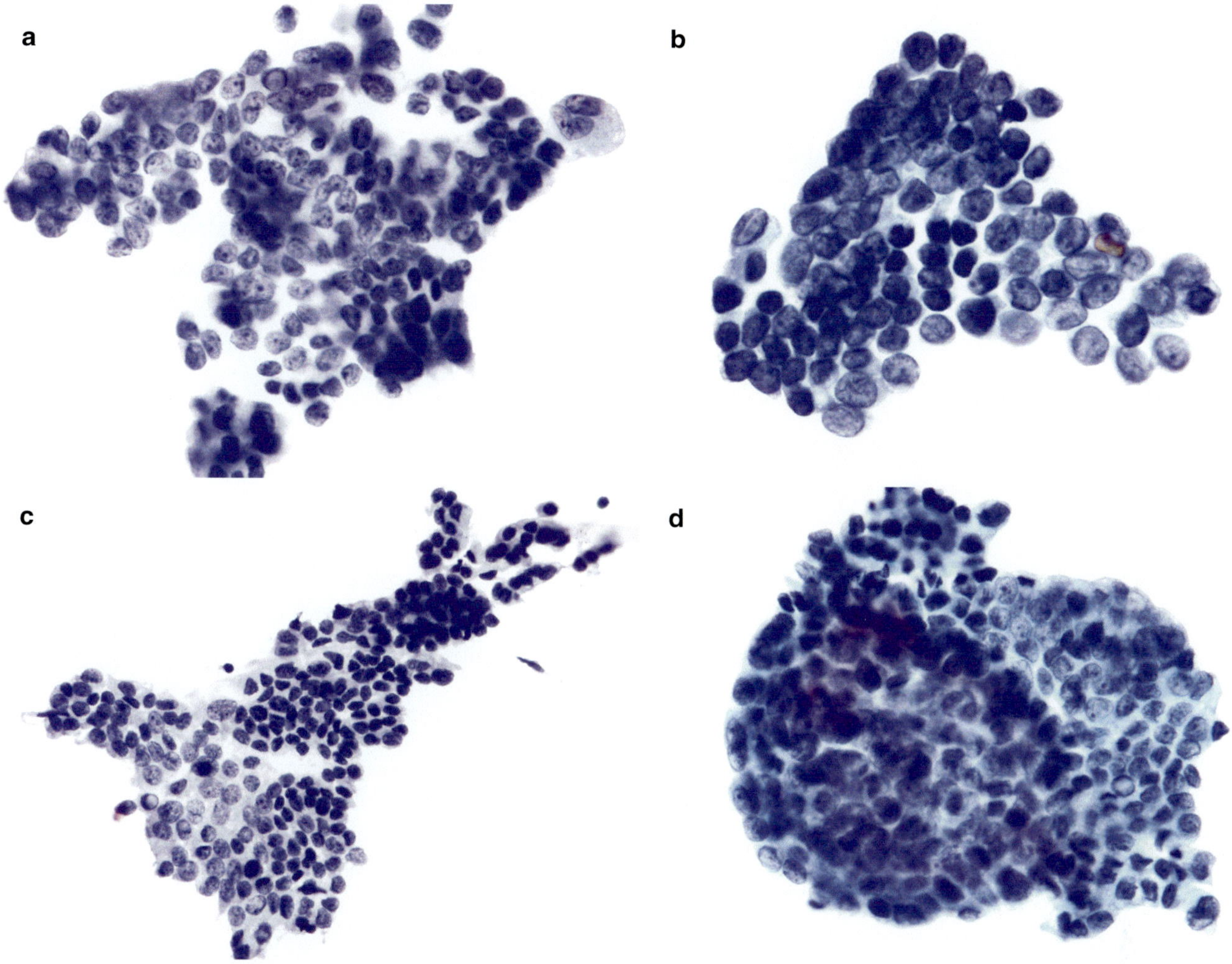

Fig. 9.4 Cytologic features of c-PTC on ThinPrep® (TP). (**a**–**d**) Four different cases of c-PTC showing architecture similar to that seen on CS, with classic nuclear features of c-PTC including enlarged and elongated or oval nuclei with overlapping, nuclear membrane irregularity, fine pale chromatin, grooves, INPI, and small nucleoli (TP, Pap stain)

- Although LBP give better cytomorphology for follicular cells, the papillary structures do appear smaller (fragmented) or may not be seen at all (*see* Fig. 9.6).
- The identification of both nuclear features and papillary structures with psammoma bodies is suggested to render a PTC diagnosis in liquid-based and CS cytology. (See the definition of PTC above.)

Differential Diagnosis of c-PTC

- *Benign follicular nodule:* Monolayered syncytial fragments may mimic benign follicular cells. Close inspection will see nuclear overlapping/crowding and molding in c-PTC.
- *Hashimoto's thyroiditis:* This may show subtle nuclear clearing and grooves, but other nuclear features of PTC are not present.

Histologic Variants of PTC that Can Be Diagnosed on FNA

- Follicular
- Macrofollicular
- Oncocytic or oxyphilic
- Clear cell
- Warthin-like
- "Hobnail"
- Tall cell
- Columnar cell
- Cribriform-morular

Molecular Profile of PTC

- *BRAF*V600E mutation is the most common genetic alteration seen in PTC; it occurs in 40–45% of cases. It is also specific to PTC.

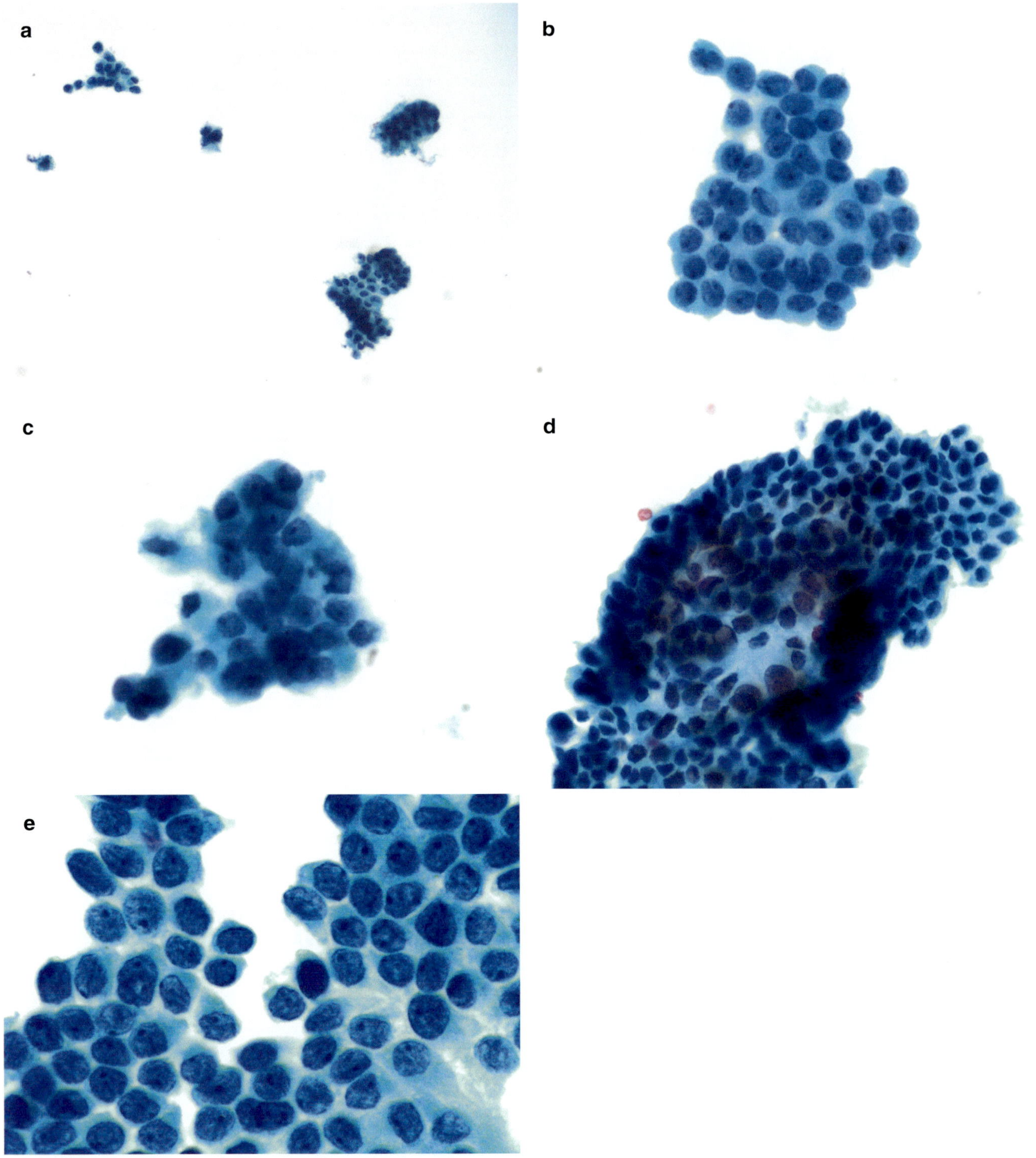

Fig. 9.5 Cytologic features of c-PTC on SurePath™ (SP). (**a–e**) Three different cases (**a–c**) of c-PTC showing architecture similar to that seen on CS and TP, with the classic nuclear features of c-PTC as described above. Note good cellularity in (**a**). (SP, Pap stain)

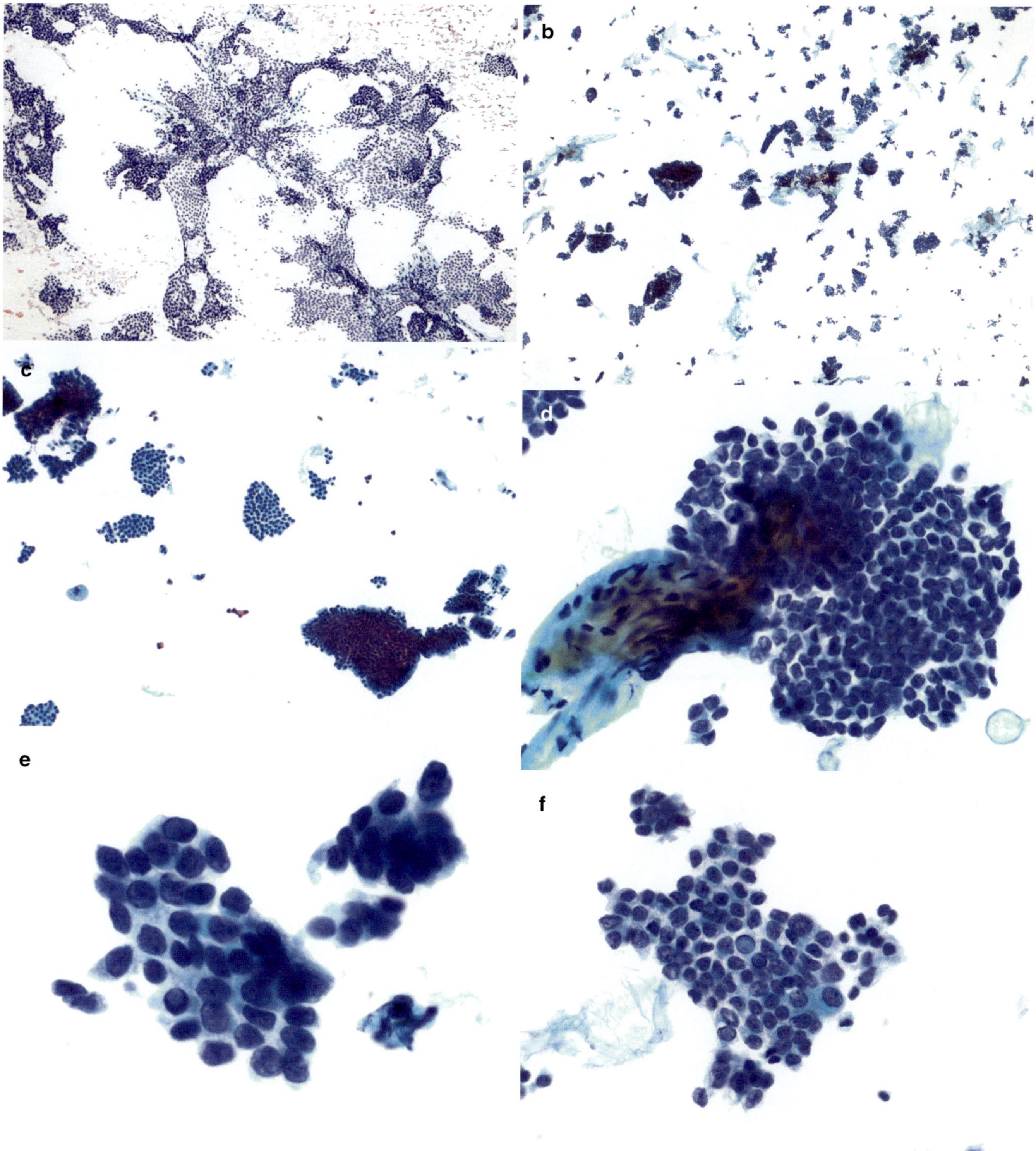

Fig. 9.6 Gross, cytologic, and histologic features of c-PTC. (**a**) The Pap-stained CS shows monolayered, large syncytial and branching sheets and some papillary structures. (**b**, **c**) On TP, the same case shows high cellularity with fragmentation of papillary structures and of large syncytial, monolayered sheets. Papillae are present (Pap stain). (**d**) One intact papillary structure was retained (TP, Pap stain). (**e**, **f**) Classic nuclear features of PTC with crisp morphology (TP, Pap stain). (**g**) Immunostain for CK19 showed strong positivity. (**h**) Pap-stained CS with PTC nuclei. Note that the nuclear features are better preserved on TP. (**i**) Gross picture of this c-PTC shows a discrete but ill-defined mass. The mass is predominantly solid with focal cystic change. The cut surface is tan- brown to yellow with a granular appearance, which reflects the underlying papillary architecture. (**j**, **k**) Typical c-PTC showing well-formed, complex, branching and ramifying papillae with fibrovascular core with characteristic nuclear morphology (H&E stain)

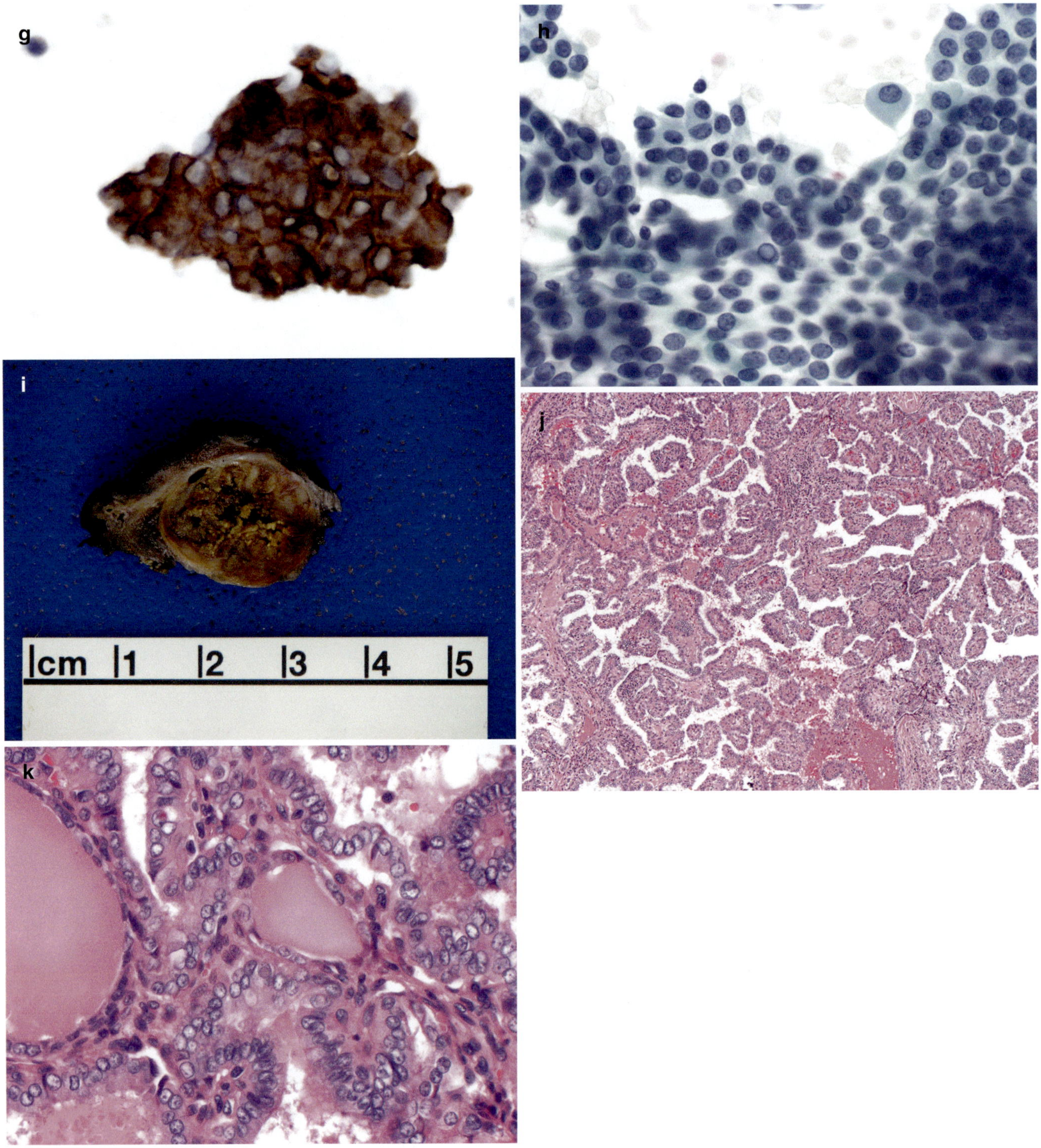

Fig. 9.6 (continued)

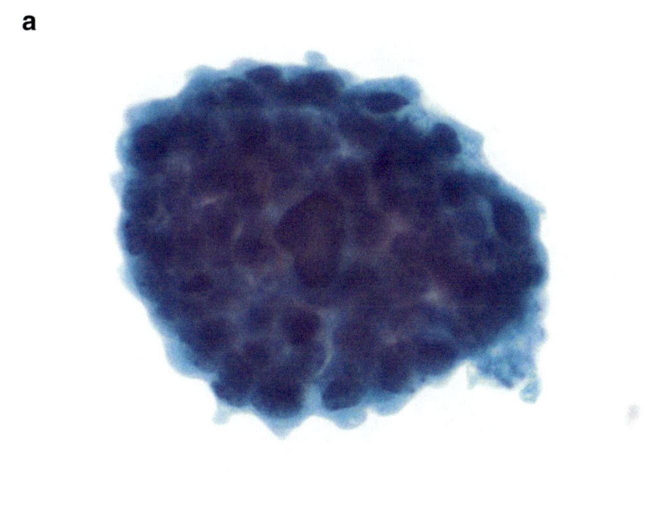
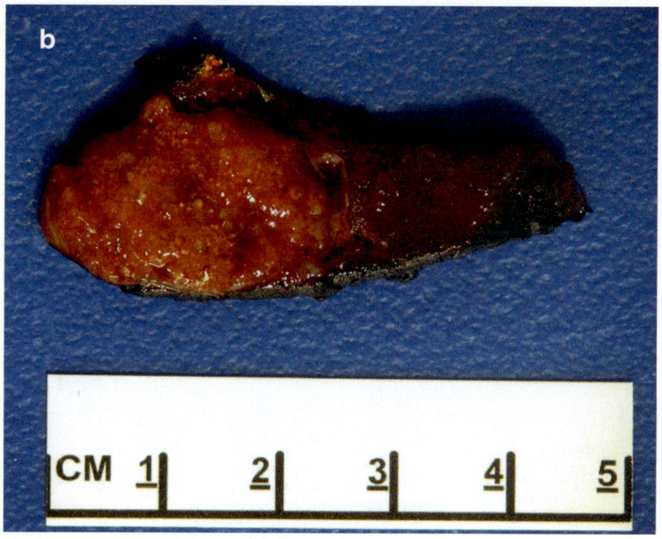

Fig. 9.7 Psammoma bodies in c-PTC. Psammoma bodies are less frequently seen in FNA than in histology and should be associated with abnormal cells to be significant. (**a**) A psammoma body in the middle of a cell cluster of PTC (Pap stain, TP). (**b**) Gross image shows a well-delineated mass with a tan-red cut surface. Minute calcifications can be appreciated

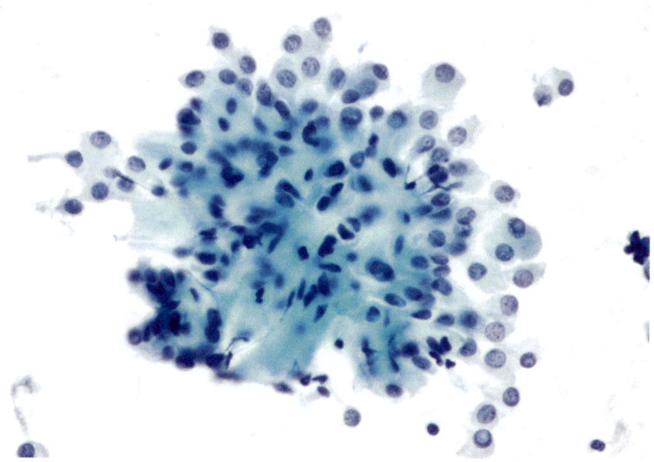

Fig. 9.8 "Hobnail" cells of c-PTC. "Hobnail" cells have eccentric nuclei attached to a fibrovascular core (Pap stain, TP)

- The other common mutation is in the *RAS* gene.
- Other genes are also involved, but with a lower frequency.
- More detailed analyses of molecular abnormalities in PTC are found in the 2019 book by Nikiforov et al., *Diagnostic Pathology and Molecular Genetics of the Thyroid* [4].

Follicular Variant of PTC (FVPTC)

- FVPTC is the second-most-common variant of PTC, accounting for about 18–30% of all PTC.

Classification of FVPTC

- FVPTC is classified into two categories:
  - **Follicular Variant, Infiltrative**
    - Irregular infiltrative border, lacks a capsule
    - Clinical and biologic behavior similar to classic PTC
    - Molecular alterations similar to c-PTC, such as *BRAF*V600E; *RAS* mutations are rare.
  - **Follicular Variant, Encapsulated/Well-Demarcated**
    - Tumors with a capsule or well-demarcated border
    - Molecular and clinical features similar to follicular carcinoma, but with moderate to well-developed nuclear features of PTC
    - *Follicular variant, encapsulated/well-demarcated with capsular invasion:* These tumors show invasion, either capsular or vascular.
    - *Follicular variant, encapsulated/well-demarcated, noninvasive:* This category is for the rare tumors

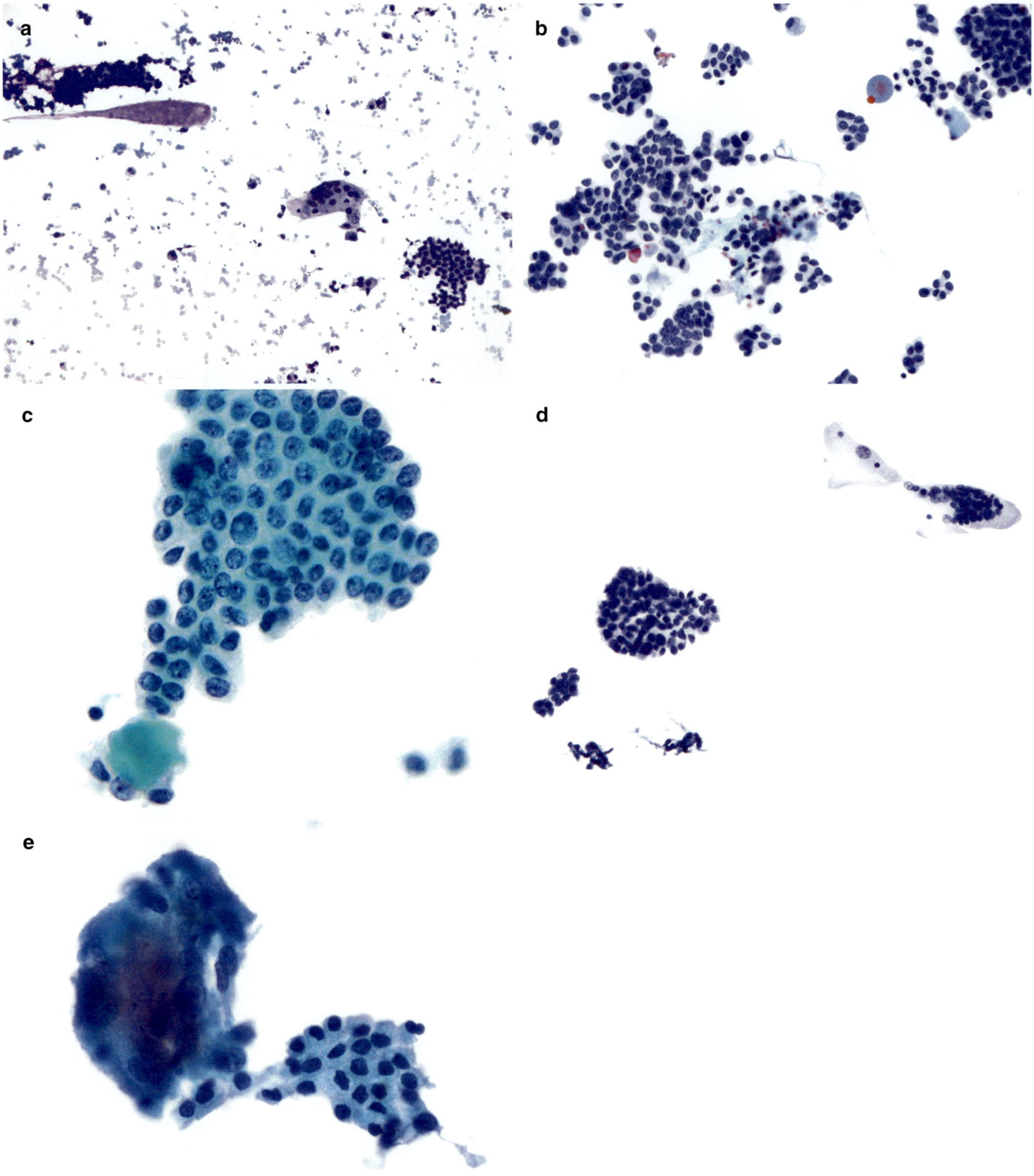

Fig. 9.9 Colloid and multinucleated giant cells in c-PTC. (**a**) DQ-stained CS shows magenta-staining, ropy colloid and multinucleated giant cells. (**b**) Pap-stained TP shows bluish, ropy colloid in the middle and bubble-gum colloid at top right. (**c**) Pap-stained SP shows bubble-gum colloid. (**d**, **e**) Pap-stained TP shows multinucleated giant cells

Table 9.1 Consensus diagnostic criteria for diagnosing NIFTP on histology (Endocrine Pathology Society)

Major inclusion criteria
Encapsulation/well demarcated
Follicular growth (<1% papillae)
Nuclear features of PTC
No papillae
Exclusion criteria
Invasion (vascular and/or capsular)
Solid/trabecular growth >30%
Tall cell, columnar, or cribriform-morular morphology
"True" papillae >1%
Psammoma bodies
Tumor necrosis
High mitotic activity (>3/10HPF)

HPF high-power field, *NIFTP* noninvasive follicular thyroid neoplasm with papillary-like nuclear features, *PTC* papillary thyroid carcinoma

that lack invasion but do not completely fulfill the criteria for NIFTP (>30% solid/trabecular/insular growth pattern, or high-grade features).

- A subset of noninvasive follicular variants can be reclassified as NIFTP if they meet the inclusion criteria shown in Table 9.1.

Clinical and Imaging Features of FVPTC

- The tumors involve younger patients and are often larger than c-PTC.
- Ultrasonography shows oval to round, isoechoic to hypoechoic nodules with or without a hypoechoic rim (Fig. 9.10a). In contrast, nodules of c-PTC are taller than wide and appear markedly hypoechoic.
- The hypoechoic rim is also more commonly encountered in FVPTC than in c-PTC.
- The imaging features of FVPTC show a greater degree of overlap with follicular lesions such as nodular hyperplasia and follicular adenoma.

Pathological Features of FVPTC

- Grossly, encapsulated invasive FVPTC is similar to NIFTP. The lesions appear well-circumscribed and solid, with an average size of about 2–4 cm (Fig. 9.10b). Infiltrative FVPTC also appears predominantly solid but shows gross invasion (Fig. 9.10c).
- On histology, the tumors can be minimally invasive or widely invasive and composed of small to medium-sized follicles lacking papillae (Fig. 9.10d, e). The cells lining the follicles show enlarged, oval and pale nuclei with nuclear overlap and intranuclear grooves. INPI are present but markedly less in number than in c-PTC (especially with the minimally invasive FVPTC) and are very similar to NIFTP.

Cytological Features of FVPTC: Application to LBP

- As described above, two variants of FVPTC are observed, the encapsulated (invasive) variant and the infiltrative variant. The encapsulated variant is more common than the infiltrative variant. The encapsulated, noninvasive variant of FVPTC is now referred to as NIFTP and will be discussed separately.
- Cytology cannot distinguish between these various FVPTC categories.
- The aim of this chapter is to highlight features of FVPTC.
- Cytologic features of FVPTC mirror histology in that the aspirate smears show thick colloid, prominent microfollicles with enlarged nuclei, pale chromatin, nuclear grooves, and occasional pseudoinclusions. Syncytial clusters can also be seen. Psammoma bodies or papillary structures are generally lacking (Figs. 9.11, 9.12, 9.13, and 9.14).
- The features of FVPTC on LBP are fairly similar to CS. FVPTC lack papillary structures, and almost all cases of FVPTC show a microfollicular pattern and nuclear grooves.
- The infiltrative variant of FVPTC tends to show more INPI.
- In some cases, the features can be subtle and focal, leading to FVPTC being diagnosed as one of three indeterminate Bethesda categories, categories III, IV, and V.
- If FVPTC is suspected on cytology (suspicious for malignancy), an optional note such as "The cytomorphologic features are suspicious for FVPTC or its recently described indolent counterpart, NIFTP" is recommended per TBSRTC.
- The sensitivity of a diagnosis of FVPTC on FNA is approximately 42%, and specificity is 83%.
- In a study by Lin et al. [9], the sensitivity for a diagnosis of FVPTC on FNA was 25%, compared with 74% for conventional PTC.

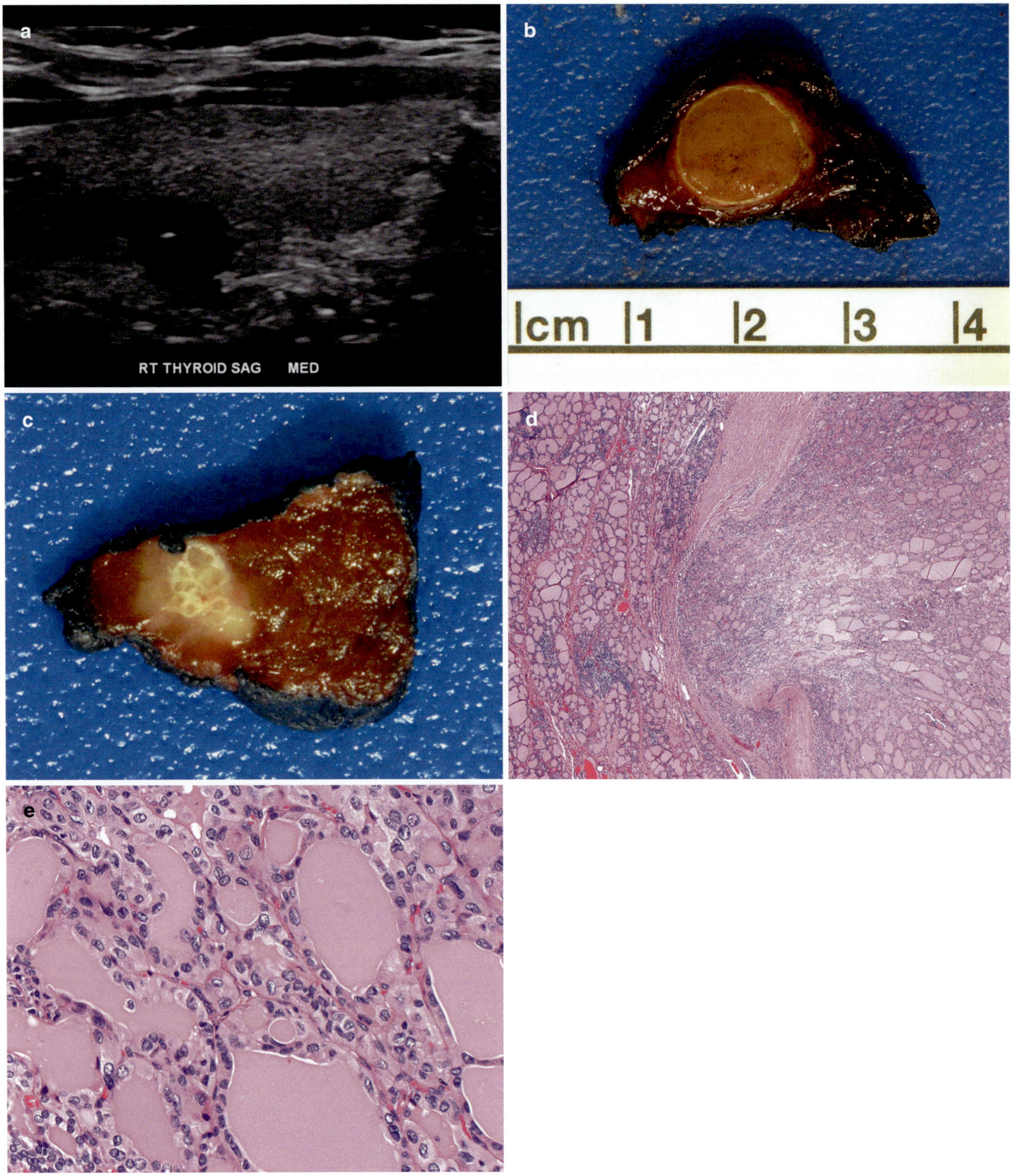

Fig. 9.10 Follicular variant of PTC (FVPTC). (**a**) Ultrasound image of a case of FVPTC showing an oval, predominantly hypoechogenic nodule with an irregular abutting border inferiorly, corresponding to invasion. (**b**) Grossly, the encapsulated, invasive FVPTC appeared well-circumscribed, encapsulated, and solid, with an average size of about 2–4 cm. (**c**) The infiltrative FVPTC appears predominantly solid but shows gross invasion, corresponding to the ultrasound image in (**a**). (**d**, **e**) Histology showing an encapsulated lesion composed of irregularly shaped follicles with nuclei showing features of PTC. (**d**) shows evidence of capsular invasion (H&E stain)

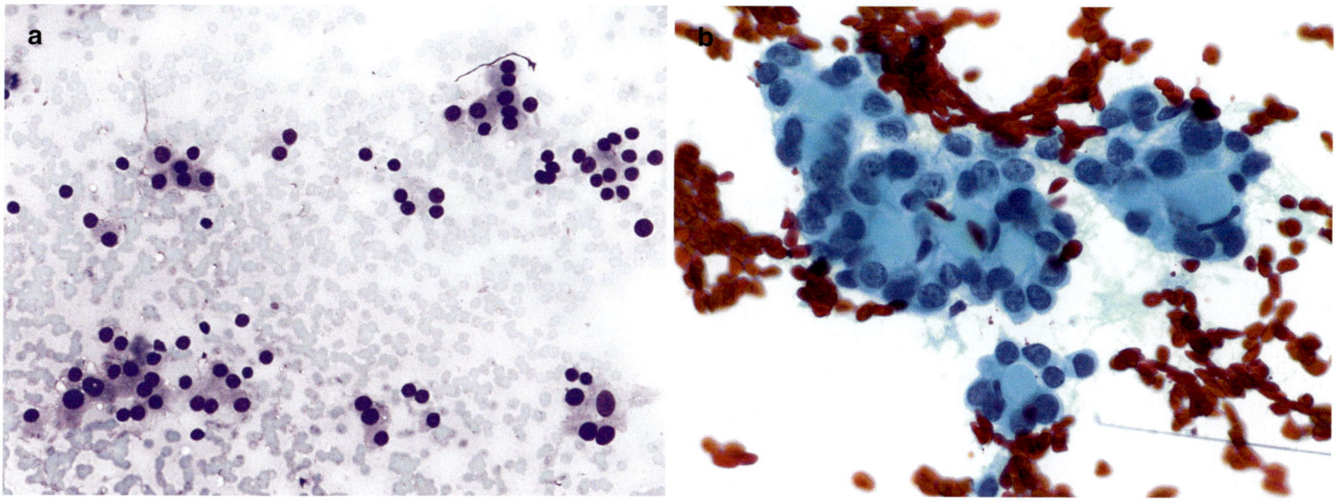

Fig. 9.11 FVPTC: Appearance on CS. (**a**) Air-dried smear shows a cellular aspirate with mostly loose or fragmented microfollicles, with some nuclear enlargement (DQ stain, CS). (**b**) Alcohol-fixed smear shows the striking microfollicular architecture, with nuclei showing features of PTC such as nuclear enlargement, pallor, and peripherally placed nucleoli. Note the elongate nuclei, (some with angulation), in contrast to round and regular nuclei of follicular adenoma. The microfollicles show thick colloid in the lumen (Pap stain, CS)

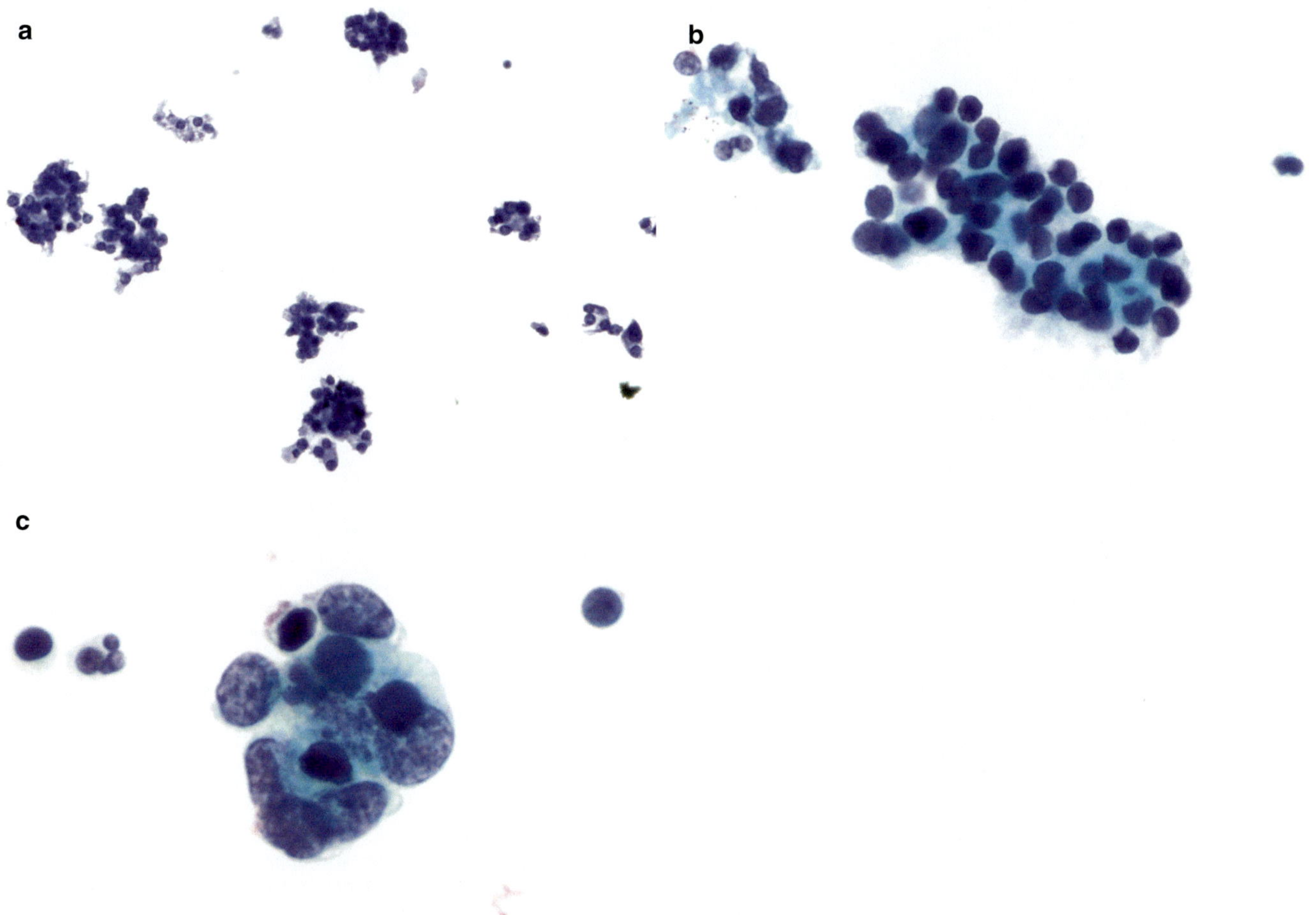

Fig. 9.12 FVPTC: Appearance on LBP. (**a**) LBP showing a cellular sample composed of loose microfollicles (Pap stain, TP). (**b, c**) Higher magnification of the microfollicles. (**b**) shows compacted but irregularly shaped microfollicles; (**c**) shows appreciable nuclear atypia, in which the nuclei appear paler than the adjacent lymphocyte and are significantly enlarged in comparison to the lymphocytes and red blood cells (Pap stain, TP)

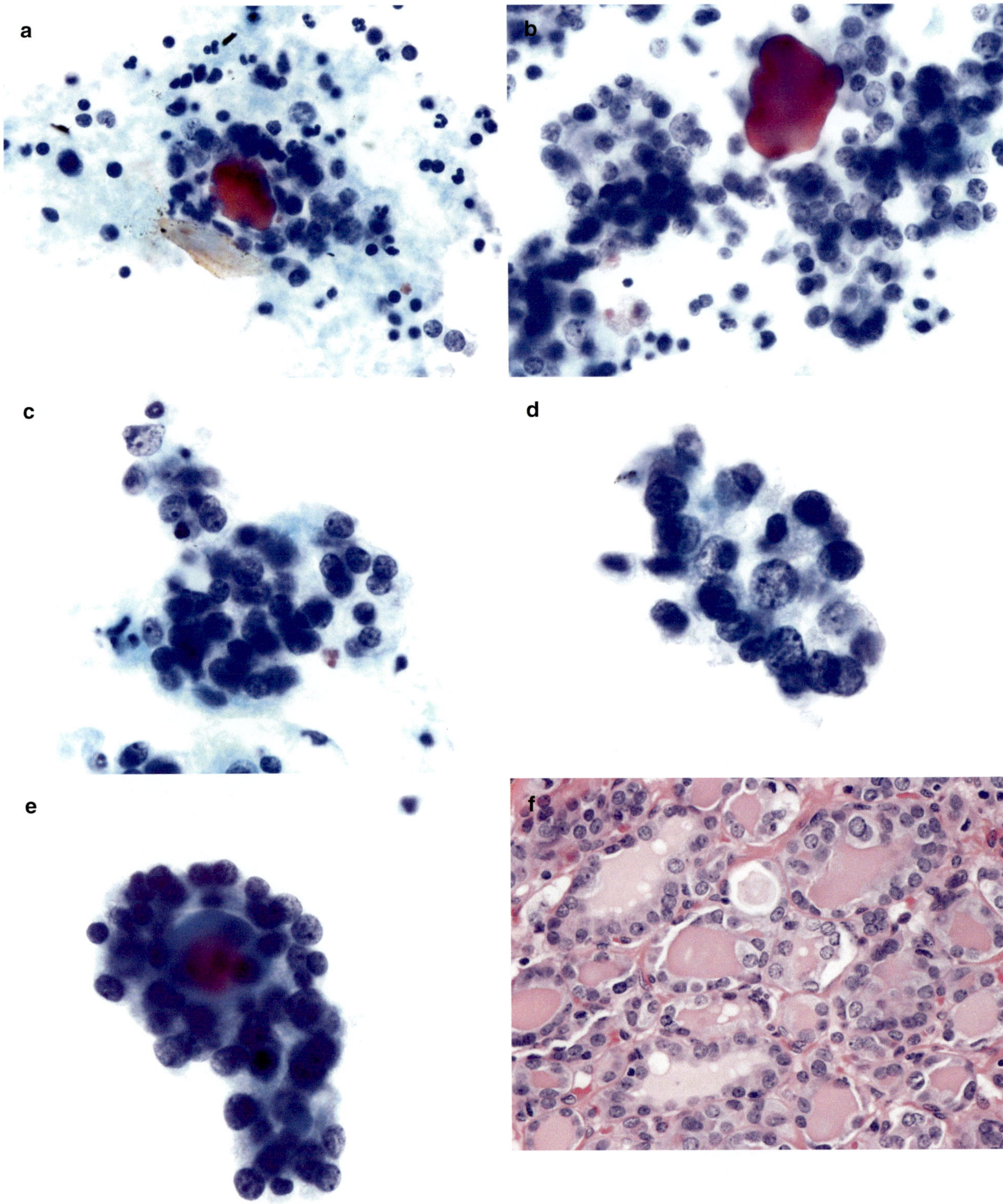

Fig. 9.13 FVPTC: Appearance on LBP. In these two other cases of FVPTC, the sample was sent only in TP preservative solution. (**a–c**) In this case, LBP shows a cellular aspirate composed of microfollicles. In (**a**) the follicular cell nuclei are loosely clustered around a central thick fragment of colloid. In (**b**, **c**) we can see a cellular area composed of compacted but loose microfollicles, with nuclei showing enlargement, pallor, and overlap. In (**b**) the thick fragment of colloid is extruded from the microfollicle and displaced away from the lumen. In both (**b**, **c**) the nuclear enlargement and pallor are striking when compared with the adjacent lymphocytes. We can also appreciate the peripherally placed nucleoli. The increased cellularity and the nuclear features help in a diagnosis of FVPTC. In this case, FVPTC was suspected, and the case was reported as "Suspicious for PTC" with an optional note "The cytomorphologic features are suspicious for a FVPTC or its recently described indolent counterpart NIFTP" (Pap stain, TP). (**d**, **e**) In this case, note the microfollicle with the nuclear features as described above and dense luminal colloid (Pap stain, TP). (**f**) Histology showed FVPTC, with histologic findings similar to the cytologic findings (H&E stain)

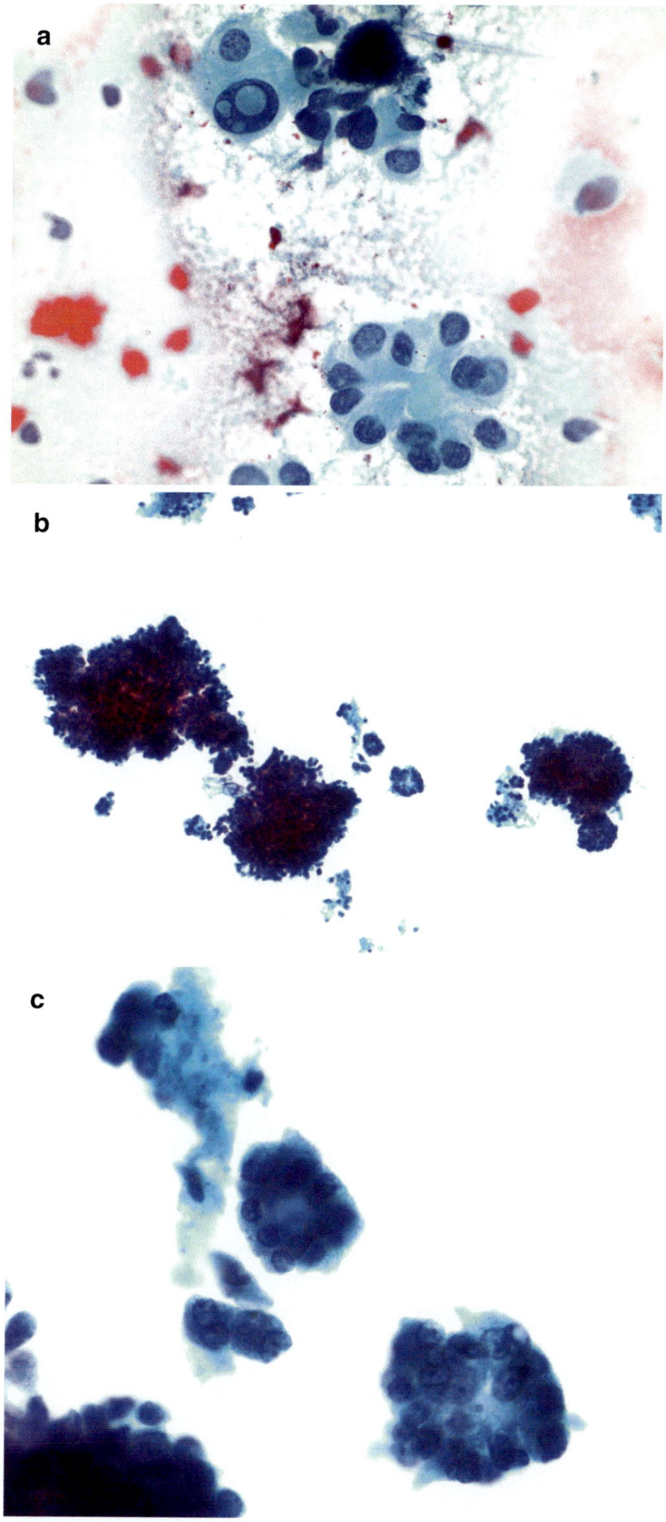

Fig. 9.14 FVPTC: Appearance on CS and SP. (**a**) This example of the cytology of an infiltrative FVPTC shows microfollicles and follicular cell nuclei with prominent intranuclear inclusions. Intranuclear inclusions are not so common in the encapsulated variant or NIFTP, but can be seen readily in the widely infiltrative FVPTC (Pap stain, CS). (**b, c**) FVPTC on a SP specimen, showing high cellularity with dense cellular clusters or cell balls and some individual microfollicles, which on higher magnification show nuclear features of PTC including INPI (Pap stain, SP)

Molecular Profile of FVPTC

- The molecular profile of encapsulated invasive FVPTC is similar to that of NIFTP in that it is closer to that seen in the follicular adenoma/carcinoma group of tumors, characterized by general lack of *BRAF*V600E and by the prevalence of *RAS* mutations (and in some cases, *PPAR*γ rearrangement). It tends to have an excellent prognosis.
- Infiltrative FVPTC, on the other hand, is similar to c-PTC, with lymph node metastases. It can show mutation in *BRAF*V600E.

Noninvasive Follicular Thyroid Neoplasm with Papillary-Like Nuclear Features (NIFTP)

- The tumor (described by Nikiforov et al. [18]) represent a distinct class of thyroid tumor that were previously referred to as the "encapsulated noninvasive variant of FVPTC." They have very low risk of adverse outcome and have a set of reproducible histologic criteria (Table 9.2). The encapsulated invasive and diffusely infiltrative types of FVPTC are discussed separately.
- In thyroid cytopathology, the introduction of NIFTP is a diagnostic challenge, as follicular-patterned lesions (including adenomatous nodule, follicular adenoma, follicular carcinoma, and FVPTC) have overlapping cytological features and cannot be reliably distinguished.
- In particular, it is extremely challenging to make a definitive diagnosis of FVPTC and NIFTP, and it is even more challenging to distinguish FVPTC and NIFTP on cytology alone. The degree to which the nuclear features are displayed in FVPTC and NIFTP vary from case to case and between observers.

Table 9.2 Diagnostic criteria for NIFTP

1. ***Yes*** for encapsulation or clear demarcation
2. ***Yes*** for follicular growth pattern with
<1% papillae
<30% solid/trabecular/insular
No psammoma bodies
3. ***Yes*** for nuclear features of PTC (Nuclear score 2–3)[a]
4. ***No*** invasion
5. ***No*** high mitotic activity
6. ***No*** tumor necrosis

[a]Nuclear score dependent on *(a)* size and shape (enlargement, elongation, and overlap); *(b)* membrane irregularities (grooves, folds, irregular contours, INPIs); and *(c)* chromatin characteristics ("glassy" nuclei; powdery, delicate chromatin; chromatin margination to the membrane; and clearing). Two of the above three categories must show adequate features (i.e., score 2 of 3) to allow for cytomorphologic diagnosis of NIFTP

- The nuclear features also can be extremely subtle, especially in NIFTP, thus allowing for these cytologic samples to be diagnosed as one of the indeterminate categories: Suspicious for Malignancy (SM, 18–35%), FN/SFN (25–30%), or AUS/FLUS (10–35%).
- NIFTP has also had the most impact on the TBSRTC implied risk of malignancy (ROM). The introduction of NIFTP as nonmalignant has produced an appreciable decrease in the ROM, in the indeterminate categories of TBSRTC.
- Faquin et al. [16] reported that the impact on the ROM of reclassifying noninvasive FVPTC as NIFTP was most pronounced and statistically significant in the three indeterminate categories. The ROM for AUS/FLUS decreased from 31% to 18%, for FN/SFN from 33% to 18%, and for SM from 83% to 59%.
- Zhou et al. [20] recently demonstrated similar findings of a decrease in ROM with the reclassification of NIFTP in a large, multi-institutional study. They also found the greatest decrease in ROM in the indeterminate categories (8.7% for AUS/ FLUS, 7.9% for FN/SFN, and 10.9% for SM), but the impact overall (especially on the SM category) was far less in this study than in prior studies, highlighting the variability in pathologists' cytologic and histopathologic diagnostic thresholds and clinicians' management thresholds.
- The introduction of NIFTP also reduced the PPV of the malignant category for thyroid FNA from 99% to about 94–96%.
- The decreases in the ROM and the PPV have raised some concerns in the cytology community about the classification of follicular-patterned lesions with focal features of PTC and the effect of changes in the cytologic interpretation on downstream patient management.
- Because of its lower ROM, NIFTP can be successfully treated by lobectomy alone. Total thyroidectomy and subsequent radioiodine ablation are not necessary.

Imaging Features of NIFTP

- On ultrasonography, NIFTP usually appears as round to oval, well-circumscribed nodule, varying in echogenicity from hypoechoic to isoechoic to hyperechoic, with a hypoechoic rim (Fig. 9.15a).

Pathological Features of NIFTP

- Gross findings include a well-circumscribed, solid nodule with an average size of about 2–4 cm (Fig. 9.15b). The nodule can be completely to partially encapsulated or may lack a capsule. It can occasionally grow larger.
- On histology, NIFTP must be well-demarcated, with or without a capsule, showing no evidence of capsular and/or vascular invasion (Fig. 9.15c). The tumor is composed largely of follicles (predominantly microfollicular) with nuclei showing features like PTC. No "true" papillae or psammoma bodies are identified (*see* Tables 9.1 and 9.2).

Cytological Features of NIFTP

- Cytologic features of NIFTP largely mirror histology except for capsulation and demarcation, which are impossible to assess on cytology alone. The aspirate of NIFTP is a follicular-patterned aspirate composed of microfollicles. The nuclei show features of PTC that include overlap, pallor, membrane irregularity, and peripherally placed nucleoli, but intranuclear inclusions are rare to absent (Fig. 9.16a–d).
- By definition (as on Table 9.2), cytologic features noted in c-PTC such as psammoma bodies, papillae, and prominent INPI should be absent.
- A prospective study by Strickland et al. [19] showed that the presence of a microfollicular architecture and the absence of papillae, psammomatous calcifications, and INPI help in distinguishing potential NIFTP cases from c-PTC.
- As previously mentioned, cytological distinction between potential NIFTP and FVPTC may be more challenging. As per Legesse [17], infiltrative FVPTC may occasionally show architectural features typical of papillae, irregular branching linear and swirling sheets, and INPI, in comparison to NIFTP. Most cases of NIFTP lack INPI; those present were very few.
- Although all the above cytologic features can be recognized in LBP, currently data on the cytomorphology of NIFTP on LBP are limited.
- Similar to what is seen on CS, NIFTP lack prominent papillary structures on LBP. Bizzarro et al. [15] in the largest published series on the cytomorphologic features of FVPTC on LBP, showed that almost all cases of FVPTC show a microfollicular pattern and nuclear grooves. In particular, NIFTPs showed minimal nuclear size enlargement (14 μm to 20 μm) when compared with infiltrative FVPTC or c-PTC. The presence or absence of colloid in the background appeared to be an insignificant finding. As in CS, prominent papillae, psammoma bodies, and increased INPI should not be present (Figs. 9.16e–h and 9.17).
- Presence of high mitotic rate, tumor necrosis, and more than one-third of solid growth excludes a tumor from the NIFTP category.
- As many of these follicular patterned lesions fall under the indeterminate category, adding an immunohistochemical panel of CK19, HBME-1, and galectin-3 may reduce the indeterminate diagnosis in about 95% of cases, categorizing them rightfully as FVPTC and not benign.
- Cytopathologists need to be aware of the cytological criteria that may suggest NIFTP, although it cannot be accurately diagnosed on FNA alone. It requires histopathologic

examination to exclude features such as frank invasion, capsular or vascular invasion, papillary architecture, mitotic activity, necrosis, or solid growth.

Molecular Profile of NIFTP

- Molecular testing appears to play a role in further characterizing the variants of PTC. NIFTP tends to harbor the *RAS* mutation and *PAX8/PPARγ* gene rearrangement and lack *BRAF*V600E.
- Strickland et al. [19], in their study on molecular testing of a cohort of 56 thyroid FNAs already stratified as NIFTP/FVPTC or c-PTC, showed that seven of eight cases favored to be NIFTP/FVPTC showed molecular results supporting conservative management (*NRAS-1*, wild type-6).

TBSRTC Recommendations for FVPTC and NIFTP

- Given the ensuing challenges in diagnosing NIFTP on cytology alone and its placement in the indeterminate categories, TBSRTC recommends optional notes explaining the conundrum in ruling out NIFTP or FVPTC based on cytology alone.
- If a lesion is diagnosed as a follicular neoplasm, TBSRTC recommends an optional note such as "Although the architectural features suggest a follicular neoplasm, some nuclear features raise the possibility of an invasive FVPTC or its recently described indolent counterpart, NIFTP; definitive distinction among these entities is not possible on cytologic material."

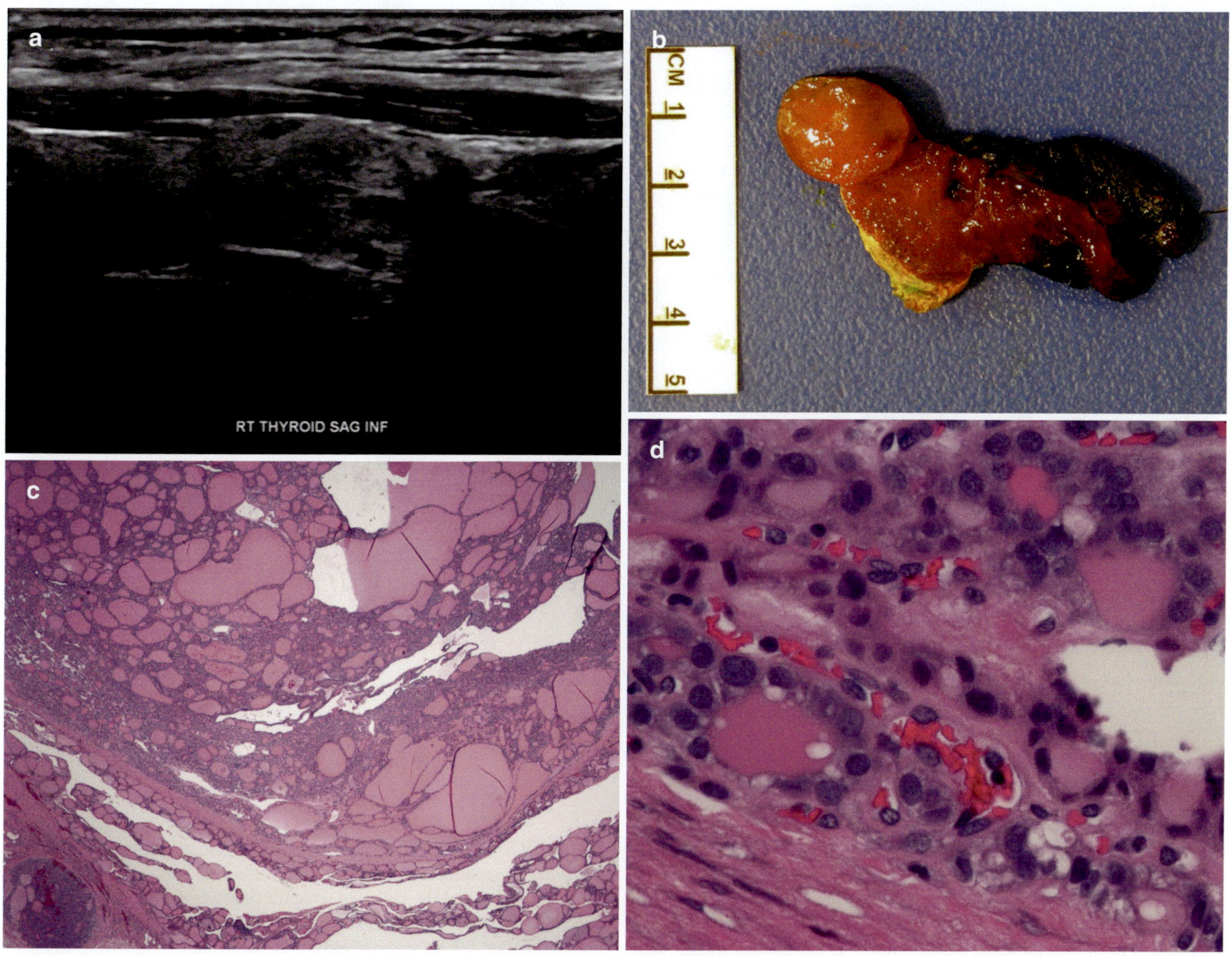

Fig. 9.15 NIFTP: Imaging, gross, and histologic findings. (**a**) Ultrasound image of NIFTP, showing a round to oval, well-circumscribed, predominantly solid nodule with mostly isoechoic areas punctuated with some hypoechoic to hyperechoic areas. A hypoechoic rim is not conspicuous here. (**b**) Grossly, NIFTP can grow larger, but on average are about 2–4 cm in size. This image of NIFTP shows a well-circumscribed and encapsulated solid nodule. The capsule surrounding the tumor may be thin to thick, and it may be well to partially encapsulated or unencapsulated, as long there is a discrete interface between the tumor and the surrounding thyroid parenchyma. The nodule in this image shows a thin capsule. The nodule must be well sampled, with sectioning along the tumor-capsular-parenchymal interface to rule out any invasion, either capsular or vascular. (**c**) The corresponding histology shows a well-circumscribed, thinly encapsulated nodule that is well delineated from the surrounding thyroid parenchyma (H&E). (**d**) High magnification of the tumor (H&E)

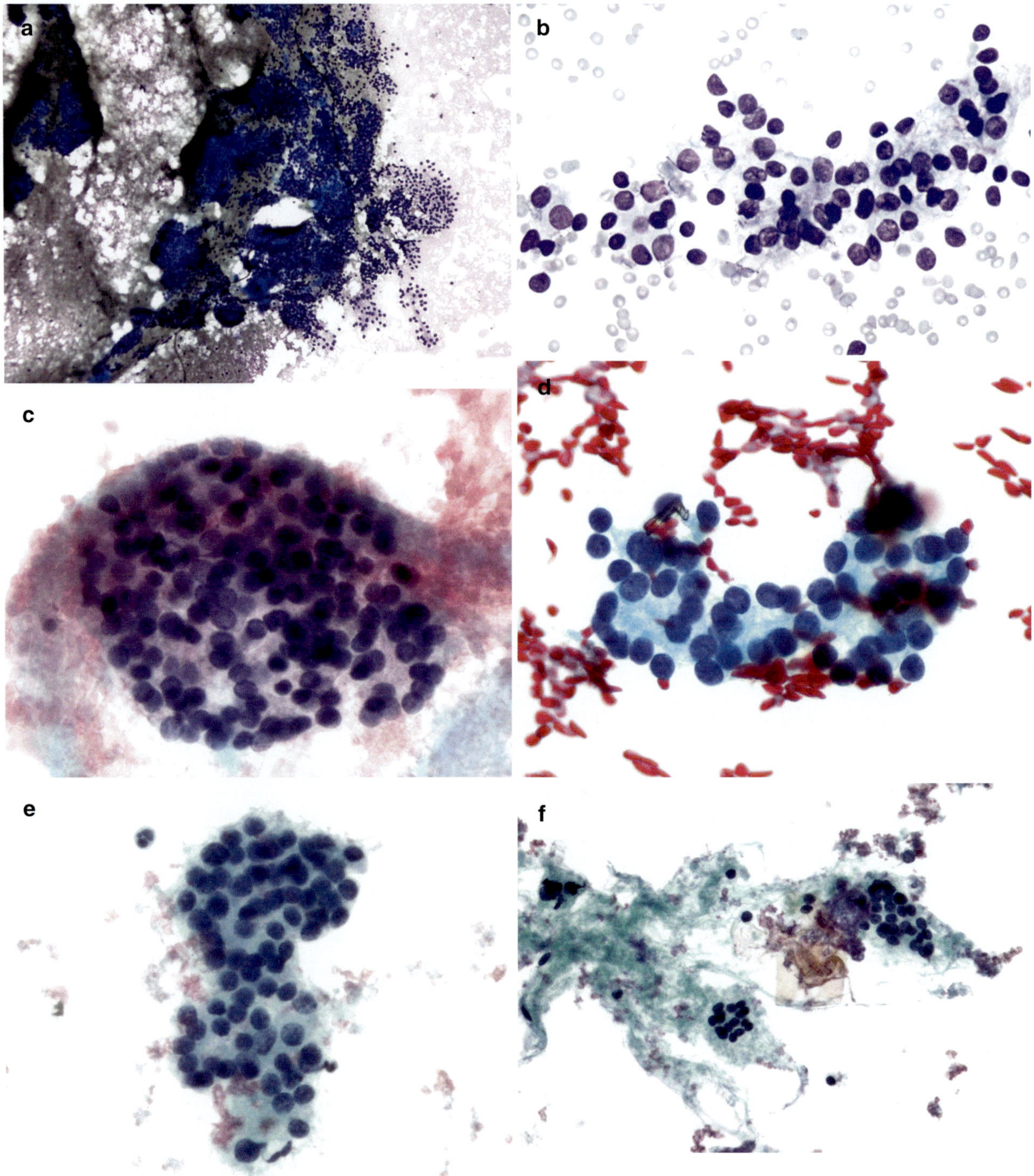

Fig. 9.16 NIFTP: Cytologic and histologic findings. This is a case of a well-circumscribed 2-cm nodule in the right lower lobe. (**a**) The air-dried smear is cellular, composed mostly of compacted and loose microfollicles. The background shows mostly blood and lacks colloid. (**b**) Higher magnification of the air-dried smear shows loose microfollicles with nuclear enlargement and nuclear sizes ranging from 2 to 4 times the size of the adjacent red blood cells. Even on this DQ stain, the nuclei look pale and show overlapping in some foci. Although nuclear abnormalities are noted here, it is best to use alcohol-fixed smears to appreciate these nuclear features (**a**, **b**, DQ stain, CS). (**c**, **d**) Alcohol-fixed smears showing microfollicles with considerable nuclear enlargement when compared with the adjacent red blood cells. In (**c**) a group of microfollicles are admixed with blood, but the nuclear features are still well appreciated, including crowding, nuclear enlargement, and pallor (**c**, **d**, Pap stain, CS). (**e**, **f**) LBP from the same case show similar nuclear alterations as seen on the smear preparations. In LBP, the clusters appear much tighter and more cohesive, and the cell size appears smaller. Nevertheless, the presence of irregularly shaped microfollicles with nuclear enlargement, overlap, and pallor can be appreciated. In all these slides (including smears), no prominent INPIs are evident. The cytomorphologic features in this case warranted a call of follicular neoplasm/suspicious for a follicular neoplasm (FN/SFN, Bethesda IV) (Pap stain, TP). (**g**, **h**) Histology showed a well-circumscribed, encapsulated nodule composed of follicles. On higher magnification, the nodule is composed of a follicular growth pattern (predominantly microfollicles), with nuclear features of PTC such as enlargement, overlap, grooves, pale chromatin, and irregular membranes. INPIs are not readily identified (H&E stain)

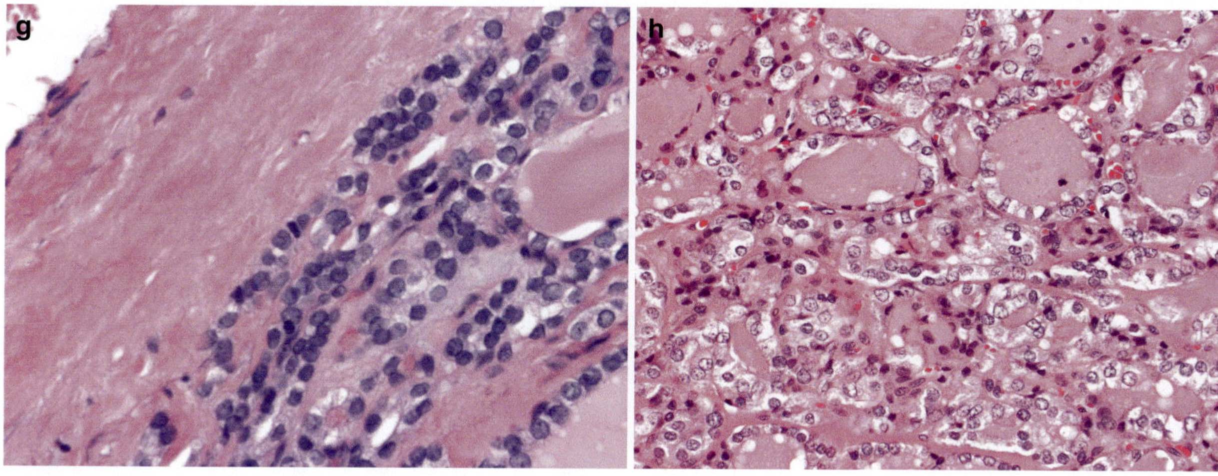

Fig. 9.16 (continued)

- If a FVPTC is suspected on cytology (suspicious for malignancy), TBSRTC recommends an optional note such as "The cytomorphologic features are suspicious for a FVPTC or its recently described indolent counterpart, NIFTP."

Salient Points for FVPTC and NIFTP

- Introduction of NIFTP as nonmalignant and the modified ROM that followed has led to some changes in how we approach follicular-patterned lesions on cytology.
- The key is to avoid diagnosing follicular-patterned PTC as overtly malignant. Some helpful features on cytology include a follicular-patterned lesion with microfollicles showing nuclear features of PTC such as crowding, slight enlargement, overlap, and grooves, and lacking prominent intranuclear inclusions.
- Cytological characteristics of NIFTP on LBP are less understood. Nevertheless, the cytologic features of NIFTP on LBP are similar to what is seen on CS, with less evidence of pseudoinclusions and less bloody background (*see* Fig. 9.17).
- The recommendation is to use the "SM" or "FN/SFN" category with a note of the possibility that it may be FVPTC or NIFTP.
- Sampling for molecular testing is always recommended in follicular-patterned lesions mimicking PTC. If molecular testing determines a *RAS* mutation over a *BRAF*, a likelihood of NIFTP can be entertained.
- Preoperative determination of the likelihood of NIFTP is important, as lobectomy is the treatment of choice, not total thyroidectomy.
- In summary, NIFTP is a noninvasive thyroid tumor of follicular origin and nuclear features of PTC, with a potential for invasion to invasive encapsulated FVPTC. It is therefore considered a precursor of carcinoma, with low rates of recurrence and metastatic potential. Imaging findings and preoperative cytology are not definitive.

Tall Cell Variant of PTC (TCV-PTC)

- TCV-PTC, an aggressive variant of PTC, comprises 3–11% of all PTC.
- Originally reported by Hawk and Hazard in 1976, this variant includes tumor cells with nuclear features of PTC that are two to three times as tall as they are wide, which are therefore referred to as "tall cells."

Clinical and Imaging Features of TCV-PTC

- TCV-PTC commonly presents at an older age (about 55 years) and with increasing rates of lymph node metastasis and extrathyroidal extension (ETE). Its 5-year disease-free survival (81%) is poorer than that of conventional PTC (98%).
- On ultrasound imaging, TCV-PTC appears as markedly hypoechoic, predominantly solid nodule with frequent internal microcalcifications, ETE, and lymph node metastasis (Fig. 9.18a).

Pathological Features of TCV-PTC

- Grossly, the tumors are usually large with extrathyroidal extension, solid, firm, pale tan to white.
- On histology, for a diagnosis of TCV-PTC, at least 30% of the tumor must be composed of tall cells. This percentage is controversial, as it has been noted that tumors with even 10% of tall cells (so-called PTC with tall cell features) carry a relatively aggressive prognosis (Fig. 9.18b, c).

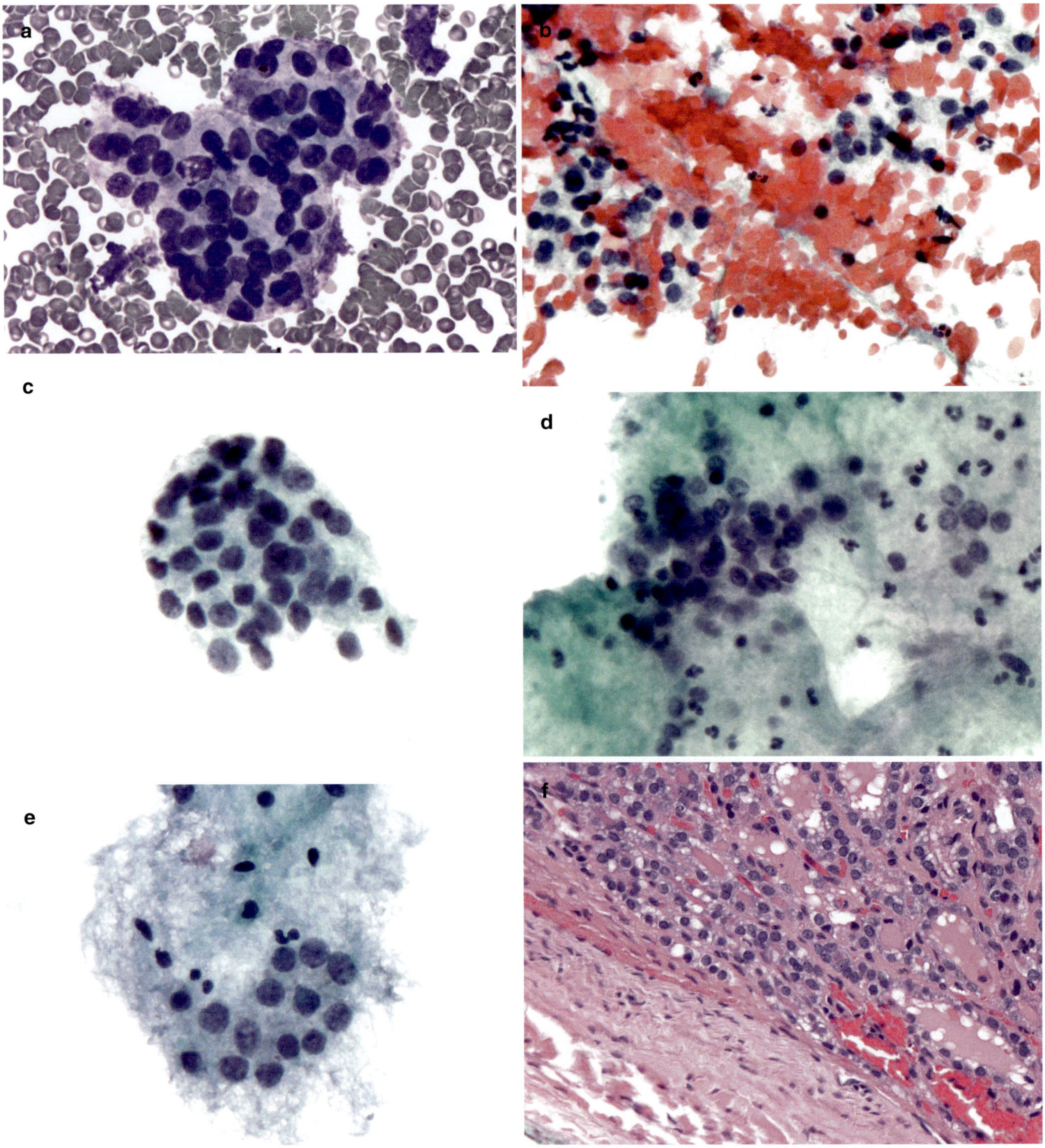

Fig. 9.17 NIFTP: Cytomorphology, with emphasis on LBP. (**a–f**) illustrate a case of a solid, 2.7-cm nodule with a previous diagnosis of follicular lesion of undetermined significance (FLUS). (**a**), The air-dried smear shows a compact group of microfollicles with nuclear enlargement, crowding, and pallor (Diff-Quik, CS). (**b**) An alcohol-fixed smear shows similar features of loose clusters of follicular cells with nuclear atypia as described above. Note the left lower group, showing a follicular cell nucleus with grooves (Pap stain, CS). (**c–e**) LBP show nuclear features similar to the aspirate smears. The background is less bloody (**c**). INPIs are rare in NIFTP, but (**d**) shows a group of follicular cells on the right with an INPI; the background shows blood. (**e**) shows a microfollicle with nuclear features as described above. A diagnosis of FLUS was rendered. Molecular testing showed an *NRAS* mutation (**c–e**, Pap stain, TP). (**f**) The corresponding histology was NIFTP; note the thin capsule surrounding the lesion. The nuclear features on histology mirror those on cytology (H&E stain). (**g–i**) LBP from another case of NIFTP, with a cytologic diagnosis of FN/SFN (Bethesda IV), showing a cellular sample composed of microfollicles with nuclear enlargement, pallor, overlap, and peripherally placed nucleoli. Note the presence of thick colloid (scant in **i**) (**g–i**, Pap stain, TP)

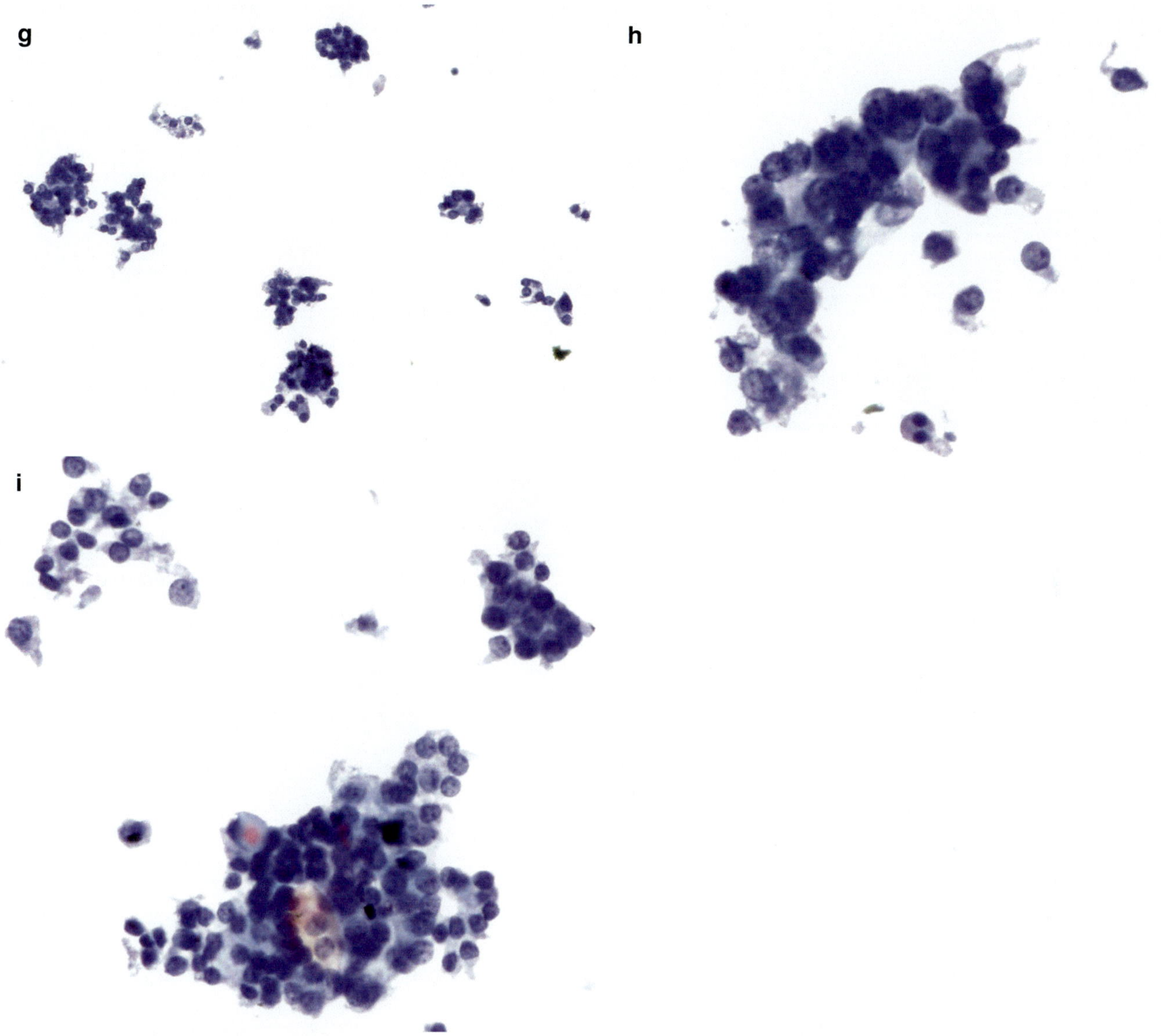

Fig. 9.17 (continued)

Cytology of TCV-PTC: Application to LBP

- FNA can aid in the preoperative identification of the tall cells. The aspirates show tall cells with increased oncocytic cytoplasm, with a low N:C ratio, prominent cell outlines, and nuclear features of PTC with multiple intranuclear "soap bubble–like" pseudoinclusions when compared with conventional PTC (Figs. 9.18d–i and 9.19).
- Kaw [23] described tissue fragments with scalloped outer borders on conventional smears of TCV-PTC.
- Features are similar on LBP, but LBP is superior in the detection of tall cells because cellular preservation is better than on CS.
- Lee et al. [24], in their study on SurePath™ (SP) samples of TCV-PTC, showed findings such as tall cells with oncocytic cytoplasm and distinct cell borders well appreciated in LBP samples. In dense clusters, these tall cells were better appreciated in the periphery of the cell cluster.
- Our group's study of TCV-PTC on ThinPrep® (TP) [21] showed that cytologic features of these tall cells, as described on CS, could readily be identified on TP, and TP appeared to have better cellular preservation. The most helpful diagnostic feature included increased numbers of tall cells arranged as both single cells and in the periphery of the cell groups, with oncocytic cytoplasm, distinct cell borders, and cytoplasmic tails. We first described "cytoplasmic cuff"—the peripheral rim of cytoplasm noted on some monolayered and syncytial groups—as a feature of TCV-PTC.
- The "soap bubble–like" INPIs described as a notable feature of TCV-PTC on CS are present in TP samples but may be less appreciated.

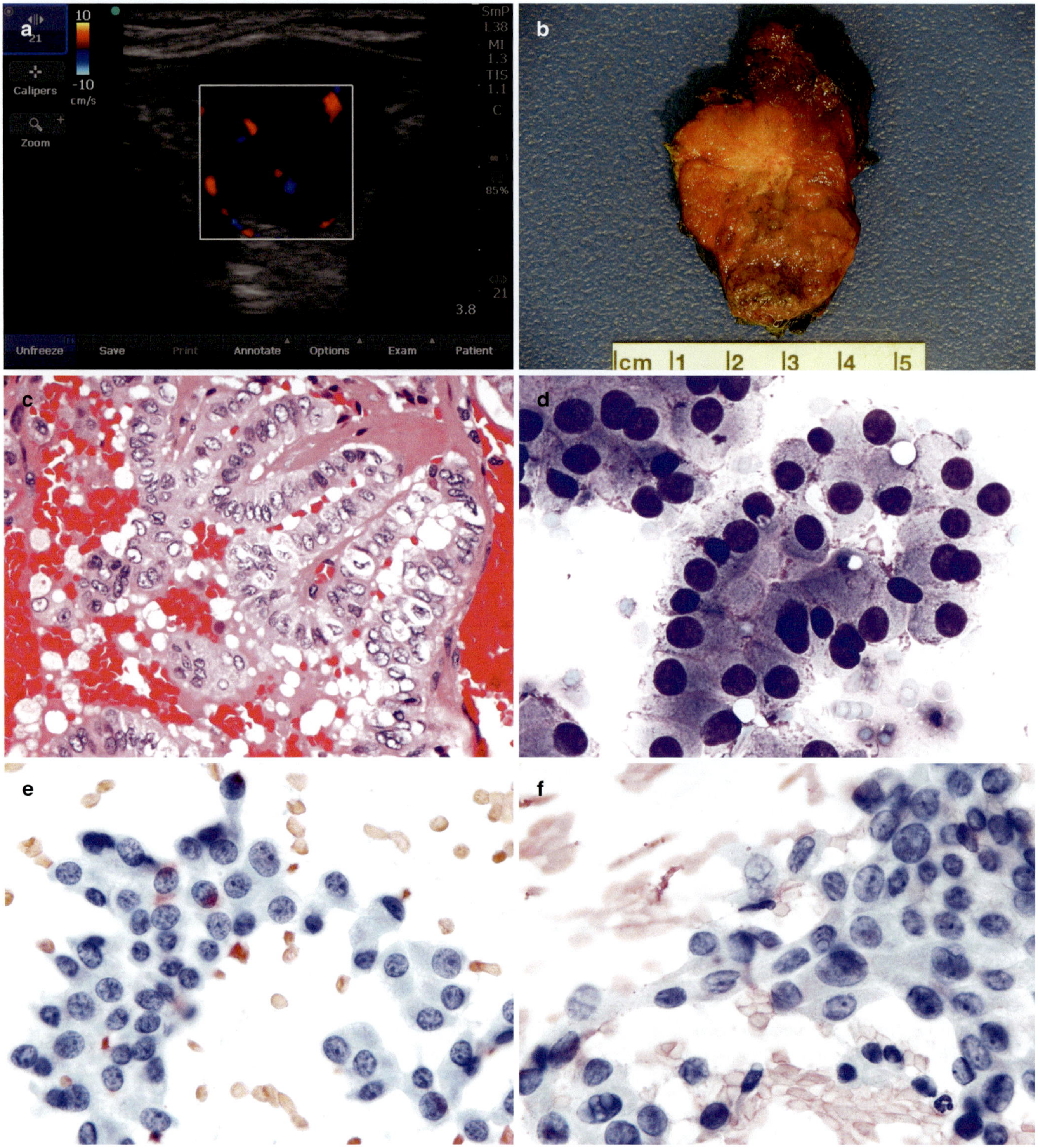

Fig. 9.18 Tall cell variant of PTC (TCV-PTC): Imaging, gross, and histologic findings. (**a**) Ultrasound image of TCV-PTC, showing a markedly hypoechoic but predominantly solid nodule with internal vascularity. Compared with classic PTC, TCV-PTC tends to show frequent internal microcalcifications, extrathyroidal extension, and lymph node metastasis. (**b**) Gross image of TCV-PTC showing a predominantly tan-brown solid nodule with some cystic foci; it is poorly circumscribed, with blurring of the borders between the nodule and the adjacent thyroid parenchyma. (**c**) Histology of the nodule shows tumor cells arranged as tall cells (with length at least 2–3 times the width) and moderately abundant cytoplasm. The nuclear features appear similar to the classic PTC (H&E). (**d**) Preoperative FNA cytology. This air-dried aspirate smear shows tumor cells with decreased N:C ratio, abundant oncocytic cytoplasm, and enlarged nuclei. Compare the nuclear sizes of the tumor cells to that of the adjacent RBCs. The cell borders appear to be well defined (DQ stain, CS). (**e**, **f**) The alcohol-fixed smears show all nuclear features similar to PTC, such as nuclear enlargement, pallor, membrane irregularity, grooves, overlap, and INPIs; an occasional cell (*bottom left*) shows multiple "soap bubble"–like INPIs (Pap stain, CS). (**g**–**i**) LBP from this aspirate shows tumor cells that appear to have more cytoplasm and are "tall" (better appreciated at the edges of the cluster). The nuclear features are similar to those of c-PTC. Note the laminated psammoma body (Pap stain, TP)

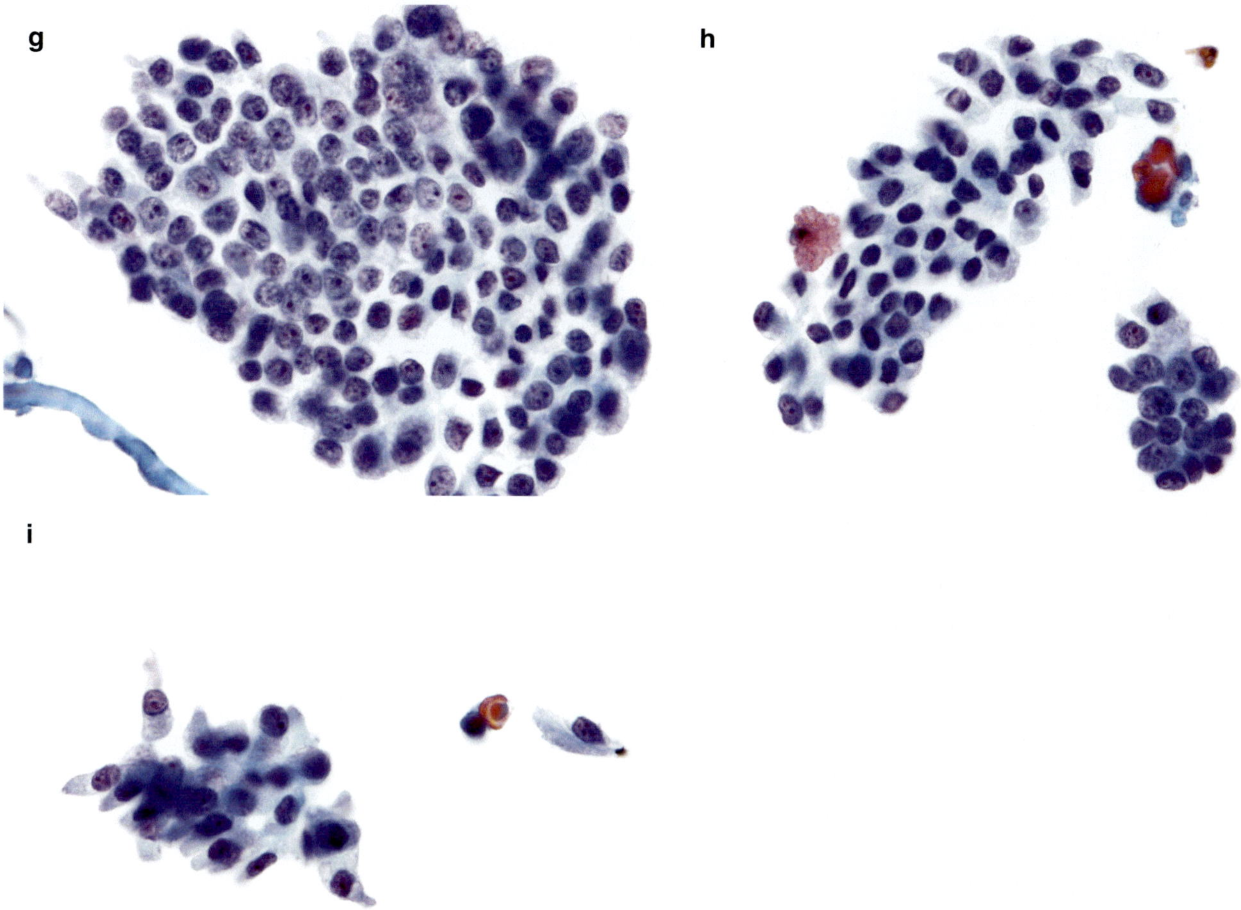

Fig. 9.18 (continued)

Molecular Profile of TCV-PTC

- Notable molecular alterations include *BRAF*V600E mutations; TCV-PTC shows the highest frequencies when compared with c-PTC.
- Also seen are loss of heterozygosity for chromosome 1 (D1S243) and the *p53* gene (TP53) and *RET*/*PTC3* rearrangement.

Cystic PTC

- Partially cystic thyroid nodules (PCTNs) are commonly seen on ultrasound.
- Li et al. [30] published a detailed ultrasonographic assessment of PCTNs.
- Most cystic thyroid nodules are a result of degenerative changes arising in underlying lesions. A true epithelial cyst of the thyroid is rare.
- 4.6–17.6% of PCTNs are malignant.
- Among malignant neoplasms, cystic change is the second most common in PTC. Up to 50% of PTC lesions are at least partially cystic, and about 10% are predominantly cystic.
- The guidelines of the American Thyroid Association (ATA) [28] recommend that PCTNs with suspicious ultrasound features or nodules with the greatest dimension >1.5 cm should undergo FNA and follow-up.

Imaging Features of Cystic PTC

- Li et al. [30] described suspicious features of a PCTN:
  - Irregular and eccentrically located solid component within the cyst, comprising at least 50% of the lesion
  - Microcalcifications
  - Increased vascularity in the solid component or cyst wall
- Based on these features, ultrasound differentiated malignant from benign PCTN with 84.6% sensitivity, 84.0%

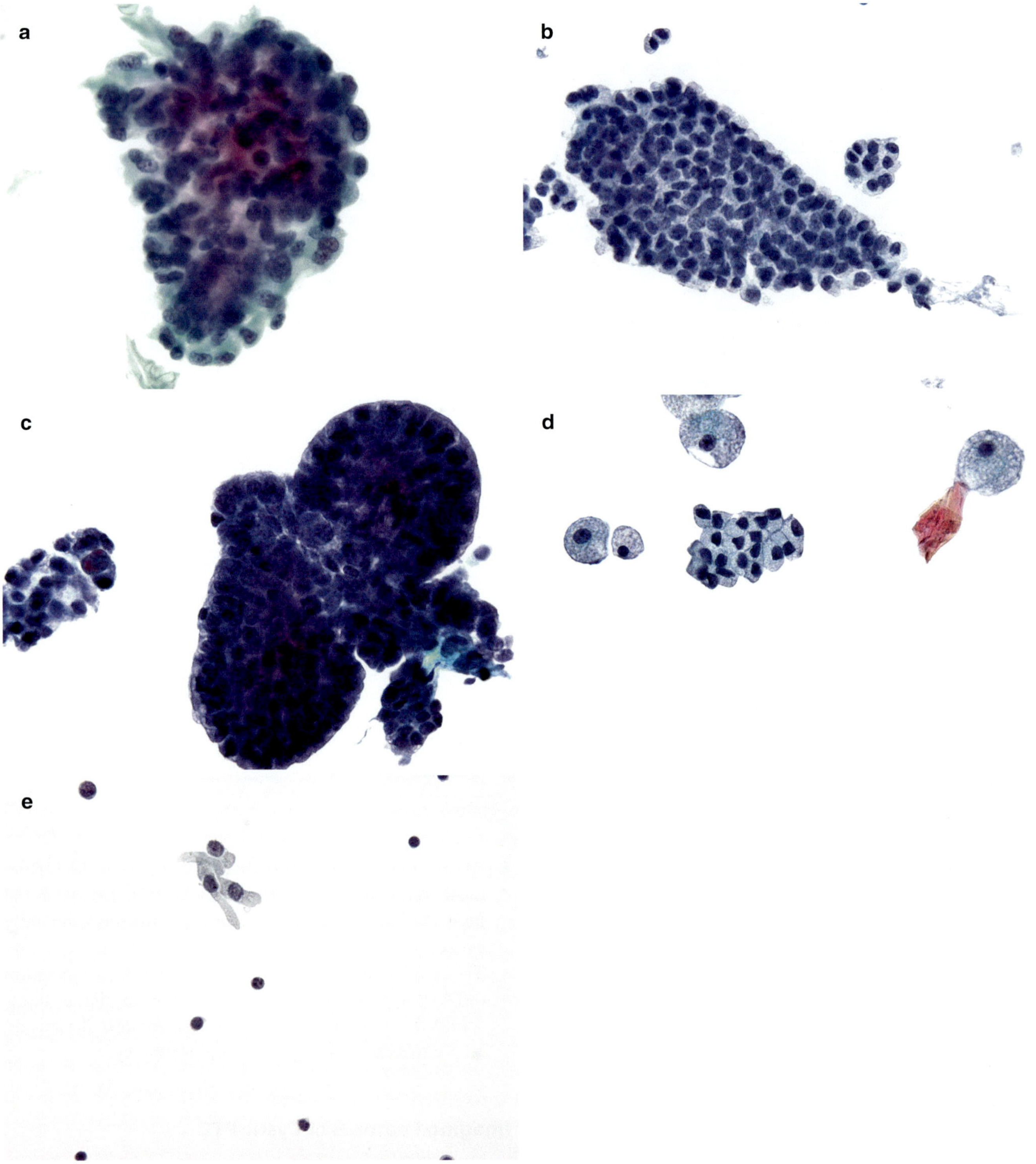

Fig. 9.19 TCV-PTC: Cytologic findings on LBP. These images show examples of TCV-PTC on LBP (Pap stain, TP). (**a**) The cluster of tumor cells from a case of TCV-PTC. Note the soap bubble–like (multiple) INPIs in a few of these nuclei. (**b**, **c**) These are tighter, flat sheets and dense cellular branching clusters of tumor cells. Cells arranged in the periphery of these sheets show a cytoplasmic "palisade" with apical cytoplasm and basal nuclei showing features of PTC. Baum et al. [21] highlighted this feature in LBP of TCV-PTC, referring to it as "cytoplasmic cuff." (**d**) Similar cytoplasmic cuffing; well-defined cell outlines and moderately abundant oncocytic cytoplasm can be seen in TCV-PTC on LBP. LBP appear to preserve the cell outlines better than CS. (**e**) This example shows single tall cells, better appreciated on LBP. Note that the nuclear sizes of the tumor cells are fairly enlarged when compared with the lymphocytes in the background

specificity, and 84.0% accuracy; the positive predictive value (PPV) was 20.4% and the negative predictive value (NPV) was 99.1%.

Pathological Features of Cystic PTC

- PTC may undergo cystic change.
- Grossly, a multicystic tumor can be seen.
- Histologically, papillary structures are noted facing the lumen of the cyst (Fig. 9.20).

Cytopathology of Cystic PTC: Application to LBP

- Cystic PTC is predominantly cystic; the nodule contains thin, watery fluid accompanied by abundant histiocytes and vacuolated (histiocytoid) tumor cells.
- Specimens are usually hypocellular.
- Faquin et al. [27] and the 2nd edition of TBSRTC [25]) outlined cytological features of cystic PTC, and Mokhtari et al. [31] outlined newer cytological features, discussed below. All the cytological features were described on CS but are equally applicable to LBP.
- Cystic PTC shows a cystic background with numerous hemosiderin-laden macrophages, thin watery colloid, cystic debris, large epithelioid giant cells with many nuclei, and rare psammoma bodies.
- Epithelial cells are sparse, composed of cells with nuclear features of PTC. Hypervacuolated cells with a "histiocytoid cell" morphology are also present.
- Cells appear as isolated plasmacytoid cells with occasional signet-ring forms, and also may be arranged in syncytial fragments, small groups with irregular borders, small clusters with a radial distribution of cells (cartwheel pattern), small ball-like cellular clusters (cellular swirls), papillae or follicles, and clusters of "histiocytoid" cells with scalloped, well-defined borders.
- Although all nuclear features of PTC are present, nuclear grooves are prominent, "powdery" chromatin may be less prominent, and INPIs may be occasional. Cytoplasm is abundant, vacuolated, and granular or dense (Figs. 9.21, 9.22, 9.23, 9.24, and 9.25).

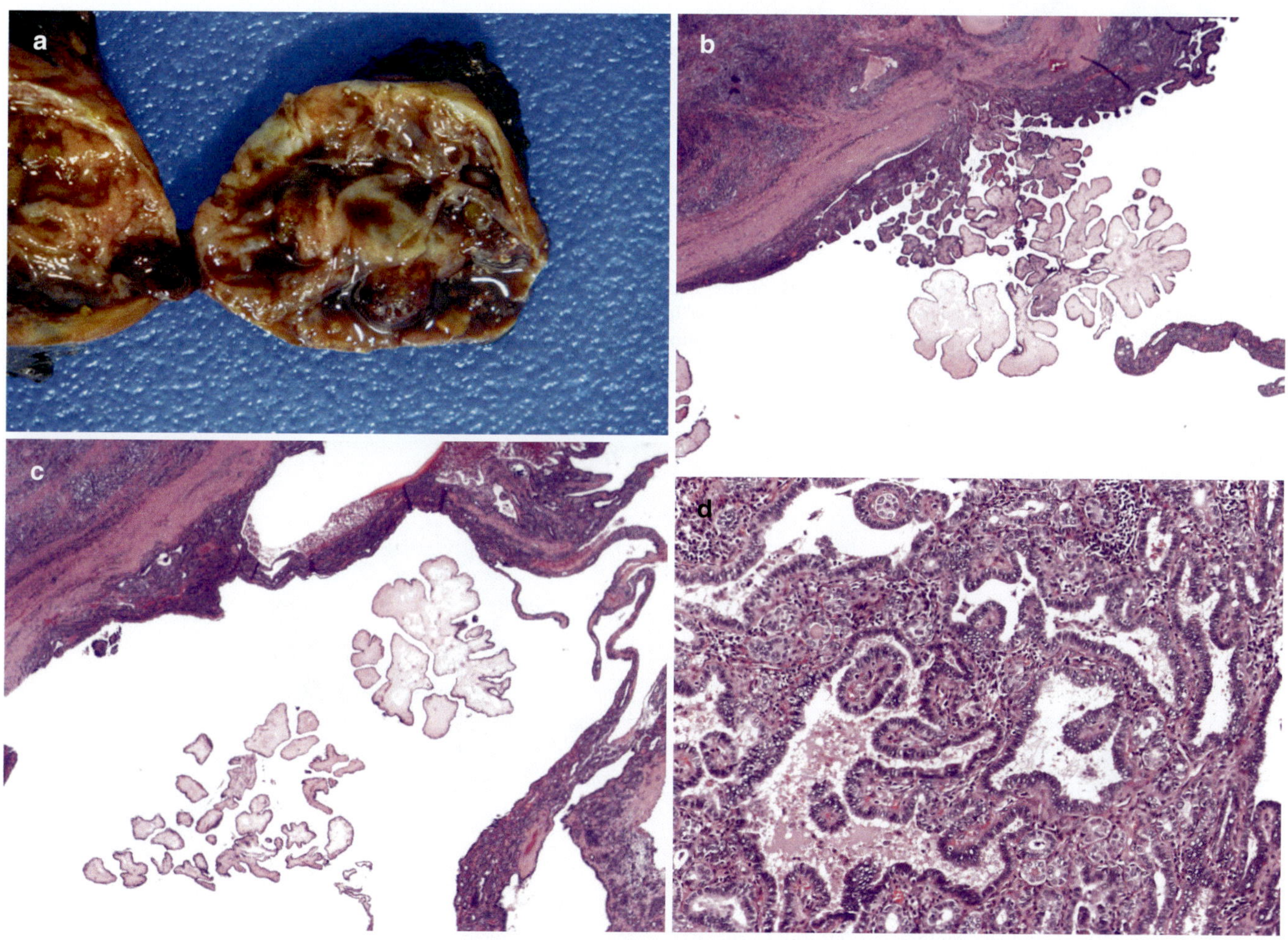

Fig. 9.20 Cystic PTC: Gross and histologic features. (**a**) Gross appearance of a cystic PTC. (**b**, **c**) Histology of cystic PTC. Note the attached and dislodged papillary structures. (**d**) High magnification shows all nuclear features of PTC (**b**–**d**, H&E stain)

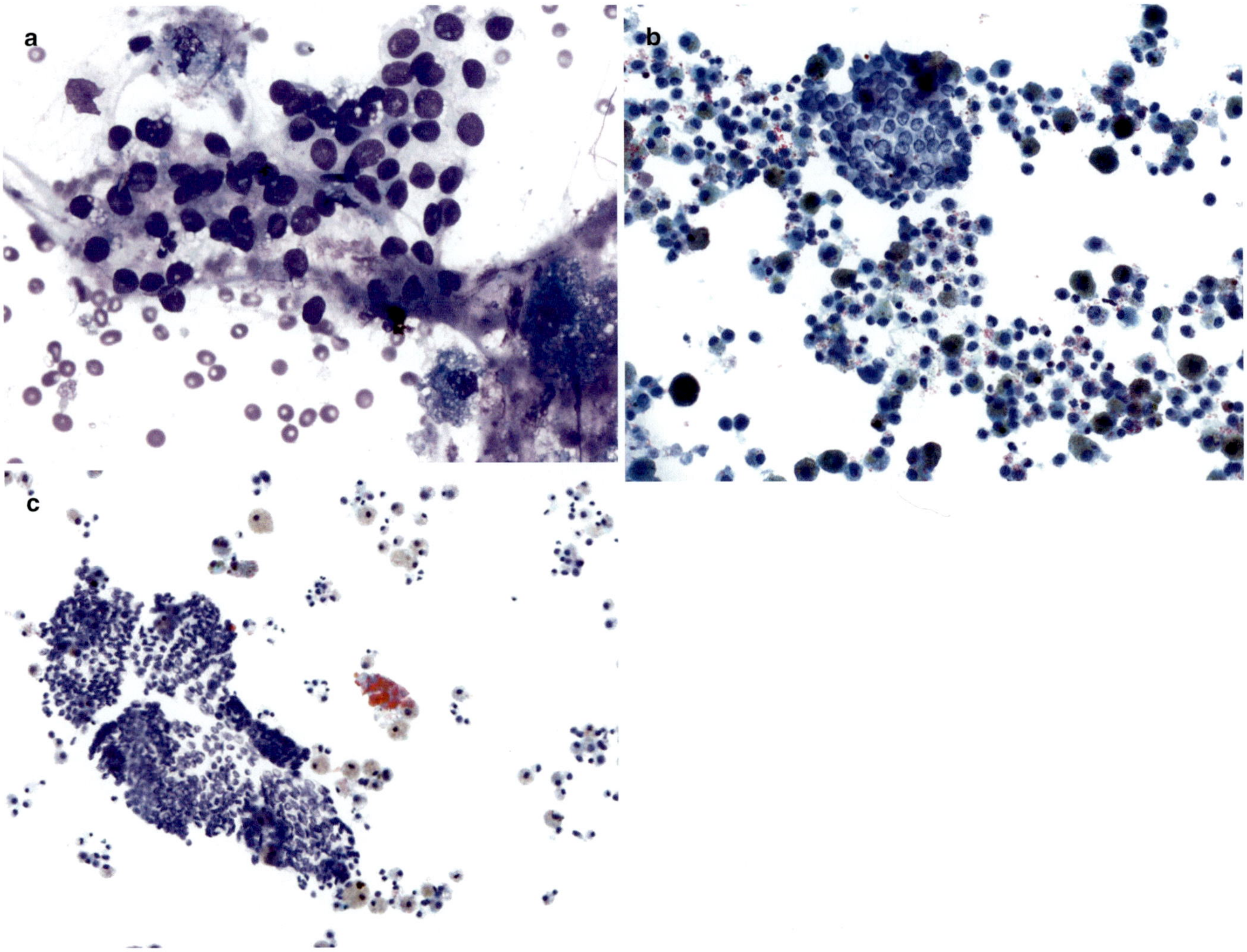

Fig. 9.21 Cystic PTC: Cytologic findings. (**a**, **b**) CS shows an irregular sheet and small, ball-like cellular clusters (cellular swirls) in a cystic background with many hemosiderin-laden macrophages (**a**, DQ stain, CS; **b**, Pap stain, CS). (**c**) On the same case, TP shows similar findings. Even in the irregular sheet of tumor cells, some cell swirling is visible (Pap stain)

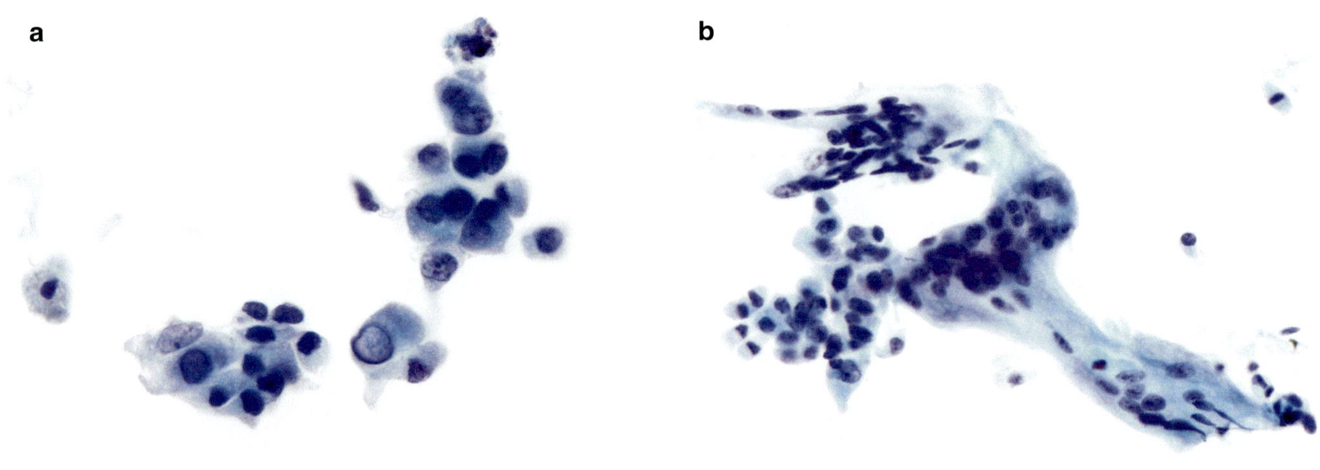

Fig. 9.22 Cystic PTC: Cytologic findings on TP. (**a**) Cystic PTC showing enlarged cells with granular cytoplasm and well-defined cell walls. Note focal radial distribution of cells (cartwheel pattern) on bottom left. All nuclear features of PTC, including a well-formed INPI (*middle*) are evident. (**b**) Cystic PTC with a giant multinucleated cell (**a**, **b**, Pap stain, TP)

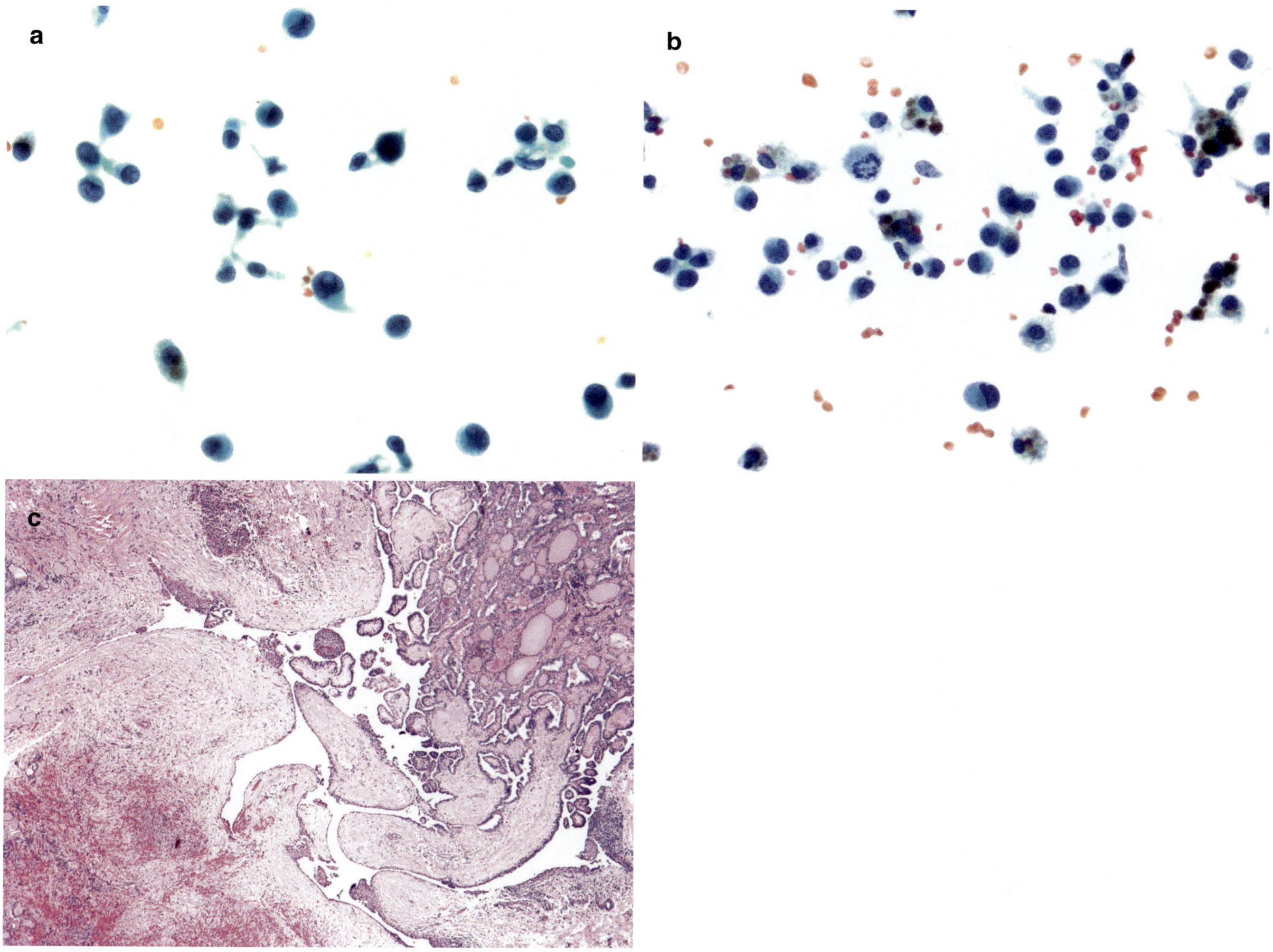

Fig. 9.23 Cystic PTC: Cytologic and histologic findings on LBP. (**a**) Isolated, enlarged plasmacytoid cells in comparison to RBCs in the background. Note the well-formed INPI (*middle*) (Pap stain, SP). (**b**) Isolated, enlarged plasmacytoid cells in comparison to RBCs. Note the cystic background with many hemosiderin-laden macrophages (Pap stain, TP). (**c**) Histology of cystic PTC (H&E stain)

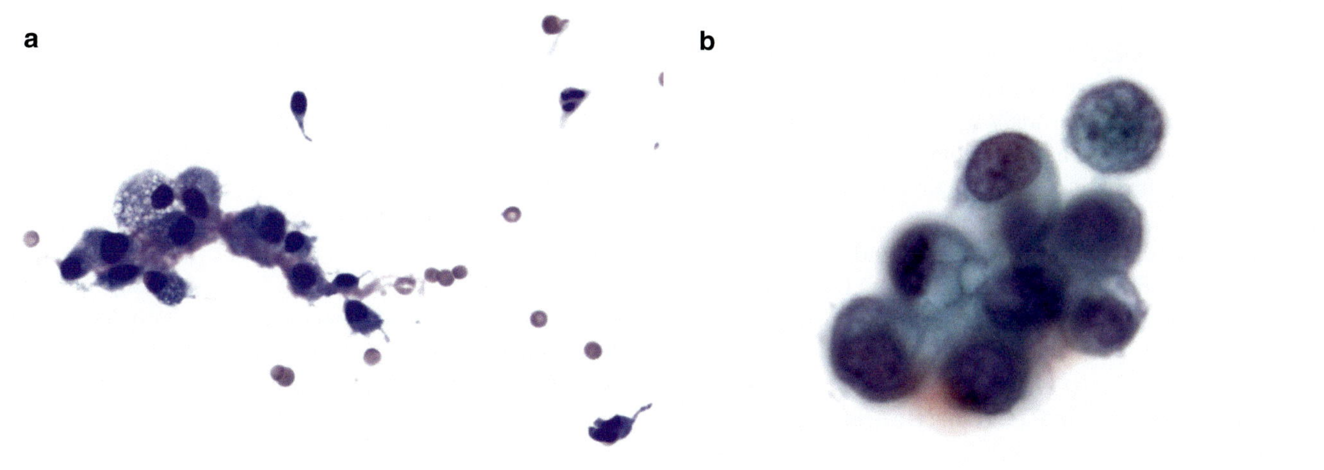

Fig. 9.24 Cystic "histiocytoid" PTC: Pathologic features. (**a**) DQ-stained CS shows a cluster of cells with "histiocytoid" morphology and scalloped borders. Cells and nuclei are enlarged (compare with RBCs) and cytoplasm is granular. (**b–e**) TP images of various cell groups from this case show also clusters of cells with "histiocytoid" morphology and scalloped borders. Cells and nuclei are enlarged (compare with RBCs) and cytoplasm is granular to vacuolated to dense, with distinct cell outlines. An occasional signet-ring form (**c**) can be seen. All nuclear features of PTC are apparent, including an INPI in (**c**). (**f**) Histology of this case shows crisp "histiocytoid" morphology at the top of the field and similar morphology in the detached papillary structures (H&E stain)

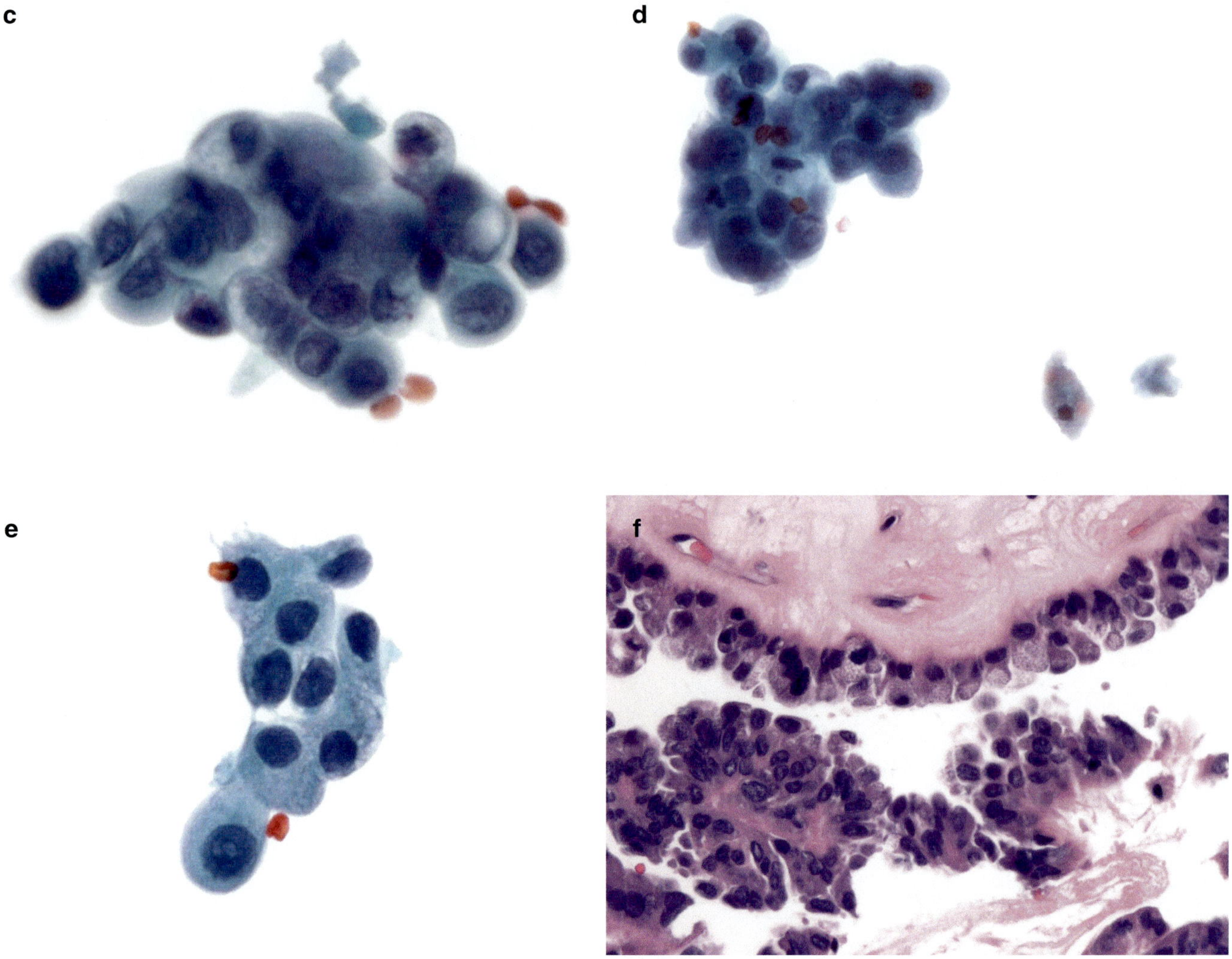

Fig. 9.24 (continued)

Diagnostic Pitfalls of Cystic PTC

- A pitfall of cystic PTC is that aspirates may be sparsely cellular and interpreted as nondiagnostic, leading to false negative results. In the study by Li et al. [30] of PCTNs, 7.8% had a nondiagnostic cytology result. The risk of malignancy for nondiagnostic thyroid nodules varies between 2% and 15%.
- Another pitfall is that many benign and non-neoplastic lesions may undergo cystic degeneration; benign cyst lining cells may mimic PTC and lead to false positive results.

Distinguishing Cystic PTC from Benign Cystic Nodules

- Faquin et al. [27] and Mokhtari et al. [31] have also indicated some cytological features that may help in distinguishing cystic PTC from benign cystic nodules:
  - Presence of large and irregular multinucleated giant cells with many nuclei and dense cytoplasm
  - Psammoma bodies
  - Isolated plasmacytoid cells
  - Dense cytoplasm and dusty chromatin
  - Cells with PTC nuclear features arranged as papillae
  - Clusters with scalloped borders lined by enlarged cells and nuclei
  - Cellular swirls
  - Clusters with a cartwheel pattern.
- Cystic PTC shows cell crowding and overlapping, whereas cells in benign cystic lesions usually occur in small, flat, cohesive and polarized sheets with distinct cell borders and windows between cells.
- See Chaps. 4 and 5 for distinguishing features and images of benign cyst lining cells and cystic PTC.

Oncocytic Variant of PTC (OV-PTC)

- Carr et al. [32] published a detailed analysis on OV-PTC.
- Oncocytic thyroid cells, also known as Hürthle or oxyphilic cells, are generally larger than normal follicular

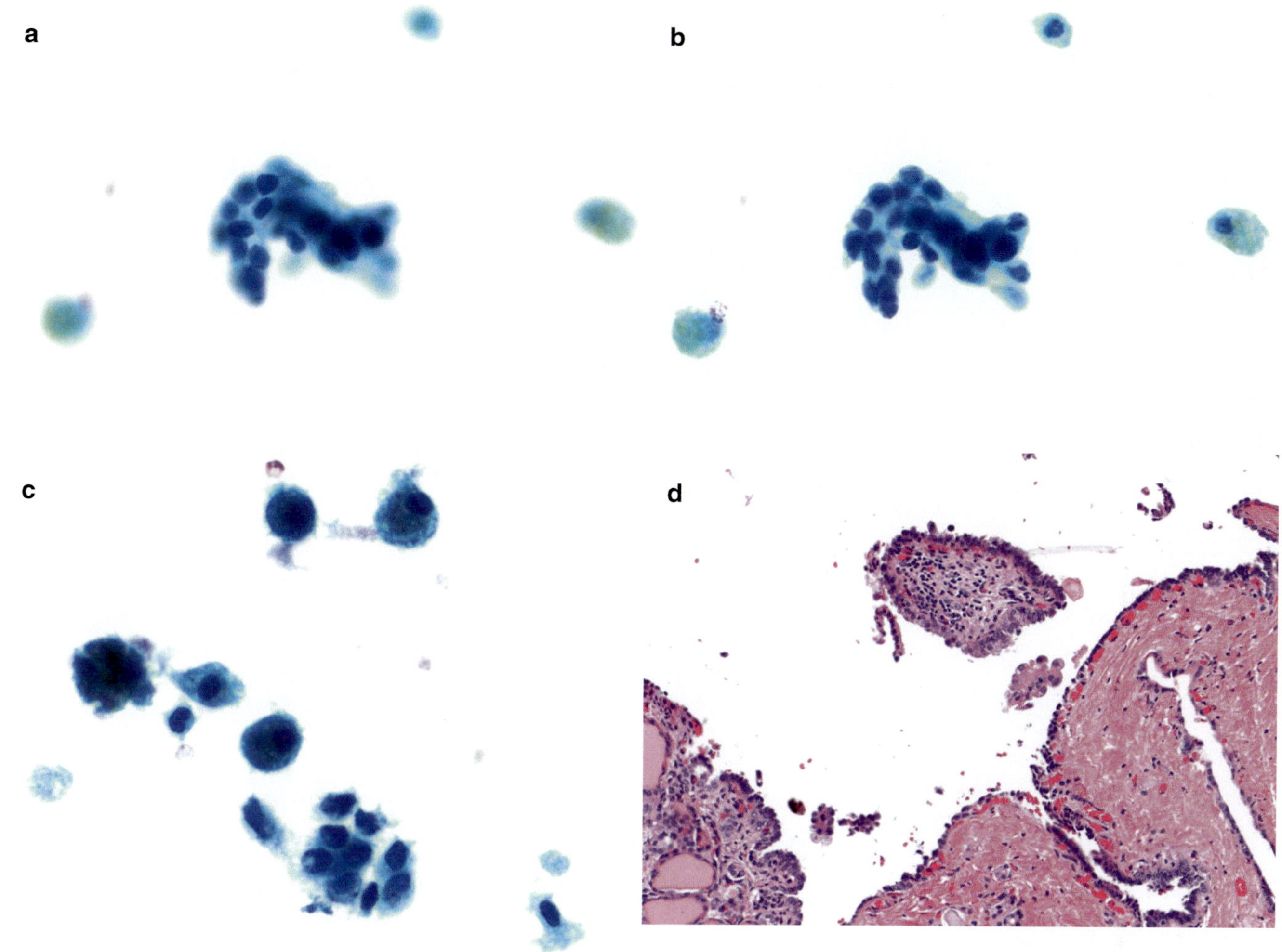

Fig. 9.25 Cystic PTC: Cytologic and histologic findings on SP. (**a**, **b**) Both images show the same small "histiocytoid" cell cluster in a cystic background. Cells can be focused in different planes, showing subtle nuclear features of PTC, particularly grooves, chromatin changes, and small nucleoli. (**c**) Another example of cystic PTC on SP shows PTC nuclei, including an INPI, in a cystic background with many hemosiderin-laden macrophages (**a–c**, Pap stain). (**d**) Histology showing several detached "histiocytoid" cell clusters, which appear in FNA specimens (H&E stain)

cells. They are polygonal and are characterized by abundant eosinophilic cytoplasm due to the accumulation of numerous abnormal mitochondria.

- Oncocytic changes may be seen in both benign and malignant thyroid neoplasms. (See Chaps. 4, 6, and 7.)
- To be histologically considered an OV-PTC, oncocytic change should apply to at least 75% of the tumor.

Clinical Behavior and Prognosis of OV-PTC

- The incidence of OV-PTC has been reported to be 1–11%.
- Clinical behavior and prognosis are variable. In their study, Carr et al. concluded that when matched with c-PTC of similar stage and age, OV-PTC does not appear to have worse histopathologic characteristics or a significantly worse prognosis. Some studies have suggested a more aggressive behavior of OV-PTC, with extrathyroidal extension and higher rates of disease recurrence and mortality.
- According to Carr et al. [32], the pure form of OV-PTC is very rare and must be differentiated from TCV-PTC, which also has abundant eosinophilic cytoplasm but is characterized by cells that are two to three times as tall as they are wide.

Gross and Histologic Features of OV-PTC

- Grossly, OV-PTC shows a well circumscribed mass with a mahogany-brown cut surface (Fig. 9.26a).
- The histologic criteria used for the diagnosis of OV-PTC include a predominant papillary pattern of growth with the same nuclear morphological features

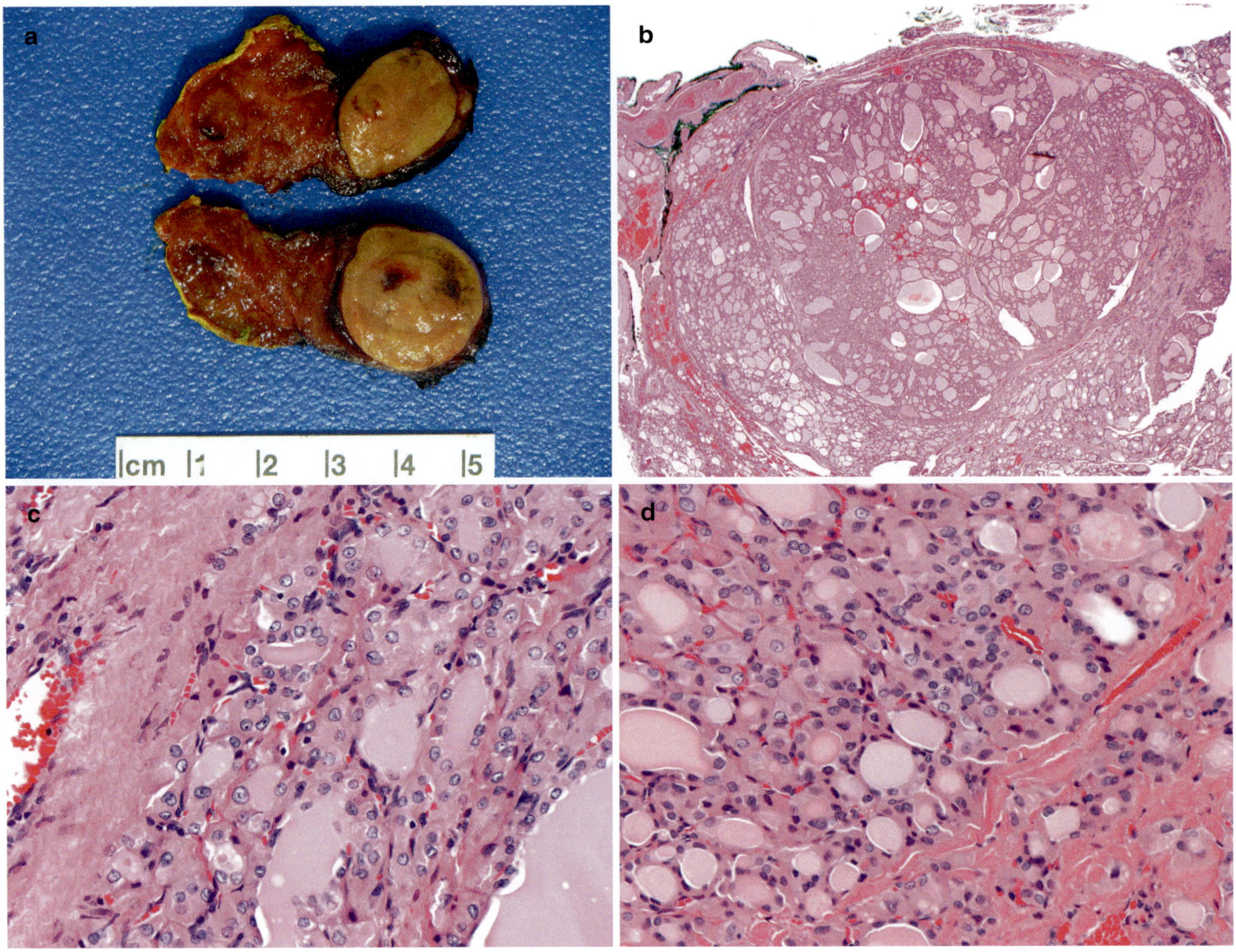

Fig. 9.26 Oncocytic variant of PTC (OV-PTC): Gross and histologic features. (**a**) OV-PTC showing a well-circumscribed mass with a brown cut surface. (**b–d**) Though the predominant pattern of growth is usually papillary, follicular growth pattern can be seen. On high power, the tumor cells have a granular eosinophilic cytoplasm. Nucleoli are generally present but are not prominent. The nuclei show classic nuclear features of PTC (H&E stain)

seen in c-PTC, such as irregularly shaped, elongated, and crowded nuclei with chromatin clearing, prominent grooves, and pseudoinclusions. Nucleoli are generally present but are not prominent. The majority of cells should exhibit granular eosinophilic (oncocytic) cytoplasm (Fig. 9.26b–d).

- Follicular growth pattern can also be seen.

Cytological Features of OV-PTC

- Aspirates comprise oncocytic cells arranged in papillae, sheets, and microfollicles, and also singly dispersed (Figs. 9.27, 9.28, and 9.29).
- All nuclear features seen in c-PTC are present.
- Background lymphocytes are generally absent.
- Cytological differential diagnosis of OV-PTC includes Hürthle cell carcinoma, oncocytic variant of follicular carcinoma and medullary thyroid carcinoma (MTC), and metastatic tumors with oncocytic differentiation.
- As per TBSRTC, if the constellation of nuclear features of PTC are not evident, the case is best diagnosed as Follicular Neoplasm of Hürthle cell type or Suspicious for a Follicular Neoplasm of Hürthle cell type (FNHCT/SFNHCT).

Warthin-Like Variant of PTC (WLV-PTC)

- WLV-PTC is a rare variant of PTC with a clinical presentation and prognosis similar to classic PTC.

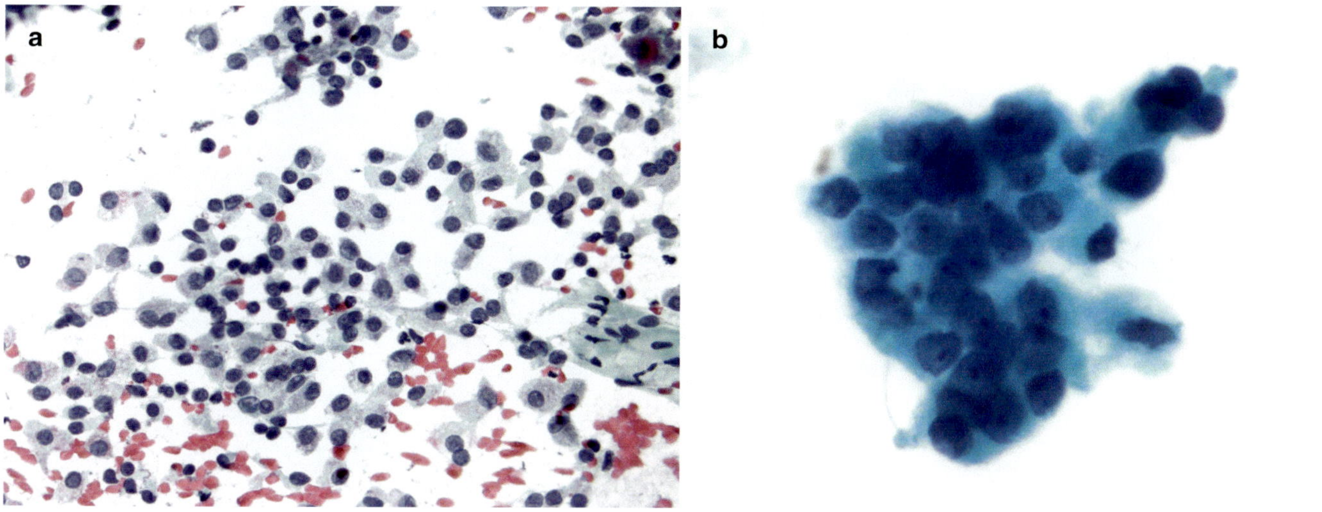

Fig. 9.27 OV-PTC: Cytological features on CS and SP. (**a**) Pap-stained CS shows loosely cohesive, enlarged oncocytic cells with a moderate amount of granular basophilic to eosinophilic cytoplasm, with round to oval, eccentrically placed nuclei with nuclear features of PTC. Some cells are binucleated, and small nucleoli are visible. (**b**) Pap-stained SP of the same case shows a cluster of cells with all nuclear features of PTC and dense to granular cytoplasm. Nucleoli are a bit more prominent than on CS

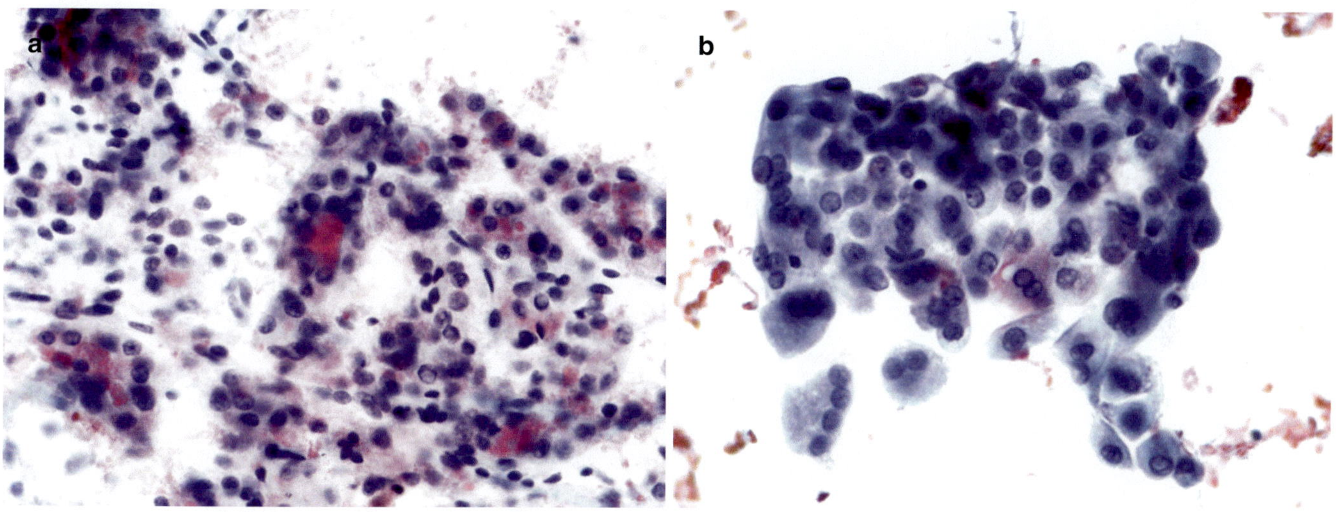

Fig. 9.28 OV-PTC: Cytological features on CS and TP. (**a**) Pap-stained CS of another case shows features similar to the case of OV-PTC in Fig. 9.27. (**b**) Pap-stained TP from this case shows distinct oncocytic cytoplasm and all nuclear features of PTC

- Apel et al. [35] first described the tumor and named it "Warthin-like" because it resembles Warthin tumor of salivary glands, histologically comprising oncocytic and lymphocytic cells.

Imaging and Pathological Features of WLV-PTC

- The most common ultrasound features of WLV-PTC are a solid and hypoechoic appearance, with a wider-than-tall shape [38].
- Grossly, the tumor appears solid, well-circumscribed, and brown (Figs. 9.30a and 9.32a).
- Histologically, WLV-PTC shows a papillary architecture lined by oncocytic cells with nuclear features of PTC and dense lymphoplasmacytic infiltration of the papillary stalks. Lymphoid follicles can also be seen (Fig. 9.30b–d).

Cytological Features of WLV-PTC

- Preoperative diagnosis of WLV-PTC on FNA is challenging because chronic lymphocytic thyroiditis (CLT, Hashimoto thyroiditis) also shows abundant lymphocytes and oncocytic (Hürthle) follicular epithelial cells, and also because WLV-PTC can arise in a background of CLT.
- CS and TP samples of WLV-PTC show irregular and papillary clusters with oncocytic cytoplasm and many lymphocytes within the tumor clusters and background (Figs. 9.31 and 9.32b).

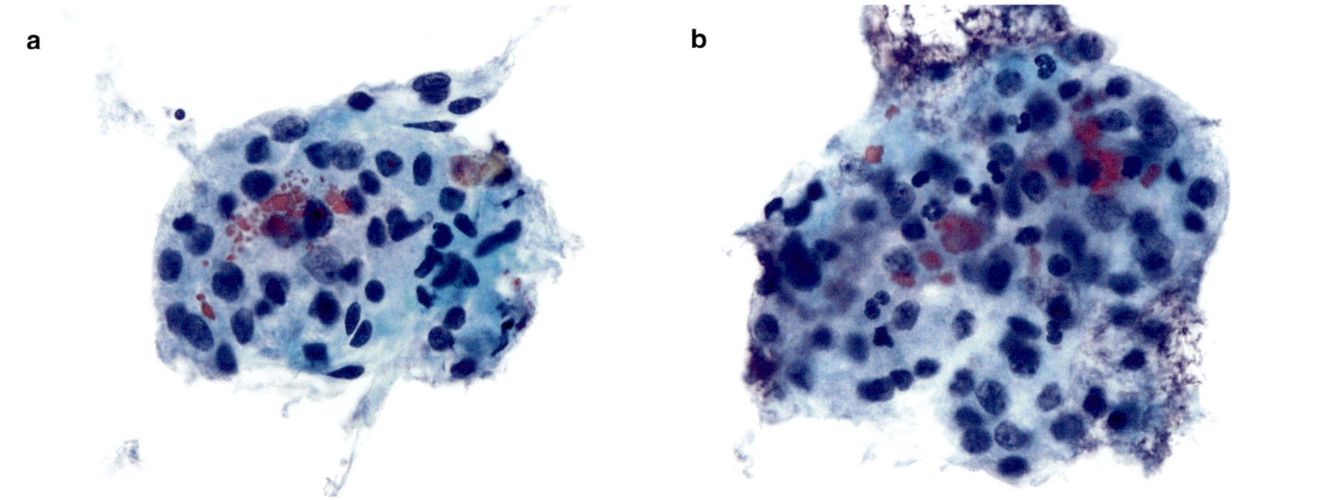

Fig. 9.29 OV-PTC: Cytological features on TP. (**a**, **b**) Another case of OV-PTC showing PTC nuclear features; a small INPI can be seen in (**b**) (Pap stain, TP)

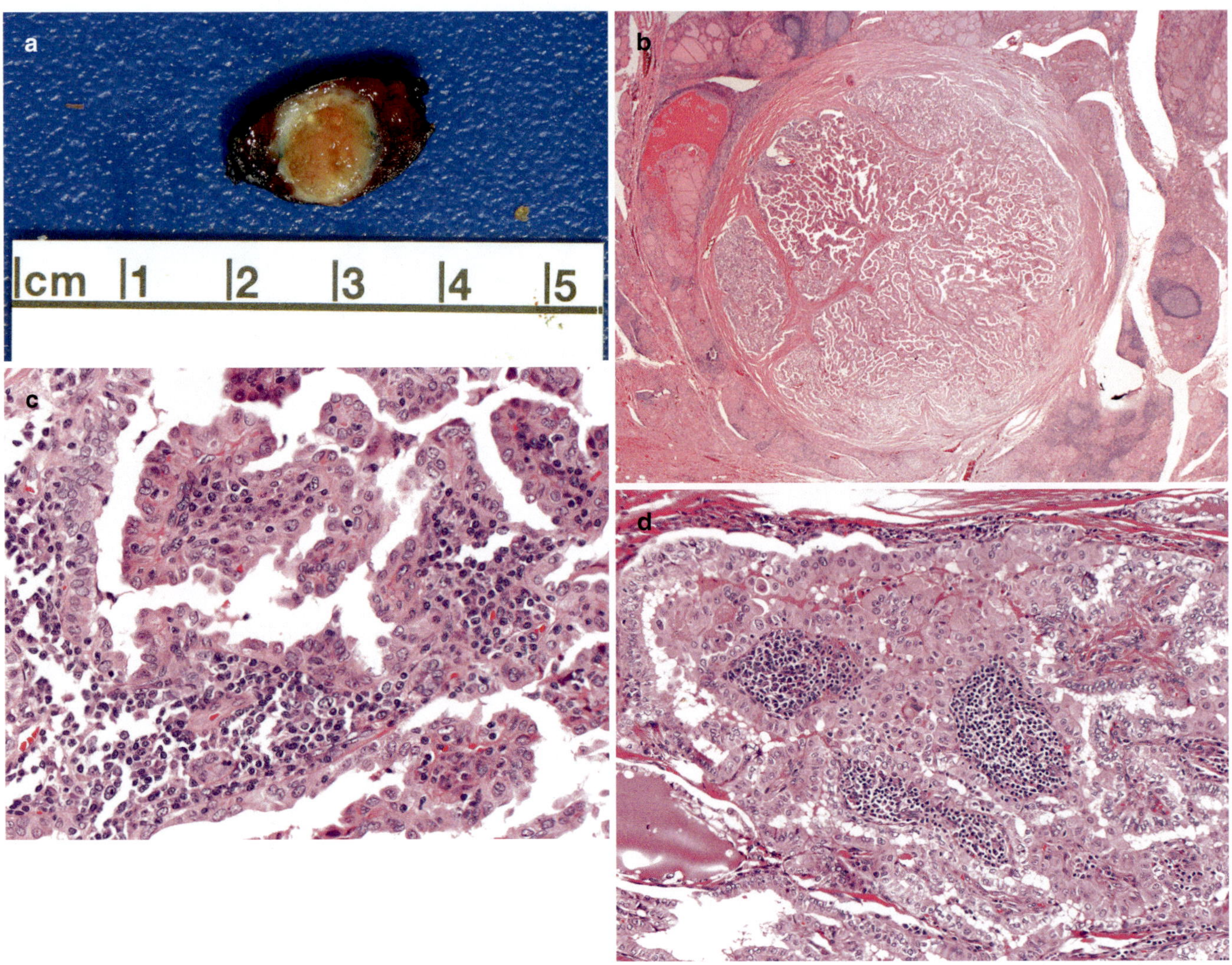

Fig. 9.30 Warthin-like variant of PTC (WLV-PTC): Gross and histologic features. (**a**) Gross of a WLV-PTC showing a well-circumscribed mass with a tan-brown cut surface. (**b**) Whole-mount histologic section shows that the tumor is arising in the background of chronic lymphocytic thyroiditis. (**c**, **d**) On higher power, a papillary growth pattern is prominent. The papillae are lined by follicular cells with abundant eosinophilic cytoplasm. Nuclear features of PTC are evident. The fibrovascular cores are expanded by a lymphoplasmacytic infiltrate (**b–d**, H&E stain)

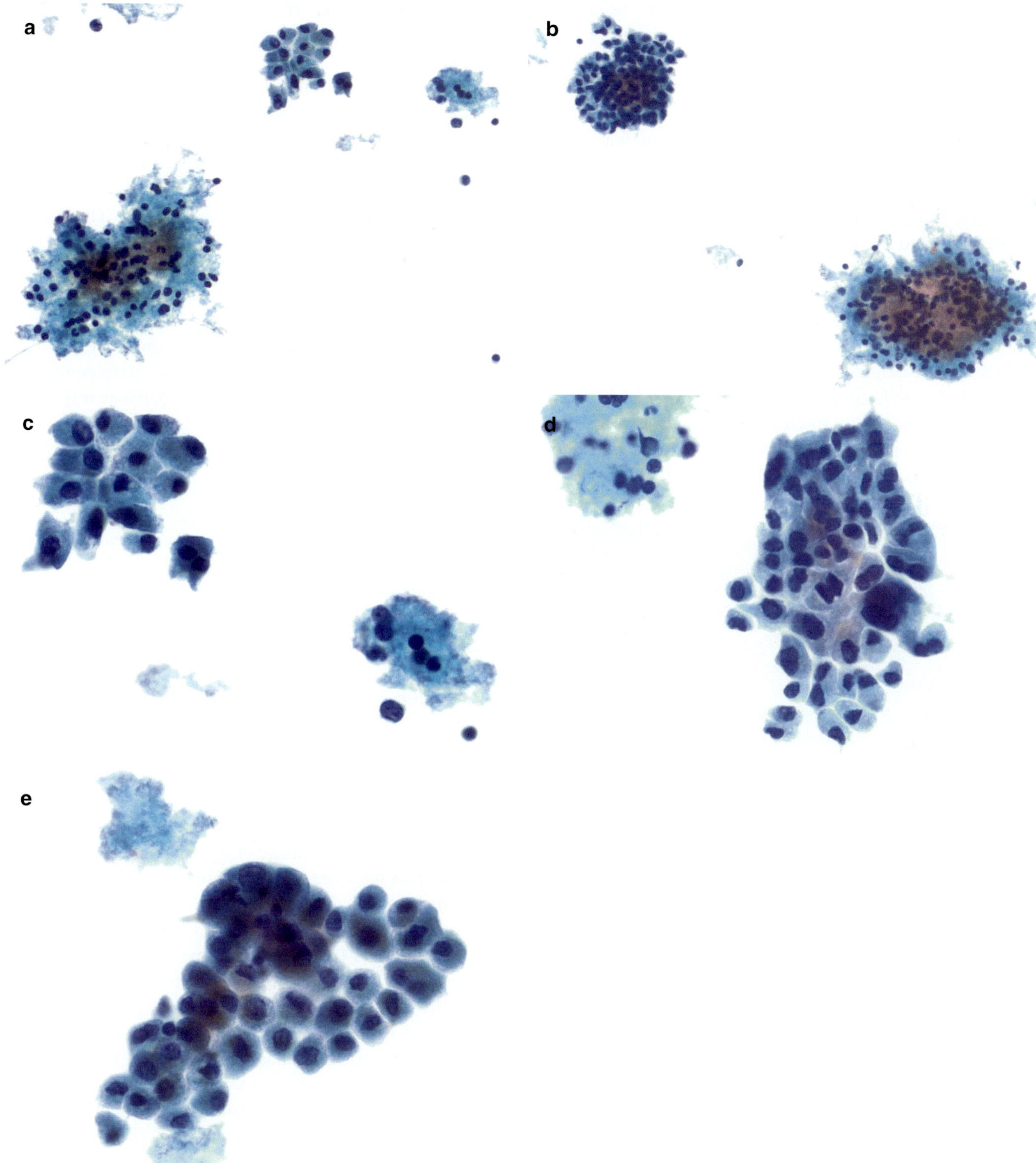

Fig. 9.31 WLV-PTC: Cytological features on TP. (**a**–**d**) TP shows round and irregular clusters of oncocytic cells with nuclear features of PTC closely associated with lymphocytic infiltrate. (**e**) Only this image shows lymphoid cells within the tumor cell clusters, unlike the finding by Kim et al. [39], which showed many of them. Unlike the 2014 study by Chong et al., which used SP, the TP slides in our case retained the background lymphocytes (**a**–**e**, Pap stain, TP)

- Yousef et al. [41] first described cytologic features of WLV-PTC. Since then, nuclear features typical of PTC, combined with oncocytic cytoplasm and lymphocytic background, have been considered to be the cytologic features of WLV-PTC
- In 2018, Kim et al. published cytological features of WLV-PTC on CS and TP, and indicated that the lymphocytic smear pattern was similar in both.
- Chong et al. [36] published a case report on WLV-PTC using CS and SP. They reported that conventional preparations showed low cellularity, with mainly isolated follicular cells and some small, irregular clusters in a lymphocyte-rich background. The follicular cells displayed an abundant polygonal morphology and contained well-defined cytoplasm and centrally or eccentrically located, round to oval nuclei with fine chromatin and inconspicuous nucleoli or micronucleoli. The tumor cells showed many nuclear grooves and occasional INPIs, which were highly suggestive of PTC. On the SP preparation, the cellularity was higher, there were few or no INPIs, and background lymphocytes were absent.
- Cytologic differential diagnosis of WLV-PTC includes c-PTC with CLT (PTC-CLT), CLT, OV-PTC, and follicular neoplasm with oncocytic features. WLV-PTC can be distinguished from PTC-CLT by the presence in WLV-PTC of an increased number of lymphocytes within cell clusters and in the background. This feature can be seen in both CS and TP. In CLT, the nuclei are round with prominent nucleoli, and they may show subtle chromatin clearing and grooves, but they lack papillary architecture and INPI. Paker et al. [40] indicated that the most important differential point that may help in the recognition of WLV-PTC is the mixture of lymphocytes and oncocytic follicular cells, tissue fragments, and papillary structures.

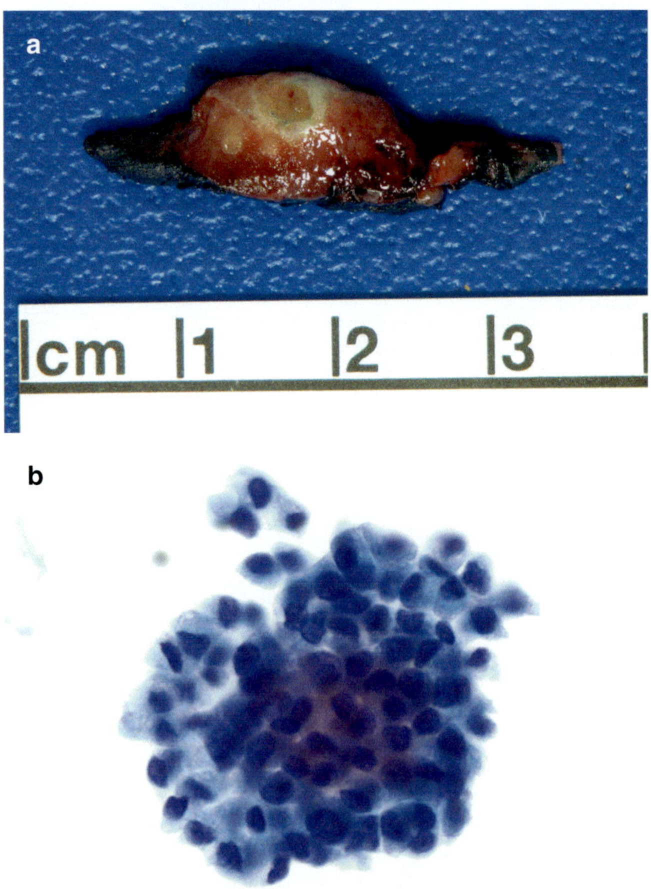

Fig. 9.32 WLV-PTC: Cytological features on SP. (**a**) Gross of a WLV-PTC, showing a well-circumscribed mass with a tan-brown cut surface and small focus of cystic change. (**b**) Cluster of atypical follicular cells with abundant oxyphilic cytoplasm and some nuclear features of PTC. Lymphoid stroma is not evident. A few lymphoid cells were seen in a different plane of focus (**b**, Pap stain, SP)

Genetic Profile of WLV-PTC

- This tumor harbors *RET/PTC* fusions, indicating that it is a variant of PTC.

Cribriform-Morular Variant of PTC (CMV-PTC)

- Cameselle-Teijeiro et al. [42] published a detailed overall analysis of CMV-PTC.
- CMV-PTC is classically associated with familial adenomatous polyposis (FAP), but it can also occur as a sporadic neoplasm.
- It has a marked female preponderance (F:M ratio of 31:1), particularly affecting those of a young age.
- In FAP patients, extracolonic manifestation includes thyroid tumors. The prevalence of thyroid cancer in FAP is 12%.
- In patients with FAP, CMV-PTC is generally multifocal and/or bilateral (multinodular appearance), whereas the tumors in sporadic cases tend to occur as single nodules.
- Prognosis is good.
- Preoperative cytologic diagnosis of CMV-PTC is possible based on cytological features and immunohistochemistry (Table 9.3), which may lead to the early detection of FAP and correct clinical management.

Pathologic Features of CMV-PTC

- Grossly, the tumors are well delimited (Fig. 9.33).
- Histology is characteristic and shows a variety of patterns, including cribriform, morular, papillary, trabecular, solid, and follicular. Tumor cells are tall, cuboidal, or spindled and pseudostratified. Cytoplasm is abundant. Nuclei are

Table 9.3 Characteristic features of the Cribriform-morular variant of PTC (CMV-PTC)

Histology	
	Cribriform, solid, trabecular, papillary, follicular, columnar
	Squamous morules
	Focal PTC features
Immunostains	
	Thyroid transcription factor-1 (TTF-1)
	Thyroglobulin
	Aberrant nuclear staining with β-catenin
	Estrogen receptor (ER)
	Progesterone receptor (PR)

generally hyperchromatic, with the occasional nuclear features of c-PTC such as grooves, chromatin clearing, INPI, and overlapping. Usually in the solid areas, there are interspersed nodular squamoid whorls (morules), which show cells with peculiar nuclear clearing (Figs. 9.34 and 9.35).

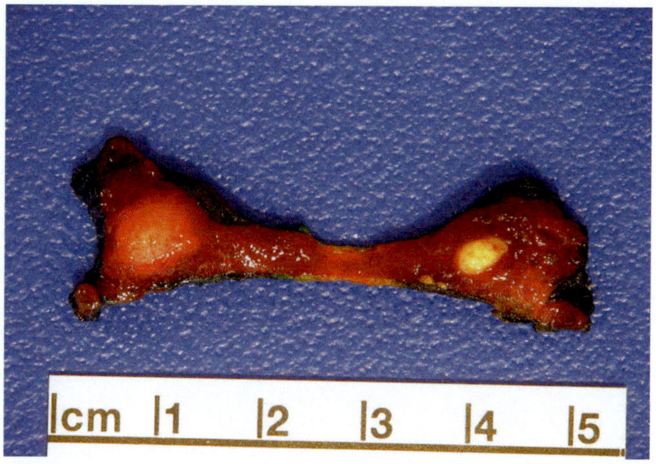

Fig. 9.33 Cribriform-morular variant of PTC (CMV-PTC): Gross appearance. This total thyroidectomy specimen shows two well-demarcated tumors. The cut surface of the right-sided nodule is tan; it appears to have a capsule

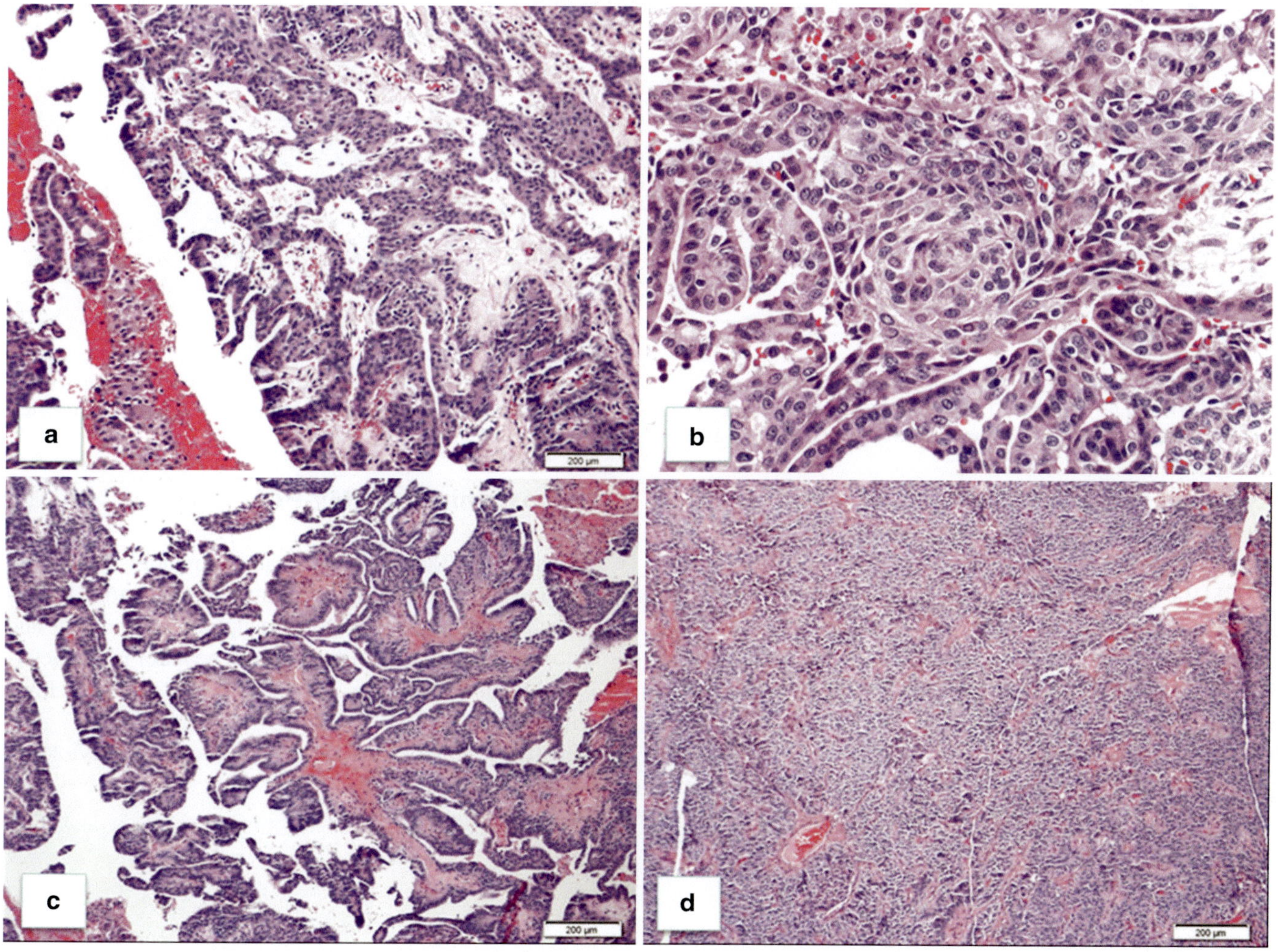

Fig. 9.34 CMV-PTC: Histologic features. Tumors show a mixture of growth patterns: cribriform and trabecular (**A**); morular (**B**); papillary (**C**), and solid (**D**) (H&E stain)

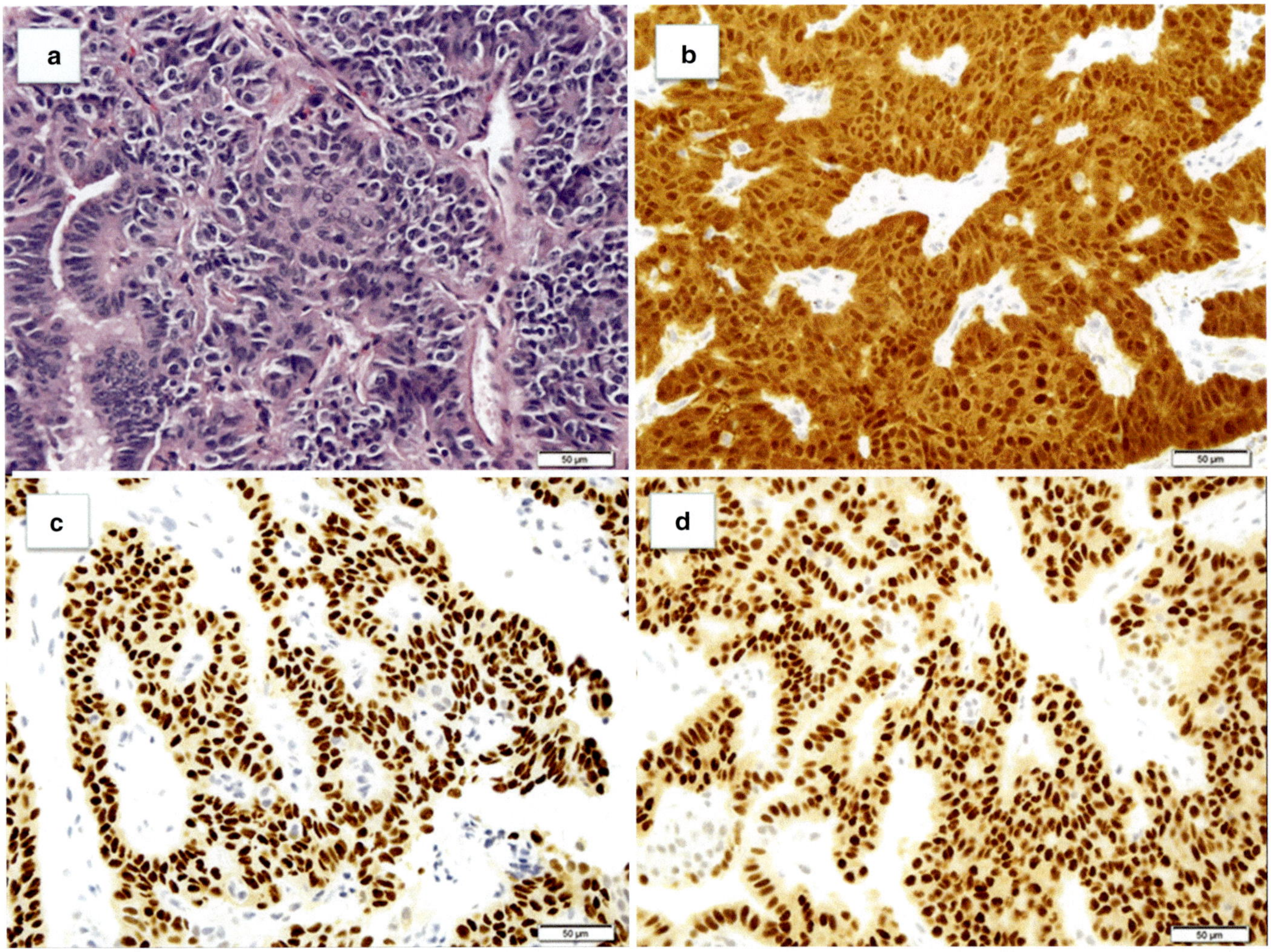

Fig. 9.35 CMV-PTC: Histologic and immunohistochemical features. (**a**) Histology of CMV-PTC showing a morule that lacks keratinization (H&E stain). (**b–d**) Tumor shows cytoplasmic and nuclear immunoreactivity for β-catenin (a hallmark for this tumor) and intense nuclear positivity for estrogen receptor (ER) and progesterone receptor (PR)

Cytologic Features of CMV-PTC: Application to LBP

- CMV-PTC can be diagnosed on FNA using a combination of cytologic findings and immunostaining, particularly for TTF-1 and β-catenin [43].
- All cytological features seen on CS are also present in LBP.
- The samples are usually hypercellular, showing most of the architectural patterns and cytological features seen in histology (Figs. 9.36, 9.37, 9.38, 9.39, and 9.40).
- Typical nuclear features of c-PTC are not present.

Immunostaining for CMV-PTC

- As shown in Table 9.3, the main immunohistochemical positivity is seen for thyroid transcription factor-1 (TTF-1), estrogen and progesterone receptors, and nuclear and cytoplasmic staining for β-catenin. The latter is characteristic of this tumor type and may be performed in FNA with features of CMV-PTC.
- Negative immunostains include calcitonin and cytokeratin 20.

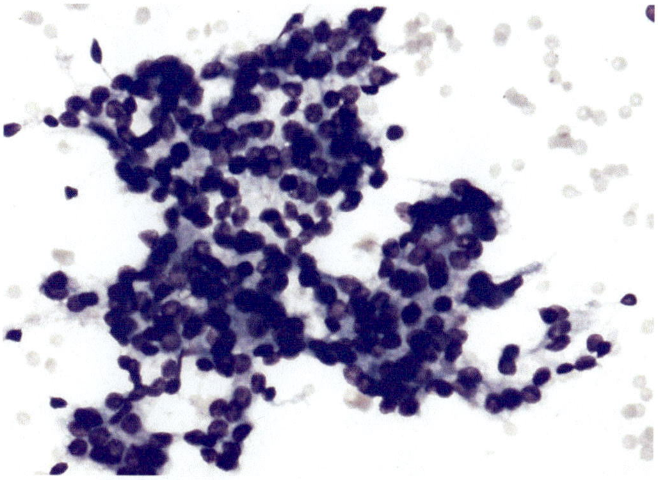

Fig. 9.36 CMV-PTC: Cytological features. This 25-year-old woman presented with multiple bilateral thyroid nodules. A diagnosis of "suspicious for malignancy, suspect CMV-PTC" was rendered. Material was not submitted for molecular testing. Familial adenomatous polyposis (FAP) was clinically suspected. The patient underwent a total thyroidectomy based on cytology diagnosis and immunohistochemical analysis. The DQ-stained smear shows a cribriform appearance comprising cells with faint, indistinct cytoplasm and small round-to-oval, overlapping nuclei with tiny nucleoli

Differential Diagnosis of CMV-PTC

- Differential diagnoses with overlapping pathologic patterns include MTC, poorly differentiated thyroid carcinoma, and metastatic breast and colonic tumors.
- Immunohistochemical positivity for TTF-1 and β-catenin in CMV-PTC help in distinguishing between them.

Molecular Profile of CMV-PTC

- Patients with FAP have a germline mutation in the *APC* gene that works as an antagonist of the WNT/β-catenin signaling pathway. This is a non-*BRAF*-non-*RAS* subtype of the molecular classification of thyroid tumors [42].

Management of CMV-PTC

- Clinicians should be alerted to the possibility of FAP when a diagnosis of CMV-PTC is made.

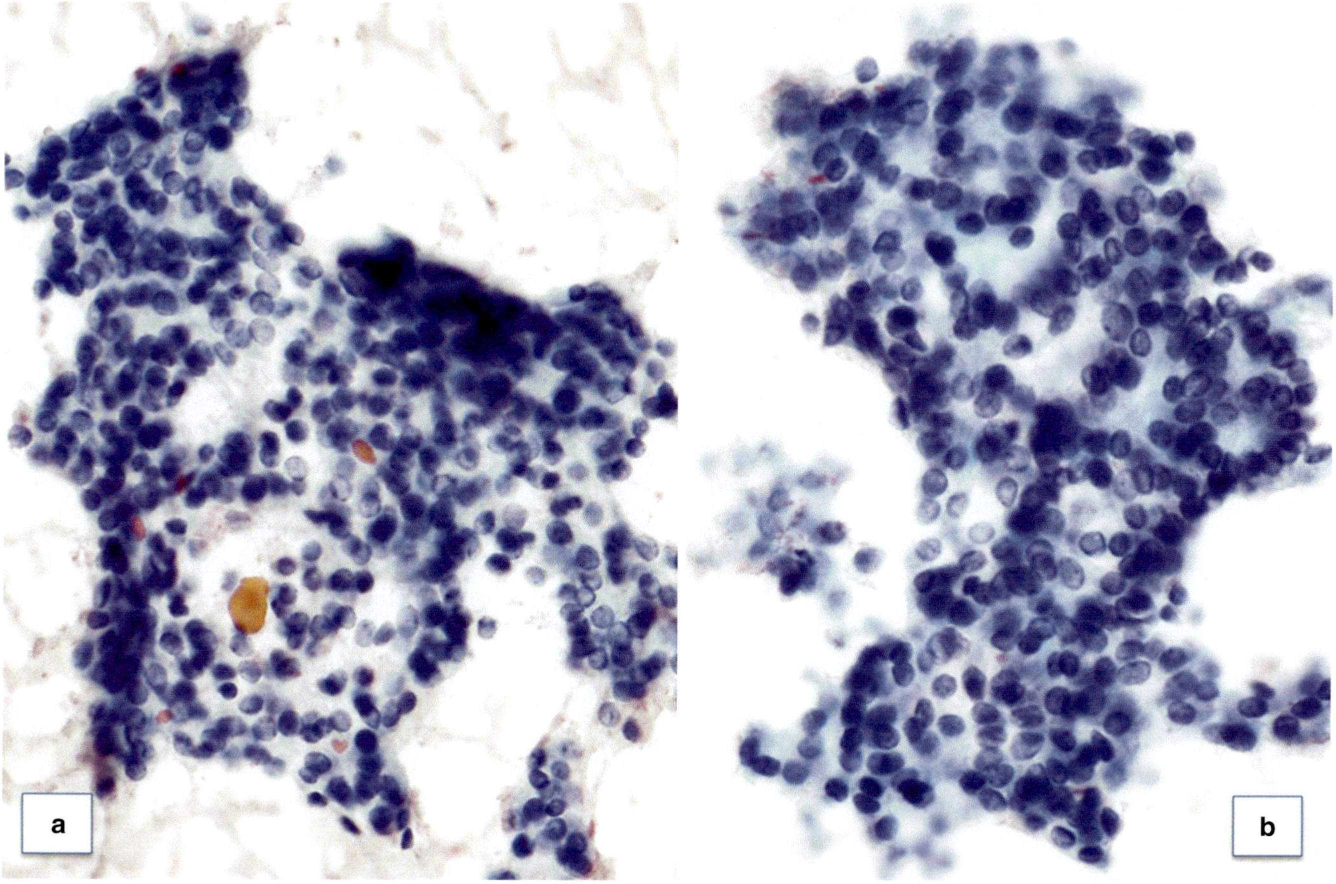

Fig. 9.37 CMV-PTC: Cytological features on CS and TP. Pap-stained CS (**a**) and TP (**b**) show a cribriform appearance with round empty spaces within large cell clusters or formed by anastomosing bars and arches of cells without fibrovascular stroma. Tumor cells have faint, indistinct cytoplasm and small round-to-oval, overlapping nuclei with grooves, tiny nucleoli, and peculiar chromatin clearing

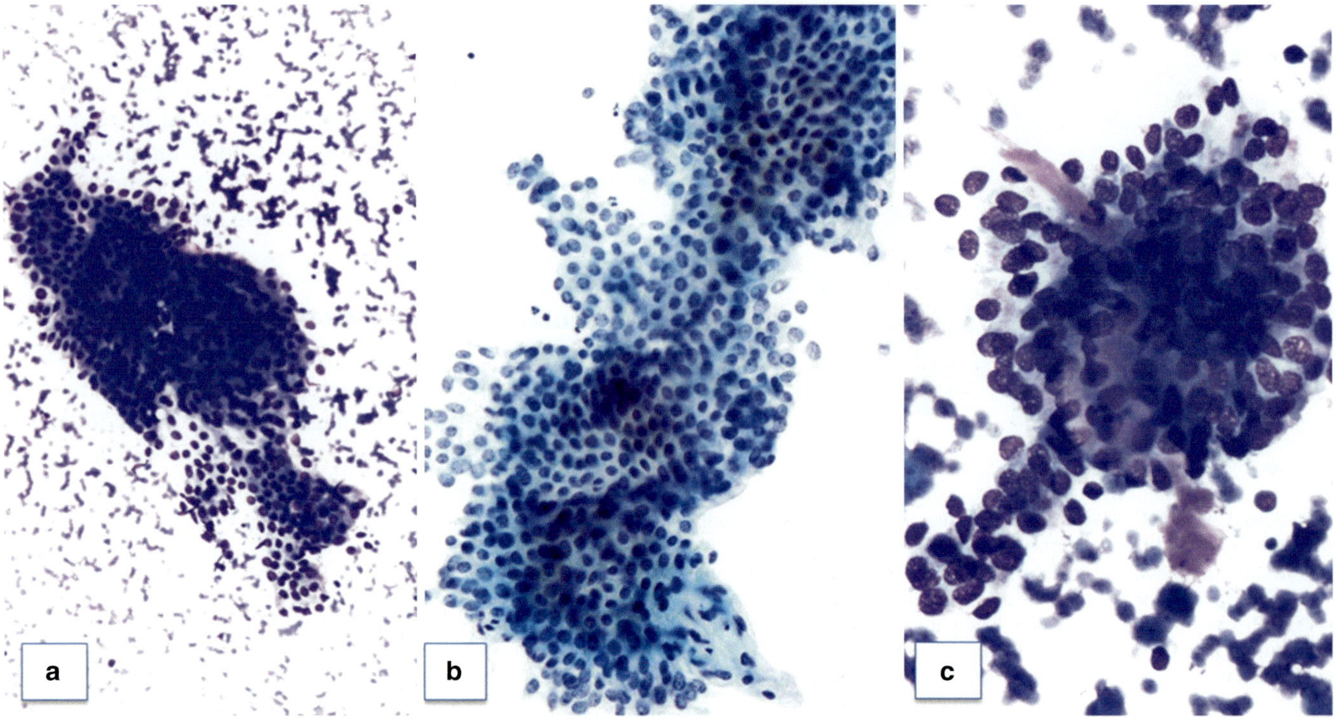

Fig. 9.38 CMV-PTC: Cytological features on TP and CS. (**a**–**c**) Morula formation. Hyaline globules are visible in (**c**). Note the cuboidal nuclei, peculiar chromatin clearing, and clean background. Columnar cells were not seen in our case (**a**, **c**, DQ stain, CS; **b**, Pap stain, TP)

- The 2015 ATA guidelines recommend total thyroidectomy.
- Elevated expression of estrogen and progesterone receptors and activation of the WNT/β-catenin pathway may prove useful as putative therapeutic targets in cases that do not respond to conventional therapy.

Columnar Cell Variant of PTC (CCV-PTC)

- CCV-PTC is an aggressive but uncommon variant of PTC, which was first described by Evans in 1986.
- It occurs predominantly in women.
- Because its behavior is more aggressive, preoperative diagnosis of this type of PTC is important so that effective surgical treatment can be instituted early.

Pathological Features of CCV-PTC

- Grossly, the tumor is usually large, ovoid, tan, and firm, with a fleshy or granular cut surface (Fig. 9.41a, b).
- Histologically, CCV-PTC demonstrates papillae or gland-like structures lined by columnar cells with prominent nuclear stratification. Cytoplasm is scant, and nuclei are elongated and lack INPI and grooves (Fig. 9.41c, d).

Cytological Features of CCV-PTC: Application to LBP

- CCV-PTC lacks classic nuclear features of PTC, so it is a challenge to identify this subtype of PTC in FNA.
- Specimens are usually hypercellular and show papillary structures with fibrovascular cores lined by elongated cells with nuclear pseudostratification, syncytial fragments, clusters, and single cells. Complex branching architecture of the cellular fragments, rosette-like formation, and acinar formation may also be seen (Fig. 9.42).
- Cells are monotonous, small to medium in size, columnar, and spindle-shaped.
- Cytoplasm is wispy and scant. Cytoplasm may also appear as elongated cytoplasmic tails.

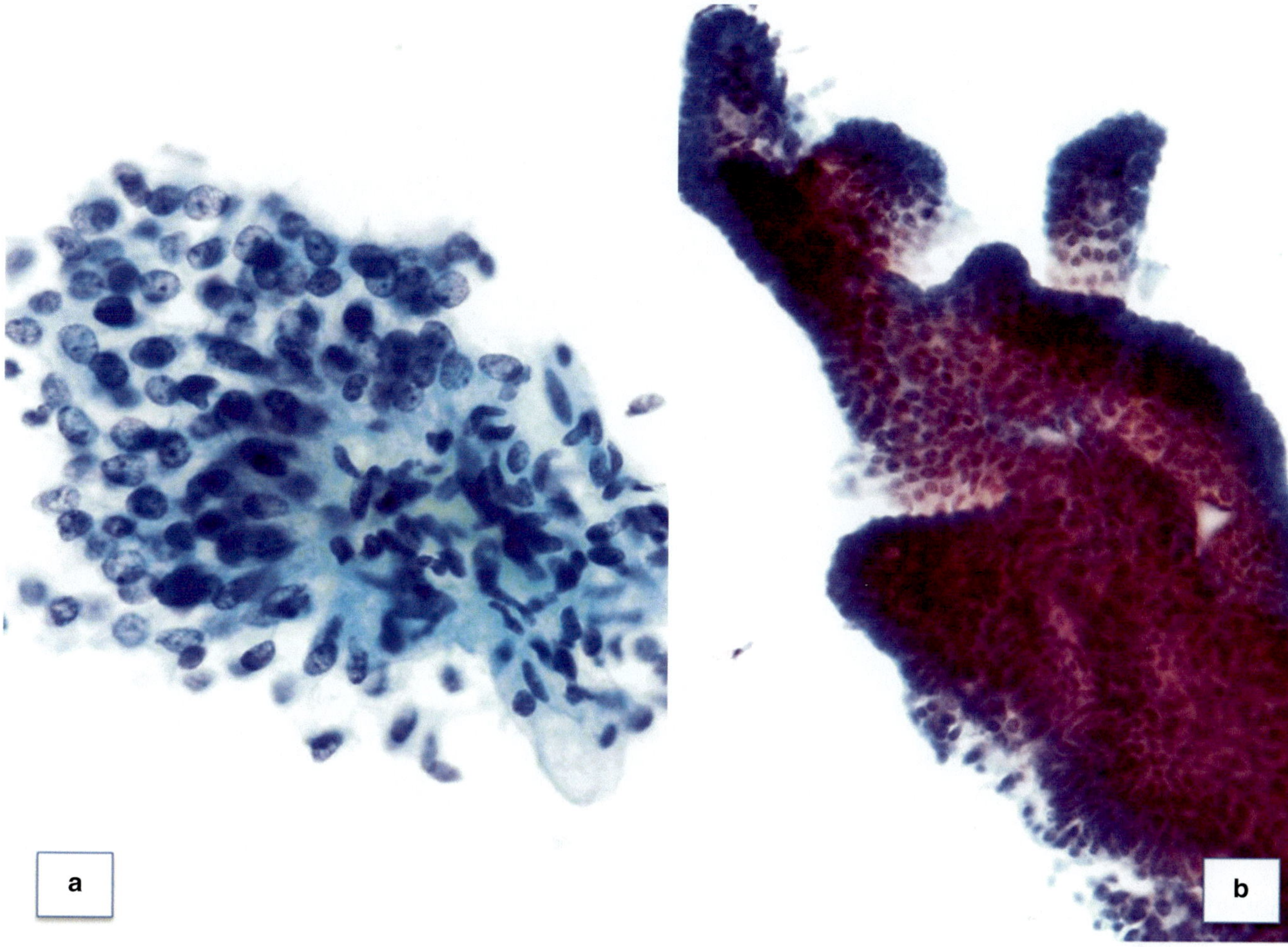

Fig. 9.39 CMV-PTC: Cytological features on TP. (**a**, **b**) Pap-stained TP shows complex papillae. Note nuclear features that are suggestive but not characteristic of c-PTC

- Nuclei show little or no atypia, pseudostratification, are oval to spindled with finely granular or darker chromatin, and rare or absent INPI and grooves.
- Colloid may be minimal, and psammoma bodies are absent.

Immunohistochemistry of CCV-PTC

- The tumor cells in both columnar cell and tall cell areas have demonstrated the following immunohistochemical staining profile:
  - Positive for TTF-1, CK19, galectin, Hector battifora mesothelial-1 (HBME-1) (focal), and thyroglobulin (focal)
  - Negative for synaptophysin, calcitonin, monoclonal CEA, and caudal-type homeobox gene 2 (*CDX-2*)

Differential Diagnosis of CCV-PTC

- *TCV-PTC* in cytology specimens can be distinguished from CCV-PTC by the cytoplasmic oxyphilia of the tumor cells, the absence of nuclear pseudostratification, and the presence of nuclear features of PTC, including "soap bubble"–like nuclear pseudoinclusions.
- *MTC* can be distinguished from CCV-PTC by immunohistochemical positivity for calcitonin and neuroendocrine markers.
- *Metastatic adenocarcinomas* from an intestinal, endometrial, or pulmonary primary can be distinguished from CCV-PTC by immunohistochemical positivity for both thyroglobulin and TTF-1 in the latter and by pertinent immunohistochemical markers for the suspected metastatic tumor.

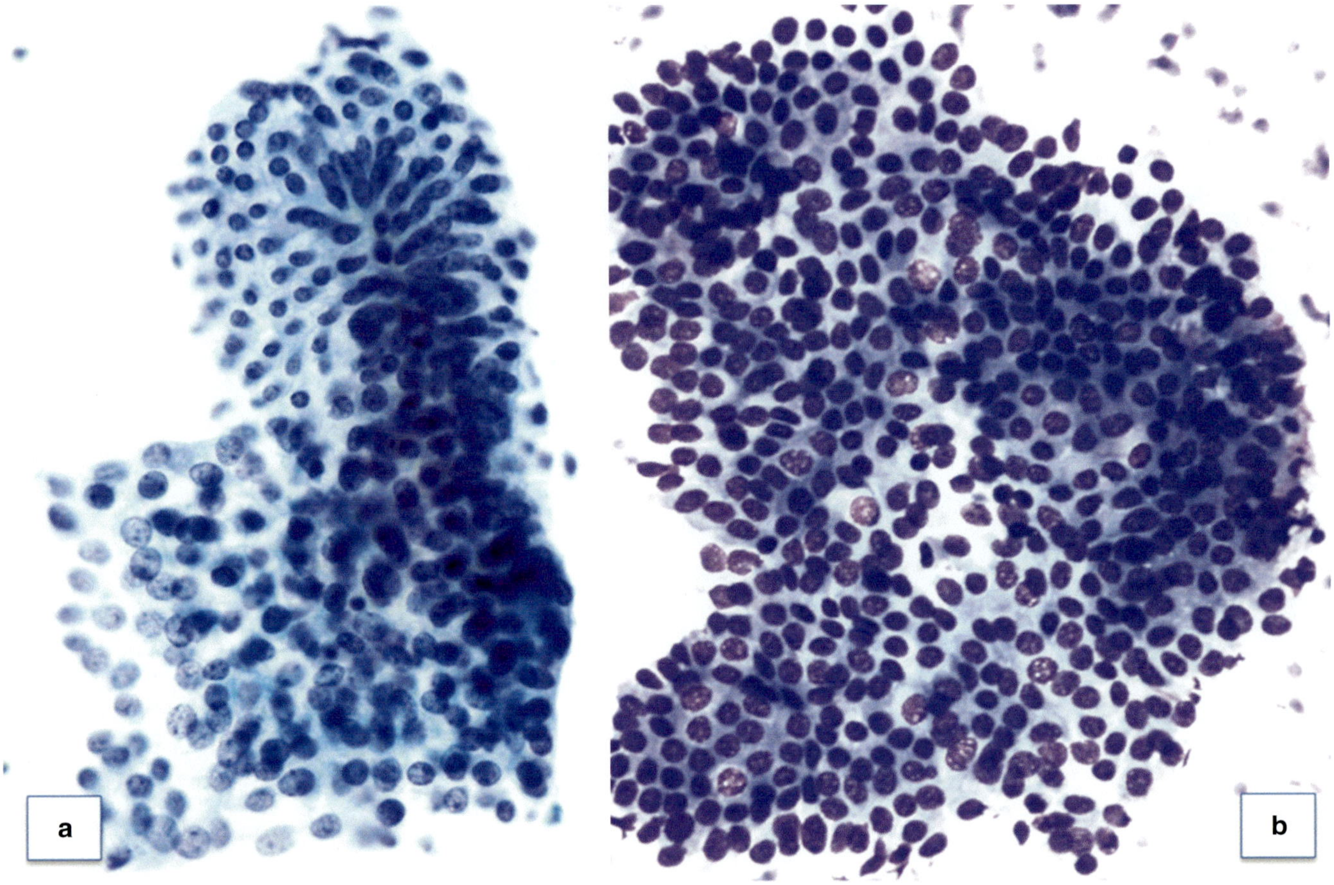

Fig. 9.40 CMV-PTC: Cytological features on TP and CS. (**a**, **b**) Pap-stained TP and DQ show solid architectural features

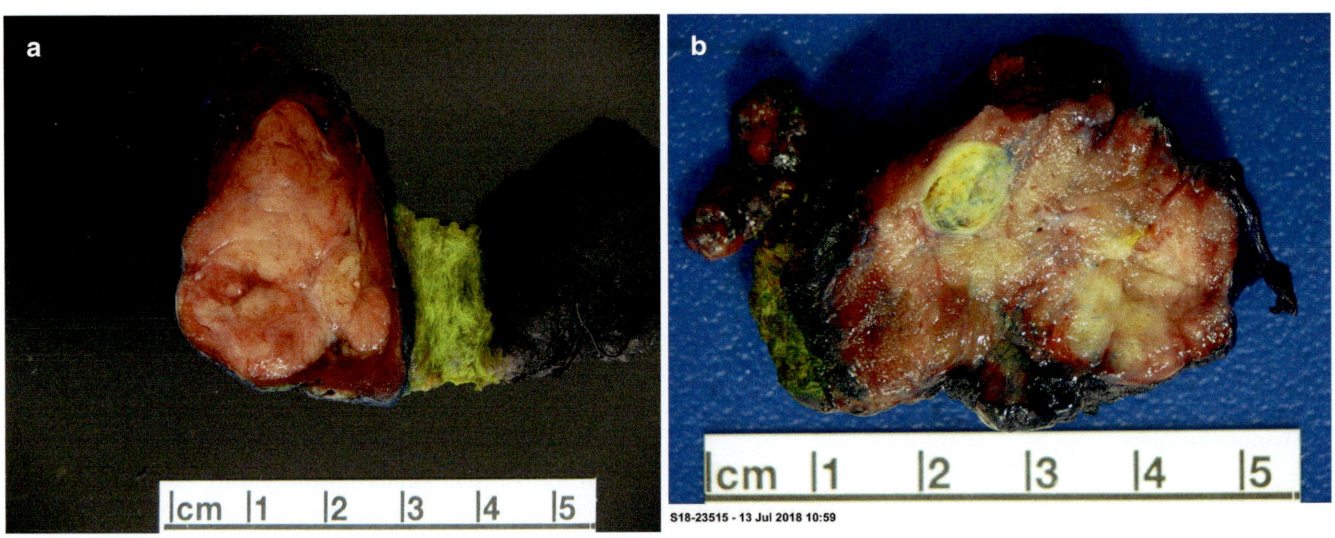

Fig. 9.41 Columnar cell variant of PTC (CCV-PTC): Gross and histologic features. Grossly, CCV can present as a well-circumscribed mass or widely invasive tumor. (**a**, **b**) These gross specimens from two different cases of CCV-PTC show infiltrative tumors with a tan-white cut surface, which replaced the majority of the affected lobes. (**c**) Histologic section of CCV-PTC shows elongated and tightly packed follicles. (**d**) The nuclei are pseudostratified and hyperchromatic. Nuclear features of PTC are lacking (**c**, **d**, H&E stain)

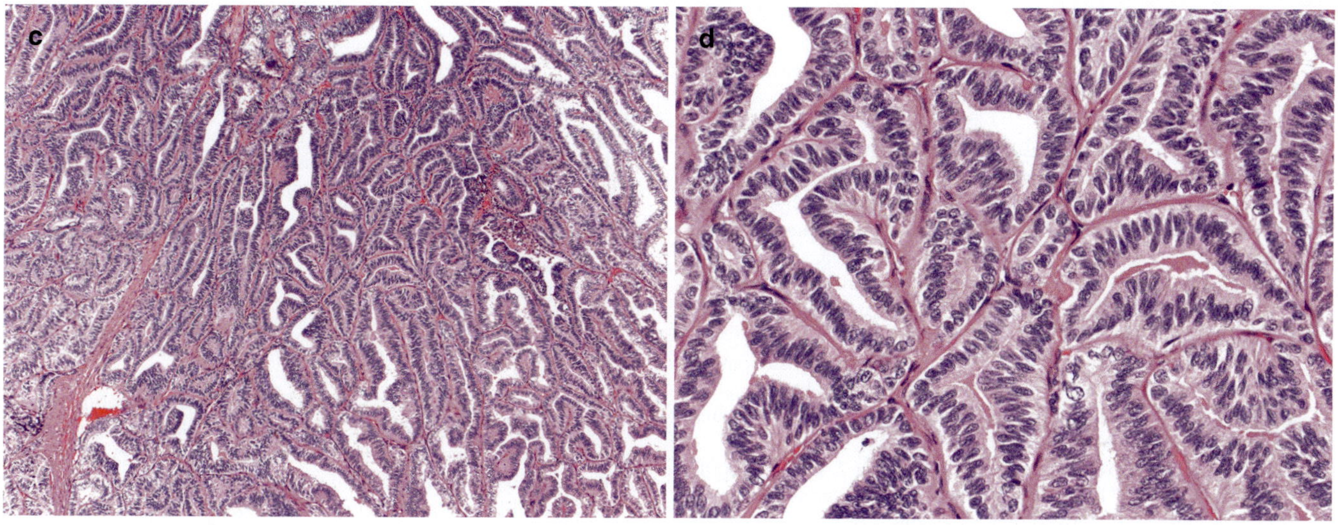

Fig. 9.41 (continued)

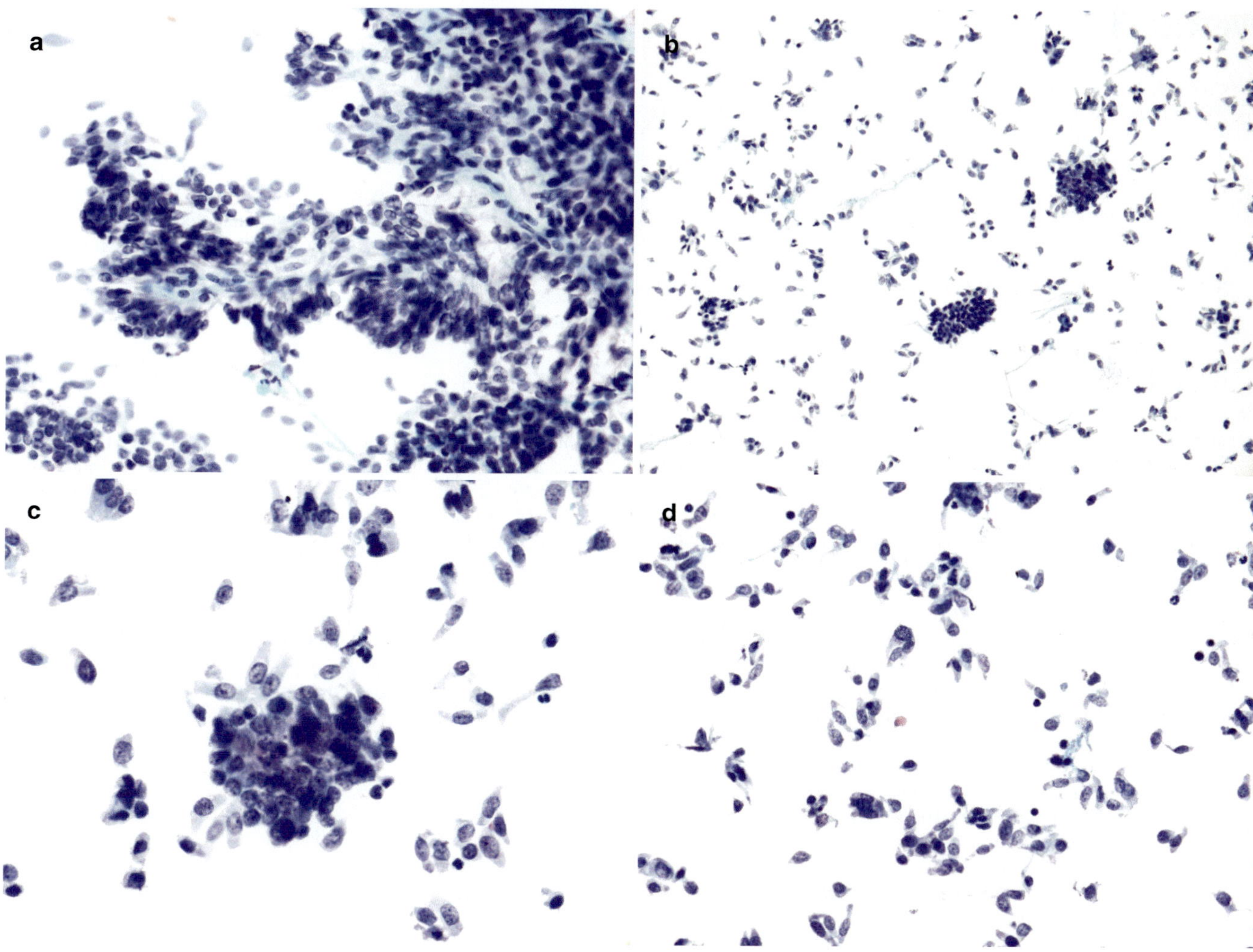

Fig. 9.42 CCV-PTC: Cytologic features on CS and TP. (**a**) CS shows a papillary structure with an inner fibrovascular core. Elongated cells at the periphery show pseudostratification. Nuclei show minimal atypia and are round to oval, overlapping or crowded, with slightly granular to clear chromatin and small nucleoli. INPI and grooves were not observed. The specimen was hypercellular (Pap stain). (**b**) The TP slide is also hypercellular but shows fragmentation of the bigger papillary structures that were seen in the CS, flat sheet, and numerous singly dispersed columnar/spindled cells. (**c**, **d**) Note cell clusters and dispersed single cells. Nuclear features are similar to those described for the CS (**b**–**d**, Pap stain, TP)

Suggested Reading

Classic PTC

1. Ali SZ, Cibas ES. The Bethesda system for reporting thyroid cytopathology II. Acta Cytol. 2016;60:397–8.
2. Ali SZ, Cibas ES. The Bethesda system for reporting thyroid cytopathology; definitions, criteria, and explanatory notes. 2nd ed. Cham: Springer International Publishing AG; 2018a.
3. Cibas ES, Ali SZ. The 2017 Bethesda system for reporting thyroid cytopathology. Thyroid. 2017;27:1341–6. https://doi.org/10.1089/thy.2017.0500.
4. Nikiforov YE, Biddinger PW, Thompson LDR. Diagnostic pathology and molecular genetics of the thyroid: a comprehensive guide for practicing thyroid pathology. 3rd ed. Philadelphia: Wolters Kluwer/Lippincott Williams & Wilkins; 2019.
5. Sahpaz A, Önal B, Yeşilyurt A, Han Ü, Delibaşı T. BRAF(V600E) mutation, RET/PTC1 and PAX8-PPAR gamma rearrangements in follicular epithelium derived thyroid lesions – institutional experience and literature review. Balkan Med J. 2015;32:156–66. https://doi.org/10.5152/balkanmedj.2015.15101.

FVPTC

6. Chai YJ, Kim SJ, Kim SC, Koo do H, Min HS, Lee KE, et al. BRAF mutation in follicular variant of papillary thyroid carcinoma is associated with unfavourable clinicopathological characteristics and malignant features on ultrasonography. Clin Endocrinol. 2014;81:432–9. https://doi.org/10.1111/cen.12433.
7. Hahn SY, Shin JH, Lim HK, Jung SL, Oh YL, Choi IH, et al. Preoperative differentiation between noninvasive follicular thyroid neoplasm with papillary-like nuclear features (NIFTP) and non-NIFTP. Clin Endocrinol. 2017;86:444–50. https://doi.org/10.1111/cen.13263.
8. Hung YP, Barletta JA. A user's guide to non-invasive follicular thyroid neoplasm with papillary-like nuclear features (NIFTP). Histopathology. 2018;72:53–69. https://doi.org/10.1111/his.13363.
9. Lin HS, Komisar A, Opher E, Blaugrund SM. Follicular variant of papillary carcinoma: the diagnostic limitations of preoperative fine-needle aspiration and intraoperative frozen section evaluation. Laryngoscope. 2000;110:1431–6.
10. Manimaran D, Karthikeyan TM, Khan DM, Thulasi RR. Follicular variant of papillary thyroid carcinoma: cytological indicators of diagnostic value. J Clin Diagn Res. 2014;8:46–8. https://doi.org/10.7860/JCDR/2014/7477.4103.
11. Point du Jour K, Schmitt AC, Chen AY, Griffith CC. Application of strict criteria for noninvasive follicular thyroid neoplasm with papillary-like nuclear features and encapsulated follicular variant papillary thyroid carcinoma: a retrospective study of 50 tumors previously diagnosed as follicular variant PTC. Endocr Pathol. 2018;29:35–42. https://doi.org/10.1007/s12022-018-9537-4.
12. Tallini G, Tuttle RM, Ghossein RA. The history of the follicular variant of papillary thyroid carcinoma. J Clin Endocrinol Metab .2017;102:15–22. https://doi.org/10.1111/his.13363.
13. Trabzonlu L, Paksoy N. Cytomorphological analysis of thyroid nodules diagnosed as follicular variant of papillary thyroid carcinoma: a fine needle aspiration study of diagnostic clues in 42 cases and the impact of using Bethesda system in reporting—an institutional experience. Endocr Pathol. 2018;29:351–6. https://doi.org/10.1007/s12022-018-9550-9.
14. Wu HH, Jones JN, Grzybicki DM, Elsheikh TM. Sensitive cytologic criteria for the identification of follicular variant of papillary thyroid carcinoma in fine-needle aspiration biopsy. Diagn Cytopathol. 2003;29:262–6.

NIFTP

15. Bizzarro T, Martini M, Capodimonti S, Straccia P, Lombardi CP, Pontecorvi A, et al. Young investigator challenge: the morphologic analysis of noninvasive follicular thyroid neoplasm with papillary-like nuclear features on liquid-based cytology: some insights into their identification. Cancer Cytopathol. 2016;124:699–710. https://doi.org/10.1002/cncy.21777.
16. Faquin WC, Wong LQ, Afrogheh AH, Ali SZ, Bishop JA, Bongiovanni M, et al. Impact of reclassifying noninvasive follicular variant of papillary thyroid carcinoma on the risk of malignancy in the Bethesda system for reporting thyroid cytopathology. Cancer Cytopathol. 2016;124:181–7. https://doi.org/10.1002/cncy.21631.
17. Legesse T, Parker L, Heath J, Staats PN. Distinguishing non-invasive follicular thyroid neoplasm with papillary-like nuclear features (NIFTP) from classic and invasive follicular-variant papillary thyroid carcinomas based on cytologic features. J Am Soc Cytopathol. 2019;8(1):11–7. https://doi.org/10.1016/j.jasc.2018.07.004.
18. Nikiforov YE, Seethala RR, Tallini G, Baloch ZW, Basolo F, Thompson LD, et al. Nomenclature revision for encapsulated follicular variant of papillary thyroid carcinoma: a paradigm shift to reduce overtreatment of indolent tumors. JAMA Oncol. 2016;2:1023–9. https://doi.org/10.1001/jamaoncol.2016.0386.
19. Strickland KC, Eszlinger M, Paschke R, Angell TE, Alexander EK, Marqusee E, et al. Molecular testing of nodules with a suspicious or malignant cytologic diagnosis in the setting of non-invasive follicular thyroid neoplasm with papillary-like nuclear features (NIFTP). Endocr Pathol. 2018;29:68–74. https://doi.org/10.1007/s12022-018-9515-x.
20. Zhou H, Baloch ZW, Nayar R, Bizzarro T, Fadda G, Adhikari-Guragain D, et al. Noninvasive follicular thyroid neoplasm with papillary-like nuclear features (NIFTP): implications for the risk of malignancy (ROM) in the Bethesda system for reporting thyroid cytopathology (TBSRTC). Cancer Cytopathol. 2018;126:20–6. https://doi.org/10.1002/cncy.21926.

TCV-PTC

21. Baum JE, Soong L, Scognamiglio T, Margolskee EM, Hoda RS, Rao R. Cytological diagnosis of papillary thyroid carcinoma with tall cells on ThinPrep liquid-based cytology. Diagn Cytopathol. 2019;47:541–6. https://doi.org/10.1002/dc.24146.
22. Hawk WA, Hazard JB. The many appearances of papillary carcinoma of the thyroid. Cleve Clin Q. 1976;43:207–15.
23. Kaw YT. Fine needle aspiration cytology of the tall cell variant of papillary carcinoma of the thyroid. Acta Cytol. 1994;38:282.
24. Lee SH, Jung CK, Bae JS, Jung SL, Choi YJ, Kang CS. Liquid-based cytology improves preoperative diagnostic accuracy of the tall cell variant of papillary thyroid carcinoma. Diagn Cytopathol. 2014;42:11–7.

Cystic PTC

25. Ali SZ, Cibas ES. The Bethesda system for reporting thyroid cytopathology; definitions, criteria, and explanatory notes. 2nd ed. Cham: Springer International Publishing AG; 2018b.
26. Clark DP, Faquin WC. The thyroid cytopathology. 2nd ed. New York: Springer; 2010.
27. Faquin WC, Cibas ES, Renshaw AA. "Atypical" cells in fine-needle aspiration biopsy specimens of benign thyroid cysts. Cancer. 2005;105:71–9.
28. Haugen BR, Alexander EK, Bible KC, Doherty GM, Mandel SJ, Nikiforov YE, et al. 2015 American Thyroid Association man-

agement guidelines for adult patients with thyroid nodules and differentiated thyroid cancer: the American Thyroid Association Guidelines Task Force on Thyroid Nodules and Differentiated Thyroid Cancer. Thyroid. 2016;26:1–133. https://doi.org/10.1089/thy.2015.0020.

29. Hoda RS, VandenBussche C, Hoda SA. Diagnostic liquid-based cytology. New York: Springer; 2017.
30. Li W, Zhu Q, Jiang Y, Zhang Q, Meng Z, Sun J, et al. Partially cystic thyroid nodules in ultrasound-guided fine needle aspiration: prevalence of thyroid carcinoma and ultrasound features. Medicine (Baltimore). 2017;96:e8689. https://doi.org/10.1097/MD.0000000000008689.
31. Mokhtari M, Kumar PV, Hayati K. Fine-needle aspiration study of cystic papillary thyroid carcinoma: rare cytological findings. J Cytol. 2016;33:120–4.

OV-PTC

32. Carr AA, Yen TWF, Ortiz DI, Hunt BC, Fareau G, Massey BL, et al. Patients with oncocytic variant papillary thyroid carcinoma have a similar prognosis to matched classical papillary thyroid carcinoma controls. Thyroid. 2018;28:1462–7. https://doi.org/10.1089/thy.2017.0603.
33. Hong JH, Yi HS, Yi S, Kim HW, Lee J, Kim KS. Implications of oncocytic change in papillary thyroid cancer. Clin Endocrinol. 2016;85:797–804. https://doi.org/10.1111/cen.13115.
34. Lloyd RV, Buehler D, Khanafshar E. Papillary thyroid carcinoma variants. Head Neck Pathol. 2011;5:51–6. https://doi.org/10.1007/s12105-010-0236-9.

WLV-PTC

35. Apel RL, Asa SL, LiVolsi VA. Papillary Hürthle cell carcinoma with lymphocytic stroma. "Warthin-like tumor" of the thyroid. Am J Surg Pathol. 1995;19(7):810–4.
36. Chong Y, Suh S, Kim TJ, Lee EJ. Fine needle aspiration cytology of Warthin-like papillary thyroid carcinoma: a brief case report. Korean J Pathol. 2014;48:170–3. https://doi.org/10.4132/KoreanJPathol.2014.48.2.170.
37. Evranos B, Polat SB, Baser H, Ozdemir D, Kilicarslan A, Yalcin A, et al. Bethesda classification is a valuable guide for fine needle aspiration reports and highly predictive especially for diagnosing aggressive variants of papillary thyroid carcinoma. Cytopathology. 2017;28:259–67. https://doi.org/10.1111/cyt.12384.
38. Kim GR, Shin JH, Hahn SY, Ko EY, Oh YL. Ultrasonographic features and clinical characteristics of Warthin-like variant of papillary thyroid carcinoma. Endocr J. 2016;63:329–35. https://doi.org/10.1507/endocrj.EJ15-0620.
39. Kim J, Lim BJ, Hong SW, Pyo JY. Preoperative cytologic diagnosis of Warthin-like variant of papillary thyroid carcinoma. J Pathol Transl Med. 2018;52:105–9. https://doi.org/10.4132/jptm.2017.12.26.
40. Paker I, Kokenek TD, Yılmazer D, Seker GE, Alper M. Oncocytic variant of papillary thyroid carcinoma with lymphocytic stroma (Warthin-like variant): report of a case with fine needle aspiration cytology and review of the literature. Cytopathology. 2012;23:408–10. https://doi.org/10.1111/j.1365-2303.2011.00877.x.
41. Yousef O, Dichard A, Bocklage T. Aspiration cytology features of the Warthin tumor-like variant of papillary thyroid carcinoma. A report of two cases. Acta Cytol. 1997;41(4 Suppl):1361–8.

CMV-PTC

42. Cameselle-Teijeiro JM, Peteiro-González D, Caneiro-Gómez J, Sánchez-Ares M, Abdulkader I, Eloy C, et al. Cribriform-morular variant of thyroid carcinoma: a neoplasm with distinctive phenotype associated with the activation of the WNT/β-catenin pathway. Mod Pathol. 2018;31:1168–79. https://doi.org/10.1038/s41379-018-0070-2.
43. Hirokawa M, Maekawa M, Kuma S, Miyauchi A. Cribriform-morular variant of papillary thyroid carcinoma--cytological and immunocytochemical findings of 18 cases. Diagn Cytopathol. 2010;38:890–6. https://doi.org/10.1002/dc.21309.

CCV-PTC

44. Bongiovanni M, Mermod M, Canberk S, Saglietti C, Sykiotis GP, Pusztaszeri M, et al. Columnar cell variant of papillary thyroid carcinoma: Cytomorphological characteristics of 11 cases with histological correlation and literature review. Cancer Cytopathol. 2017;125:389–97. https://doi.org/10.1002/cncy.21860.
45. Evans HL. Columnar cell carcinoma of the thyroid: a report of two cases of an aggressive variant of thyroid carcinoma. Am J Clin Pathol. 1986;85:77–80.
46. Tranchida P, Bernacki E, Budev H, Giorgadze T. Preoperative cytologic diagnosis of papillary thyroid carcinoma with mixed columnar cell and tall cell features. Diagn Cytopathol. 2012;40(Suppl 1):E4–7. https://doi.org/10.1002/dc.21616.

Medullary Thyroid Carcinoma

10

Rema Rao, Theresa Scognamiglio, and Rana S. Hoda

Introduction to Medullary Thyroid Carcinoma

- Medullary thyroid carcinoma (MTC) represents 1–2% of thyroid carcinomas.
- MTC occurs in sporadic and familial forms; sporadic MTC accounts for 75% of cases.
- Familial cases occur in the setting of multiple endocrine neoplasia (MEN) 2A/2B and familial MTC.
- Activating point mutations in the *RET* proto-oncogene located on chromosome 10 are responsible for familial forms of MTC and can also occur in up to 80% of sporadic cases.
- Sporadic MTC usually presents as a single, solitary nodule. Patients are usually in their 5th or 6th decade
- Familial MTC tends to present in the 2nd or 3rd decade and is usually multifocal.
- Grossly, MTC nodules appear circumscribed and unencapsulated (Fig. 10.1a, b). Histologically, MTC can demonstrate various growth patterns and cytologic features; a number of variants have been described (Fig. 10.1c, d).

TBSRTC Definition of MTC

- The Bethesda System for Reporting Thyroid Cytopathology (TBSRTC) defines MTC as a malignant neuroendocrine tumor arising from C cells (parafollicular cells) of the thyroid gland.

R. Rao · T. Scognamiglio
Department of Pathology and Laboratory Medicine, New York Presbyterian Hospital, Weill Cornell Medical College, New York, NY, USA

R. S. Hoda (✉)
CBLPath, Rye Brook, NY, USA
e-mail: rhoda@cblpath.com

Cytologic Criteria for Diagnosis of MTC on Conventional Smears (CS)

- On fine needle aspiration (FNA), MTC is typically categorized as suspicious for malignancy (Bethesda V) or malignant (Bethesda VI), and rarely as Atypia of Undetermined Significance (AUS, Bethesda III) or benign (Bethesda II).
- In a study of 28 cases of FNA aspirates of MTC with surgical follow-up, Dyhdalo and Chute [5] showed one case interpreted as benign, four as AUS/FLUS, one as FN/SFN, five deemed suspicious for malignancy, and 17 as positive for malignancy. The few discordant cases tended to show air-drying artifact and lacked typical features of MTC, such as plasmacytoid appearance and dyshesion.
- In CS, the aspirates show moderate to high cellularity and are composed of groups and clusters and single tumor cells. The tumor cells show round to oval nuclei with nuclear pleomorphism and a neuroendocrine-type salt-and-pepper chromatin. The tumor cells typically show eccentrically placed nuclei and granular cytoplasm imparting a "plasmacytoid" appearance, although spindled, oncocytic, or clear cell types can be seen.
- The cells can also be arranged as trabeculae or in microfollicles (Fig. 10.2a–d). The tumor cells can frequently be binucleate or multinucleate and can exhibit intranuclear cytoplasmic pseudoinclusions (INPI) as well (Fig. 10.2e).
- Occasional bizarre neuroendocrine type atypia can be noted (Fig. 10.2f). The background can show colloid in some cases but typically shows dense, amorphous, stromal material composed of "amyloid", which is also well identified on smears and cell block sections (Fig. 10.2g, h). Among rare findings are cytoplasmic stippling, nuclear budding, and lymphoma-like cells.
- A cell block preparation is extremely helpful for ancillary confirmatory studies (Fig. 10.2h, i). Immunohistochemistry

R. S. Hoda et al. (eds.), *Atlas of Thyroid Cytopathology on Liquid-Based Preparations*,
https://doi.org/10.1007/978-3-030-25066-9_10

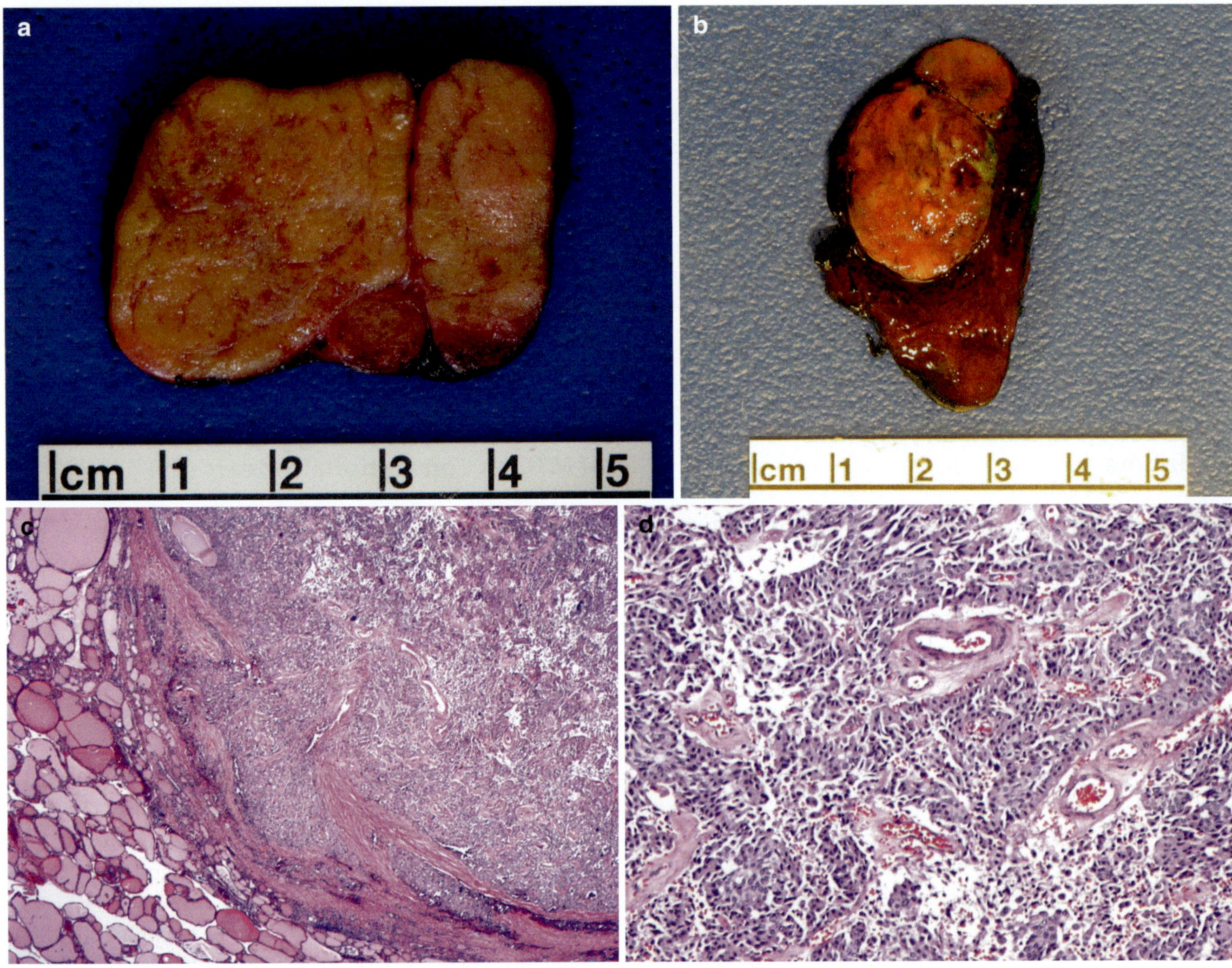

Fig. 10.1 Gross appearance of medullary thyroid carcinoma (MTC). (**a**, **b**) Grossly, two cases of MTC appear as well-circumscribed, unencapsulated nodules, which can occasionally have an infiltrative border. The cut surface is tan-white or pink to gray. Hemorrhage and necrosis are usually absent. Calcifications may be seen. (**c**, **d**) Low-power view of the histology of MTC, showing the circumscribed edge of the tumor. Higher magnification shows the spindle cell type of MTC (H&E stain)

can be strongly immunoreactive for calcitonin, CEA and other neuroendocrine markers (synaptophysin, chromogranin), and for TTF-1. Thyroglobulin is negative, and staining with PAX8 is variable (Fig. 10.2j).

Cytologic Criteria for Diagnosis of MTC on LBP

- The cytologic features of MTC are fairly similar on LBP and CS.
- A few subtle differences include the appearance of tumor cell clusters and groups that are smaller and more fragmented on LBP than on CS. Also, single tumor cells are more prominent on LBP.
- In LBP, the presence of many small, singly dispersed spindle or plasmacytoid cells should raise suspicion for MTC (Figs. 10.3 and 10.4).
- Occasionally, in LBP, the cytoplasm may appear finely vacuolated and granularity may be inconspicuous.
- The background is relatively clean on LBP. Fragments of amyloid can appear fibrillary or dense on LBP, rather than only dense, as seen in CS (*see* Fig. 10.3d, e).

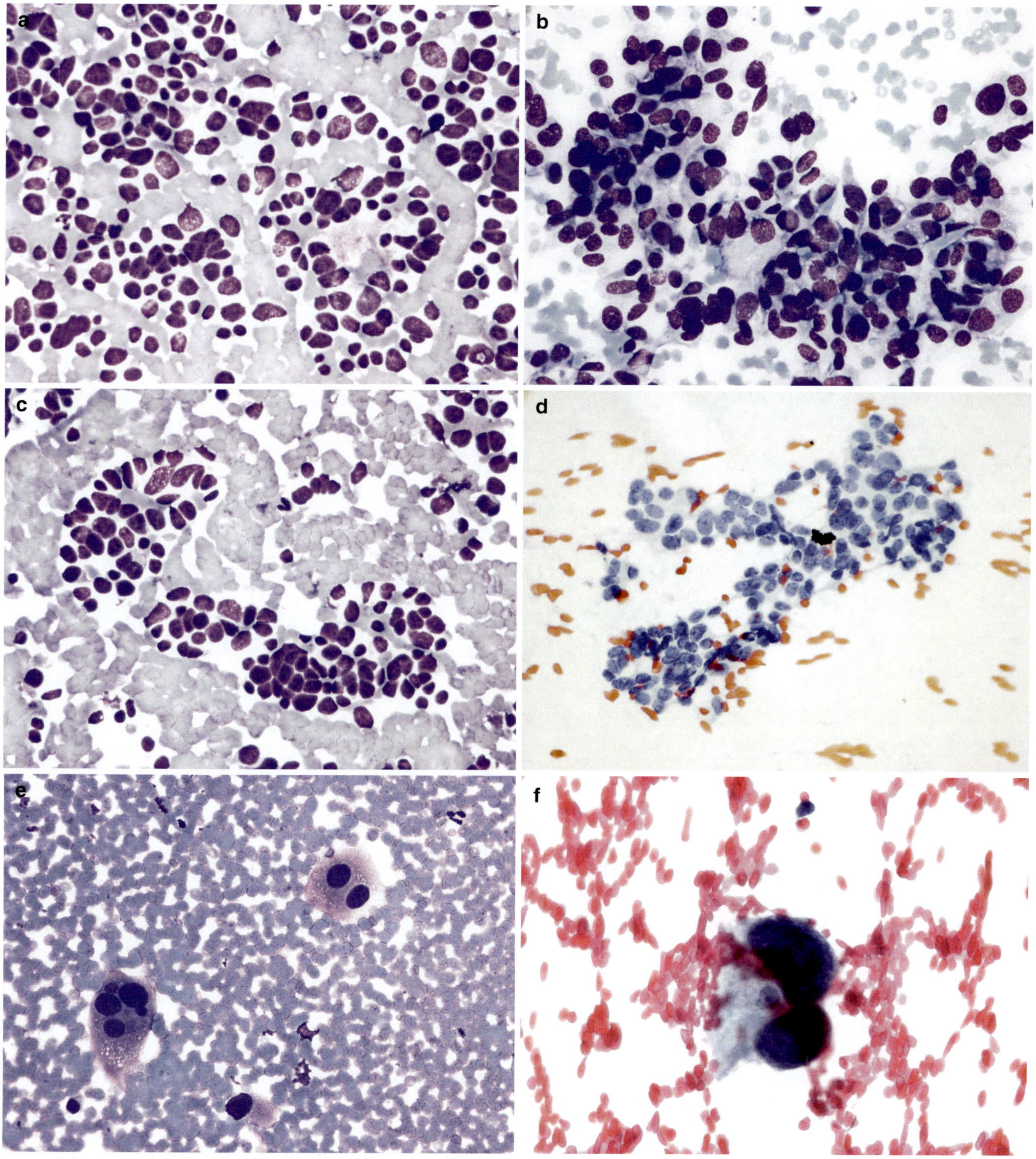

Fig. 10.2 Fine needle aspiration (FNA) of MTC on conventional smears (CS). (**a–c**) On CS, aspirates of MTC show moderate to high cellularity and are composed of groups, clusters, and single tumor cells. The tumor cells show round to oval to spindled nuclei, with nuclear pleomorphism arranged predominantly as single cells and as loose trabeculae (**a–c**, Diff Quik [DQ] stain). (**d, e**) Nuclei have a neuroendocrine-type, salt-and-pepper chromatin pattern. The aspirate shows binucleate and multinucleate tumor cells, which can be seen in cases of MTC. (**d**, Pap stain; **e**, Diff Quik). (**f**) MTC can show "bizarre"-type neuroendocrine atypia (Pap stain). (**g**) Amyloid appears dense and acellular and mixed with abundant background blood (Pap stain). (**h, i**) Cell block preparations of MTC shows amyloid as a cellular dense material closely associated with tumor cells. Amyloid can be identified by staining with special stain for Congo Red and using polarizing light microscopy which shows apple-green birefringence (**h, i**, H&E). (**j**) Immunostaining for calcitonin highlights these tumor cells by staining the cytoplasm. Almost all MTC stains positive for calcitonin. In calcitonin negative cases, the possibility of metastases and even a rare paraganglioma must be ruled out

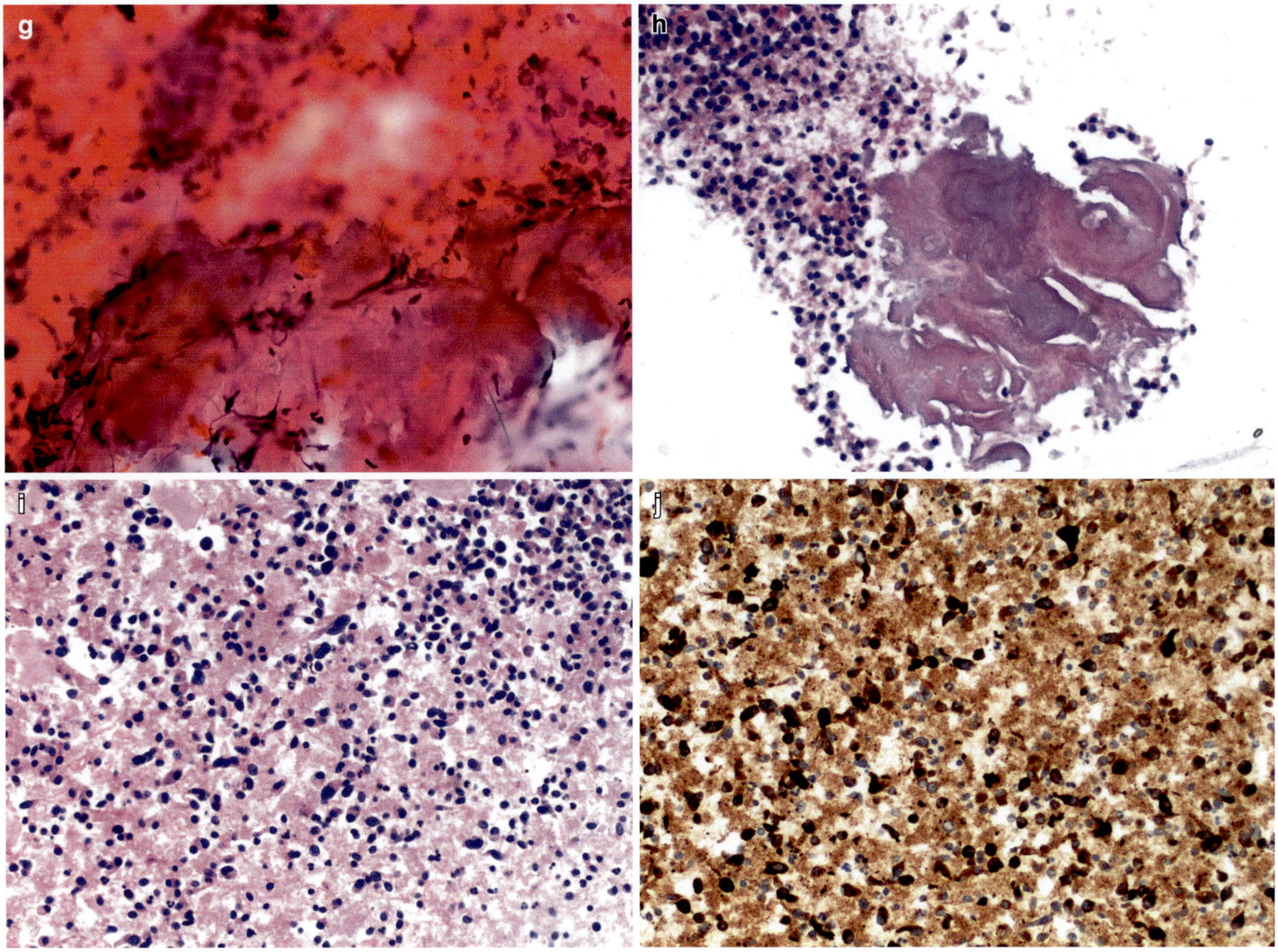

Fig. 10.2 (continued)

Variants and Differential Diagnosis of MTC

- Although most cases of MTC display a characteristic cytomorphology, MTC can demonstrate a variety of growth patterns and cytologic features.
- A number of variants have been described, as listed on Table 10.1 and illustrated in Fig. 10.5: Papillary (pseudopapillary), oncocytic, follicular, giant cell, small cell, paraganglioma-like, spindle cell, clear cell, squamous cell, melanin-producing, angiosarcoma-like, and amphicrine (mucin-producing).
- Variable tumor morphology can make the diagnosis challenging; each of these variants can mimic other primary and secondary tumors.
- Diagnostic accuracy for MTC is not as high as for papillary thyroid carcinoma (PTC) because of the diverse cytologic appearance. A large meta-analysis showed that FNA could detect only about 50% of cases of MTC.
- Diagnostic accuracy can be increased by the use of immunohistochemistry (IHC) and calcitonin assays in needle rinse.

Oncocytic Variant of MTC (MTC-OV) vs Hürthle Cell Neoplasm

- The oncocytic variant of MTC (MTC-OV) tends to show a monomorphic proliferation of tumor cells with enlarged, eccentrically placed nuclei showing salt-and-

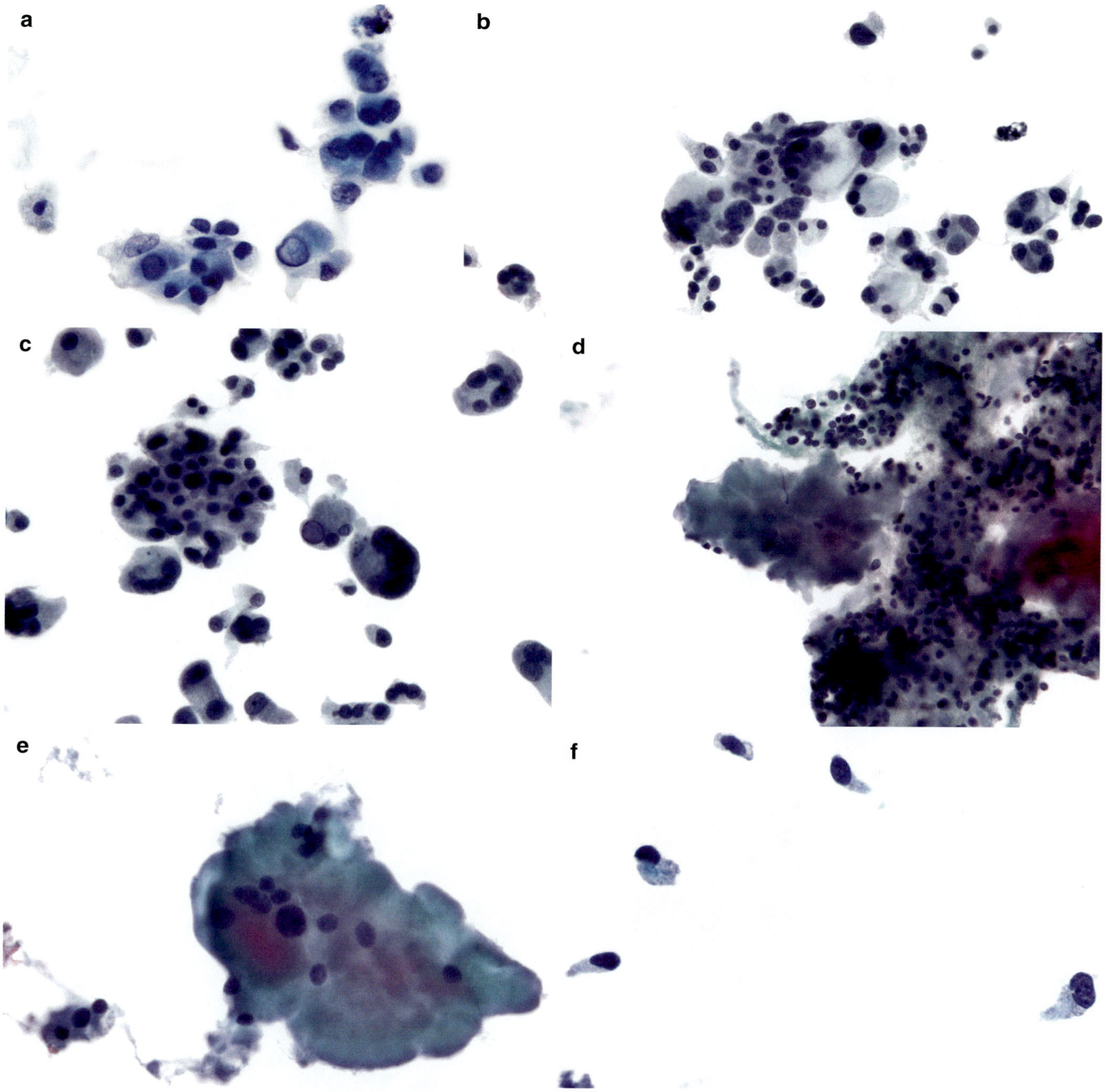

Fig. 10.3 Cytology of MTC on ThinPrep®. (**a**) Intranuclear pseudoinclusions can be seen in MTC and can be well recognized on TP as in CS. Therefore, INPI are not entirely specific for papillary thyroid carcinoma (PTC). (**b**, **c**) Just as in CS, the binucleate and multinucleate tumor cells can be prominent on TP. (**c**) One of the multinucleate cells shows an INPI and a few other tumor cells show bizarre nuclear atypia. (**d**, **e**) show appearances of "amyloid" on TP as dense amorphous stromal material appearing separate or intermixed with tumor cells. In LBP, amyloid can appear fibrillary or dense. In these examples they appear dense. Images from two different cases of MTC (**f–l** and **m–p**) processed with TP, showing tumor cells predominantly single, in trabeculae, and in clusters, similar to CS. Tumor cells are small and plasmacytoid to spindly in appearance. The cytoplasm of these cells on LBP shows microvacuolations and granularity (Pap stain, TP). When many small spindled to oval cells with spindled to oval nuclei are noted in LBP, it should raise a suspicion for MTC (Pap stain, TP)

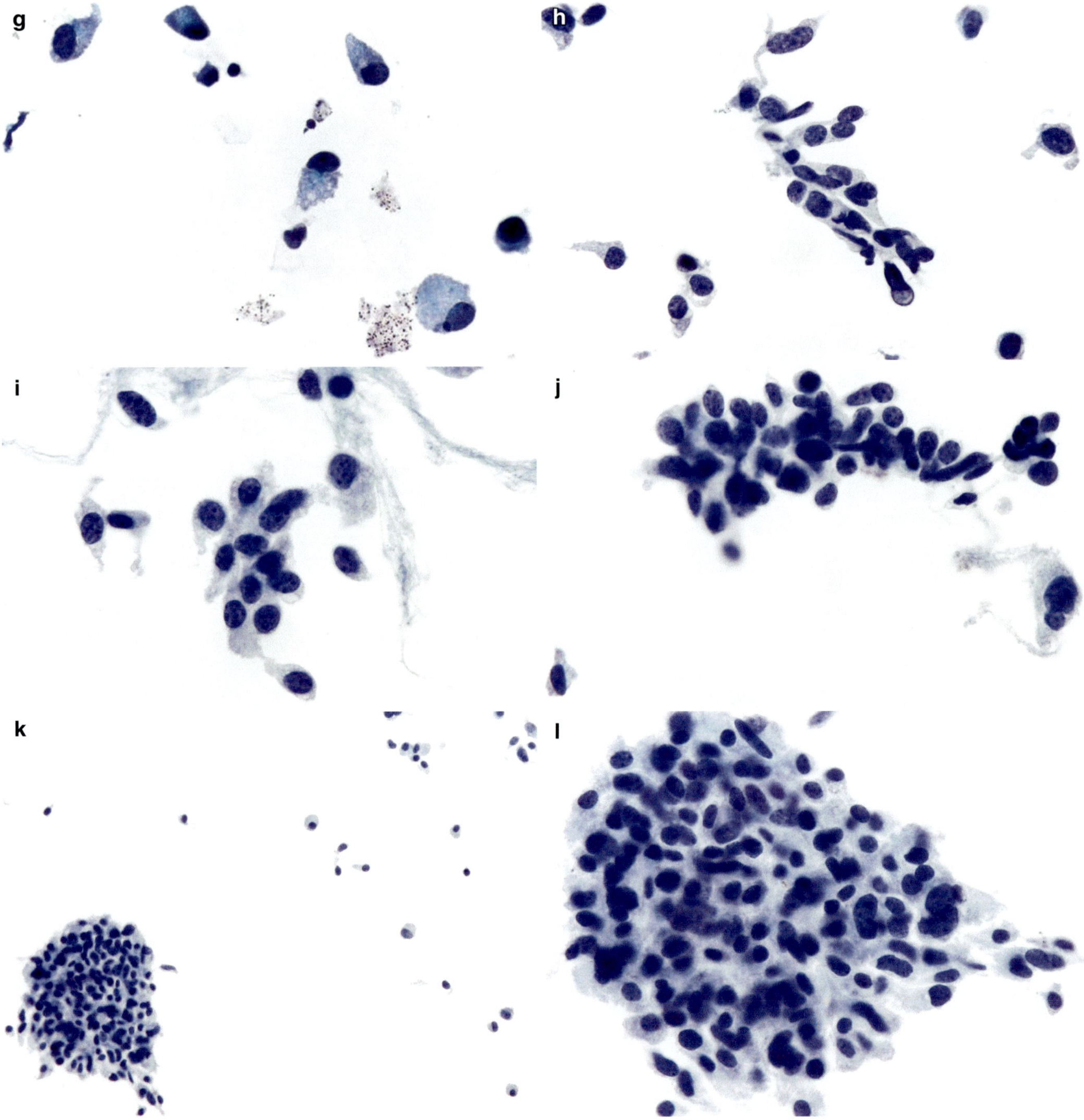

Fig. 10.3 (continued)

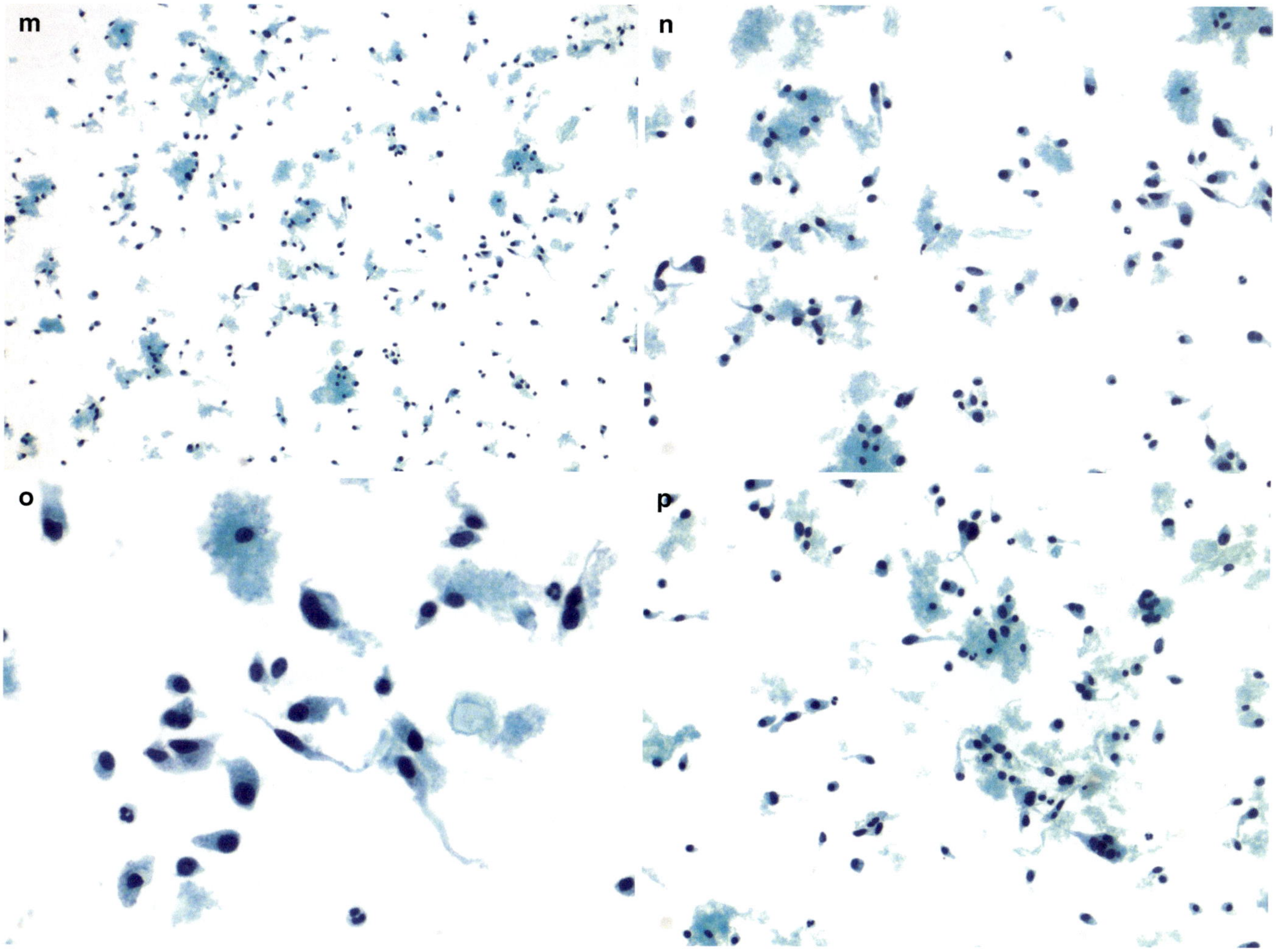

Fig. 10.3 (continued)

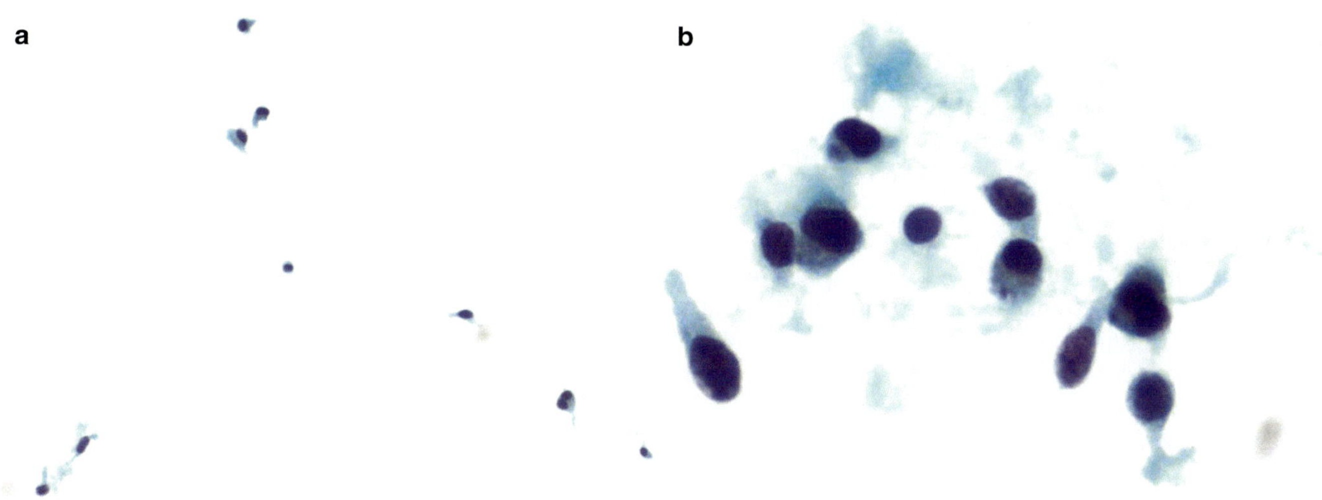

Fig. 10.4 Cytology of MTC on SurePath™ (SP). (**a**–**d**) Images from a case of MTC processed as SP show mostly single tumor cells and loosely cohesive groups. Tumor cells are spindly in appearance, with plasmacytoid to spindly nuclei. Occasional cells are binucleated. The cytoplasm is also spindled. Note that some cells appear in a different plane of focus, and nuclear morphology is less well-preserved than on TP. In both types of LBP, the presence of singly dispersed small, spindled cells should raise suspicion for MTC (Pap stain, SP)

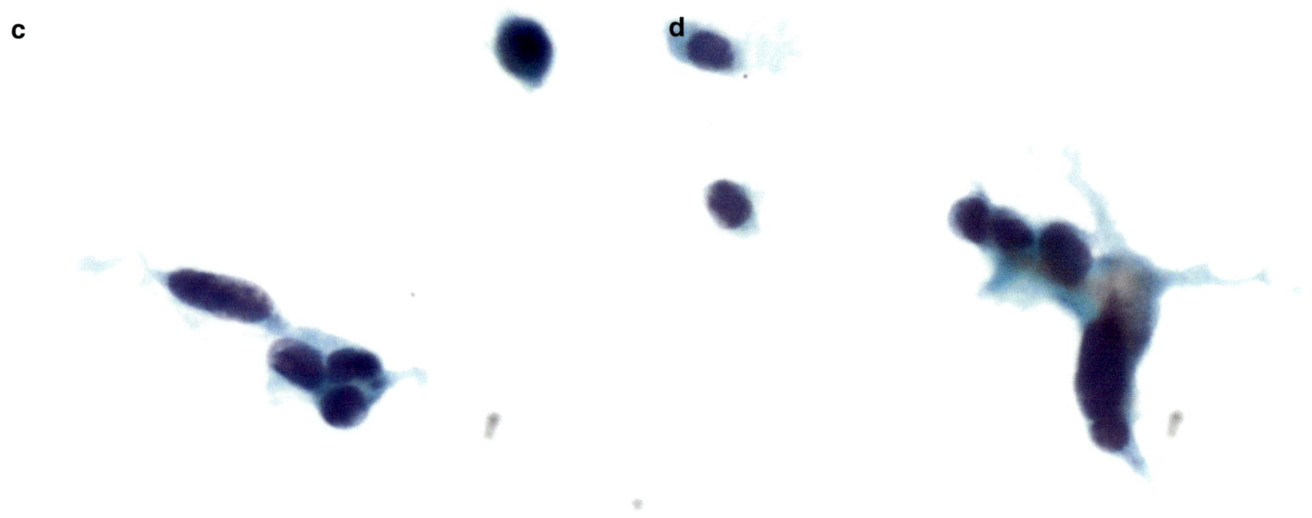

Fig. 10.4 (continued)

Table 10.1 Medullary thyroid carcinoma (MTC) variants: differential diagnosis and their immunohistochemical profile

		Immunohistochemistry (IHC)	
Variant	Differential diagnosis	Positive	Negative
Papillary/pseudopapillary	Papillary thyroid carcinoma (PTC)	TTF-1, PAX8, TG	Calcitonin, NE markers
Oncocytic	Oncocytic neoplasm PTC, oncocytic type	TTF-1, PAX8, TG	Calcitonin, NE markers
Follicular/glandular	Follicular neoplasm	TTF-1, PAX8, TG	Calcitonin, NE markers
Giant cell	Anaplastic thyroid carcinoma (ATC)	TTF-1 (variable), PAX8 (variable)	Calcitonin, TG, NE markers
Small cell	Metastatic small cell carcinoma	NE markers	Calcitonin
Paraganglioma-like	Hyalinizing trabecular tumor (HTT)	TTF-1, TG, Ki67 (membranous)	Calcitonin, NE markers
	Paraganglioma	NE markers, S100	Calcitonin, TTF-1, CK
Spindle cell	Sarcoma	Variable	Calcitonin, TTF-1, CK
Clear cell	Follicular neoplasm with clear cells	TTF-1, PAX8, TG	Calcitonin, NE markers
Squamous cell	Anaplastic thyroid carcinoma (ATC)	TTF-1 (variable), PAX8 (variable)	Calcitonin, NE markers, TG
	PTC with squamous differentiation	TTF-1, PAX8, TG	Calcitonin, NE markers
	Squamous cell carcinoma (SCC)	P63, p40	Calcitonin, NE markers
Melanin-producing/pigmented	Melanoma	S100, HMB45, A103, SOX-10	Calcitonin, TG, CK, NE markers
Angiosarcoma-like	Angiosarcoma	CD34, CD31, ERG	Calcitonin, TG, CK
Amphicrine	Metastatic adenocarcinoma	Variable depending on location	Calcitonin, TG

CK cytokeratin, *NE* neuroendocrine, *TG* thyroglobulin

pepper nuclear chromatin and oncocytic cytoplasm, with granularity and cytoplasmic vacuolization (Fig. 10.6a–f). These oncocytic variants can be misdiagnosed as Hurthle cell neoplasms (HCN), especially if they appear cohesive and lack the plasmacytoid appearance.

- MTC can be cytologically distinguished from HCN by the presence of a variable population of plasmacytoid and spindle cells, salt-and-pepper granular chromatin, and lack of prominent nucleoli.
- HCN shows round nuclei, small nucleoli, and lack the neuroendocrine type of chromatin (Fig. 10.6g–i).
- Confirmation of the diagnosis of MTC can be facilitated with positive staining for calcitonin and negative thyroglobulin staining.

Hyalinizing Trabecular Tumor/Adenoma

- Hyalinizing trabecular tumor (HTT) also known as hyalinizing trabecular adenoma (HTA) is a follicular-derived neoplasm that may resemble MTC both cytologically and histologically. (*See* Chap. 6 for more information on the hyalinizing trabecular tumor [HTT].)

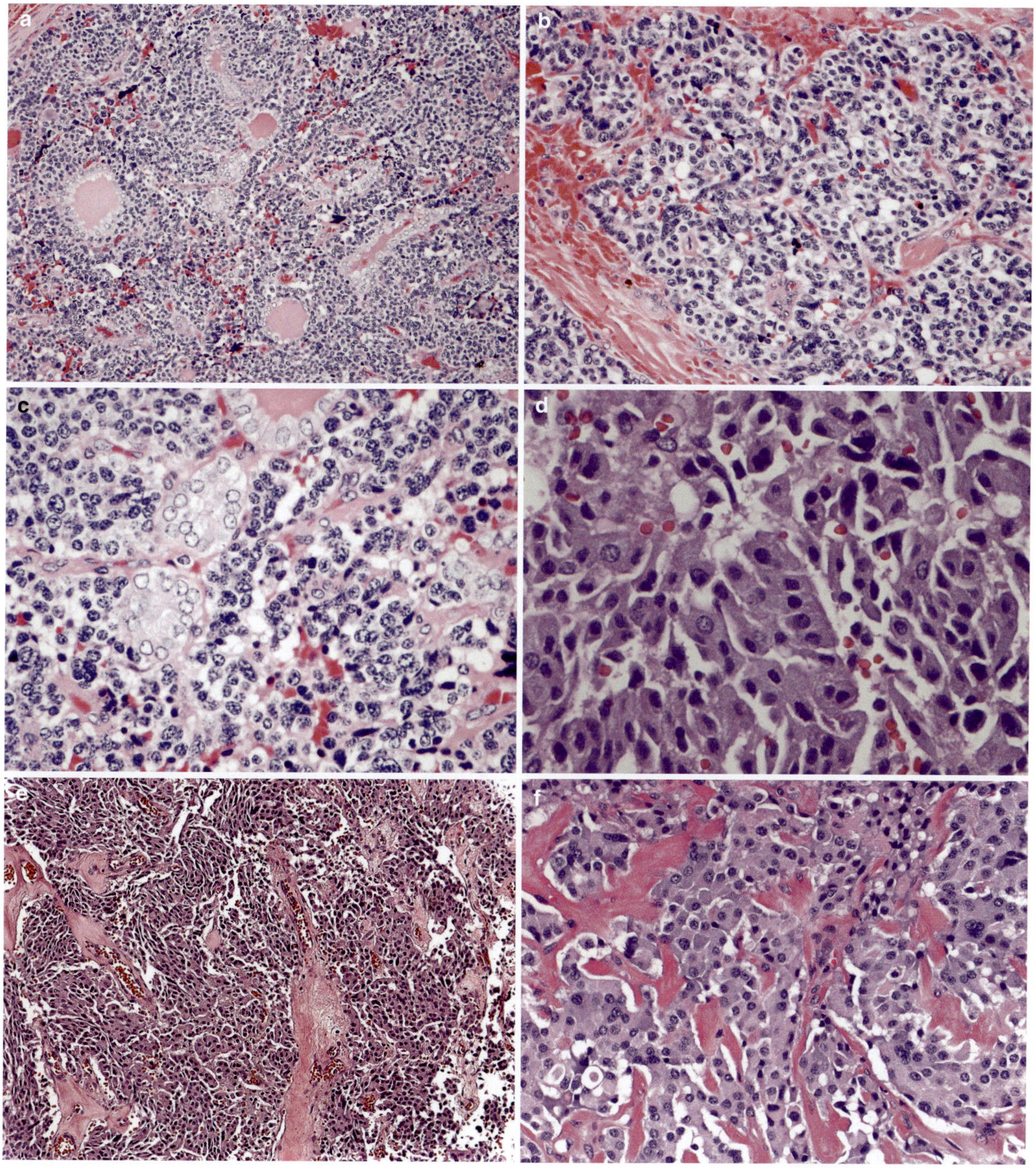

Fig. 10.5 Histology of MTC. The tumor may have a variable histologic appearance. Typical features include a combination of solid, nested, follicular, and trabecular growth pattern. The tumor cells show a combination of spindle, epithelioid, and plasmacytoid morphology. The nuclei have a salt-and-pepper chromatin pattern and may contain inclusions. (**a–c**) Histologic sections of a case of MTC showing syncytial and trabecular patterns of growth. Tumor cells show nuclei with "salt-and-pepper" neuroendocrine pattern and infiltrating preexisting follicles. (**d**) In this MTC, the tumor cells tend to show varying cytomorphology, with some cells having a glandular appearance and some having a plasmacytoid appearance and low nuclear-cytoplasmic (N:C) ratio. The cytoplasm appears granular. (**e, f**) Histologic sections of MTC with prominent plasmacytoid tumor cells. (**g**) In this histologic section of MTC, the tumor cells appear spindled and are growing in a sheet-like manner interspersed by plasmacytoid cells in nests. (**h**) The corresponding aspirate is cellular with markedly spindled cells with features very similar to that seen in the histologic section. Note the neuroendocrine chromatin pattern, which is readily appreciated on both cytology and histology. (Compare CS with the spindle cell morphology seen in TP in Fig. 10.3.) (**i**) Amyloid deposits are present in up to 80% of cases; they appear as amorphous hyaline material and strongly suggest MTC, but because they can be seen in other thyroid lesions not involving cancer cells they are not diagnostic of MTC but rather are a helpful feature in the presence of MTC cytology. (**j**) Histologic section of MTC with strong staining for calcitonin in the cytoplasm of the tumor cells. (**k**) Histologic section of MTC showing negative staining for thyroglobulin

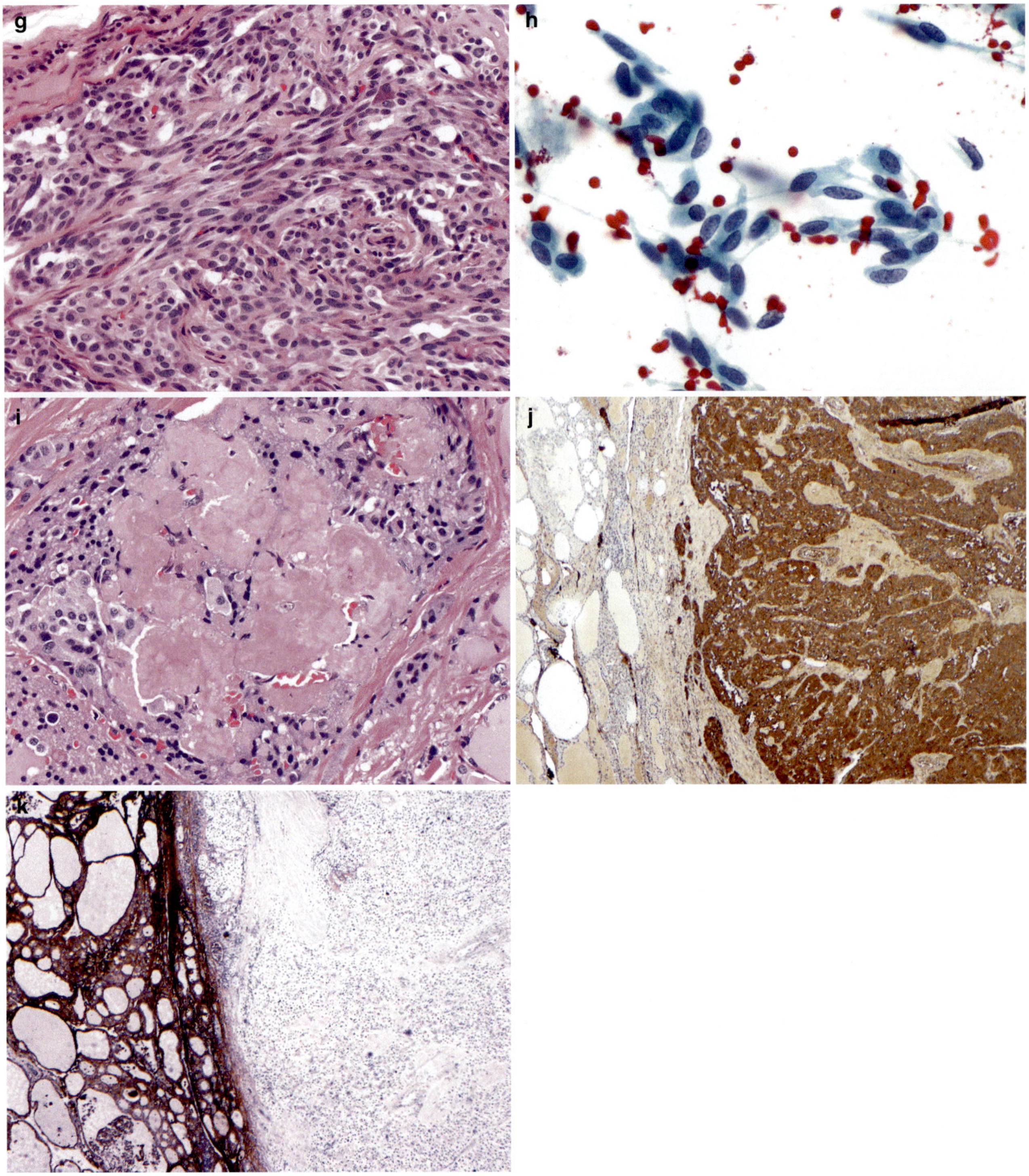

Fig. 10.5 (continued)

- Both neoplasms may show isolated cells in loose cohesive clusters, spindle-shaped cells, and acellular hyaline material. MTC can be distinguished from HTT by the presence of both plasmacytoid and spindle cells, frequent binucleation and multinucleation, and salt-and-pepper granular chromatin, as opposed to the PTC-like nuclei of HTT (Fig. 10.7; *see* Fig. 6.14).
- Immunohistochemical stains for calcitonin and thyroglobulin can aid in the distinction. MIB-1 immunostain has a distinct cytoplasmic and membranous staining in HTT unlike any other lesion/tumor.

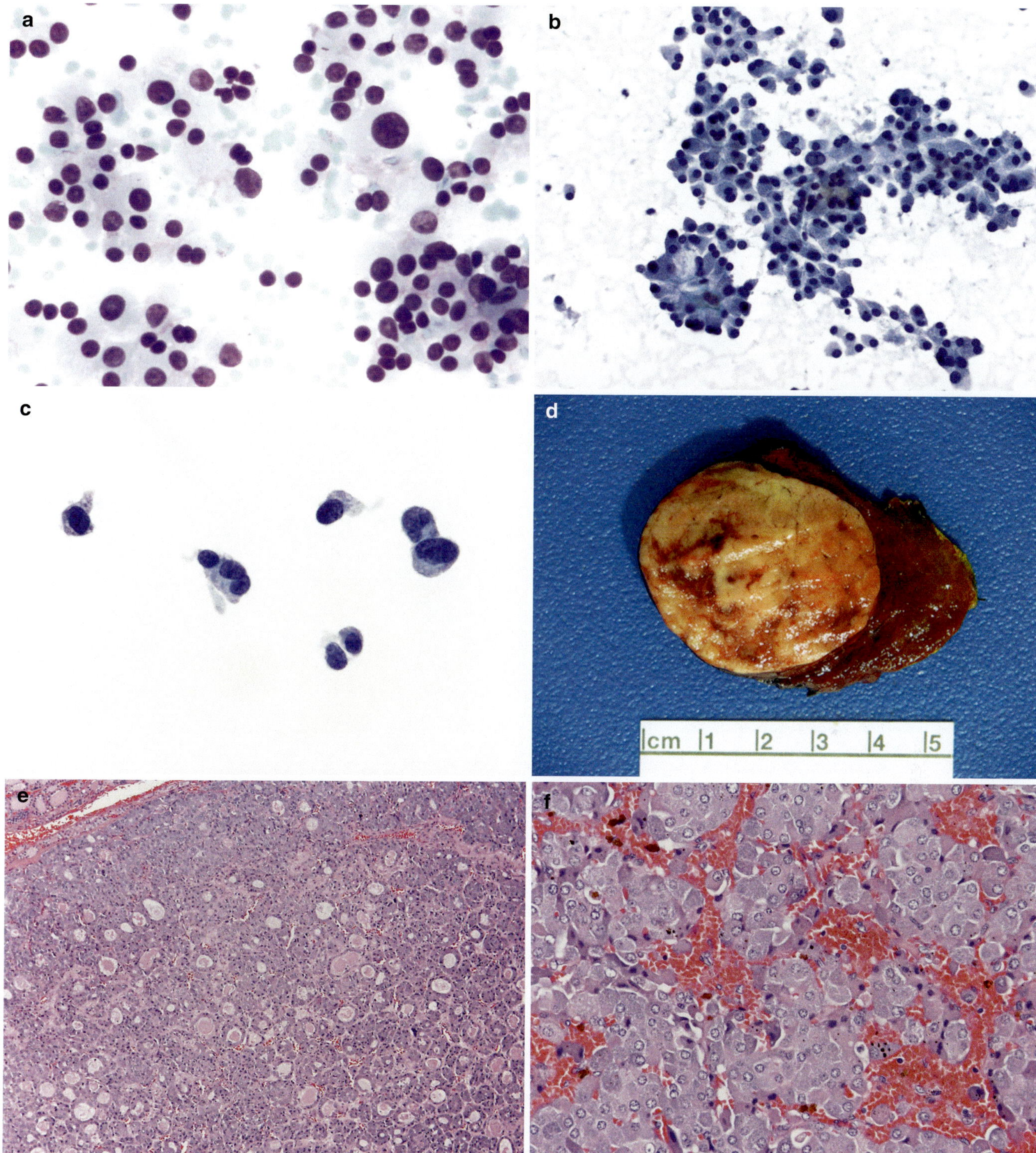

Fig. 10.6 Oncocytic variant of MTC (MTC-OV). (**a**, **b**) CS of MTC-OV show more granular cytoplasm and plasmacytoid nuclei on both DQ-stained CS (**a**) and Pap-stained CS (**b**). (**c**) Same case processed as TP shows similar features. (**d**) Gross image of MTC-OV shows a large (about 4 cm), single, circumscribed, and non-encapsulated tumor with minute areas of hemorrhage. (**e**, **f**) Histologic section of MTC-OV showing oncocytic tumor cells with granular cytoplasm and characteristic salt-and-pepper neuroendocrine chromatin; this notable feature is absent in other oncocytic tumors of the thyroid gland, such as Hürthle cell tumors (H&E stain). (**g**, **h**) This case of Hürthle cell adenoma shows follicular cells with oncocytic cytoplasm in DQ-stained CS (**g**) and Pap-stained TP (**h**). In most cases, it may be difficult to distinguish HCN from MTC-OV on DQ stain. The Pap-stained slides are more helpful in distinguishing HCN from MTC-OV because the nuclear features are well preserved. The nuclei on TP lack the characteristic neuroendocrine pattern of chromatin of MTC and also show nucleoli. Immunostaining for calcitonin and neuroendocrine markers and molecular testing, if performed, will help in rendering a definitive diagnosis. (**i**) Histologic section of Hürthle cell adenoma

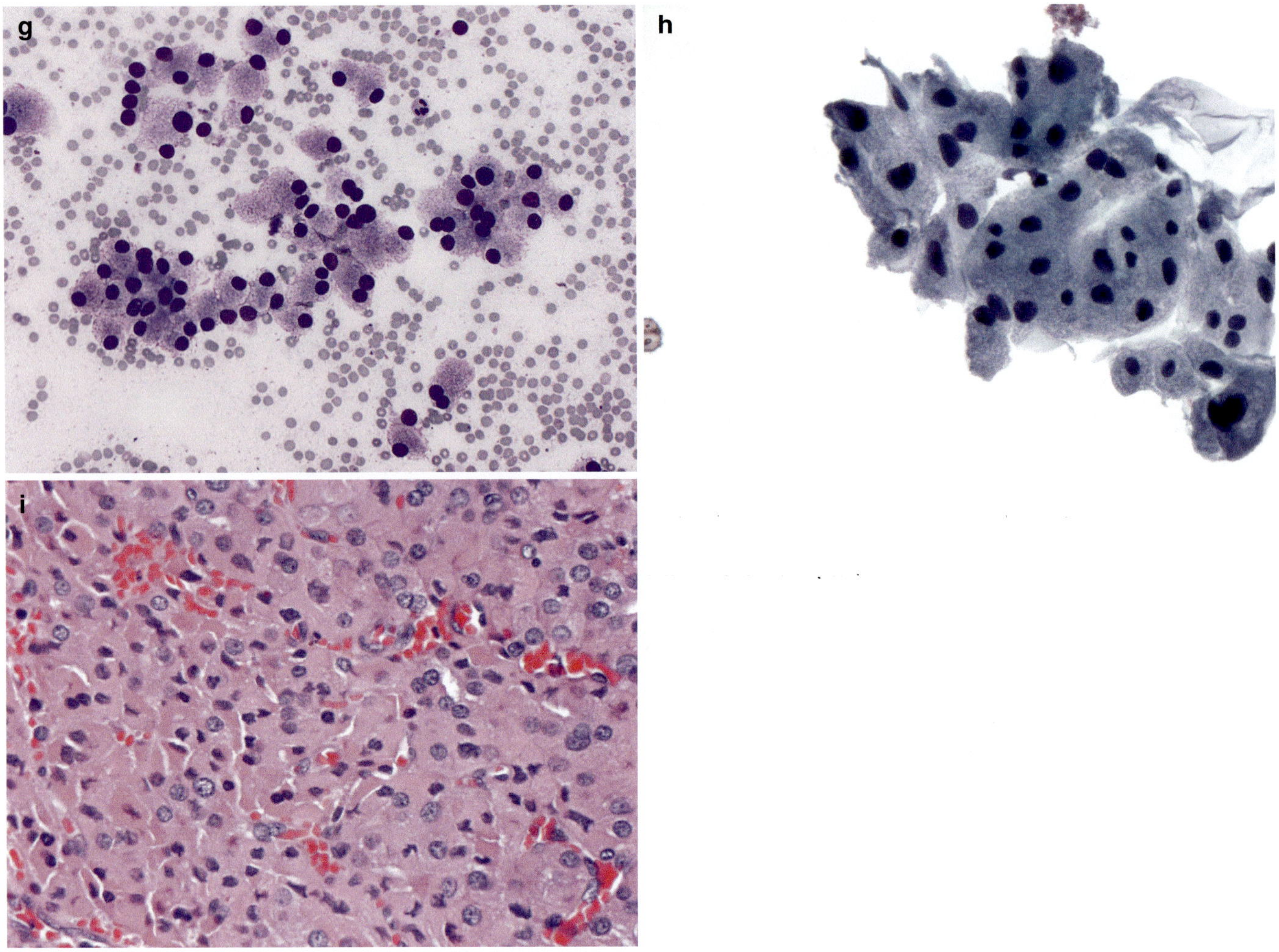

Fig. 10.6 (continued)

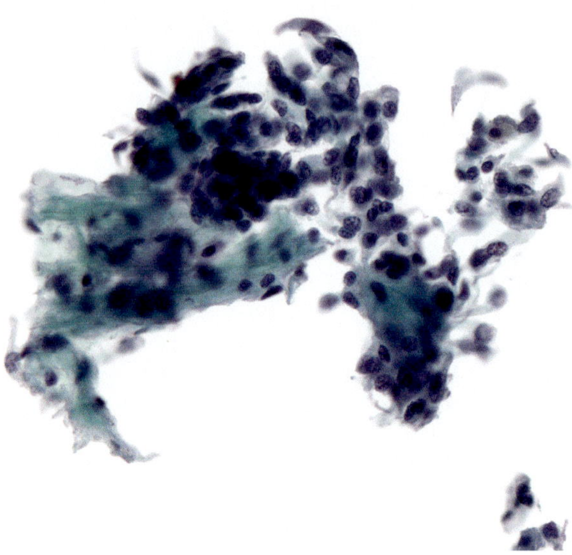

Fig. 10.7 Hyalinizing trabecular tumor (HTT) or adenoma (HTA). HTT or HTA showing loose, cohesive clusters of spindled cells with spindled to oval nuclei, few small INPI, closely associated hyaline material surrounding cells in image. This material can be mistaken for dense colloid. The nuclear pallor, grooves, INPI, and membrane irregularities mimic PTC rather than the neuroendocrine-type pattern of MTC (Pap stain, TP)

Parathyroid Adenoma

- A PTH assay performed on the FNA sample or positive staining for parathyroid hormone on smears or cell block preparations can confirm the presence of parathyroid cells. (*See* Chap. 13 on Parathyroid Gland Cytology.)

Paraganglioma

- MTC may have a paraganglioma-like pattern.
- Paragangliomas are rarely intrathyroidal.
- The salt-and-pepper chromatin and trabecular appearance resemble MTC.
- Fine, metachromatic, neurosecretory granules are noted in the cytoplasm.
- Cell block preparation is helpful for ancillary studies, for a definite distinction: S100 and neuroendocrine markers are positive; staining for calcitonin, TTF-1, and thyroglobulin are negative.
- Lesions are cytokeratin (CK)–negative, although 30% can express it.

Poorly Differentiated Thyroid Carcinoma

- The small cell variant of MTC, which consists of small uniform cells, may be difficult to distinguish from poorly differentiated thyroid carcinoma (PDTC) (Fig. 10.8). (See Chap. 11 for more information.)
- Unlike PDTC, necrosis and increased mitotic activity are usually absent in MTC aspirates.

Anaplastic (Undifferentiated) Thyroid Carcinoma

- The spindle cell pattern of MTC with pleomorphic cells may be misinterpreted as anaplastic thyroid carcinoma.
- Anaplastic thyroid carcinomas generally are more cellular and show nuclear pleomorphism and associated necrosis (Fig. 10.9).

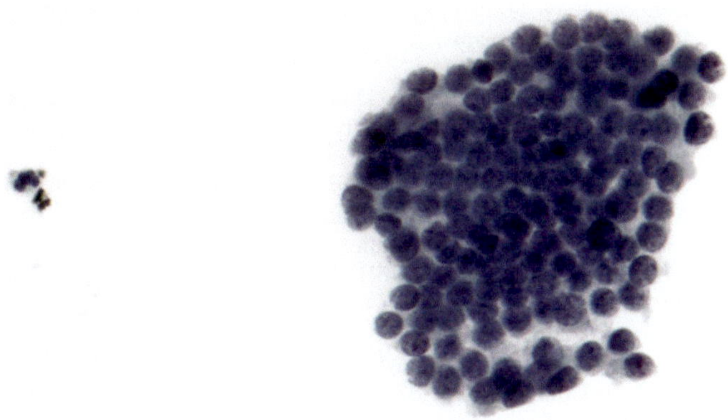

Fig. 10.8 Poorly differentiated thyroid carcinoma. LBP of a case of poorly differentiated thyroid carcinoma, showing a cellular cluster with conspicuous follicular architecture, granular chromatin and nuclei (Pap stain, TP)

- Immunostain for calcitonin may be necessary to confirm the diagnosis.

Metastatic Carcinoma Mimicking MTC

- Metastatic tumors considered in the differential diagnosis include renal cell carcinoma, melanoma, and metastatic neuroendocrine tumors.
- Immunohistochemical stains, as well as an underlying history of tumor, are useful in distinguishing MTC from its metastatic mimics.

Ultrasound features of MTC

- On ultrasonography, MTC appears as a hypoechoic, ovoid to round, solid mass with or without microcalcifications (Fig. 10.10). Lesions are read mostly as "suspicious" for malignancy.

Molecular/Genetic Alterations in MTC; the Role of Molecular Tests

- *RET* gene mutations (chromosome 10)

Management of MTC

- Total thyroidectomy and central lymph node dissection
- Lateral neck dissection may be performed, depending on imaging and calcitonin levels.

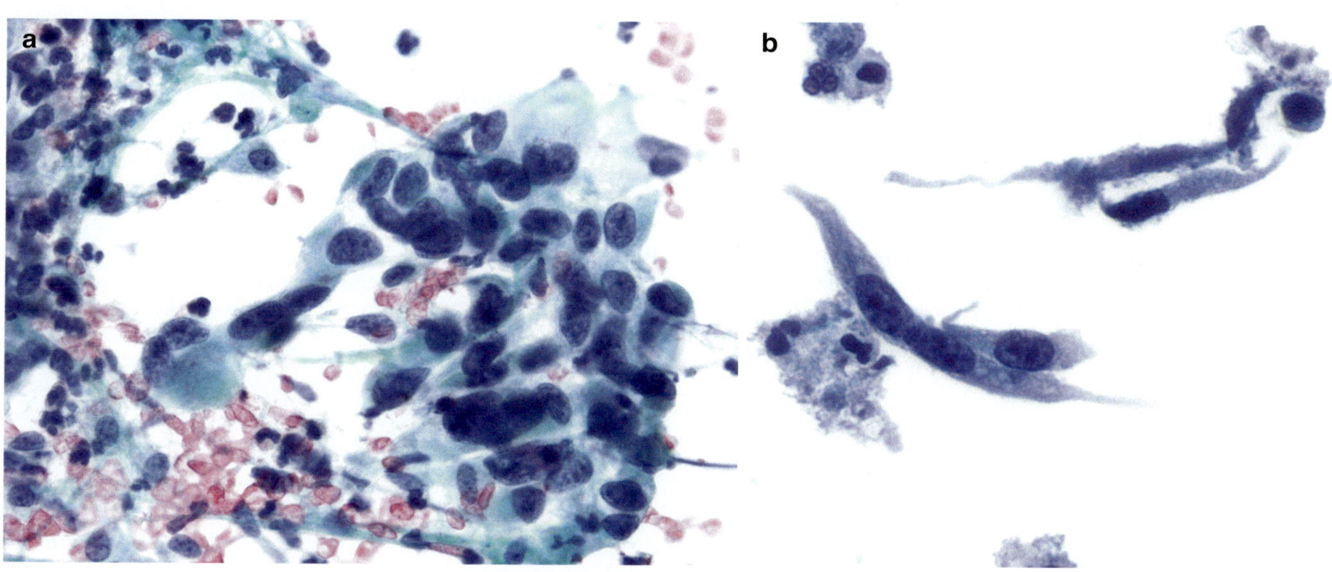

Fig. 10.9 Anaplastic thyroid carcinoma. (**a**, **b**) This case of anaplastic thyroid carcinoma shows nuclear pleomorphism and a chromatin pattern that is not the typical neuroendocrine pattern noted in MTC. Note the coarse chromatin and multiple nucleoli in the enlarged, spindled nuclei (**a**, Pap stain, CS; **b**, Pap stain, TP)

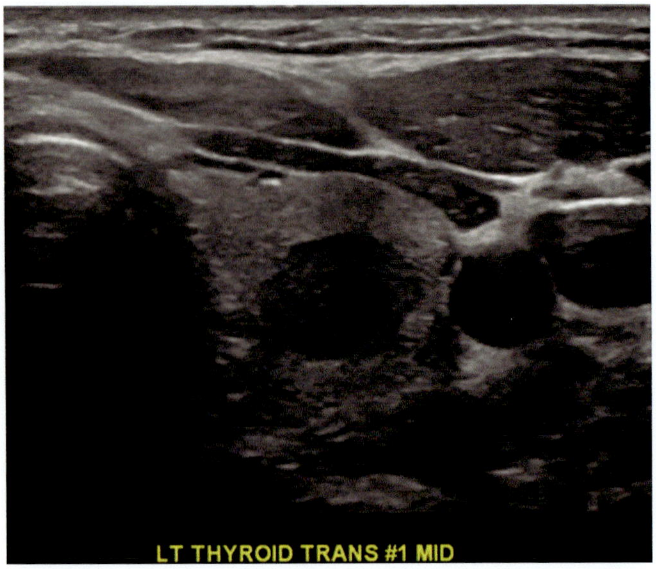

Fig. 10.10 Ultrasound features of MTC. This ultrasound image shows solid internal content, an ovoid to round shape, marked hypoechogenicity, and calcifications, findings suspicious of malignant nodules

- Genetic testing for germline *RET* mutations should be performed in patients with newly diagnosed MTC, according to the recently updated ATA management guidelines (Haugen et al.)
- Tyrosine kinase inhibitors are available for advanced disease.

Suggested Reading

1. Ali SZ, Cibas ES, editors. The Bethesda system for reporting thyroid cytopathology; definitions, criteria, and explanatory notes. 2nd ed. Cham: Springer International Publishing AG; 2018.
2. Canberk S, Onenerk M, Gunes P, Sayman E, Kilicoglu G. Oncocytic variant of medullary thyroid carcinoma. Endocr Pathol. 2015;26:320–3.
3. Chang TC, Wu SL, Hsiao YL. Medullary thyroid carcinoma: pitfalls in diagnosis by fine needle aspiration cytology and relationship of cytomorphology to RET proto-oncogene mutations. Acta Cytol. 2005;49:477–82.
4. Cibas ES, Ali SZ. The 2017 Bethesda system for reporting thyroid cytopathology. Thyroid. 2017;27:1341–6. https://doi.org/10.1089/thy.2017.0500.
5. Dyhdalo KS, Chute DJ. Barriers to the recognition of medullary thyroid carcinoma on FNA: implications relevant to the new American Thyroid Association guidelines. Cancer Cytopathol. 2018;126:397–405. https://doi.org/10.1002/cncy.21990.
6. Elisei R, Bottici V, Luchetti F, Di Coscio G, Romei C, Grasso L, et al. Impact of routine measurement of serum calcitonin on the diagnosis and outcome of medullary thyroid cancer: experience in 10,864 patients with nodular thyroid disorders. J Clin Endocrinol Metab. 2004;89:163–8.
7. Fadda G, Rossi ED. Liquid-based cytology in fine-needle aspiration biopsies of the thyroid gland. Acta Cytol. 2011;55:389–400. https://doi.org/10.1159/000329029.
8. Harach HR, Bergholm U. Medullary (C cell) carcinoma of the thyroid with features of follicular oxyphilic cell tumours. Histopathology. 1988;13:645–56.
9. Haugen BR, Alexander EK, Bible KC, Doherty GM, Mandel SJ, Nikiforov YE, et al. 2015 American thyroid association management guidelines for adult patients with thyroid nodules and differentiated thyroid cancer: the American thyroid association guidelines task force on thyroid nodules and differentiated thyroid cancer. Thyroid. 2016;26(1):1–133.
10. Hoda RS. Non-gynecologic cytology on liquid-based preparations: a morphologic review of facts and artifacts. Diagn Cytopathol. 2007;35:621–34.
11. Hoda RS, VandenBussche C, Hoda SA. Diagnostic liquid-based cytology. New York: Springer; 2017.
12. Kaushal S, Iyer VK, Mathur SR, Ray R. Fine needle aspiration cytology of medullary carcinoma of the thyroid with a focus on rare variants: a review of 78 cases. Cytopathology. 2011;22:95–105.
13. Papaparaskeva K, Nagel H, Droese M. Cytologic diagnosis of medullary carcinoma of the thyroid gland. Diagn Cytopathol. 2000;22:351–8.
14. Sams SB, Tompkins KD, Mayson S, Raeburn CD, Mehrotra S. Oncocytic variant of medullary thyroid carcinoma; a rare tumor with numerous diagnostic mimics by fine needle aspiration. Diagn Cytopathol. 2017;45:1148–52. https://doi.org/10.1002/dc.23790.
15. Seningen JL, Nassar A, Henry MR. Correlation of thyroid nodule fine-needle aspiration cytology with corresponding histology at Mayo Clinic, 2001-2007: an institutional experience of 1,945 cases. Diagn Cytopathol. 2012;40:E27–32. https://doi.org/10.1002/dc.21566.
16. Suzuki A, Hirokawa M, Takada N, Higuchi M, Ito A, Yamao N, et al. Fine-needle aspiration cytology for medullary thyroid carcinoma: a single institutional experience in Japan. Endocr J. 2017;64:1099–104. https://doi.org/10.1507/endocrj.EJ17-0238.
17. Tranchida P, Estigarribia J, Sethi S, Giorgadze T. Cytologic diagnosis of recurrent medullary thyroid carcinoma with oncocytic change twenty-one years post thyroidectomy: case report & review of the literature. Diagn Cytopathol. 2011;39:641–6.
18. Trimboli P, Cremonini N, Ceriani L, Saggiorato E, Guidobaldi L, Romanelli F, et al. Calcitonin measurement in aspiration needle washout fluids has higher sensitivity than cytology in detecting medullary thyroid cancer: a retrospective multicentre study. Clin Endocrinol. 2014;80:135–40.
19. Trimboli P, Treglia G, Guidobaldi L, Romanelli F, Nigri G, Valabrega S, et al. Detection rate of FNA cytology in medullary thyroid carcinoma: a meta-analysis. Clin Endocrinol. 2015;82:280–5.

Other Malignant Tumors of the Thyroid and Metastatic Tumors to the Thyroid

11

Rema Rao, Theresa Scognamiglio, and Rana S. Hoda

Other Malignant Tumors of the Thyroid

- This chapter discusses three other malignant tumors affecting the thyroid:
  - Anaplastic thyroid carcinomas (ATC)
  - Poorly differentiated thyroid carcinoma (PDCa)
  - Primary thyroid lymphoma

Anaplastic (Undifferentiated) Thyroid Carcinoma

- Anaplastic thyroid carcinomas (ATC) classically present as a rapidly growing thyroid mass in an elderly patient. Because of the rapid growth, patients can present with symptoms of compression or involvement of structures adjacent to the thyroid. The symptoms therefore include dysphagia, hoarseness, and dyspnea.
- ATC has an aggressive course, with frequent extrathyroidal extension (ETE) and metastases to regional lymph nodes and distant sites. The mortality rate is over 95% and the mean survival is 6 months from presentation.
- On ultrasonography, ATC appears as large, infiltrative thyroid mass with marked hypoechogenicity, necrosis, hemorrhage, dense calcifications, infiltration into surrounding structures, and cervical lymph node involvement in most cases (Fig. 11.1a).
- Grossly, ATC appears as a large, firm, tan-white to brown mass, with areas of necrosis and/or hemorrhage (Fig. 11.1b). The lesions are widely invasive, often replacing thyroid parenchyma and infiltrating the surrounding structures of the neck.
- On histology, ATC is heterogenous, with a mixture of spindled, squamoid/epithelioid, and pleomorphic giant cells; the dominant pattern varies between these cell types. The spindled variant is the commonest, accounting for about 50% of these tumors. Rare variants include paucicellular, rhabdoid, and small cell.
- Common features for all variants include invasion, extensive tumor necrosis, marked pleomorphism, and high mitotic activity. The tumor grows predominantly as solid sheets and lacks follicles. Colloid is absent; if seen, it is noted in the well-differentiated component (if present) or in pre-existing non-neoplastic follicles infiltrated by the tumor.
- On immunohistochemistry, low molecular weight cytokeratins are probably the most helpful marker, with at least weak or focal staining of the tumor cells.
- There is controversy in the interpretation of thyroglobulin immunoreactivity in ATC. Reactivity for thyroglobulin has been reported in up to 50% of cases and has been described as weak and focal, but this positivity is generally considered to be overinterpretation of positivity in entrapped non-neoplastic follicular cells, well-differentiated components, or diffusion of the stain from normal surrounding thyroid tissue. As such, thyroglobulin is of limited use in the evaluation of ATC. TTF-1 is rarely expressed in ATC.
- Like histology, on cytology, spindled cells are the commonest cell type in ATC. The spindled cells appear enlarged and pleomorphic, with high-grade nuclei, and they show mitotic activity. Usually the spindled cells are admixed with pleomorphic giant cells and/or epithelioid/squamoid–type cells; occasionally, these other cell types may be dominant (Fig. 11.1c–p).
- The presence of spindled cells in the aspirate raises a differential diagnosis that includes medullary thyroid carcinoma (MTC), Reidel thyroiditis, high-grade sarcoma,

R. Rao · T. Scognamiglio
Department of Pathology and Laboratory Medicine, New York Presbyterian Hospital, Weill Cornell Medical College, New York, NY, USA

R. S. Hoda (✉)
CBLPath, Rye Brook, NY, USA
e-mail: rhoda@cblpath.com

R. S. Hoda et al. (eds.), *Atlas of Thyroid Cytopathology on Liquid-Based Preparations*,
https://doi.org/10.1007/978-3-030-25066-9_11

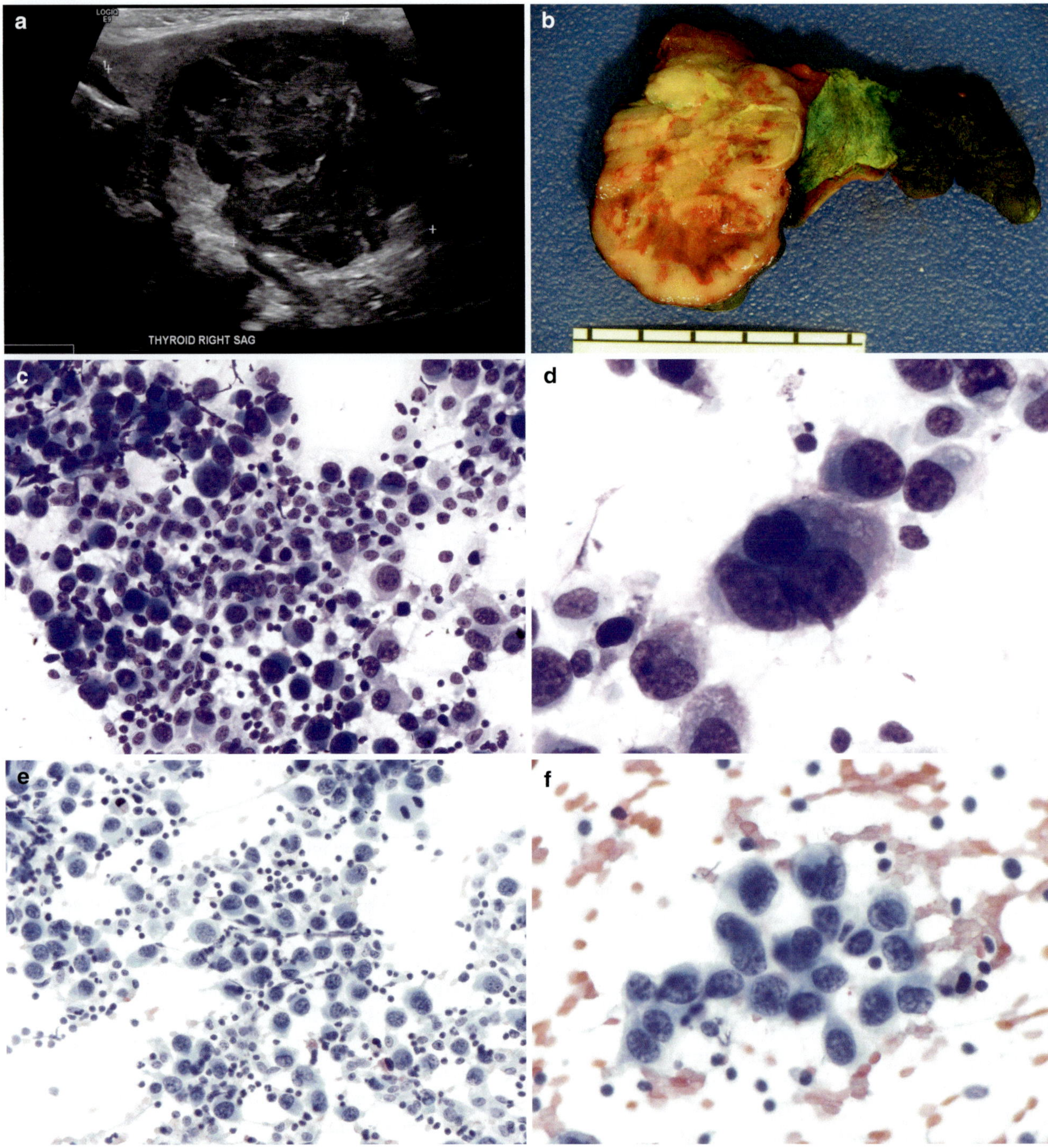

Fig. 11.1 Anaplastic thyroid carcinoma (ATC): Imaging, gross, and cytohistologic findings. (**a**) This ultrasound image of a case of ATC shows a large thyroid mass with ill-defined borders and mixed echogenicity. Prominent areas of marked hypoechogenicity are noted, in addition to areas of necrosis and dense calcifications. (**b**) Grossly, ATC appears as a large, firm, tan-white to brown mass, with areas of necrosis and/or hemorrhage. (**c**, **d**) Air-dried aspirate smears from the same case show a dyshesive population of pleomorphic cells, many showing a multinucleate giant cell morphology. The pleomorphism is marked, with nuclear sizes ranging from 1 to >10. The cytoplasm appears granular to mostly vacuolated (Diff Quik, CS). (**e**, **f**) Alcohol-fixed aspirates show similar findings as the air-dried smears, but with better nuclear details. The nuclear chromatin appears dense, coarse, and irregular, with prominent nucleoli. Note the nuclear size comparison of the tumor cells with the adjacent lymphocytes. In this case, the pleomorphic cell type is the most dominant (Pap stain, CS). (**g–l**) These images represent the cytologic features of ATC of the pleomorphic giant cell type on a liquid-based preparation (LBP), ThinPrep® (TP). Figures **g** and **i** clearly depict the difference in the background when compared with CS. In LBP, the background appears to have less blood, and in LBP the blood elements appear more granular and contain neutrophils and fibrin material; they can cling to the tumor cells, as seen on images **j** and **k**. The clusters appear tighter on LBP than on CS, as seen in image **h**. The nuclear morphology overall looks like that of the CS (**g–l**, Pap stain, TP). (**m–p**) The histologic findings seen in image (**m**) mirror that of the cytologic findings. Image (**m**) shows a dyshesive population of pleomorphic cells with vacuolated to granular cytoplasm. The tumor stains for LMWCK (**n**), and shows most tumor cells staining for PAX 8 (**o**). In (**p**), some tumor cells stain for TTF-1, but the adjacent group shows negativity. TTF-1 staining can be positive or negative in ATC; if present, it does not stain as diffusely as PAX 8 (**m–p**, Pap stain, TP)

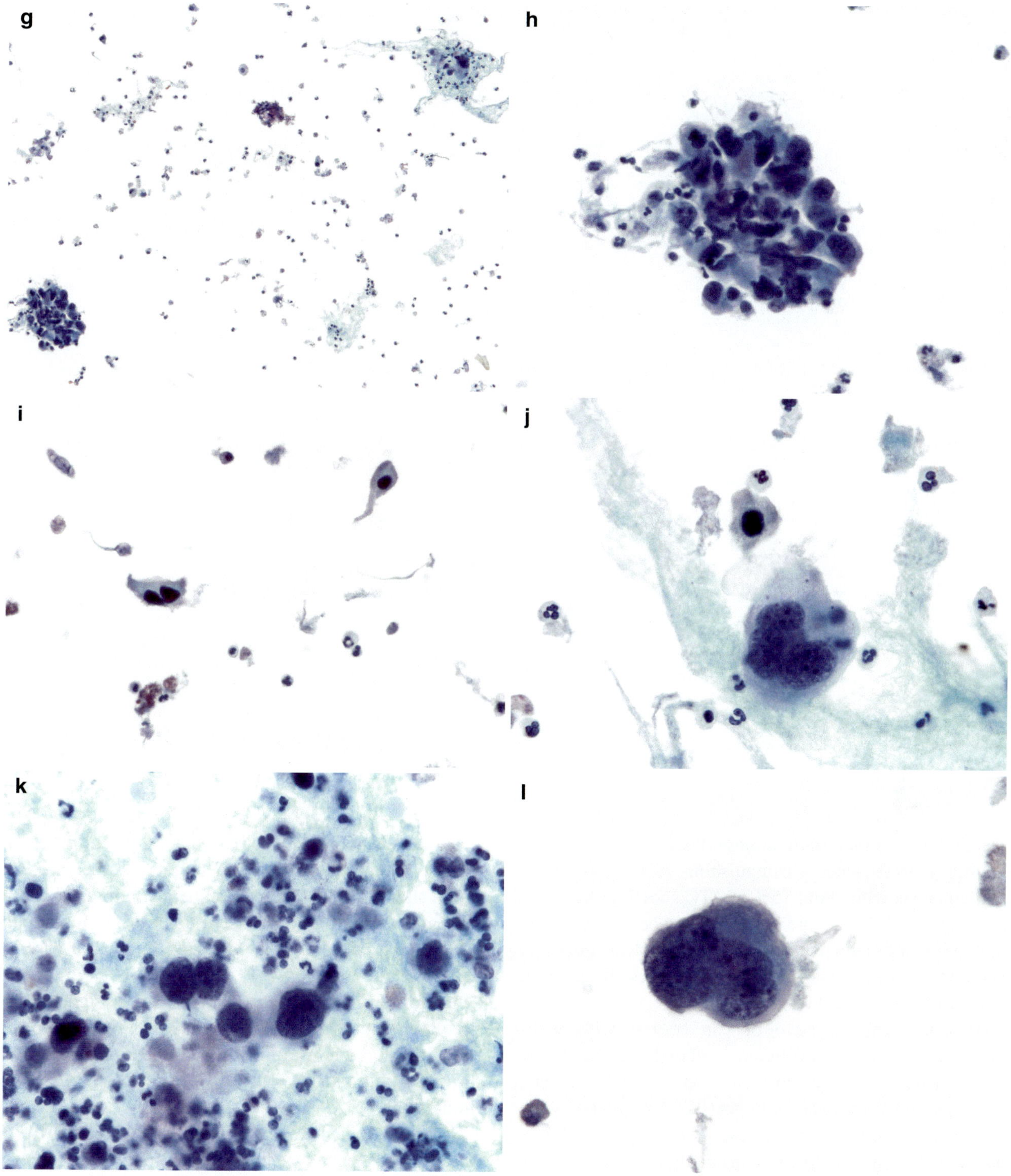

Fig. 11.1 (continued)

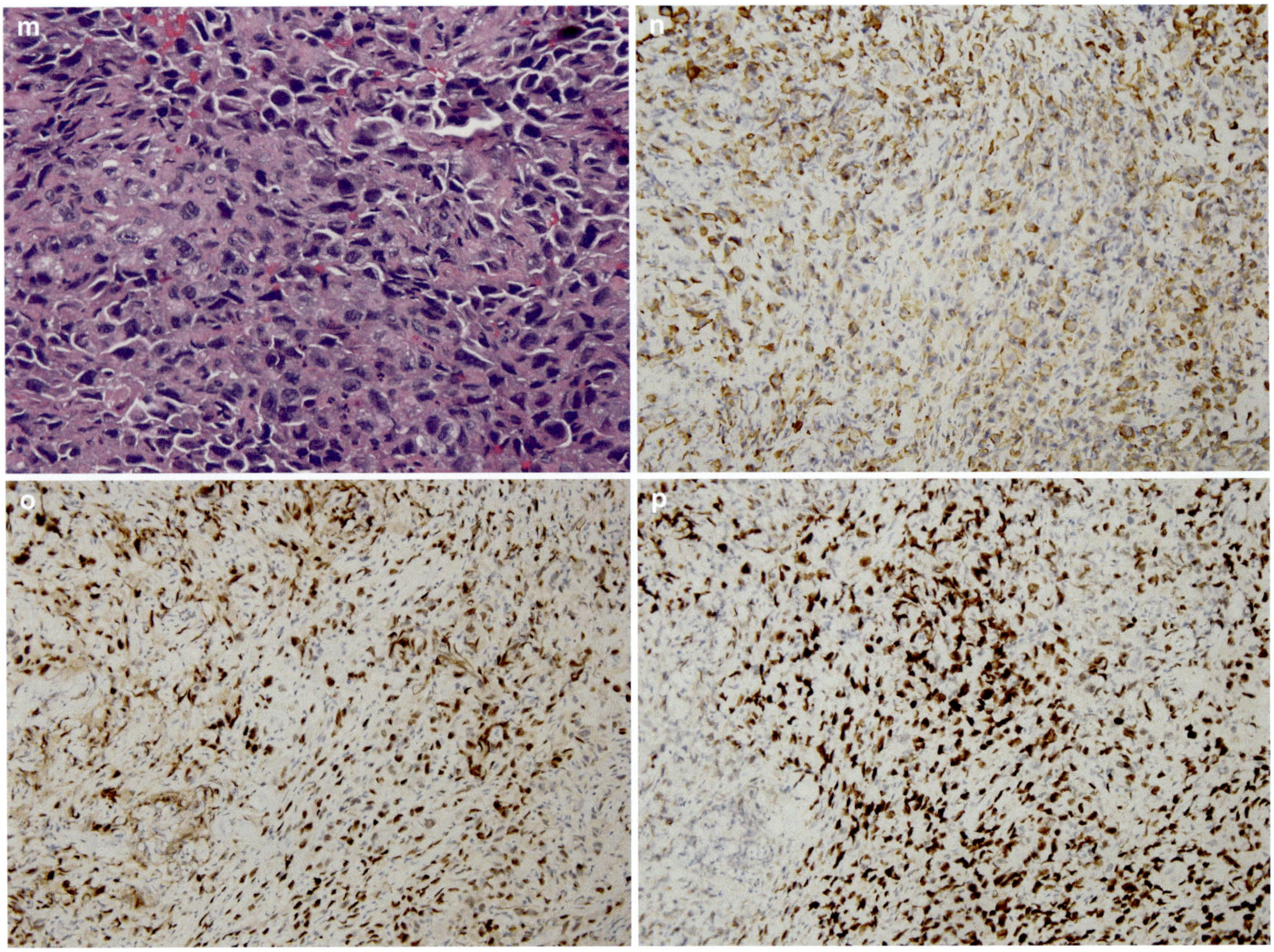

Fig. 11.1 (continued)

melanoma, and metastatic tumors. PAX 8 proves to be a helpful marker when distinguishing ATC from other malignancies with about 75% of ATC showing reactivity (*see* Fig. 11.1). The expression seems to be related to the predominant growth pattern: More than 90% of squamoid variants show reactivity, but reactivity is less frequent in other variants (Table 11.1)

- ATC can occur de novo or can coexist with well-differentiated or poorly differentiated malignancies in the thyroid (Fig. 11.2). The most common is the tall cell variant of papillary thyroid carcinoma (PTC), followed by the oncocytic variant of follicular carcinoma; a poorly differentiated thyroid carcinoma is less likely.
- ATC is characterized by accumulation of several different genetic alterations. Compared with differentiated thyroid carcinomas, ATC tends to have at least two or more mutations. *BRAF*V600E and *RAS* mutations, the most common alterations in well-differentiated thyroid carcinomas, remain the mutually exclusive main driver mutations in ATC, with *BRAF*V600E occurring in 29% of cases and *RAS* mutations in 23%.
- In addition, ATC is associated with a higher rate of telomerase reverse transcriptase (TERT) promoter mutations, seen in almost 73% of cases; these TERT promoter mutations tend to occur with *BRAF* or *RAS* mutations.
- In general, the coexistence of *BRAF/RAS* and TERT promoter mutations is synergistic and confers an aggressive potential to the malignancy and a trend towards greater mortality in ATC.

Table 11.1 Differential diagnosis of anaplastic thyroid carcinoma on FNA

Diagnosis	Cytology	Immunohistochemistry
Anaplastic thyroid carcinoma (ATC)	Spindled cells with high-grade nuclei, pleomorphism, mitoses (includes atypical) Usually admixed with pleomorphic or squamoid cells	*Positive:* LMWCK, PAX 8 *Negative:* Thyroglobulin *Positive or negative:* TTF-1
Squamous cell carcinoma	Lacks extreme pleomorphism Desmoplastic stromal spindle cells lack atypia	*Positive:* LMWCK *Negative:* PAX 8, thyroglobulin, TTF-1
Medullary thyroid carcinoma (MTC)	Spindled and/or plasmacytoid with "salt and pepper" chromatin. Bland nuclei. Endocrine-type atypia. Background can show amyloid.	*Positive:* CEA, calcitonin, neuroendocrine (NE) markers
High-grade sarcoma	Primary or metastatic Depends on the line of differentiation	*Positive:* SMA, desmin (if smooth muscle); CD34, ERG, CD31, FLI1 (if angiosarcoma)
Reidel thyroiditis	Bland-appearing fibroblasts and reactive myofibroblasts admixed with non-granulomatous–type inflammatory cells Can be cellular to paucicellular	*Positive:* SMA *Negative:* CK, EMA
Spindle epithelial tumor with thymus-like differentiation (SETTLE)	Rare Low-grade, bland-appearing spindled cells admixed with glandular epithelial cells No high-grade features such as necrosis, pleomorphism, or increased mitoses	*Positive:* AE1/AE3, CAM 5.2, CK7, vimentin, CD117

LMWCK low molecular weight cytokeratins

- Inactivating mutations in *TP53* play a major role in the tumorigenesis of ATC, with the overall prevalence in some studies being close to 60%.
- The efficacy of conventional treatments is limited in ATC because of the aggressive nature of the malignancy. Whenever possible, a multimodality approach with surgery, adjuvant chemotherapy, and radiation should be used.

Poorly Differentiated Thyroid Carcinoma (PDCa)

- PDCa is rare, about 4–7% of all thyroid cancers. It is biologically intermediate between well-differentiated and undifferentiated (anaplastic) thyroid carcinoma, with a mean survival rate of about 50%.
- It is imperative to distinguish PDCa from other well-differentiated thyroid cancers. Its aggressive nature presents increased chances of early recurrence and metastasis compared to its well-differentiated counterparts, necessitating aggressive therapy.
- On imaging, PDCa occurs as a solitary, large, solid, predominantly hypoechoic oval to round nodule that is mostly well circumscribed and has rich internal vascularity, with or without microcalcifications (Fig. 11.3a).
- Grossly, PDCas are large masses (often exceeding 5.0 cm in size) with a firm, solid, gray-white to brown cut surface with focal areas of necrosis. These tumors often show evidence of gross invasion (Fig. 11.3b).
- On cytology, PDCa shows a highly cellular aspirate composed of small cells arranged in a follicular, solid, syncytial, insular, or trabecular architecture with abundant single cells and bare nuclei on a background of blood. The cytoplasm is scant, and the nuclei are round and regular with granular chromatin and small nucleoli. There is no evidence of colloid and no nuclear features of PTC (Fig. 11.3c, d).
- The findings on liquid-based preparations (LBP) are similar to those on conventional smears (CS). The background may show reduced bare nuclei and necrosis, compared with CS (Fig. 11.3e, f). No studies to date have specifically identified the cytologic features of PDCa on LBP.
- Histologically, the commonest growth pattern is the insular growth pattern, recognized by well-defined nests or insulae with a fibrovascular outline. This can be the dominant pattern, or it can be intermixed with other patterns such as solid, trabecular, and follicular. The tumor cells appear monotonous, with round nuclei, scant cytoplasm, a high N:C ratio, granular chromatin, and small nucleoli. No features of PTC should be noted. Mitoses and necrosis can be observed (Fig. 11.3g, h).

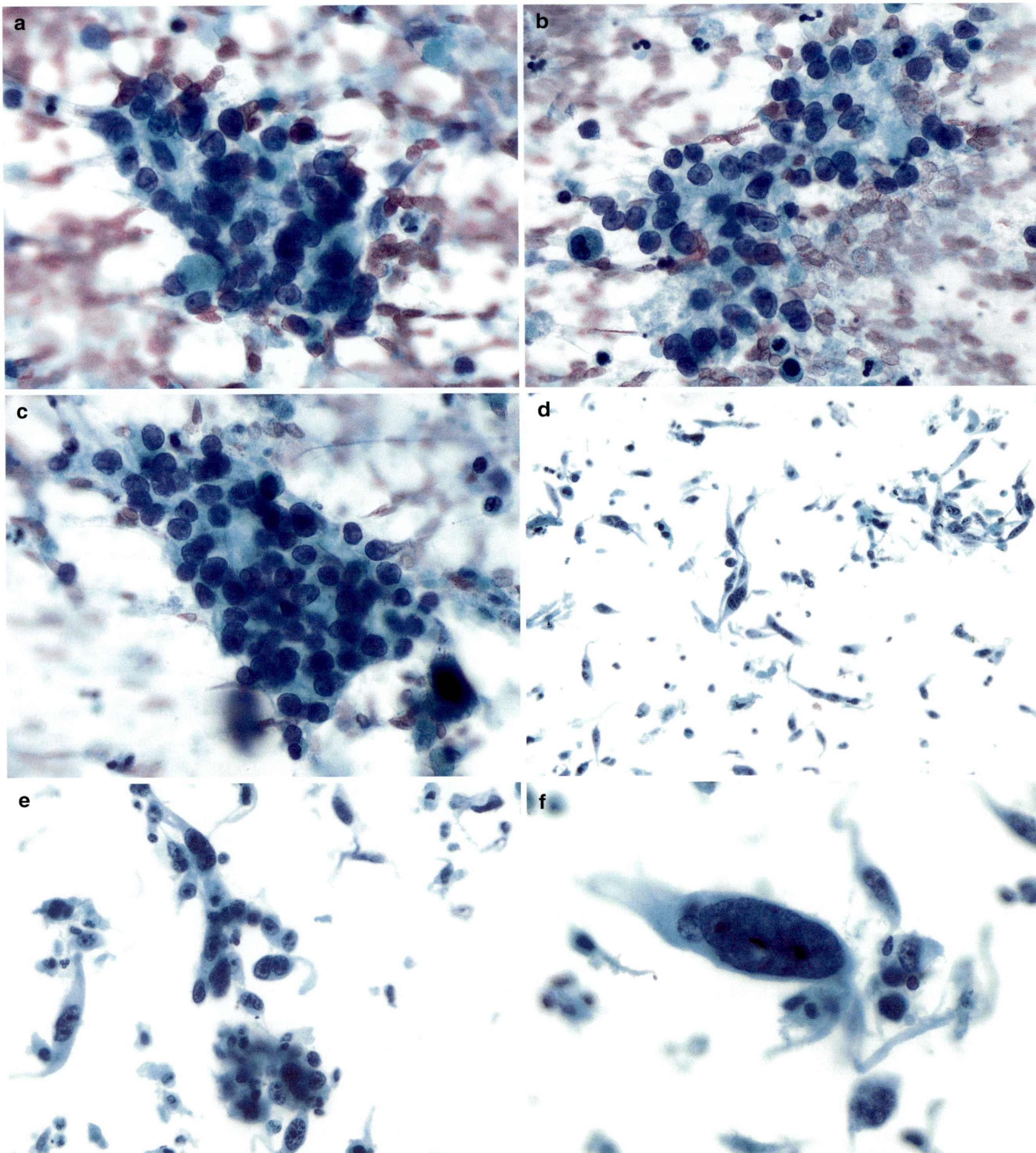

Fig. 11.2 ATC: Appearance on LBP. These images show an example of the spindled-cell variant of ATC on LBP (both TP and SurePath™ [SP]), associated with a well-differentiated component, papillary thyroid carcinoma (PTC). (**a–c**) These alcohol-fixed aspirates show the well-differentiated component, which was a PTC, as identified by the constellation of nuclear features, including nuclear overlap, grooves, membrane irregularity, pallor, and nuclear pseudoinclusions (**a–c**, Pap stain, CS). (**d–f**) The SP slides show the ATC component with prominent spindled cells showing high-grade nuclei. In these SP images, you can appreciate the dimensionality of the aspirate with blurring of some cells in the background. Just as on TP, the background in SP shows less blood (**d–f**, Pap stain, SP). (**g–j**) Compared with SP, TP is a monolayered preparation, which lacks dimensionality. The nuclear morphology otherwise looks fairly similar. On LBP, the single tumor cells appear more in number because of the preparatory technique (**g–j**, Pap stain, TP). (**k**) The surgical pathology follow-up of the tumor shows the prominent spindled cells with nuclear features similar to those seen in the SP and TP images. Note the high mitotic activity (H&E)

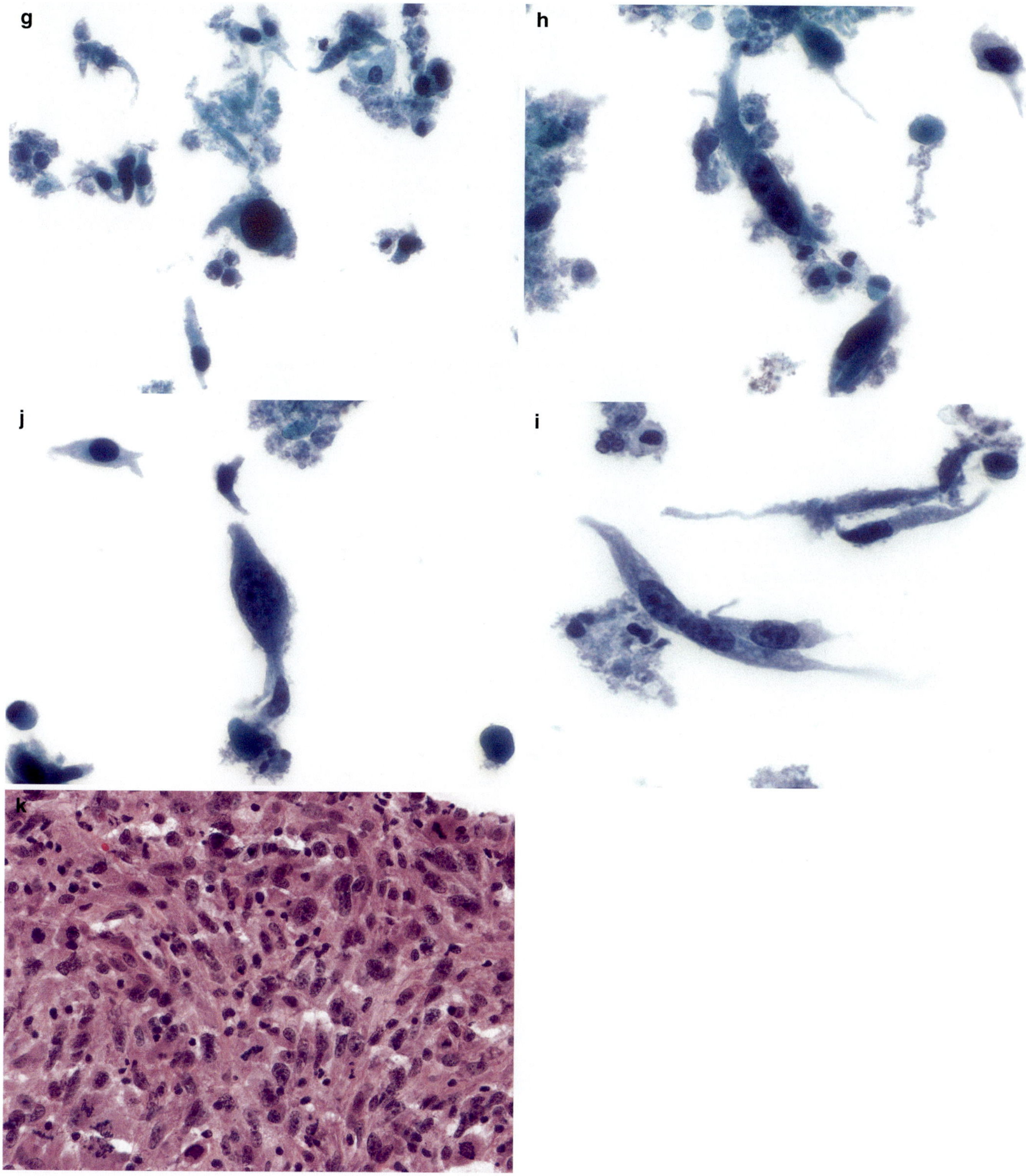

Fig. 11.2 (continued)

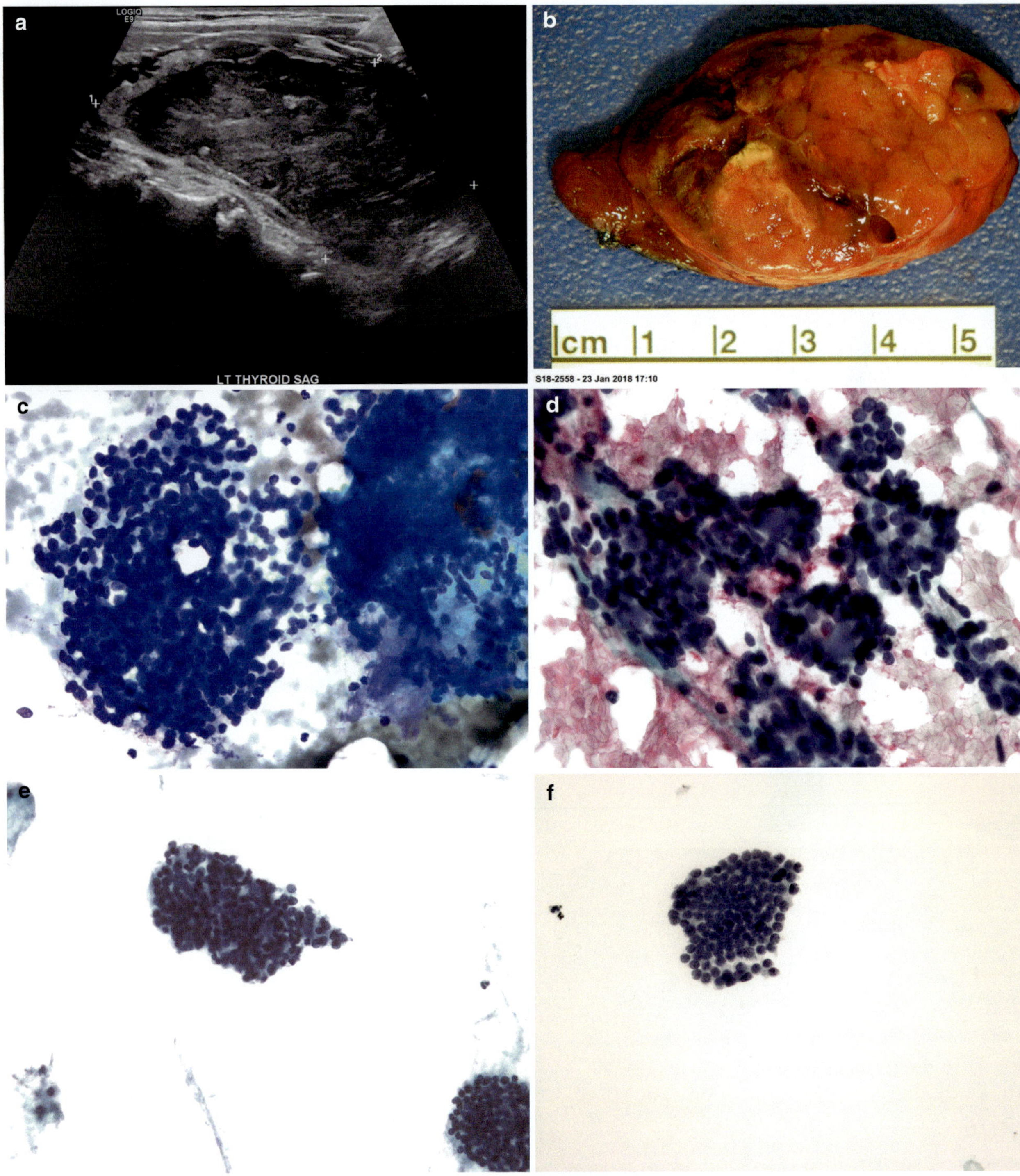

Fig. 11.3 Poorly differentiated thyroid carcinoma (PDCa): Imaging, gross, and cyto-histologic findings. (**a**) Ultrasonography shows a large mass in the thyroid with irregular borders and evidence of invasion. The mass shows mixed echogenicity with hypoechoic foci, possible areas of necrosis, and calcifications. (**b**) Grossly, the mass shows a firm, solid tan-brown to yellow cut surface; focal areas of necrosis and hemorrhage are noted. The borders of this mass appear lobulated in some areas and irregular in other areas. (**c**) This air-dried aspirate shows small cells arranged in a microfollicular architecture on a background of blood. The cytoplasm is scant and the nuclei are round and regular, with granular chromatin and small nucleoli. There is no evidence of colloid and no nuclear features of PTC (Diff-Quik, CS). (**d**) This alcohol-fixed aspirate shows similar features as seen on the air-dried aspirate. The nuclear chromatin is granular, and no nuclear features of PTC are seen (Pap stain, CS). (**e**, **f**) LBP of the same case with cytologic features similar to CS. Unlike the CS, the background here is cleaner. The cell groups show microfollicular architecture and appear to be tighter than the groups in the alcohol fixed aspirates. The chromatin details are similar to that of CS (**e**, **f**, Pap stain, TP). (**g**, **h**) Histology images of the mass showing features similar to those noted in cytology, such as microfollicular architecture. The nuclei appear round and regular; small nucleoli are seen. Wide areas of invasion are noted (H&E). (**i**, **j**) Another case of PDCa with an insular growth pattern. On this LBP, the clusters appear tighter and the background is clean. Note that the cells are small, with round nuclei. The cytoarchitectural pattern here is key in helping with the diagnosis of poorly differentiated thyroid carcinoma (Pap stain, TP)

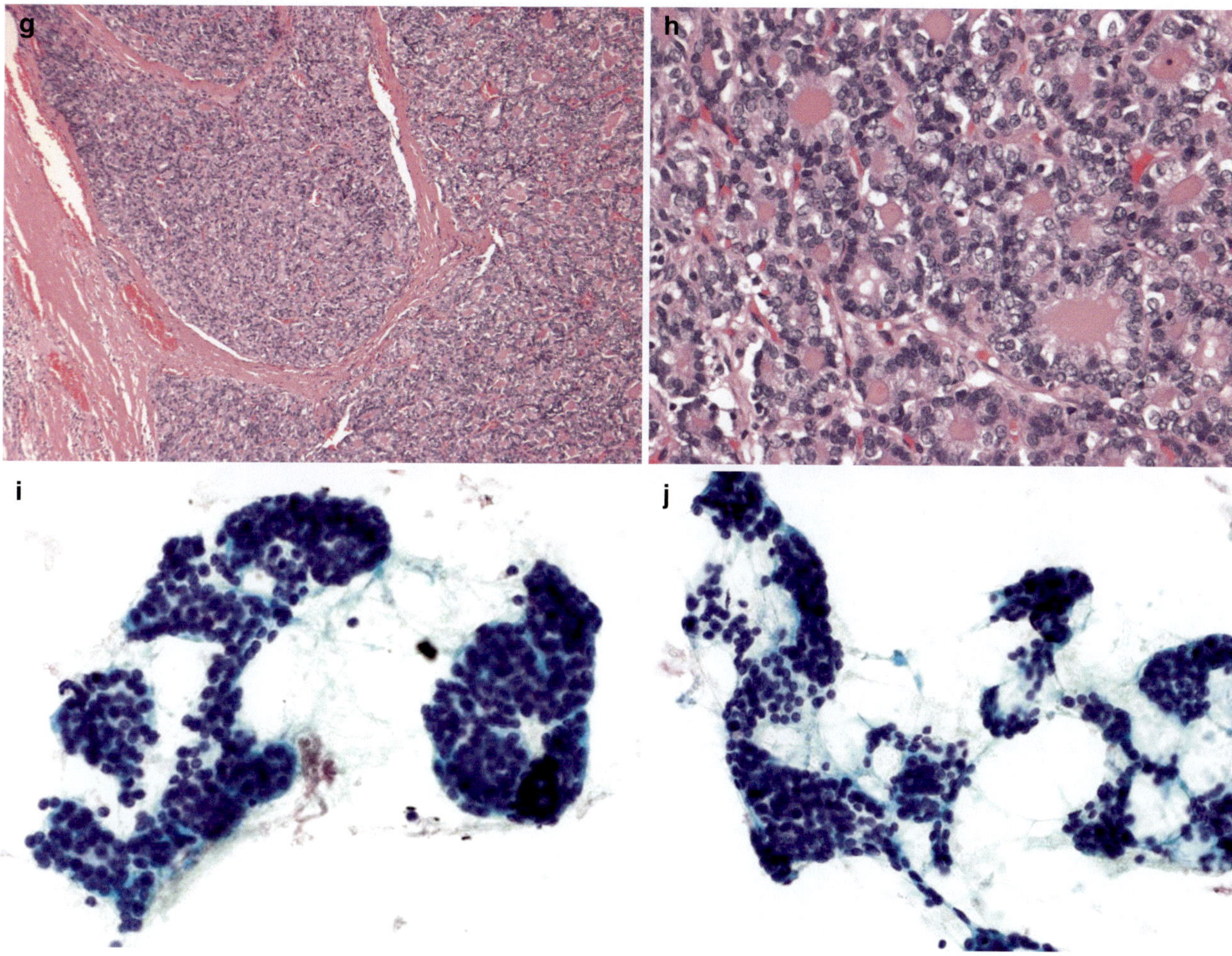

Fig. 11.3 (continued)

- Studies so far indicate that solid, trabecular, insular (STI) cytoarchitectural patterns and high cellularity are strong cytologic indicators in diagnosing PDCa (Fig. 11.3i, j), in addition to small cells, single cells, high N:C ratio, granular chromatin, severe crowding, and mitotic activity are strong cytologic indicators in aspirates.
- Bongiovanni et al. [5] noted that the combined presence of an STI cytoarchitectural pattern, single cells, high N:C ratio, and severe crowding was highly predictive of PDCa.
- Because of the prominent follicular architecture in some cases and the lack of obvious papillary-like nuclear features, PDCa is often classified as a follicular neoplasm (Bethesda IV/VI).
- The differential diagnosis of PDCa include follicular neoplasms, MTC, ATC, lymphoma, and metastases. The variable cytoarchitectural patterns, markedly increased cellularity, granular chromatin, presence of mitoses and necrosis, and lack of colloid help distinguish PDCa from other follicular neoplasms. The cytoarchitectural patterns and the lack of "salt and pepper" chromatin, along with a lack of immunoreactivity to calcitonin, CEA, and neuroendocrine markers, help distinguish it from MTC. The cytoarchitectural pattern of PDCa and the lack of immunoreactivity to lymphoid markers helps to distinguish it from lymphoproliferative neoplasms. Immunoreactivity to thyroglobulin, TTF-1, and PAX 8 as a panel helps to distinguish PDCa from other secondary malignancies to the thyroid.
- These tumors frequently carry *RAS* or *BRAF* mutations. Additional TERT promoter, *TP53*, and *EIF1AX* mutations have also been observed and are implicated in the aggressive nature of the malignancy and the associated worse prognosis.

Lymphomas Involving the Thyroid Gland

- Primary thyroid lymphoma (PTL) is a rare malignancy. It accounts for approximately 1–5% of all thyroid malignancies.
- It is most common in middle-aged to older women, with a mean age of 60–65.

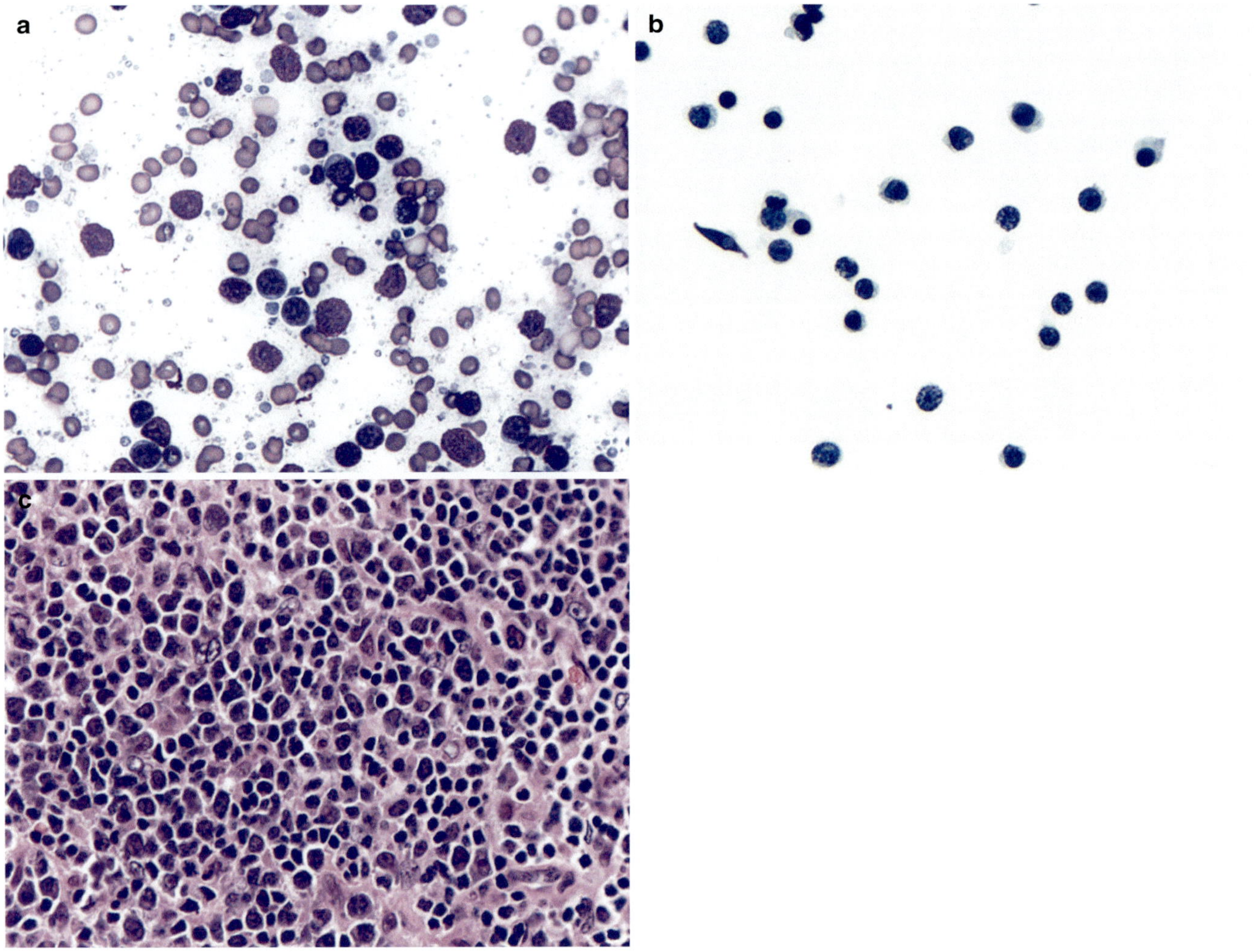

Fig. 11.4 Diffuse large B-cell lymphoma in the thyroid gland: Cytohistologic findings. (**a**) Air-dried aspirates are the best for lymphoid lesions. The background here shows red blood cells and lymphoglandular bodies (bits of bluish-gray cytoplasmic material). The malignant lymphoid cells appear enlarged (with nuclear sizes two to three times that of a red blood cell), with virtually no cytoplasm, and prominent nucleoli. Fewer intermediate-sized lymphoid cells are also noted in the background (Diff Quik, CS). (**b**) On LBP, the cells appear smaller than on the air-dried aspirate, but note that the malignant lymphoid cells show virtually no cytoplasm and appear larger, with prominent nucleoli. The background is very clean, devoid of lymphoglandular bodies or blood (Pap stain, TP). (**c**) The surgical follow-up showed a diffuse large B-cell lymphoma (H&E)

- Patients usually present with a mass that has rapidly enlarged. Compressive symptoms due to mass effect may be reported. Most patients are either euthyroid or hyperthyroid.
- Lymphomas are most frequently of the B-cell type. The most common subtypes are diffuse large B-cell lymphoma (DLBCL, 60–70%) (Fig. 11.4) and extranodal marginal zone lymphoma of mucosa-associated lymphoid tissue (MALT lymphoma, 20–30%).
- Almost all cases of PTL arise in the setting of Hashimoto thyroiditis, with an estimated relative risk of 67 to 80.
- On ultrasound imaging, the mass appears hypoechoic and asymmetrical.
- Grossly, the tumor can vary in size, and it may involve one lobe or both lobes. Tumors are lobular, multinodular, or diffuse and have a bulging, tan to white-grey cut surface.
- Microscopic appearance depends on the lymphoma subtype. The lymphoma usually effaces the normal thyroid parenchyma.
- Sheets of large, atypical lymphoid cells with destruction of thyroid parenchyma characterize DLBCL, the most common lymphoma subtype. The lymphocytic infiltrate often extends into adjacent fat and skeletal muscle. The cells have the appearance of centroblasts or immunoblasts. The tumor can be divided into germinal center–like and non-germinal center–like.
- Immunohistochemically, the tumor cells are positive for CD20, CD79a, and PAX-5.
- MALT lymphoma can demonstrate a nodular to diffuse pattern. It is composed predominantly of small cells, including marginal zone cells, monocytoid-like B cells,

and plasma cells. Scattered large cells resembling centroblasts or immunoblasts can be seen.

- Lymphoepithelial lesions consisting of glandular epithelium infiltrated by lymphoma cells, with destruction of the epithelium, are frequently seen. Lymphoma cells may colonize the germinal centers of reactive follicles and mimic follicular lymphoma.
- Immunohistochemically, MALT lymphoma is characterized by CD20, CD79a, and BCL-2 positivity; the tumor cells are negative for CD10, BCL-6, and CD5.
- Treatment usually consists of adjuvant chemotherapy and radiation. Prognosis varies depending on the subtype. Patients with MALT lymphoma have a higher 5-year disease-specific survival.
- Sensitivity for diagnosing PTL in cytology has varied from 39% to 72%.
- Aspirates are generally cellular and consist of noncohesive cells. Lymphoglandular bodies can be seen in the background.
- FNA of large B-cell lymphomas are highly cellular and consist of large cells with coarse chromatin, prominent nucleoli, and basophilic cytoplasm. Necrotic debris may be seen.
- Aspirates from low-grade lymphomas such as MALT lymphoma show predominantly small lymphocytes and plasma cells. The small cells have vesicular chromatin, small nucleoli, and a moderate amount of cytoplasm. Occasionally, larger cells with prominent nucleoli may be seen (Fig. 11.5).

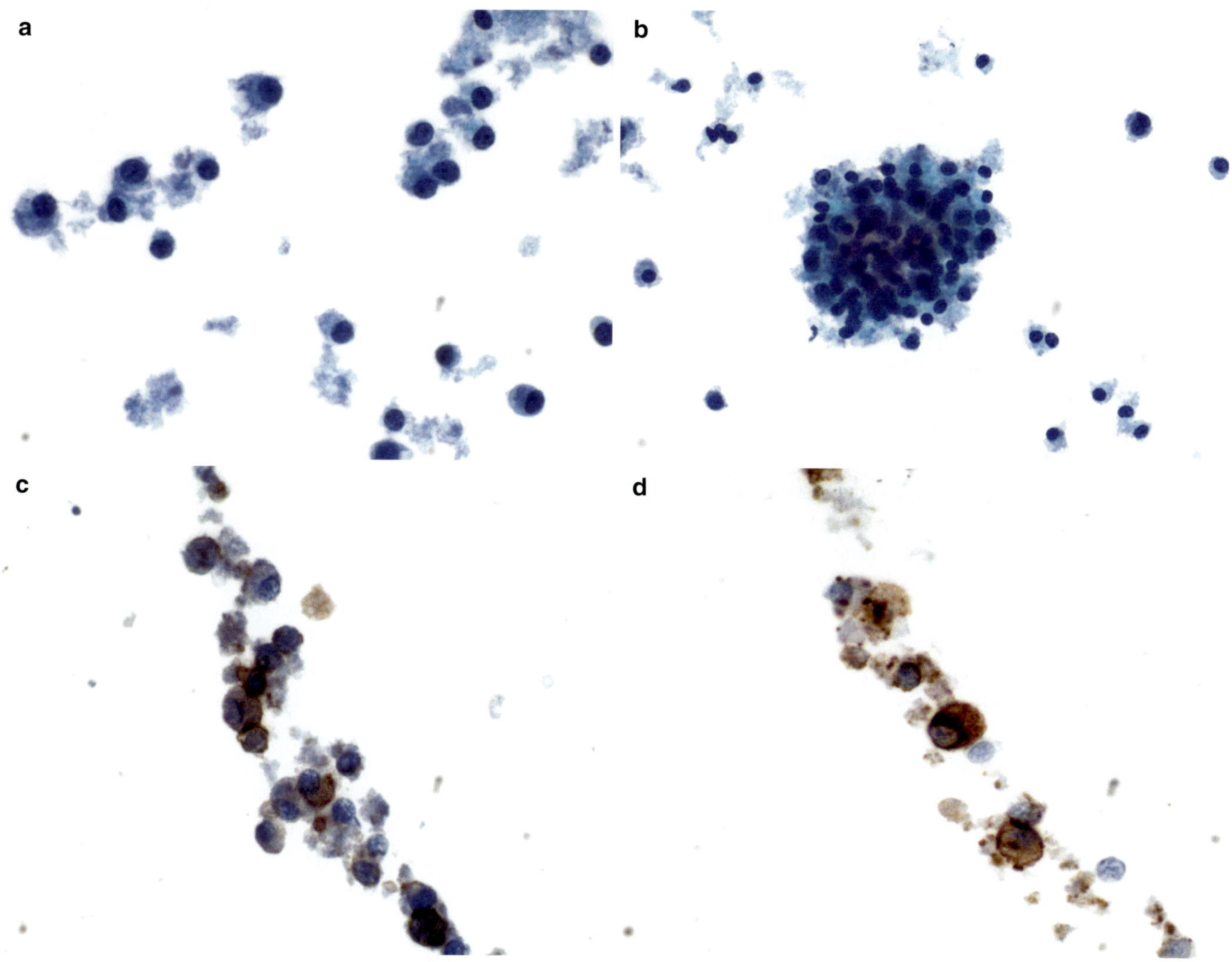

Fig. 11.5 Lymphoplasmacytic lymphoma involving the thyroid gland: Cyto-histologic findings. (**a**, **b**) LBP showing small to intermediate-sized lymphoid cells; the majority show a plasmacytoid morphology. The cell outlines appear poorly defined (Pap stain, TP). (**c**) Immunostain for leukocyte common antigen (LCA) is positive, highlighting these plasmacytoid lymphoid cells (IHC). (**d**) Immunostain for CD38 is positive in lymphoplasmacytic lymphoma (IHC)

- Because PTL typically arises in the background of Hashimoto thyroiditis, it may be difficult to make a diagnosis on FNA. The absence of oncocytes and follicular cells can help to distinguish lymphoma from Hashimoto thyroiditis.
- In equivocal cases, flow cytometry and immunohistochemical studies are helpful.

Metastatic Tumors to the Thyroid Gland

- Metastatic tumors to the thyroid are uncommon but not rare, encompassing about 1.4–3% of all thyroid malignancies, increasing to 24% in autopsy studies.
- The interval from the diagnosis of the primary to the diagnosis of metastases can vary from months to years; some have been reported more than 20 years after the diagnosis of the primary.
- In patients with prior malignancies, metastases should be entertained in the differential diagnosis of any nodular enlargement in the thyroid.
- As always, FNA is the effective first step in managing thyroid nodules and ruling out the possibility of metastases to the thyroid. Nevertheless, diagnosing metastases without the history of a known primary could be challenging on FNA.
- Although FNA has been shown to achieve diagnostic accuracy of >90% in diagnosing metastases to the thyroid, some studies report lower accuracy rates (~58%) than when diagnosing a primary thyroid malignancy (90%). This difference could be due in part to the difficulty in ruling out metastases in aspirates that are rich in spindled, clear, or pleomorphic (anaplastic) cells.
- The pathway of tumor seeding in the thyroid gland is through the lymphovascular route or through direct extension. The mechanism of tumor seeding in the thyroid is controversial at best. Some studies postulate that the high blood flow and increased velocity prevent tumors from depositing in the thyroid gland, and the high oxygen and iodine content does not cater to tumor growth in the thyroid gland, but destruction of the thyroid parenchyma by a disease process sets the stage for tumors to proliferate.
- Tumor-to-tumor metastasis can also happen in the thyroid gland; for example, tumor metastasis from other organs has been known to occur within a primary thyroid neoplasm such as a follicular adenoma.
- The most common primaries to metastasize to the thyroid gland include kidney (~34%), lung, breast, GI tract, melanoma, and head and neck cancers. Less common are metastases from gynecologic, hematopoietic, soft tissue, and genito-urinary tract malignancies.
- The overall management includes surgical resection of the metastatic lesion; patients treated surgically have longer survival than those treated using non-surgical approaches.
- The cytologic features of the metastases are similar to the primary tumors for both CS and LBP. In almost all cases, the clinical history, morphologic comparison with the patient's primary, and/or further workup using ancillary studies on cell block material are necessary for diagnostic confirmation (Table 11.2, Figs. 11.6 and 11.7).

Table 11.2 Ancillary immunohistochemical studies helpful in differentiating the metastatic tumors to the thyroid gland

Tumor	Tests
Renal cell carcinoma	*Positive:* CD10, RCC, PAX-8, CAIX (renal cell markers) *Negative:* TTF-1 and thyroglobulin (thyroid follicular cell markers); calcitonin (medullary cancer marker).
Breast carcinoma	*Positive:* GATA3, estrogen receptor (ER) *Negative:* TTF-1, PAX-8, thyroglobulin, calcitonin
Lung adenocarcinoma	*Positive:* TTF-1, napsin A, +/– P63 *Negative:* PAX-8, thyroglobulin, calcitonin
Squamous cell carcinoma (lung and other)	*Positive:* P40, P63 *Negative:* TTF-1, PAX-8, thyroglobulin, calcitonin
Colorectal primary	*Positive:* CK20, CDX2 *Negative:* CK7, TTF-1, thyroglobulin, PAX-8, calcitonin

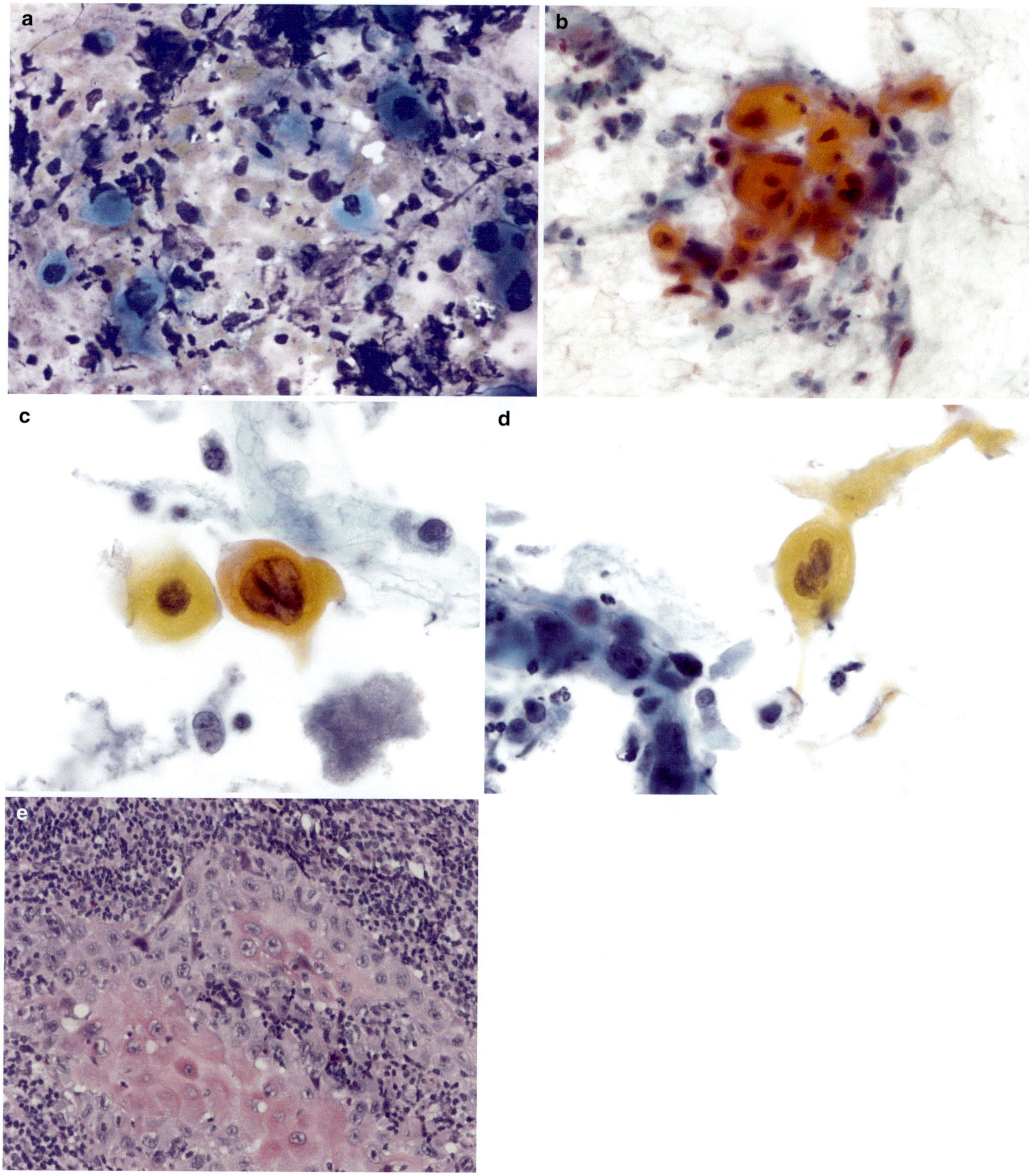

Fig. 11.6 Metastatic squamous cell carcinoma to the thyroid gland. This is an example of esophageal squamous cell carcinoma metastasizing to the thyroid gland. (**a**) This air-dried aspirate shows single cells with dense blue cytoplasm, also referred to as "Robin's egg blue" cytoplasm. This blue color is suggestive of keratinization in these tumor cells (Diff Quik, CS). (**b**) The alcohol-fixed smear shows single cells and loose clusters of malignant squamous cells with orangeophilia in the cytoplasm, compatible with keratinizing squamous cell carcinoma (Pap stain, CS). (**c**, **d**) The LBP of the same case shows keratinized malignant squamous cells, which appear fairly similar to those seen in the alcohol-fixed CS. In (**d**) we can appreciate a cluster of non-keratinized malignant squamous cells adjacent to the keratinized malignant cell. The background is less striking, with less blood. The cytoplasm can appear orange to yellow and refractile in keratinized malignant squamous cells (**c**, **d**, Pap stain, TP). (**e**) Histologic follow-up showing squamous cell carcinoma (H&E)

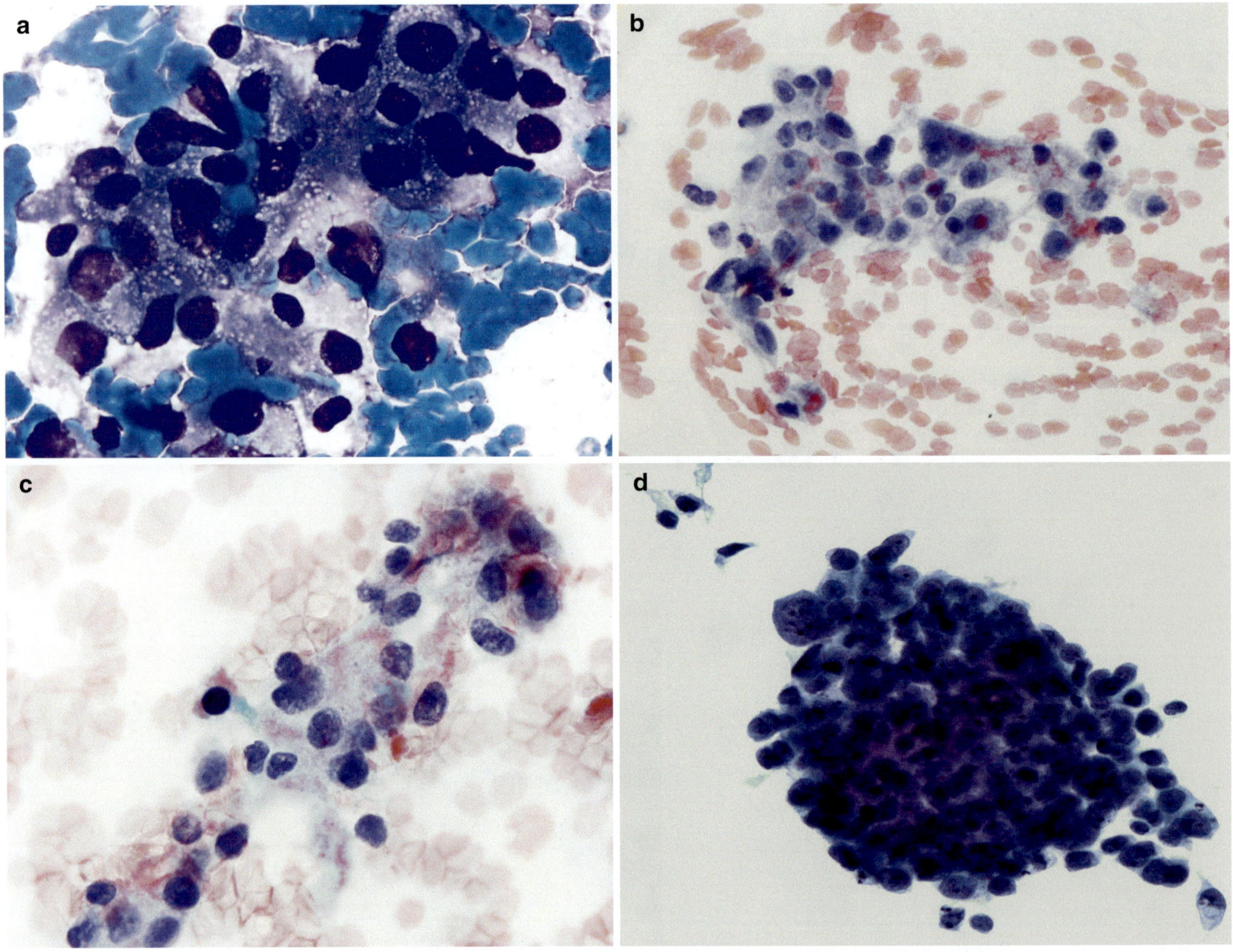

Fig. 11.7 Metastatic breast carcinoma to the thyroid gland. (**a**) Air-dried aspirate showing a loose cluster of malignant cells with vacuolated cytoplasm and markedly enlarged and hyperchromatic nuclei with nucleoli (Diff Quik, CS). (**b**, **c**) Alcohol-fixed smears showing a similar-looking cluster. The chromatin is coarse and the nucleoli appear large and prominent. The cytoplasmic details are not so clear as in the air-dried aspirate (Pap stain, CS). (**d**) On LBP, the similar clusters appear more cohesive and tighter, but the nuclear details are almost identical to those on the CS (Pap stain, TP). (**e**) The accompanying cell-block section shows cytomorphologic details similar to those noted on CS and LBP (H&E). (**f**) A GATA3 stain is positive in a breast primary and is staining the tumor cell nuclei (IHC). (**g**) The resection sample was a metastatic breast carcinoma (H&E)

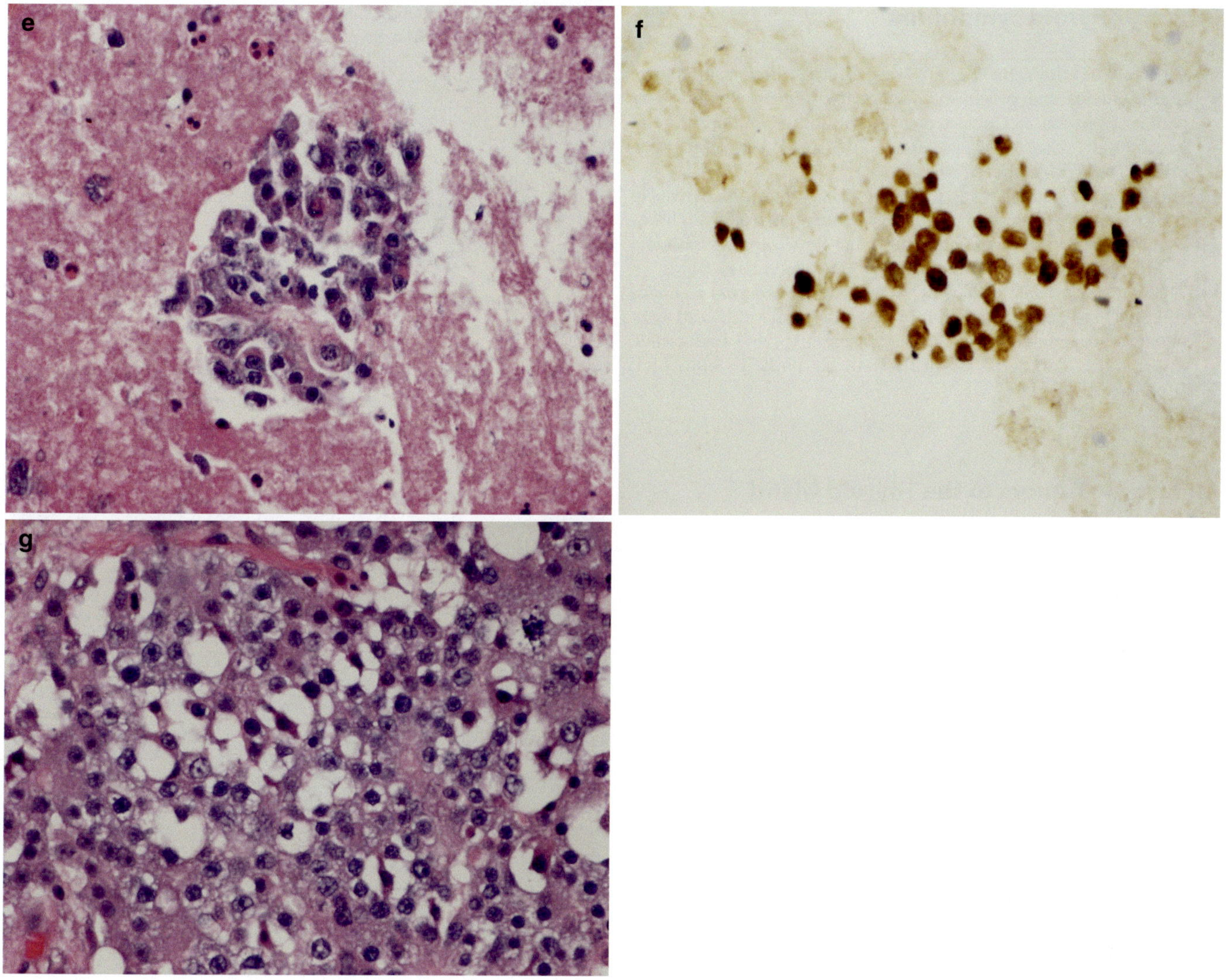

Fig. 11.7 (continued)

Suggested Reading

Anaplastic Thyroid Carcinomas

1. Molinaro E, Romei C, Biagini A, Sabini E, Agate L, Mazzeo S, et al. Anaplastic thyroid carcinoma: from clinicopathology to genetics and advanced therapies. Nat Rev Endocrinol. 2017;13:644–60. https://doi.org/10.1038/nrendo.2017.76.
2. Ragazzi M, Ciarrocchi A, Sancisi V, Gandolfi G, Bisagni A, Piana S. Update on anaplastic thyroid carcinoma: morphological, molecular, and genetic features of the most aggressive thyroid cancer. Int J Endocrinol. 2014;2014:790834. https://doi.org/10.1155/2014/790834.
3. Talbott I, Wakely PE Jr. Undifferentiated (anaplastic) thyroid carcinoma: practical immunohistochemistry and cytologic look-alikes. Semin Diagn Pathol. 2015;32:305–10. https://doi.org/10.1053/j.semdp.2014.12.012.
4. Xu B, Ghossein R. Genomic landscape of poorly differentiated and anaplastic thyroid carcinoma. Endocr Pathol. 2016;27:205–12. https://doi.org/10.1007/s12022-016-9445-4.

Poorly Differentiated Thyroid Carcinoma

5. Bongiovanni M, Bloom L, Krane JF, Baloch ZW, Powers CN, Hintermann S, et al. Cytomorphologic features of poorly differentiated thyroid carcinoma: a multi-institutional analysis of 40 cases. Cancer. 2009;117:185–94. https://doi.org/10.1002/cncy.20023.
6. Bongiovanni M, Sadow PM, Faquin WC. Poorly differentiated thyroid carcinoma: a cytologic-histologic review. Adv Anat Pathol. 2009;16:283–9. https://doi.org/10.1097/PAP.0b013e3181b50640.
7. Kane SV, Sharma TP. Cytologic diagnostic approach to poorly differentiated thyroid carcinoma: a single-institution study. Cancer Cytopathol. 2015;123:82–91. https://doi.org/10.1002/cncy.21500.
8. Saglietti C, Onenerk AM, Faquin WC, Sykiotis GP, Ziadi S, Bongiovanni M. FNA diagnosis of poorly differentiated thyroid carcinoma. A review of the recent literature. Cytopathology. 2017;28:467–74. https://doi.org/10.1111/cyt.12497.

Primary Thyroid Lymphoma

9. Chen E, Wu Q, Jin Y, Jin W, Cai Y, Wang Q, et al. Clinicopathological characteristics and prognostic factors for primary thyroid lymphoma: report on 28 Chinese patients and results of a population-based study. Cancer Manag Res. 2018;10:4411–9. https://doi.org/10.2147/CMAR.S155170.
10. Hirokawa M, Kudo T, Ota H, Suzuki A, Kobayashi K, Miyauchi A. Preoperative diagnostic algorithm of primary thyroid lymphoma using ultrasound, aspiration cytology, and flow cytometry. Endocr J. 2017;64:859–65. https://doi.org/10.1507/endocrj.EJ17-0111.
11. Zhang L, Castellana M, Virili C, Crescenzi A, Giorgino F, Zucca E, et al. Fine-needle aspiration to diagnose primary thyroid lymphoma: a systematic review and meta-analysis. Eur J Endocrinol. 2018; https://doi.org/10.1530/EJE-18-0672. pii:EJE-18-0672.R1. [Epub ahead of print].

Metastatic Tumors to the Thyroid Gland

12. Beutner U, Leowardi C, Bork U, Luthi C, Tarantino I, Pahernik S, et al. Survival after renal cell carcinoma metastasis to the thyroid: single center experience and systematic review of the literature. Thyroid. 2015;25:314–24. https://doi.org/10.1089/thy.2014.0498.
13. Hegerova L, Griebeler ML, Reynolds JP, Henry MR, Gharib H. Metastasis to the thyroid gland: report of a large series from the Mayo Clinic. Am J Clin Oncol. 2015;38:338–42. https://doi.org/10.1097/COC.0b013e31829d1d09.
14. Lee CH, Chung SY, Moon KC, Park IA, Chung YR, Ryu HS. A pilot study evaluating fine-needle aspiration cytology of clear-cell renal cell carcinoma: comparison of ancillary immunocytochemistry and cytomorphological characteristics of SurePath liquid-based preparations with conventional smears. Acta Cytol. 2015;59:239–47. https://doi.org/10.1159/000430081.
15. Magers MJ, Dueber JC, Lew M, Pang JC, Davenport RD. Metastatic ductal carcinoma of the breast to the thyroid gland diagnosed with fine needle aspiration: a case report with emphasis on morphologic and immunophenotypic features. Diagn Cytopathol. 2016;44:530–4. https://doi.org/10.1002/dc.23462.
16. Moghaddam PA, Cornejo KM, Khan A. Metastatic carcinoma to the thyroid gland: a single institution 20-year experience and review of the literature. Endocr Pathol. 2013;24:116–24. https://doi.org/10.1007/s12022-013-9257-8.
17. Stevens TM, Richards AT, Bewtra C, Sharma P. Tumors metastatic to thyroid neoplasms: a case report and review of the literature. Pathol Res Int. 2011;2011:238693. https://doi.org/10.4061/2011/238693.
18. Zhang L, Liu Y, Li X, Gao W, Zheng C. Metastases to the thyroid gland: a report of 32 cases in PUMCH. Medicine (Baltimore). 2017;96:e7927. https://doi.org/10.1097/MD.0000000000007927.

Immunocytochemistry and Immunohistochemistry on Liquid-Based Preparations of Thyroid FNA

12

Megha Joshi, Sumita Gokhale, and Rana S. Hoda

Introduction

- Immunocytohistochemistry/immunohistochemistry (ICC/IHC) has become an indispensable tool in the practice of surgical pathology and cytology. In our daily clinical practice, most specimens from thyroid fine needle aspiration (FNA) and liquid-based preparations (LBP) are diagnosed *without* the routine use of immunostain, but IHC can be used judiciously on the corresponding cell block in certain situations to confirm or rule out a diagnosis. Scraping of thick Diff-Quik (DQ)–stained smears into the CytoLyt/CytoRich Red (collection media for ThinPrep [TP] and SurePath [SP] respectively) at the time of rapid on-site evaluation (ROSE) to prepare the cell block can further enhance the yield, and multiple immunostains can be performed on the cell block if needed.
- Immunocytochemistry (ICC) on liquid-based cytology preparations (such as TP slides) has also been described and validated previously (*see* the Suggested Reading). ICC on monolayer cytology slides is much cleaner, with less background staining, than on conventional smears, and it requires smaller amounts of both the specimen and the antibody. The use of LBP for ICC is especially useful for cases in which a cell block preparation may not be feasible (such as when the specimen shows poor cellularity).
- Additional slides can be prepared for ICC from the residual liquid-based vial.

M. Joshi
Winchester Hospital, Winchester, MA, USA

S. Gokhale
Department of Cytology, Winchester Hospital, Winchester, MA, USA

R. S. Hoda (✉)
CBLPath, Rye Brook, NY, USA
e-mail: rhoda@cblpath.com

- As is true for any other site, immunostains of thyroid FNA should be interpreted in the light of cytomorphologic findings. Relying solely on immunostaining to make a diagnosis can often lead to error.
- Examples of ICC/IHC, performed on various lesions, have been shown in several chapters, including Chaps. 7, 8, 9, 10, and 11.

Papillary Carcinoma

- No single marker is sensitive or specific enough to diagnose malignant thyroid lesions. The use of a panel improves sensitivity and specificity of individual markers. Most authors recommend a panel of HBME-1 (Hector Battifora mesothelial-1), GAL-3 (Galectin-3) and CK19 (cytokeratin 19) to differentiate papillary thyroid carcinoma (PTC) from benign lesions.
- Other markers used in the above panel can include Cited-1 (Cbp/p300-interacting transactivator with Glu/Asp-rich carboxy-terminal domain, 1), or FN-1 (Fibronectin-1), CD44v6, and E-cadherin. This marker panel is also useful in differentiating the follicular variant of PTC (FVPTC) from follicular carcinoma, though a subset of follicular carcinomas can stain with HBME-1 and Galectin-3.
- TROP2 (Trophoblastic cell surface antigen 2) is a newer marker that may hold promise in identification of classic PTC and FVPTC.
- As mentioned before, HBME-1, CK19, and Galectin-3 are useful when used as a panel for the diagnosis of PTC. In general, these markers are strongest in PTC and weakest in benign thyroid nodules. Follicular carcinomas show an intermediate pattern of staining. The expression of CK19 and Gal-3 is often focal in benign epithelium and adenomatous nodules, and diffuse and strong in PTC. In one study, HBME-1 was found to be the most specific for carcinoma, and Gal-3, the most sensitive. In the same study, the expression of CK19 and HBME-1 was 100%

R. S. Hoda et al. (eds.), *Atlas of Thyroid Cytopathology on Liquid-Based Preparations*,
https://doi.org/10.1007/978-3-030-25066-9_12

specific for malignancy. Rossi et al. [10] showed that the panel of HBME-1 and Galectin-3 has an accuracy rate of 98% for the diagnosis of PTC, including the follicular variant (Fig. 12.1).

- In chronic lymphocytic thyroiditis and post-FNA reactive foci, false positive staining may be seen with CK19 and Galectin-3. It is important not to interpret this false positive staining as a sign of malignancy.

BRAF

- The BRAF V600E antibody can be used to detect the *BRAF*V600E mutation in PTC. This mutation may be associated with a higher risk of recurrent, persistent disease; lymph node metastasis; and extrathyroidal extension. The *BRAF* mutation is negative in benign conditions, medullary thyroid carcinoma (MTC), and follicular carcinoma. The *BRAF*V600E mutation has been reported in 50% of PTC, with a lower frequency in FVPTC.

Follicular Carcinoma

- Galectin-3 is a cell adhesion molecule. It is positive in a subset of follicular carcinomas, as well as in FVPTC. Though Galectin-3 may be expressed in hyperplastic nodules and follicular adenomas in a weak and focal manner, strong diffuse staining often denotes malignancy. In a prospective study of thyroid FNA samples, the sensitivity of Galectin-3 to determine who gets surgery was 78%, and the specificity was 93%. HBME-1 is also strongly positive in >40% of follicular carcinoma and PTC, and negative or focally positive in hyperplastic nodules or adenomas. p27 is one marker that is positive in benign and hyperplastic lesions and negative in follicular carcinomas and FVPTC.

Medullary Thyroid Carcinoma (MTC)

- MTC is one of those tumors in the thyroid gland where immunostaining plays a key role in its accurate diagnosis. Although quite rare, accounting for only about 5% of all thyroid carcinomas, it is important to recognize MTC, as the tumors are highly aggressive and some cases may be familial.
- Because MTC is derived from the parafollicular C cells in the thyroid gland, it is negative for thyroglobulin and stains with calcitonin—an important distinction from some of the other, more common primary thyroid neoplasms.
- These tumors usually yield cellular specimens comprising mostly of dyscohesive plasmacytoid and/or spindle cells. Based on morphology alone (depending on the predominant cell type), various tumors should be considered in its differential diagnosis: Hürthle cell neoplasms, PTC, undifferentiated carcinoma, poorly differentiated carcinoma, and metastatic tumors (*eg*, neuroendocrine carcinoma, melanoma, lymphoma).
- A useful set of immunostains to help confidently diagnose MTC and exclude others includes those that are mostly positive: calcitonin, TTF-1, chromogranin, and synaptophysin (Fig. 12.2). Those that are negative are thyroglobulin and S-100.

Poorly Differentiated and Anaplastic Carcinomas

- It should be noted that poorly differentiated and anaplastic carcinomas can be negative for TTF-1 and thyroglobulin. In fact, TTF-1 may be positive in only 18% of anaplastic carcinomas, with focal and weak thyroglobulin staining, with variability ranging from 9% to 71%. For an undifferentiated malignancy, a panel with cytokeratin, leucocyte common antigen (LCA), thyroglobulin, TTF-1, calcitonin, chromogranin, and CEA is suggested.

Metastasis

- The most common tumors that metastasize to the thyroid are carcinomas of kidney, breast, and lung origin. Elucidating a clinical history of cancer is of great importance in this instance, as thyroid FNA is a common and routine procedure, and breast and lung cancer is not uncommon in an elderly population. For known histories of malignancy, a limited number of immunostains may suffice: for renal cell carcinoma, CD10 and RCC; for breast carcinoma, GATA3; for lung, Napsin-A; for melanomas, S100, MART-1, and HMB-45; for colon cancer, CK20 and CDX2; and for lymphomas, LCA/CD45.
- In patients with no known previous malignancy, a wider panel of immunostains may be selected, based on the morphology. A good "first-round" panel may include CK7, CK20, PAX8, RCC, S-100, TTF-1, Napsin-A, and CDX2. Additional stains may be obtained depending on the morphology and immunoprofile seen on the initial staining. For example, if S-100 is positive on the first round of staining and all others are negative, positive staining with additional immunostains for HMB45, Mart-1, and MITF would help confirm a melanoma.
- It is important not to confuse a metastasis with a poorly differentiated primary thyroid carcinoma. Thyroglobulin

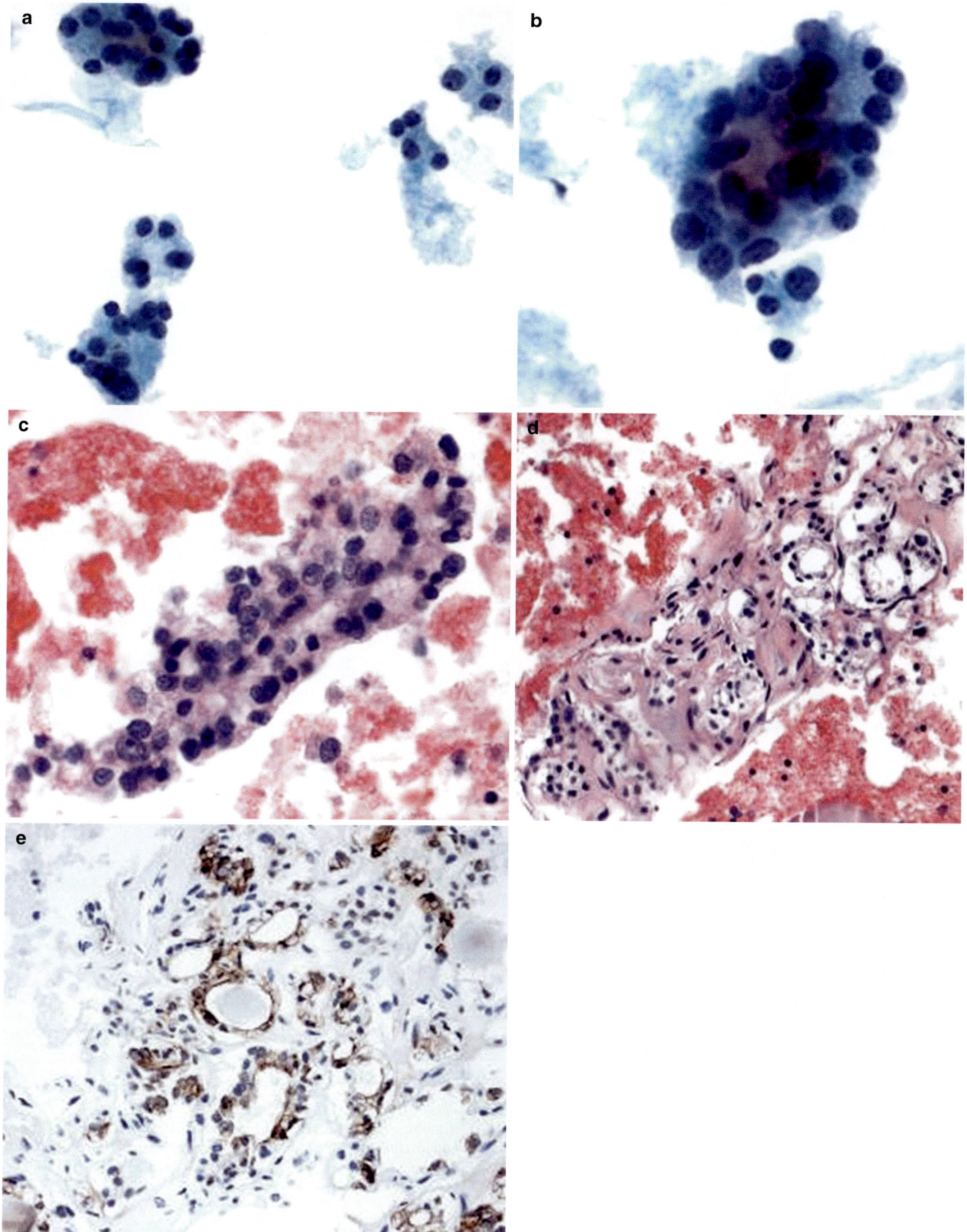

Fig. 12.1 Suspicious for follicular neoplasm. (**a–d**) ThinPrep (TP) and cell block sections showed architectural features of a follicular neoplasm with nuclear features suggestive of a follicular variant of papillary thyroid carcinoma (FVPTC). Differential diagnosis of an FVPTC was added (**a**, **b**, Pap stain, TP; **c**, **d**, H&E stain). (**e**) CK19 immunostain showed diffuse cytoplasmic positivity

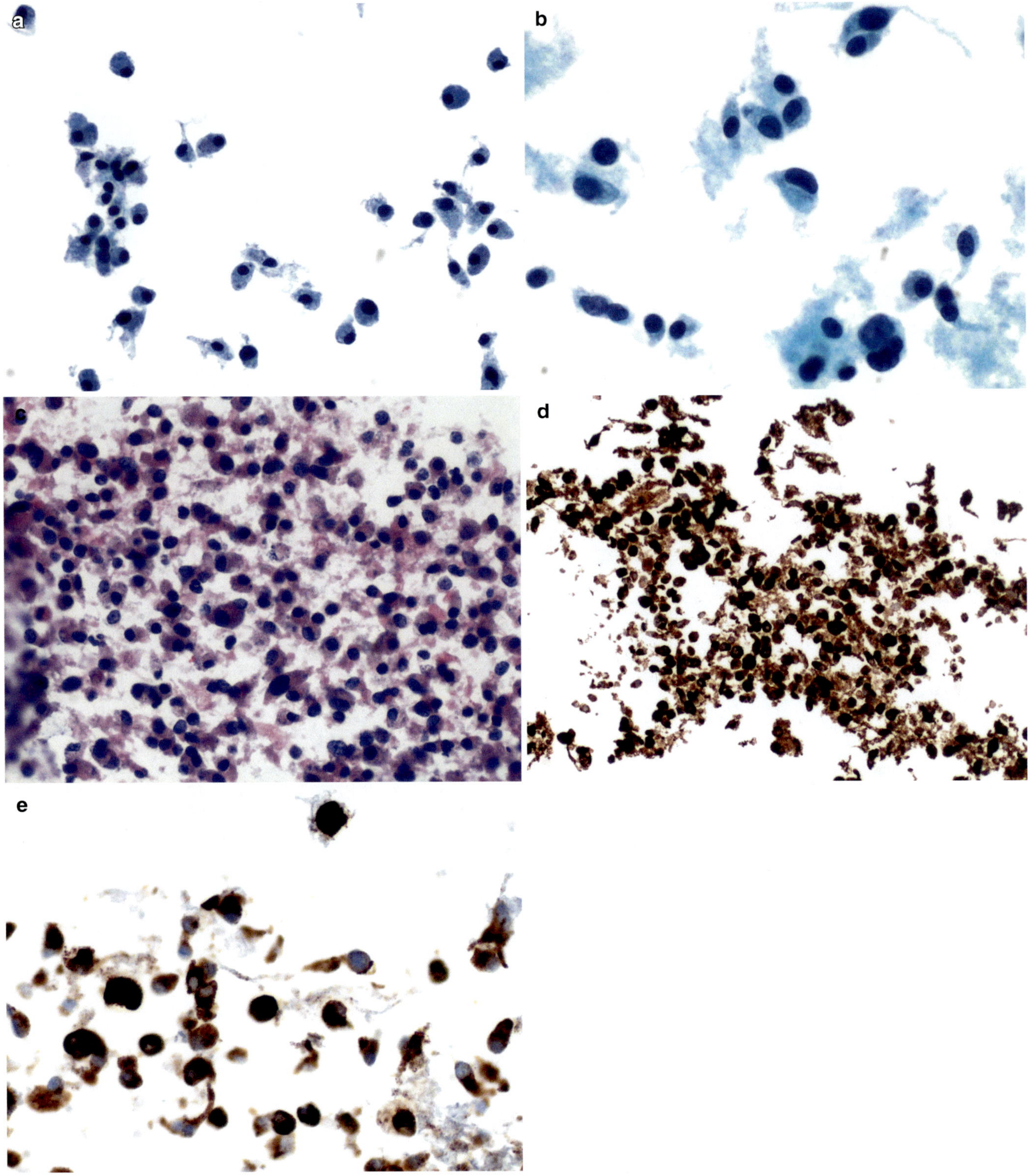

Fig. 12.2 Medullary thyroid carcinoma. (**a–c**) TP and cell block section showed features of medullary thyroid carcinoma (MTC) with large, singly dispersed, predominantly plasmacytoid cells and a few spindled cells. Nuclei were enlarged and mostly round, with some binucleated and multinucleated forms (**a**, **b**, Pap stain, TP; **c**, H&E stain). (**d**, **e**) Immunostains for calcitonin and chromogranin, performed on cell block sections, were positive and supported the diagnosis

and TTF-1 can be of help in ruling out metastases in an unusual lesion, as follicular-derived lesions usually stain for thyroglobulin and TTF-1. It should be noted, however, that especially in metastasis in female patients, thyroid carcinoma can be positive for ER and PR and negative for thyroglobulin. A TTF-1 stain may come to the rescue in such situations, though TTF-1 is positive not only in lung cancer and in the thyroid lesions but also at times in colorectal, ovarian, breast, endometrial, and endocervical carcinomas. If the 8G7G3/1 clone of TTF-1 is used, aberrant expression is less than 2%.

Lymphoma

- Lymphomas of the thyroid often arise in a background of Hashimoto's thyroiditis. Mucosa-associated lymphoid tissue (MALT) lymphomas have a distinct immunophenotype and can be differentiated from diffuse large B-cell and follicular lymphomas by IHC. If a suspicion of lymphoma arises during ROSE, a sample for flow cytometric studies can and should be collected. In the absence of flow cytometry, the initial IHC panel could include CD3, CD5, CD10, CD20, CD23, CD30, Cyclin D1, Bcl2, Bcl6, PAX5, and Ki67.
- IHC can confirm a lymphoma diagnosis. Anaplastic carcinomas can also be distinguished from lymphomas by LCA/CD45 immunostain.

Parathyroid Lesions

- Often, in a colloid-deficient microfollicular lesion, the use of immunostain for parathyroid hormone (PTH), TTF-1, and thyroglobulin can help confirm or dispute parathyroid origin. PTH is a good and reliable marker for lesions of the parathyroid, and it lends itself well for use in FNA samples, be it LBP or cell blocks. Up to 0.6% of thyroid FNAs can in actuality be parathyroid lesions. Use of the PTH marker is a simple and accurate way to avoid misdiagnosing a parathyroid sample as follicular neoplasia.

Suggested Reading

1. Clark DP, Faquin WC. Thyroid cytopathology. 2nd ed. New York: Springer; 2010.
2. Dabbs DJ, Abendroth CS, Grenko RT, Wang X, Radcliffe GE. Immunocytochemistry on the Thinprep processor. Diagn Cytopathol. 1997;17:388–92.
3. Freitag CE, Schoenfield L, Nabhan FA, Naturale RT, Jin M. Fine-needle aspiration cytology of a thyroid nodule: challenging morphologic considerations. CytoJournal. 2019;16:5. https://doi.org/10.4103/cytojournal.cytojournal_8_18.
4. Khan A. Surgical pathology of endocrine and neuroendocrine tumors. 2009. ISBN 978-1-60327-395-4. https://doi.org/10.1007/978-1-60327-396-1.
5. Kim JK, Seong CY, Bae IE, Yi JW, Yu HW, Kim SJ, et al. Comparison of immunohistochemistry and direct sequencing methods for identification of the BRAF(V600E) mutation in papillary thyroid carcinoma. Ann Surg Oncol. 2018;25:1775–81. https://doi.org/10.1245/s10434-018-6460-3.
6. Leung SW, Bédard YC. Immunocytochemical staining on ThinPrep processed smears. Mod Pathol. 1996;9:304–6.
7. Liu H, Lin F. Application of immunohistochemistry in thyroid pathology. Arch Pathol Lab Med. 2015;139:67–82. https://doi.org/10.5858/arpa.2014-0056-RA.
8. Pazaitou-Panayiotou K, Mygdakos N, Boglou K, Kiziridou A, Chrisoulidou A, Destouni C. The immunocytochemistry is a valuable tool in the diagnosis of papillary thyroid cancer in FNA's using liquid-based cytology. J Oncol. 2010;2010:963926. https://doi.org/10.1155/2010/963926.
9. Pusztaszeri MP, Bongiovanni M, Faquin WC. Update on the cytologic and molecular features of medullary thyroid carcinoma. Adv Anat Pathol. 2014;21:26–35. https://doi.org/10.1097/PAP.0000000000000004.
10. Rossi ED, Raffaelli M, Mulè A, Miraglia A, Lombardi CP, Vecchio FM, et al. Simultaneous immunohistochemical expression of HBME-1 and galectin-3 differentiates papillary carcinomas from hyperfunctioning lesions of the thyroid. Histopathology. 2006;48:795–800.
11. Rossi ED, Raffaelli M, Mulè A, Zannoni GF, Pontecorvi A, Santeusanio G, et al. Relevance of immunocytochemistry on thin-layer cytology in thyroid lesions suspicious for medullary carcinoma: a case-control study. Appl Immunohistochem Mol Morphol. 2008;16:548–53. https://doi.org/10.1097/PAI.0b013e3181690ca3.
12. Sapio MR, Guerra A, Posca D, Limone PP, Deandrea M, Motta M, et al. Combined analysis of galectin-3 and *BRAFV600E* improves the accuracy of fine-needle aspiration biopsy with cytological findings suspicious for papillary thyroid carcinoma. Endocr Relat Cancer. 2007;14:1089–97.
13. Sconamiglio T, Hyjek E, Kao J, Chen YT. Diagnostic usefulness of HBME-1, galectin-3, CK19, CITED1 and evaluation of their expression in encapsulated lesions with questionable features of papillary thyroid carcinoma. Am J Clin Pathol. 2006;126:700–8.
14. Song S, Kim H, Ahn SH. Role of immunohistochemistry in fine needle aspiration and core needle biopsy of thyroid nodules. Clin Exp Otorhinolaryngol. 2019;12:224–30. https://doi.org/10.21053/ceo.2018.01011.
15. Suzuki A, Hirokawa M, Takada N, Higuchi M, Ito A, Yanao N, et al. Fine needle aspiration cytology for medullary thyroid carcinoma: a single institutional experience in Japan. Endocr J. 2017;64:1099–104. https://doi.org/10.1507/endocrj.EJ17-0238.
16. Tripathy K, Mishra A, Singh AK, Panda PL, Mahapatra A, Lenka A. Immunocytochemistry using liquid-based cytology: a tool in hormone receptor analysis of breast cancer. J Cytol. 2018;35:260–4. https://doi.org/10.4103/JOC.JOC_23_18.
17. Wuertz FG, Kresnik E, Malle P, Hyden M, Lind P, Rogatsch H, et al. Fine-needle aspiration with immunohistochemistry using a modified scrape cell block technique for the diagnosis of thyroid and parathyroid nodules. Acta Cytol. 2016;60:118–30. https://doi.org/10.1159/000446466.

13 Parathyroid Gland Fine Needle Aspiration Cytology

Rema Rao and Rana S. Hoda

Parathyroid Gland

- Parathyroid glands are light yellow to brown and are small (about 2–7 mm). They tend to become prominent in pathological states, most commonly hyperparathyroidism. More than 80% of individuals have four parathyroid glands.
- Parathyroid glands can be located within other organs, most commonly the thyroid gland, where they are found in the perithyroidal fat.
- Normal parathyroid glands are not visible on ultrasonography and there are no specific ultrasound (US) features that distinguish an enlarged parathyroid gland from a thyroid nodule.
- The parathyroid gland is composed of three different types of cells: chief, oxyphil, and water clear cells.
- Chief cells are morphologically similar to thyroid follicular cells, and oxyphil cells are similar to Hürthle cells (Figs. 13.1 and 13.2).
- Conventional smears (CS) of parathyroid fine needle aspiration (FNA) specimens are cellular and show variable architecture, with cells arranged as disorganized, loosely cohesive two-dimensional (2-D) fragments and/or tightly cohesive 3-D fragments, as well as papillary-like structures and microfollicles. The microfollicle-like pattern may appear prominent, mimicking a follicular neoplasm (Fig. 13.3).

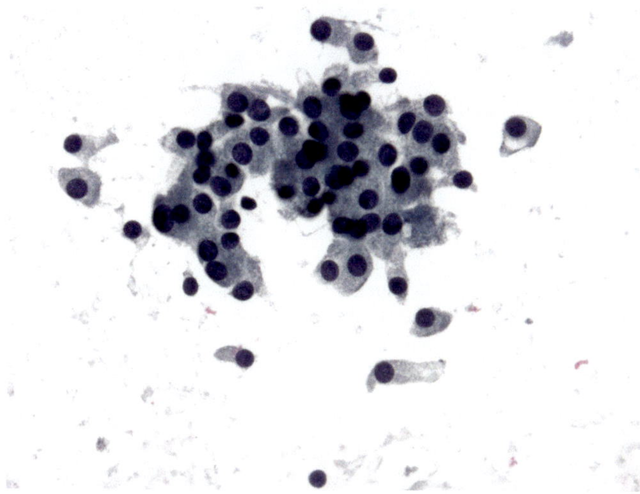

Fig. 13.1 Parathyroid Cells. ThinPrep (TP) slide showing an oxyphil cell–rich parathyroid lesion, which can mimic a Hürthle cell lesion of the thyroid follicular cells. The chromatin has a stippled, "salt and pepper" appearance, unlike Hürthle cell chromatin, which is evenly distributed, with prominent nucleoli. Hürthle cell nuclei also tend to appear larger than the parathyroid follicular cell nuclei (Pap stain)

- Nuclei are round, uniform, and overlapping, with stippled "salt and pepper" neuroendocrine-type chromatin, inconspicuous nucleoli, and a high nuclear-cytoplasmic (N:C) ratio. Cell outlines may not be well appreciated. A prominent capillary network may be noted. The background shows many naked "bare" nuclei and no obvious colloid, although colloid-like material can be observed in about 8–20% of cases (Fig. 13.4). Occasional cells with oxyphilic cytoplasm can be seen.
- In LBP, parathyroid aspirates show variable cellularity. A loose 2-D or microfollicular pattern may be commonly seen, but cells can also be seen in honeycombed sheets and clusters, as well as occasional papillary fragments (Fig. 13.5). The cell outlines are better preserved in LBP than in CS (Fig. 13.6). Nuclei tend to be smaller in LBP than in CS, although the nuclear features are fairly similar

R. Rao
Department of Pathology and Laboratory Medicine, New York Presbyterian Hospital, Weill Cornell Medical College, New York, NY, USA

R. S. Hoda (✉)
CBLPath, Rye Brook, NY, USA
e-mail: rhoda@cblpath.com

R. S. Hoda et al. (eds.), *Atlas of Thyroid Cytopathology on Liquid-Based Preparations*,
https://doi.org/10.1007/978-3-030-25066-9_13

in both CS and LBP. The "bare" naked nuclei are better appreciated in CS, as LBP tends to cluster cells and provides a clean background with reduced bare nuclei (Figs. 13.4 and 13.7; *see* Fig. 6.19 and Chap. 7).

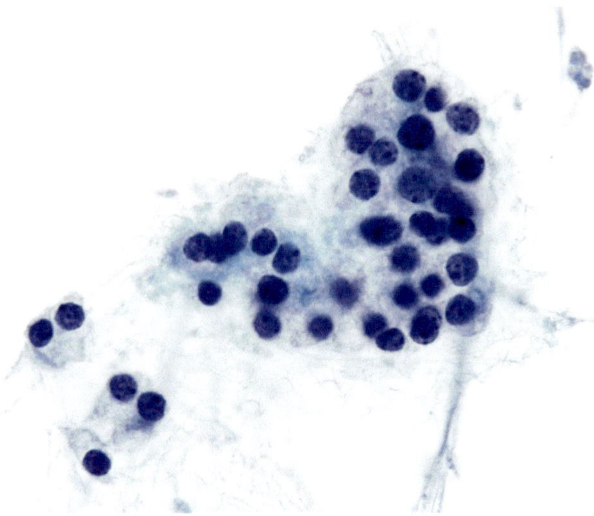

Fig. 13.2 Parathyroid Cells. Another oxyphil cell–rich parathyroid lesion, which can potentially mimic Hürthle cell lesions of the thyroid follicular cells. The stippled chromatin in this image is unlike Hürthle cell chromatin, which is evenly distributed, without prominent nucleoli (Pap stain, TP)

- In SurePath™ (SP) samples, parathyroid cells appear more 3-D than in ThinPrep® (TP), where they are monolayered and 2-D. The "bare" nuclei seem to be better observed in SP than in TP.
- In their study, Heo et al. [3] demonstrated the common features of parathyroid lesions on FNA observed on both CS and LBP, which include microfollicles, small nuclei with stippled lymphocyte-like chromatin, and naked nuclei in the background.
- Parathyroid follicular cells may be distinguished cytologically from thyroid follicular cells in Follicular Neoplasm or Suspicious for a Follicular Neoplasm (FN/SFN), although the distinction can be quite challenging. The nuclei tend to be smaller than the follicular cell nuclei of the thyroid follicles. The presence of a prominent vascular pattern, frequent "bare" naked nuclei, and "salt and pepper" nuclear chromatin are other distinguishing features favoring a parathyroid lesion over thyroid. Follicular cells also show cytoplasmic lipofuscin granules (Fig. 13.8).
- The prominent papillary configuration in parathyroid aspirates and the presence of occasional intranuclear inclusions may cause confusion with papillary thyroid carcinoma (PTC), but the absence of the constellation of nuclear features of PTC and the presence of "bare"

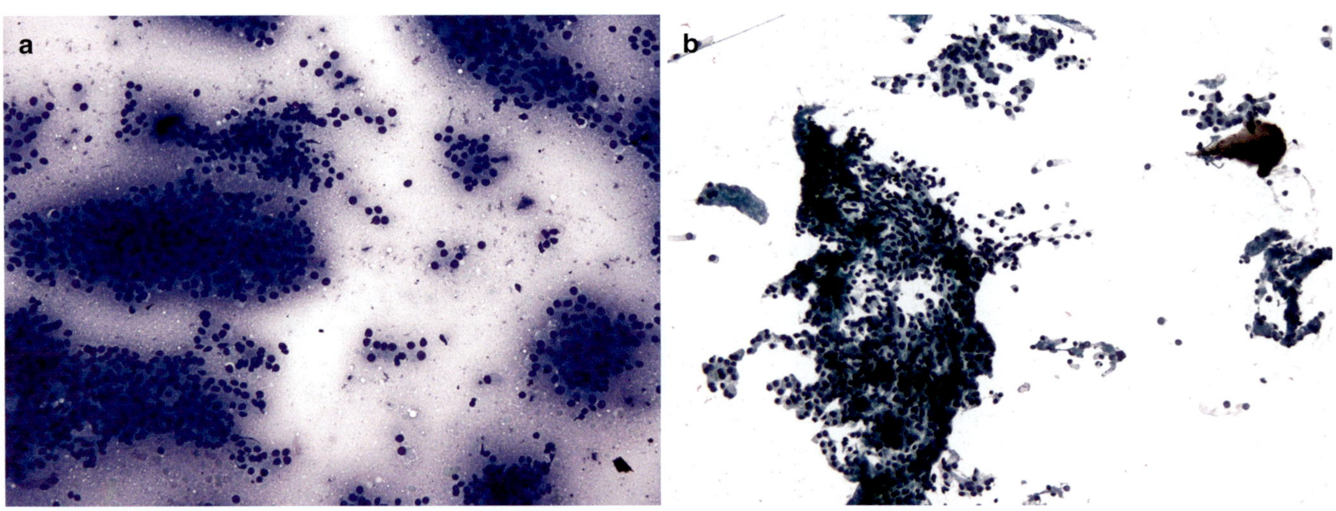

Fig. 13.3 Parathyroid Adenoma (conventional smear [CS] and liquid-based preparation [LBP]). Smears are cellular and show variable architecture, with cells arranged as disorganized, loosely cohesive 2-D fragments and/or tightly cohesive 3-D fragments, as well as papillary structures, sheets, and microfollicles. The microfollicle-like pattern may appear prominent in some cases, mimicking a follicular neoplasm. (**a**) Parathyroid adenoma showing a cellular aspirate with cells arranged in sheets and small single cells in the background (DQ stain, CS). (**b**) Alcohol-fixed Pap-stained TP slide from the same patient shows prominent vascularity and a papillary configuration, with single cells in the background

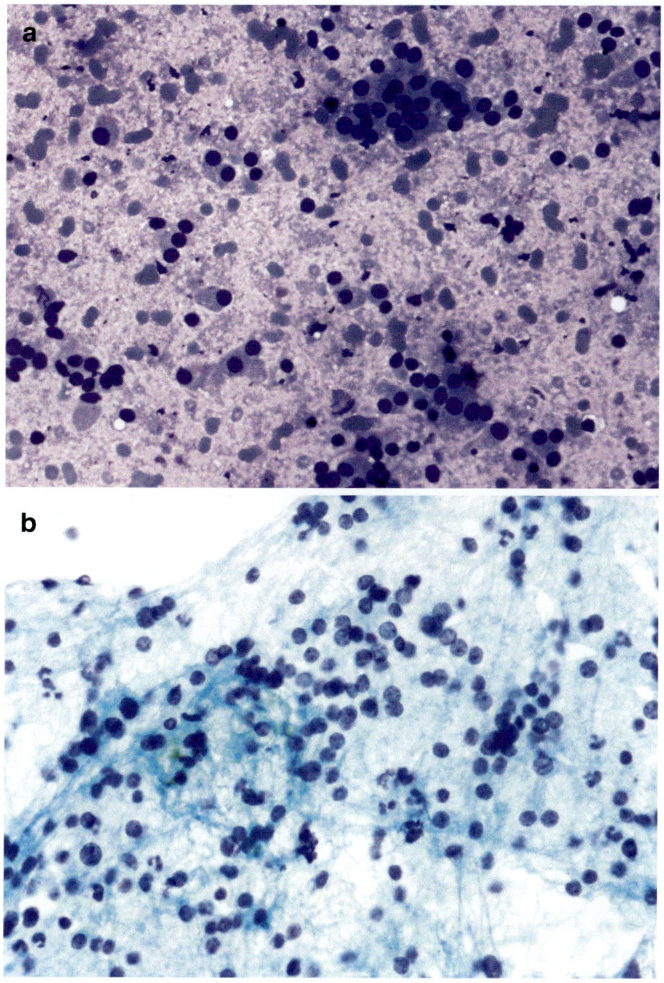

Fig. 13.4 Parathyroid Adenoma (conventional smears). Nuclei are round, uniform, and overlapping, with stippled "salt and pepper" neuroendocrine-type chromatin, inconspicuous nucleoli, and low to high nuclear-cytoplasmic (N:C) ratio. Cell outlines may not be well appreciated. (**a**) Air-dried Diff-Quik (DQ) smear of a parathyroid adenoma, showing cells in microfollicles and many single cells, with eccentrically placed nuclei and stippled chromatin. The plasmacytoid "eccentric" appearance of the nuclei can be mistaken for medullary carcinoma, which is in the differential diagnosis of a parathyroid adenoma on FNA. (**b**) Alcohol-fixed, Pap stained CS showing numerous "bare" nuclei. "Bare" nuclei are better appreciated on CS than on LBP. The presence of numerous naked nuclei can mimic lymphocytes, raising a differential diagnosis of chronic lymphocytic thyroiditis or a lymph node sampling. The stippled appearance of the chromatin is a clue towards a diagnosis of a parathyroid lesion, in addition to the other features mentioned

nuclei in the background help support a diagnosis of parathyroid cells (Fig. 13.9).

- Features of parathyroid hyperplasia, adenoma, and carcinoma are similar in both CS and LBP.
- If a parathyroid lesion is suspected clinically or on rapid on-site evaluation of adequacy, procuring material for cell block preparation can prove to be of great value. Immunostaining for parathyroid hormone (PTH) and thyroglobulin can be of diagnostic value and is used for confirmation (Fig. 13.10). PTH assay on FNA material is extremely helpful and has the highest sensitivity and

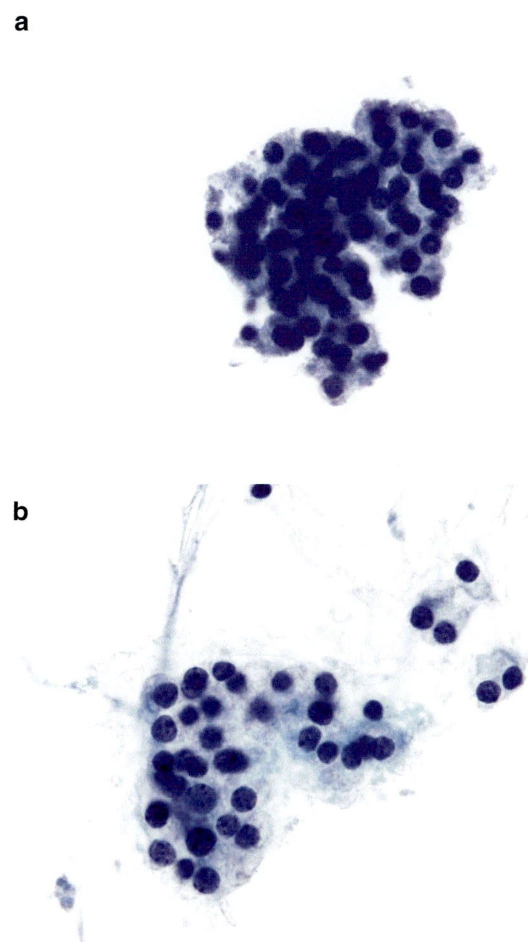

Fig. 13.5 Parathyroid Adenoma (LBP). (**a**, **b**) In LBP, parathyroid aspirates show variable cellularity. A loose 2D pattern or a microfollicular pattern may be the patterns most commonly noted in LBP, but cells also can be seen in honeycombed sheets and clusters, as well as occasional papillary fragments. Both these images show parathyroid cells in microfollicles. The stippled appearance of the chromatin, (although not diagnostic) helps in distinguishing these cells from benign thyroid follicular cells (Pap stain, TP)

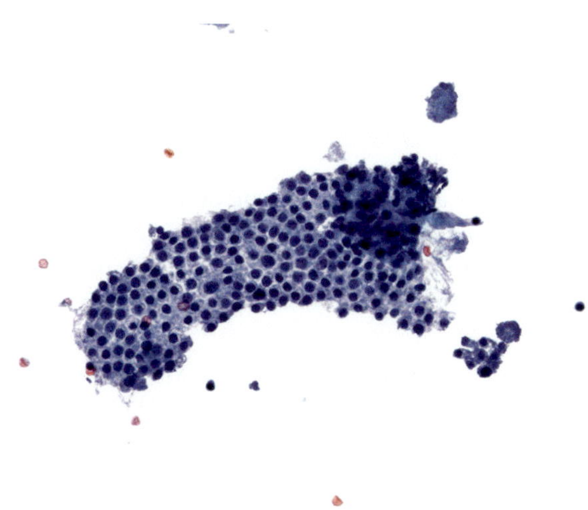

Fig. 13.6 Parathyroid (LBP). The cell outlines are better preserved in LBP than in CS (Pap stain, TP)

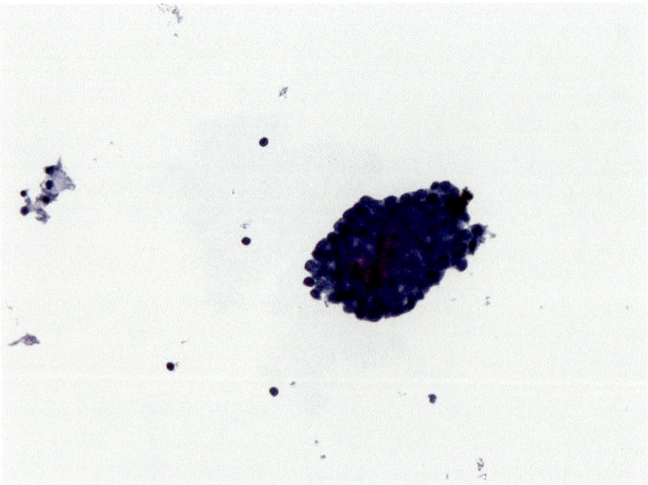

Fig. 13.7 Parathyroid (LBP). Many "bare" naked nuclei, can be seen in both CS and LBP but are better appreciated in CS (*see* Fig. 13.4). As seen here, LBP tends to cluster cells and provides a clean background with reduced "bare" nuclei in comparison to CS (Pap stain, TP)

specificity in the identification of parathyroid tissue sampling on FNA.

- Clinical correlation with PTH assay performed from the aspirated sample can also be confirmatory of parathyroid cells.
- Parathyroid lesions are usually interpreted as a Follicular Lesion of Undetermined Significance (FLUS) or FN/SFN. Subsequent molecular testing can help in further characterization. If the lesion is a parathyroid lesion, the test may detect a parathyroid gene.

Parathyroid Cyst

- Goomany et al. [2] published a case and literature search on parathyroid cysts and demonstrated that this rare entity comprises about 0.5–1% of parathyroid lesions.
- They appear as solitary and asymptomatic swellings in the neck and can be found anywhere from the angle of the mandible to the mediastinum but are most common at the antero-inferior pole of the thyroid gland, mimicking a thyroid nodule.
- About 70% are non-functioning cysts.
- FNA demonstrates clear, colorless cystic fluid with raised PTH levels. Occasionally it can be yellow or brown.
- The FNA procedure is performed primarily to confirm the PTH levels.
- Goomany et al. [2] concluded that when measuring FNA PTH levels, a C-terminal PTH (C-PTH) is preferred over intact PTH in cyst fluids due to the possibility of rapid

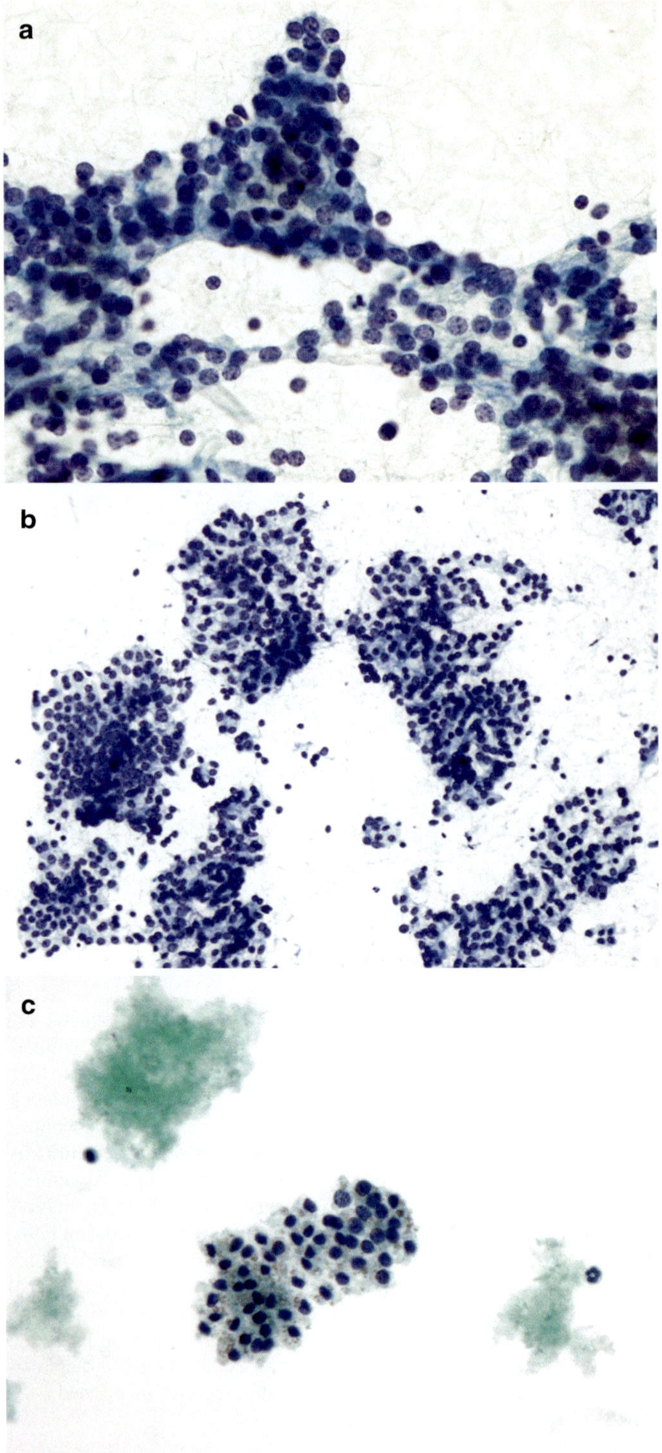

Fig. 13.8 Parathyroid Adenoma (CS and LBP). Parathyroid cells appear similar in CS (**a**, Pap stain) and in LBP (**b**, Pap stain, TP). Lipofuscin may be seen in thyroid follicular cells as yellow to light-brown granular pigment in the cytoplasm (**c**), not usually seen in parathyroid aspirates. The clinical significance of accumulation of lipofuscin in thyroid is not well understood and does not show any relation to thyroid dysfunction (Pap stain, TP)

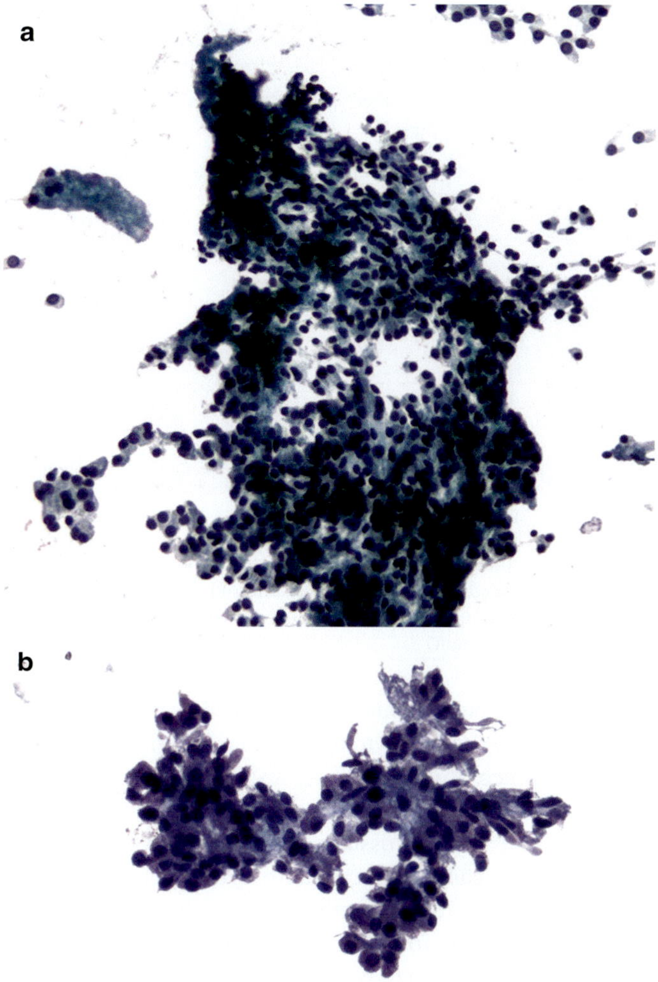

Fig. 13.9 Parathyroid Adenoma (LBP). (**a**) The prominent papillary-like configuration seen here in parathyroid aspirates and the presence of occasional intranuclear inclusions may cause confusion with PTC, but the constellation of nuclear features of PTC is absent in parathyroid aspirates. (**b**) Another example of papillary-like configuration in LBP of parathyroid aspirates (**a**, **b**, Pap stain, TP)

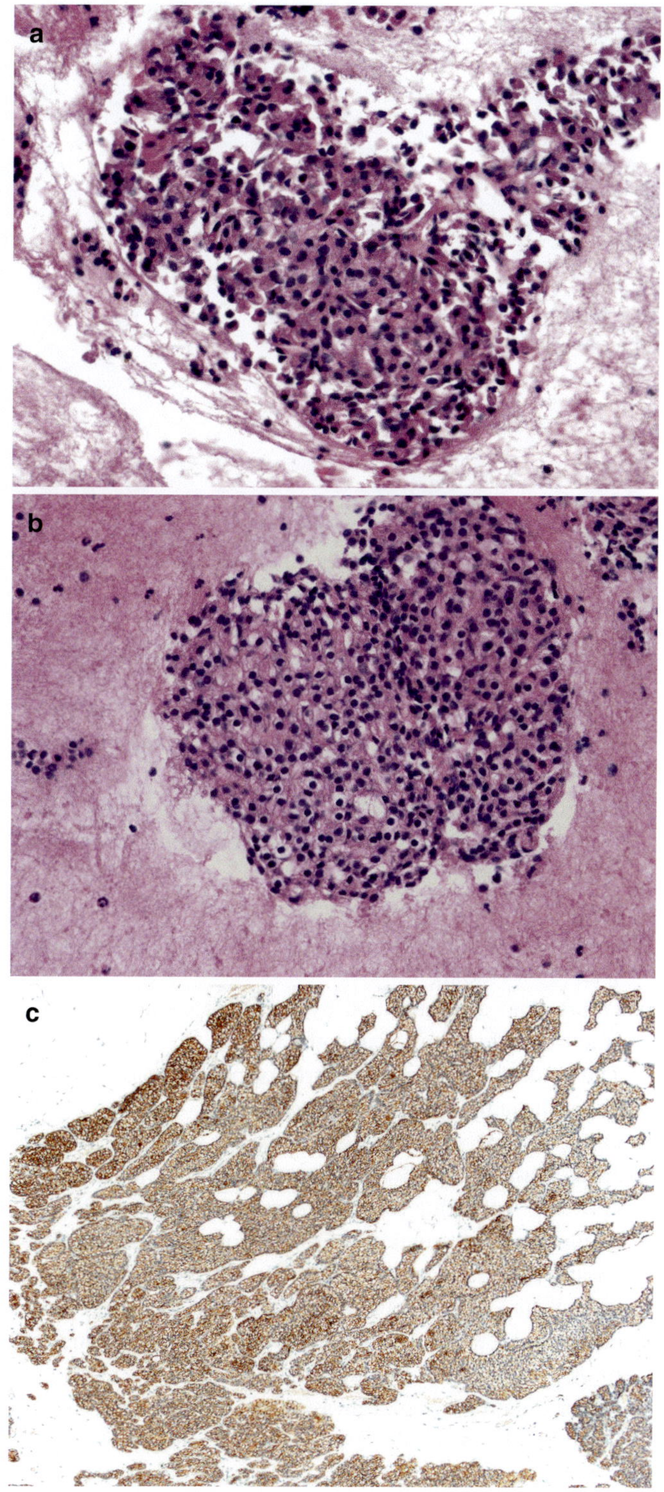

Fig. 13.10 Parathyroid Adenoma (Cytology Cell Blocks from LBP). (**a**, **b**) Images of cellblocks prepared from parathyroid aspirates. If a parathyroid lesion is suspected on rapid on-site evaluation of adequacy, acquiring material for cellblock preparation can prove to be of great value, as immunostaining for parathyroid hormone (PTH) and thyroglobulin can be performed for confirmation. A panel approach is better than using either stain alone. (**a**, **b**, H&E stain). (**c**) Histologic section of a parathyroid adenoma with follicular cells immunoreactive to PTH immunostaining

degradation of PTH into the biologically inactive C-terminal peptide.

- On histology, the cyst wall comprises a single layer of cuboidal or columnar epithelium staining positive for glycogen.

Parathyroid Adenoma/Hyperplasia

- Parathyroid adenoma is the commonest cause of primary hyperparathyroidism.
- Ultrasonographic imaging and technetium sestamibi scintigraphy are the main imaging modalities to preoperatively localize parathyroid adenomas or hyperplasia.

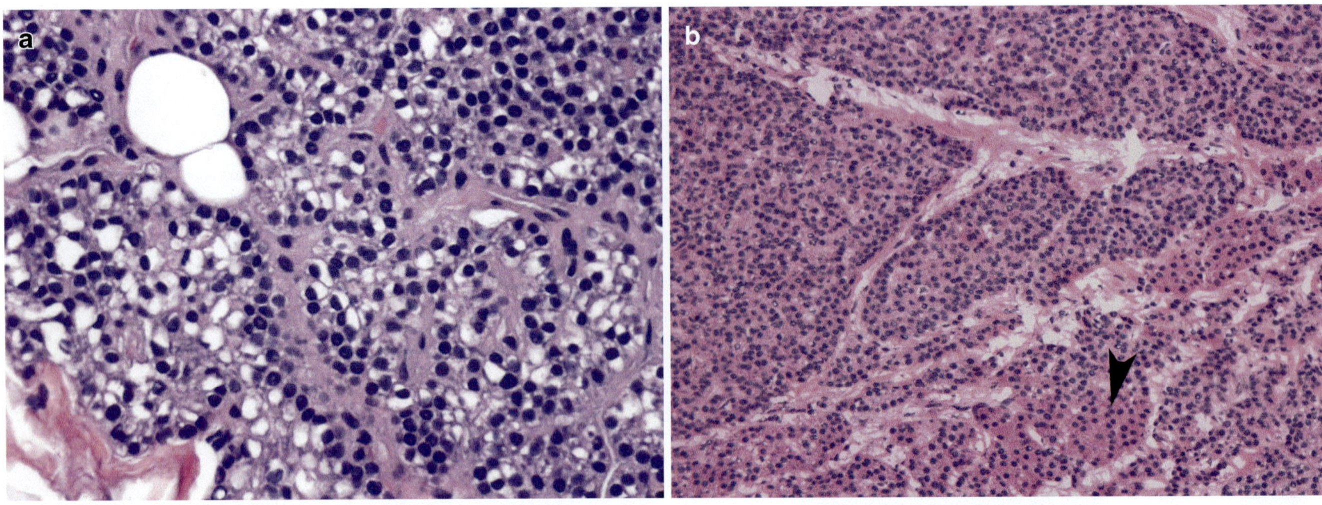

Fig. 13.11 Histology of Parathyroid Lesions. On histology, the neoplastic cells of parathyroid adenoma are arranged in nests, cords, and microfollicles surrounded by a rich capillary network, with mild nuclear pleomorphism. Mitotic figures are rare. In most parathyroid adenomas, chief cells are the dominant cell type, followed by the oxyphil cells. (**a**) Histologic section of a parathyroid adenoma composed exclusively of chief cells, as characterized by the vacuolated clear cytoplasm in these cells. (**b**) Histologic section of a parathyroid hyperplasia showing admixture of oxyphil cells (*black arrowhead*) with pink, granular cytoplasm. (**a**, **b**, H&E stain)

- Johnson et al. [4] and Cho et al. [1] published characteristic features of parathyroid adenoma on imaging, which include hypoechoic oval (or occasionally bean-shaped) lesion, with Doppler imaging showing a characteristic extrathyroidal feeding vessel and peripheral distribution of internal vascularity.
- Overall, US and sestamibi scan together have a combined sensitivity of 95%, versus either US (80%) or sestamibi scan (87%) alone.
- Parathyroid adenoma and hyperplasia are indistinguishable in cytology and histopathology.
- The cytomorphological features of parathyroid adenoma/hyperplasia have been described above.
- On histology, the neoplastic cells are arranged in nests, cords, and microfollicles surrounded by a rich capillary network, with nuclear pleomorphism, multinucleation, and giant cell formation. Mitotic figures are rare. In most parathyroid adenomas, chief cells are the dominant cell type, followed by the oxyphil cells (Fig. 13.11). Tumors composed entirely of oxyphil cells are rare and are referred to as "oxyphil adenomas."
- No capsular or vascular invasion or invasion into adjacent tissue has been noted.

Parathyroid Carcinoma

- Rodriquez et al. (2012) published histological features of parathyroid carcinoma. They indicated that macroscopically, parathyroid carcinoma is often multinodular, with a firm consistency. On histology, the tumor tends to show prominent lobular architecture separated by fibrous trabeculae, the presence of cytologic atypia, and mitotic figures. The presence of invasion is an absolute criterion for diagnosing malignancy, with vascular and/or capsular invasion, extension to adjacent tissues, or the presence of metastases.
- Parathyroid carcinoma can have cytomorphology indistinguishable from parathyroid hyperplasia/adenoma. Immunostaining for PTH and chromogranin will point toward the right diagnosis.

Suggested Reading

1. Cho M, Oweity T, Brandler TC, Fried K, Levine P. Distinguishing parathyroid and thyroid lesions on ultrasound-guided fine-needle aspiration: a correlation of clinical data, ancillary studies, and molecular analysis. Cancer Cytopathol. 2017;125:674–82. https://doi.org/10.1002/cncy.21888.
2. Goomany A, Rafferty A, Smith I. An unusual neck mass: a case of a parathyroid cyst and review of the literature. Case Rep Surg. 2015;2015:243527. https://doi.org/10.1155/2015/243527.
3. Heo I, Park S, Jung CW, Koh JS, Lee SS, Seol H, et al. Fine needle aspiration cytology of parathyroid lesions. Korean J Pathol. 2013;47:466–71. https://doi.org/10.4132/KoreanJPathol.2013.47.5.466.
4. Johnson NA, Tublin ME, Ogilvie JB. Parathyroid imaging: technique and role in the preoperative evaluation of primary hyperparathyroidism. AJR Am J Roentgenol. 2007;188:1706–15.
5. Park GS, Lee SH, Jung SL, Jung CK. Liquid-based cytology in the fine needle aspiration of parathyroid lesions: a comparison study with the conventional smear, ThinPrep, and SurePath. Int J Clin Exp Pathol. 2015;8:12160–8.
6. Rodriguez C, Nadéri S, Hans C, Badoual C. Parathyroid carcinoma: a difficult histological diagnosis. Eur Ann Otorhinolaryngol Head Neck Dis. 2012;129:157–9. https://doi.org/10.1016/j.anorl.2012.01.002.

Application of Molecular Tests in Indeterminate Thyroid FNA

14

Theresa Scognamiglio, Rana S. Hoda, Christina M. Narick, and Yuri E. Nikiforov

Introduction to Molecular Genetics in Indeterminate Thyroid Nodules

- Indeterminate diagnoses on FNA is the major limitation of thyroid cytology. The problem results from cytological features overlapping between non-neoplastic and neoplastic follicular lesions, which are reflected by the low concordance among pathologists in the indeterminate category. (*See* Chaps. 5, 6, and 7).
- The heterogeneity of the outcome in indeterminate cytology on thyroid FNA results in either repeat FNA or surgical lobectomy.
- Molecular testing helps to stratify cytologically indeterminate thyroid nodules into clinically meaningful categories. These markers can serve as cytopathologic adjuncts to improve the accuracy of diagnostic testing of thyroid nodules [1, 2].
- The revised 2015 management guidelines of the American Thyroid Association (ATA) [3] recommend performing a mutational panel in cases with indeterminate cytology. The ATA includes "Suspicious for Malignancy" in the indeterminate category.
- Because of wide acceptance by all clinical thyroid organizations, molecular tests are fast becoming an integral part of thyroid FNAs.
- They are increasingly being used as an adjunctive test for the 15–30% of thyroid FNAs falling in the indeterminate categories of The Bethesda System for Reporting Thyroid Cytopathology (TBSRTC):
  - (i) Atypia of Undetermined Significance or Follicular Lesion of Undetermined Significance (AUS/FLUS)
  - (ii) Follicular Neoplasm or Suspicious for a Follicular Neoplasm (FN/SFN) and those of the oncocytic (Hürthle cell) type (FNHCT/SFNHCT)
  - (iii) Suspicious for Malignancy (SM)
- Molecular tests will improve preoperative diagnostic accuracy of thyroid FNAs to guide clinicians in the management of patients.
- They may also be useful for noninvasive follicular thyroid neoplasm with papillary-like nuclear features (NIFTP) (*see* Chap. 9).

Commercially Available Molecular Tests

- Three molecular diagnostic tests for thyroid FNA specimens are commercially available:
  1. **Afirma Genomic Sequencing Classifier (GSC), 2017, "rule-out" test:**
     - Next-generation sequencing (NGS) analysis, developed to address limitations in detection of Hürthle cell lesions and improve specificity and positive predictive value (PPV)
     - Expanded from 142 genes to total of 10,196 genes, with 1115 core genes
     - Includes a series of classifiers: parathyroid, medullary thyroid carcinoma (MTC), *BRAF*V600E, *RET/PTC*, follicular content index, Hürthle cell index, and Hürthle cell neoplasm index
  2. **ThyroSeq v3 Genomic Classifier (GC), 2017, "rule-in" and "rule-out" test:**
     - NGS analysis

T. Scognamiglio
Department of Pathology and Laboratory Medicine, New York Presbyterian Hospital, Weill Cornell Medical College, New York, NY, USA
e-mail: ths9004@med.cornell.edu

R. S. Hoda (✉)
CBLPath, Rye Brook, NY, USA
e-mail: rhoda@cblpath.com

C. M. Narick
Interpace Diagnostics, Pittsburgh, PA, USA

Y. E. Nikiforov
Department of Pathology, Division of Molecular and Genomic Pathology, University of Pittsburgh, Pittsburgh, PA, USA

R. S. Hoda et al. (eds.), *Atlas of Thyroid Cytopathology on Liquid-Based Preparations*,
https://doi.org/10.1007/978-3-030-25066-9_14

- ThyroSeq v3 was built with three goals: (1) Expanding the ThyroSeq v2 test panel through the inclusion of recently discovered genetic markers related to thyroid nodules and cancer; (2) Enabling the analysis of additional classes of genetic alterations that were not previously tested (*ie*, copy number alterations [CNAs]); (3) Improving the test's accuracy for detecting various types of Hürthle cell (oncocytic) tumors.
- ThyroSeq v3 is an expanded assay from 56 to 112 thyroid-related genes for mutations, fusion, copy number variations, and gene expression.

3. **ThyGeNEXT/ThyraMIR, "rule-in" and "rule-out" test:**
   - *ThyGeNEXT:* Targeted NGS analysis that has been expanded from a 7-gene mutation panel to a 10-gene mutation panel, including TERT, with a 38-member mRNA fusion panel.
   - *ThyraMIR:* Measures expression level of 10 miRNAs by RT-PCR to identify low-risk and high-risk thyroid nodules.

Goals of Molecular Tests

- Avoid unnecessary surgery for benign nodules, or better predict a benign nodule.
- Distinguish between high-risk thyroid carcinoma, which would require total thyroidectomy, and low-risk carcinoma, which could be treated with a lobectomy, or better predict a high-risk malignant nodule.
- Preoperatively detect high-risk thyroid carcinoma, so that a central lymph node dissection can be performed.

Challenges of Molecular Testing

- They are expensive tests and should be used judiciously.
- Intra-laboratory monitoring of molecular test results and lack of correlation with concurrent FNA.
- Clinical follow-up of nodules with negative molecular test results has not yet established appropriate surveillance intervals.
- Molecular test results in NIFTP are not yet fully understood and documented.
- Understanding the value of second-opinion cytology review for an accurate diagnosis may reduce cost by preventing an unnecessary molecular test.
- Accurate results depends on specimen sampling and preservation.

Facts About Genomic Landscape of Thyroid Lesions

- The Cancer Genome Atlas results showed that *BRAF*, *RET*, and *RAS* mutations are the most common genetic alterations [1].
- *BRAF*V600E is the most common point mutation in classic papillary thyroid carcinoma (PTC). It can also be seen in poorly differentiated and anaplastic carcinomas of the thyroid.
- *BRAF* and TERT promoter mutations are high-risk mutations that are indicative of an adverse prognosis in PTC.
- *RAS* (*HRAS*, *NRAS* and *KRAS*) is the second most common point mutation, which occurs mostly in follicular carcinoma. *RAS* mutation can also be seen in the follicular variant of PTC (FVPTC) and follicular adenoma. Additional mutations are found in follicular carcinomas [2, 3].
- *RET/PTC* gene rearrangement may be seen in PTC and in benign thyroid nodules.
- *PAX8/PPARγ* gene rearrangement, when present, indicates follicular carcinoma.
- Hürthle cell carcinomas have a unique genomic landscape. Most common are copy number alterations (CNAs). Numerical chromosome changes involve loss and/or gain of whole chromosomes or chromosome arms. Widely invasive Hürthle cell carcinomas are polysomic, with universal duplication of chromosome 7. Most common loss is of chromosome 8.
- Most familial MTC has *RET* mutations.
- *RET* and *RAS* mutations are seen in a subset of sporadic MTC.
- Overexpression of microRNA 375 is well documented in MTC.
- Benign thyroid tumors can have mutations in the thyroid stimulating hormone (TSH) receptor, in addition to the other mutations described above.

Application of Molecular Tests in Liquid-Based Preparations (LBP)

- Krane et al. [4] demonstrated that molecular analysis can be performed on residual ThinPrep (TP) material even after prolonged storage at room temperature.
- Liquid-based FNA material allows for efficient RNA extraction for common point mutations and rearrangements.
- Molecular tests on residual LBP material can be performed routinely in a molecular cytology laboratory for commonly encountered abnormalities including *BRAF*V600E

and *RAS* point mutations and *RET/PTC* and *PAX8/PPARγ* rearrangements.

- Molecular testing on residual LBP material can also be performed if the molecular test fails because of inadequate cellularity when performed on the specimen in the molecular test preservative.

Afirma Thyroid Molecular Test

- The Afirma gene expression classifier (GEC) was introduced in 2012 to improve preoperative risk assessment of indeterminate thyroid nodules. The Afirma GEC measured the mRNA expression transcript levels of 167 genes. The expression of those genes was used to classify indeterminate aspirates as either benign or suspicious. In a large, prospective multicenter validation study, the GEC showed a specificity of 52% with a sensitivity of 92%. The GEC was designed to identify benign nodules and had a high negative predictive value (NPV) of 93%, with a PPV of 47% [5]. Nodules identified as benign could be followed; those with suspicious findings required diagnostic surgery. Additional studies demonstrated similar high sensitivity and NPV [6, 7]. The GEC performance was limited in nodules with Hürthle (oncocytic) cytology, however. These nodules frequently demonstrated an increased rate of suspicion on the GEC even though the risk of malignancy on subsequent resections was quite low [8, 9].
- A new, robust genomic sequencing classifier (GSC) was recently introduced with the aim of improving specificity while maintaining high sensitivity for malignancy. The GSC uses next-generation sequencing (NGS) and incorporates an ensemble model consisting of 12 independent classifiers. The model utilizes 10,196 genes, of which 1115 are core genes that drive the prediction model. The Afirma GSC test includes seven additional components, including a parathyroid cassette, an MTC cassette, a *BRAF*V600E cassette, a *RET/PTC1* and *RET/PTC3* fusion detection module, a follicular content index, and Hürthle cell and Hürthle neoplasm indices. The ensemble model, in addition to the follicular content index and Hürthle cell and Hürthle neoplasm indices, forms the core classifier engine for determining benign versus suspicious.
- Clinical validation of the Afirma GSC was performed in a multi-institutional prospective blinded validation study. The GSC was performed on a set of indeterminate thyroid nodules obtained by FNA samples from 49 academic and community centers from June 2009 to December 2010. Pathological review of all histology slides was performed by a panel of expert pathologists, who were blinded to the genomic and clinical data. The primary endpoint was sensitivity, specificity, NPV, and PPV in Bethesda III and IV nodules.
- The study consisted of FNA samples previously used to validate the Afirma GEC. Those samples were derived from 4812 aspirates collected from 3789 patients. 190 indeterminate thyroid nodules from 183 patients had adequate residual RNA for analysis and were examined by the GSC and compared with blinded expert pathology review, as well as the GEC.
- Of the 190 indeterminate FNA samples, 114 (60%) were Bethesda III and 76 (40%) were Bethesda IV. For Bethesda III nodules, the sensitivity was 92.9%, with a specificity of 70.9%. The PPV was 51% and NPV was 96.8%, with a cancer prevalence of 24.6%. For Bethesda IV nodules, the sensitivity and specificity were slightly lower, at 88.2% and 64.4% respectively. The PPV was 41% and NPV was 95.0%, with a cancer prevalence of 22.4%.
- Overall, for Bethesda III and IV nodules, the GSC demonstrated a sensitivity of 91% and specificity of 68%. The NPV and PPV were 96% and 47% respectively, with a cancer prevalence of 23.7%. Compared with the GEC, the GSC had a higher specificity and benign call rate, accurately classifying more indeterminate nodules as benign.
- Of the 190 indeterminate nodules, 17 (8.9%) were Hürthle cell adenomas and 9 were Hürthle cell carcinomas. The GSC had 88.9% sensitivity and 58.8% specificity for Hürthle cell lesions, which was significantly improved over the specificity of 11.8% for the Afirma GEC. A recent independent validation study evaluated 600 nodules from 563 patients and compared results of the GEC to the GSC with particular focus on the performance of these tests for nodules with Hürthle cell cytology. The study demonstrated a higher benign call rate for the GSC than for the GEC, and a decrease in the overall "suspicious" rate, predominantly among nodules with Hürthle cell cytology [10].
- In summary, GSC demonstrates a high sensitivity and high NPV for cytologically indeterminate thyroid nodules (Bethesda II and IV). The test sensitivity of the GSC is similar to that of the GEC, although the test specificity is improved (GEC specificity 50%, *vs.* 68% for GSC). The increased specificity suggests that at least 30% more indeterminate nodules (Bethesda III and IV) that are histologically confirmed benign nodules will receive a benign result. This increase in benign call rate should allow more patients to avoid unnecessary diagnostic surgery [11].

Interpace Diagnostic Testing

Introduction

- Oncogenic alterations detected in malignant thyroid nodules often involve the MAPK and PI3K/AKT signaling pathways. *BRAF*V600E point mutation has been extensively reported in PTC and also poorly differentiated and anaplastic thyroid cancers [12–14]. *RAS* mutations also have a distinct role in thyroid carcinogenesis and are found in follicular forms of thyroid carcinoma, including FVPTC and follicular thyroid carcinoma. These mutations are also associated with NIFTP and benign follicular adenomas [14–16]. Chromosomal rearrangements resulting in oncogenic gene fusions, such as RET/PTC or PAX/PPARγ, also have clear association with classic PTC and follicular neoplasms, respectively [14, 17]. TERT promoter region mutations have been extensively reported in malignant thyroid nodules and occur at high frequency in nodules with aggressive clinicopathologic behavior, particularly if coexistent with *BRAF*V600E or *RAS* mutational change [18, 19]. Gene mutations occurring at lower frequency in the PI3K/AKT pathway (*eg*, AKT1, PIK3CA, PTEN) with synergistic oncogenic effects leading to cancer progression have also been reported [14]. Based on characterization of molecular pathogenesis in thyroid lesions, both the National Comprehensive Cancer Network and ATA guidelines support molecular testing when FNA specimens are indeterminate (Bethesda category III, IV, or V) [20, 21].
- The ThyGeNEXT/ThyraMIR combination test, introduced in 2015, was originally developed by Asuragen and later acquired by Interpace Diagnostics (Parsipanny, NJ). Developed to assist clinical management decisions and surgical triage, this test includes both an NGS-based analysis of DNA and messenger RNA (ThyGeNEXT) and a PCR-based microRNA classifier (ThyraMIR). Sample evaluation is performed at one of two CLIA-approved laboratories accredited by the College of American Pathologists (CAP), in Pittsburgh, PA, or New Haven, CT. The validated sample types include FNA specimens placed directly into an RNA preservative solution (provided in sample kits), cytology slide smears, and formalin-fixed paraffin-embedded (FFPE) recuts. The original ThyGenX panel included five genes (*BRAF*V600E, *HRAS*, *KRAS*, *NRAS*, and *PIK3CA*) and three RNA fusions (PAX/PPARγ, RET/PTC1, RET/PTC3) known to have association with thyroid carcinoma. Because some mutations have a well-established strong association with malignancy, these mutations, when present, indicate surgical intervention and can also clarify the appropriate surgical approach. In contrast, other genetic alterations, such as *RAS* mutations, have a less clearly defined malignancy risk, as these changes can be found in both benign and malignant thyroid nodules. These mutations may be viewed as "weak" drivers with a complex role in neoplastic and malignant pathology. These mutations are reported in approximately 30% of all follicular adenomas, 50% of NIFTP, 30–45% of follicular forms of thyroid carcinoma, and 20% of PTC [22–24]. Thus, the presence of *RAS* mutations alone cannot be equated with malignancy; it is best assessed as a moderate risk, which can be further evaluated by a gene expression classifier (such as ThyraMIR) or diagnostic lobectomy. From our interpretive perspective, the concept of a strong driver *versus* a weak driver relates to the PPV and strength of association to malignancy. The strong driver mutations are highly specific, and identification of such mutations in an aspirate from a thyroid nodule indicates the presence of malignancy with a high degree of certainty. In contrast, detection of a weak driver mutation alone is not sufficient to affirm malignancy; this analysis may benefit from additional molecular information, such as miRNA expression profiling, to clearly and definitively discriminate between benign and malignant nodule status.

ThyraMIR miRNA Classifier

- Recognizing that not all detected mutations carry identical malignancy risk, gene expression profiles can prove beneficial to further characterize malignancy risk and can provide an independent molecular approach for cancer diagnosis [25]. ThyraMIR is a microRNA (miRNA) classifier that evaluates 10 distinct miRNAs through targeted quantitative PCR (qPCR) as surrogate markers for oncogenic or tumor suppressor activity. MicroRNAs, first identified in 1993, are small, noncoding RNAs (19–24 nucleotides in length) that act to repress translation of certain messenger RNAs, and therefore play a critical role in regulation of gene expression at the posttranslational level. These miRNAS therefore impact proliferation, differentiation, migration, apoptosis, metabolism, and stress response, clearly reflecting disease pathogenesis [26]. Numerous studies have identified the significance of miRNAs in various forms of carcinoma. miRNAS that are overexpressed (upregulated) in carcinomas are thought to function as oncogenes, promoting tumor development by negative regulation of genes that control cell differentiation or apoptosis. In contrast, miRNAs that are underexpressed (downregulated) are thought to influence tumor suppressor activity. Clinical experience indicates that strongly positive miRNA status is most highly predictive of malignancy. Additionally, qualitative aspects of RNA expression are used to reflect the specific type and degree of cellular proliferation. In this way, the miRNA expression analysis serves as an objective, highly reproducible method to characterize and discriminate between benign and malignant thyroid nodules that do not demonstrate a strong oncogenic driver on ThyGeNEXT.

Combination Testing (NGS and microRNA)

- The key advantage of combination testing is its ability to rule in malignant nodules that lack oncogenic mutations, to rule out benign nodules with somatic mutations of uncertain clinical indication, to identify those lesions that are most likely benign; the result is overall improvement in patient management by guiding the surgical approach and identifying nonsurgical patients. The combination test is a risk-assessment tool, with results designated as highly likely benign, highly likely malignant, or moderate risk of malignancy. Nodules with strong driver mutations or with weak driver mutations and strongly positive ThyraMIR status are at markedly elevated risk of malignancy [27]. Conversely, nodules that are fully negative for both NGS mutations/fusions and a negative microRNA classifier are highly likely to be benign. Because this combined test incorporates both NGS-based mutational testing and a microRNA classifier, it can be viewed as both a "rule in" and "rule out" test [28]. The combination of NGS mutational panel and miRNA analysis resulted in strong sensitivity (94%) and a calculated PPV of 74% at 32% cancer prevalence, with an NPV of 94% [26]. Additional test performance data established through clinical validation is presented in Table 14.1.

Table 14.1 Test performance of ThyGeNEXT/ThyraMIR combination testing

	Cohort	AUS/FLUS	FN/SFN
Number of cases	109	58	51
Sensitivity (%)	89 (73–97)	94 (73–100)	82 (57–96)
Specificity (%)	85 (75–92)	80 (64–91)	91 (76–98)
PPV (%)	74 (58–86)	68 (46–85)	82 (57–96)
NPV (%)	94 (85–98)	97 (84–100)	91 (76–98)

Adapted from Labourier et al. [28]; with permission

AUS/FLUS atypia of undetermined significance or follicular lesion of undetermined significance, *FN/SFN* follicular neoplasm or suspicious for a follicular neoplasm, *NPV* negative predictive value, *PPV* positive predictive value

ThyGeNEXT (Expanded NGS Panel)

- With the limited 5-gene panel of ThyGenX, and additional oncogenic mutational change reported in the literature, Interpace recognized the need to expand the platform to ensure coverage of key oncogenic alterations, to improve management decisions and optimize patient care. Although additional markers in a diagnostic NGS-based test would conceptually lead to improved test sensitivity, it is important to note that broadening a panel to include rare mutations with uncertain clinical relevance could lead to increased false positive rates. On this basis, the additional markers incorporated into the panel were carefully selected based on reported clinical relevance for carcinoma or clinicopathologic aggressiveness.
- The ThyGenX test was transitioned to an expanded panel (ThyGeNEXT) to include 10 genes and 38 mRNA fusions (Table 14.2). Markers of aggressiveness, TERT and ALK, were added, as well as the *RET* protooncogene (indicative of MTC), *PTEN*, and *GNAS*. Additional fusions, including

Table 14.2 Expanded ThyGeNEXT panel

DNA markers		mRNA fusion transcripts	
Gene	Codon range		
BRAF	598–615	NKX2–1	NTRK2/TERT
HRAS	9–20	PAX8	PRKARIA/RET
HRAS	59–76	TBP	NCOA4/RET_3
KRAS	4–15	USP33	GOLGA5/RET_5
KRAS	55–65	CCDC6/RET	ELKS/RET
NRAS	9–20	NCOA4/RET_4	TRIM24/RET
NRAS	55–67	PAX8/PPARg_1	TRIM33/RET
PIK3CA	540–551	PAX8/PPARg_2	KTN1/RET_8
PIK3CA	1038–1049	PAX8/PPARg_3	PCM1/RET_11
ALK	1191–1206	PAX8/PPARg_4	RFG9/RET_9
GNAS	843–855 (also known as 201–213)	CREB3L2/PPARg	TRIM27/RET
GNAS	864–879 (also known as 227–242)	PARG/BMSI	HOOK3/RET
RET	624–648	STRN/ALK	NCOA4/RET_3d
RET	877–889	EML4/ALK	AGK/BRAF
RET	918–930	TPM3/NTRK1	AKAP9/BRAF
PTEN	124–138	TFG/NTRK1	SPTLC2/BRAF
PTEN	134–154	TPR/NTRK1-1	THADA28/LOC389473
TERT	Promoter region	TPR/NTRK1-2	THADA29/LOC389473
		ETV6/NTRK3-1	THADA31/IGF2BP3-2
		ETV6/NTRK3-2	THADA30/IGF2BP3-3
		SLC12A6/NTRK3	TRA2A/THADA

Adapted from Ablordeppey et al. [30]

Table 14.3 Additional molecular information provided by ThyGeNEXT

Specimen	ThyGenX	ThyGeNEXT	Outcome
Smear	Negative	TERT p.C228T	FTC
Smear	BRAF p.V600E	AGK/BRAF, BRAF p.V600E	PTC
Smear	BRAF p.V600E	TERT p.C228T, BRAF p.V600E	PTC
FNA	BRAF p.V600E	TERT p.C228T, BRAF p.V600E	PTC

FNA fine needle aspiration, *FTC* follicular thyroid carcinoma, *PTC* papillary thyroid carcinoma

the NTRK and ALK fusions recently identified as possible therapeutic targets, were added to the panel.

- In a bridge study with ThyGenX, the ThyGeNEXT expanded panel demonstrated 100% concordance with the markers common to both panels (95% CI: 99.5–100%). Both panels identified 24 positive markers and 779 negative markers. As expected, ThyGeNEXT also identified additional mutations and fusions strongly associated with aggressive forms of thyroid cancer (*eg*, *TERT*, *RET*, and *ALK* genes) in four cases (Table 14.3) [29].

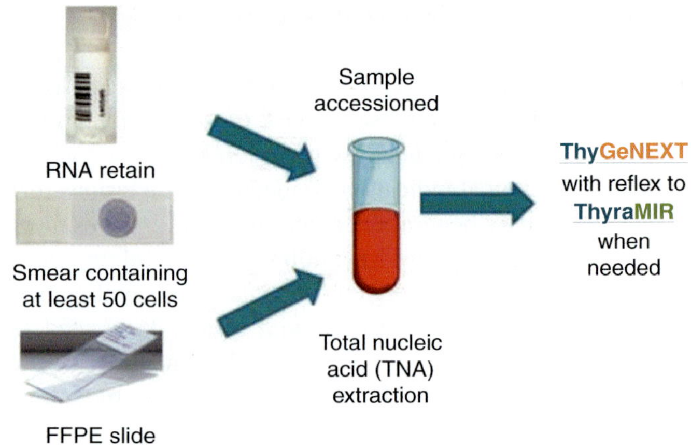

Fig. 14.1 Interpace testing sample types

Cytology Slide Smears

- Based on well-recognized interobserver variability and sample heterogeneity, the use of diagnostic cytology slide smears for molecular analysis may prove beneficial. Kumar et al. reported in abstract form [30] that 67% of cases diagnosed as "Insufficient" (Bethesda category I) proved to have adequate material for molecular analysis, and in 2 of 49 cases, a significant *BRAF*V600E mutation was identified. The proposed explanation for this finding lies not in the sensitivity of molecular analysis, but instead is likely a reflection of the known variability between each needle pass during the biopsy procedure. The actual cytology slide smear used for microscopic diagnosis thus presents an opportunity not only to ensure that molecular testing is performed on the actual cellular material used for microscopic evaluation (therefore minimizing sample variation) but also to eliminate the need for additional sampling at the time of biopsy. Cytology slide smears for molecular testing present advantages not only to the pathology laboratory, with no need for special storage of material designated for specific molecular testing, but also to the sonographer performing the biopsy and to the patient, by eliminating the need for a dedicated needle pass. Internal validation data demonstrate that nucleic acid captured from cytology slides correlates with the presence of malignancy and also correlates with the previously validated combination testing performed on FNA biopsy specimens aspirated into an RNA preservative solution. Overall results demonstrate 89% concordance between the results of NGS-based mutation sequencing and 90% concordance in miRNA expression–based testing [31].

Testing/Logistics

- The combination testing platform can be performed on FNA aspirates placed into preservative solution, on cytology slide smears (affording the opportunity to test the actual cells of concern microscopically), and on recuts from formalin-fixed paraffin-embedded (FFPE) blocks, as depicted in Fig. 14.1. The samples in preservative solution can be stored at room temperature for up to 6 weeks and require no special shipping conditions. Upon receipt at the laboratory, samples in preservative solution undergo extraction of total nucleic acid (TNA) using the standard phenol chloroform extraction method. Cytology slide smears undergo cover slip removal and microdissection into a buffer solution prior to nucleic acid extraction. Several quality assessments are in place to ensure adequate material prior to analysis. Following amplification and library prep, samples undergo targeted NGS on Illumina MiSeq analyzers (illumina, San Diego, CA) to detect alterations in 10 genes (DNA) and 38 fusions (mRNA). Each NGS run includes positive controls and negative controls, and samples are analyzed for markers of thyroid follicular cells to ensure biopsy adequacy. Each sample is run in duplicate to confirm positive findings, and variants are detected as a percentage of total reads. In cases that do not show mutational change strongly associated with malignancy (*BRAF*V600E, *TERT* promoter region, *RET/PTC*), the sample is then subjected to miRNA analysis to further characterize malignancy risk. Adequacy is first determined based on quantity of nucleic acid, and each miRNA test run includes both positive and negative controls. Specific quality parameters are used to evaluate the presence of excessive blood, the presence of parathyroid (rather than thyroid) tissue, and overall performance of each miRNA, for inclusion in the proprietary mathematical algorithm calculation. Each sample is run in duplicate and all positive findings are confirmed through repeat analysis.

- Board-certified pathologists interpret results of combination testing as shown in Fig. 14.2. Reporting incorporates consideration of the cytology diagnosis, as this denotes expected prevalence of disease based in TBSRTC. If ThyGeNEXT identifies a "strong driver" mutation, the case is then reported out as high risk, and the miRNA classifier is not necessary for risk assessment. Conversely, if ThyGeNEXT shows no mutational change, and ThyraMIR status is also negative, these nodules, fully negative for genetic alterations, are most likely benign and can confidently undergo surveillance, provided that there are no concerning patient or clinical features. The remaining nodules then represent the gray zone, with a moderate level of risk. Reflex testing to ThyraMIR is indicated only in the absence of strong driver mutations. If no mutations are detected on NGS, or a weak driver mutation is detected, the miRNA analysis can prove beneficial. The grey zone remains evident in cases that have a weak driver mutation and either negative or weakly positive ThyraMIR status. This category represents a minority of clinical cases, but it remains nonetheless as we continue to further our understanding of genetic alterations in various forms of thyroid carcinoma and neoplasia. In all cases, clinicians must use the results of molecular testing in the context of the clinical characteristics of their patients. Sonographic features, thyroid function testing, patient history, and patient preference must all be considered in management decisions. Molecular analysis, supported by guidelines of both the ATA [3] and the National Comprehensive Cancer Network (NCCN) [20], can provide additional information in cases with indeterminate cytology, for consideration by the treating physician and the patient.

ThyroSeq

Test History and Test Design

- ThyroSeq is a molecular test for indeterminate thyroid nodules designed at the University of Pittsburgh Medical Center. It is based on the detection of specific molecular alterations in DNA and RNA that are characteristic of thyroid cancer. Since the test was first introduced in 2007, it has undergone expansion and improvement based on the

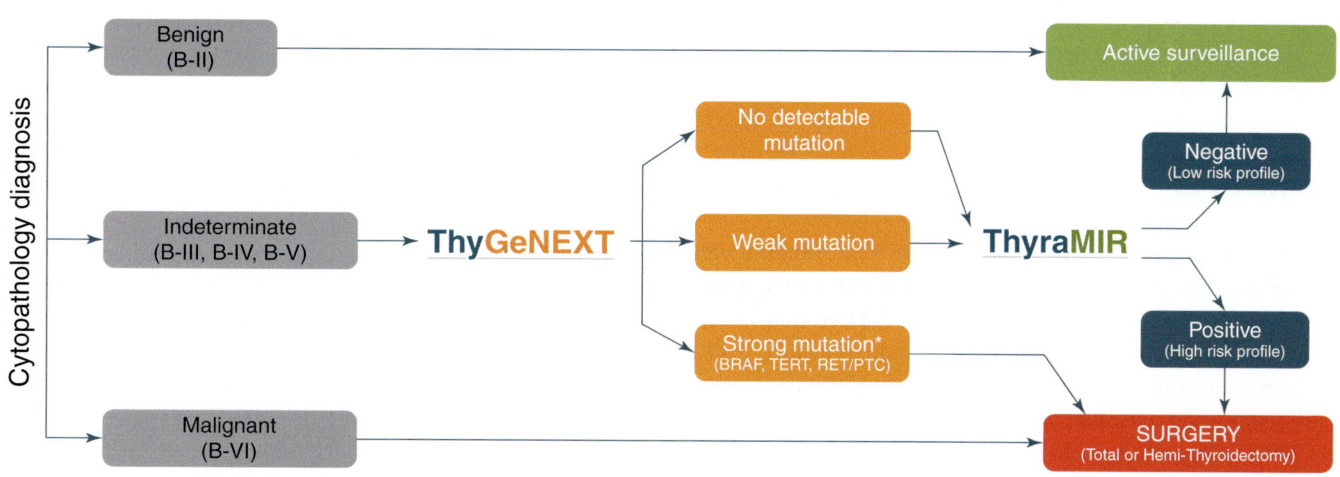

Fig. 14.2 Interpretive algorithm for combination testing. Suggested patient management scenarios based on results from combined ThyGeNEXT + ThyraMIR test and cytological diagnosis. The actual management may differ because the clinical decisions are based on comprehensive evaluation of patient characteristics, sonographic findings, and correlative clinical factors. NCCN guidelines for management of nodules with Bethesda III and Bethesda IV cytology diagnoses include consideration of molecular analysis. ∗ThyGeNEXT samples that are positive for BRAF, TERT, ALK, and RET/PTC will solely receive a ThyGeNEXT test result. ThyGeNEXT samples that test positive for markers that have a lower risk of malignancy, such as RAS, will also receive a ThyraMIR test result

advances in the understanding of genetic mechanisms of thyroid cancer and the development of novel molecular techniques applicable to thyroid FNA samples.

- The first version of the test, ThyroSeq v0, was launched for clinical use in 2007. ThyroSeq v0 was a 7-gene panel that utilized Sanger sequencing and real-time PCR assays that were available at the time. The test detected mutations in genes commonly mutated in thyroid cancer, including *NRAS*, *HRAS*, and *KRAS*, along with gene fusions *RET/PTC1*, *RET/PTC3*, and *PAX8-PPARG*. Though ThyroSeq v0 had high specificity and PPV, which made it a good "rule-in" test, it lacked sufficiently high sensitivity and NPV to be a good "rule-out" test. The test sensitivity of 62% did not allow diagnostic surgeries for mutation-negative nodules to be avoided in most clinical situations [32–34].
- The advent of next-generation sequencing (NGS) expanded diagnostic technology for thyroid cancer. NGS brought many advantages, including the ability to use a very small amount of sample, detect many types of genetic alterations in one test, and provide quantitative information on genetic alterations. ThyroSeq v1 was launched in 2013 as a 15-gene panel, with 78% sensitivity.
- The accelerated discovery of thyroid cancer markers, along with the expanding customized use of NGS technology, paved the way for ThyroSeq v2, which was launched in 2014. ThyroSeq v2 was a 56-gene panel that interrogated thyroid-specific hotspots for point mutations, insertions and deletions, gene fusions, and gene expression changes. This test version significantly increased sensitivity to 90%, as demonstrated in clinical validation studies, and similar levels were reported in independent post-validation studies [35–38].

ThyroSeq v3

- The most recent and comprehensive test version was launched in November 2017 as ThyroSeq v3 Genomic Classifier (GC). Similar to ThyroSeq v2, ThyroSeq v3 GC uses NGS technology, but it has expanded to analyze 112 genes and provide information on over 12,000 mutation hotspots and over 120 fusion types.
- The test detects five classes of alterations:
  - Mutations (single nucleotide variants, SNVs)
  - Insertion/deletion polymorphisms (indels)
  - Gene fusions
  - Gene expression alterations
  - Copy number alterations
- Additionally, ThyroSeq v3 utilizes a proprietary genomic classifier that relies on the algorithmic analysis of all detected genetic alterations to report test results as negative, currently negative, or positive.
- ThyroSeq v3 GC. is optimized for fresh thyroid FNA biopsy samples that are collected into nucleic acid preservative solution, but the test is also available for cytology cell blocks and cytology smears, as well as for FFPE thyroid tissue sections.
- ThyroSeq v3 testing has several steps, as demonstrated in Fig. 14.4:
  - The test starts with an assessment of cellularity in the FNA sample, to ensure that the amount of nucleic acid isolated from the sample is sufficient for testing.
  - If the sample is adequate (as are about 97% of cases), the sample's cellular composition is evaluated, to ensure that there is an adequate proportion of thyroid follicular cells. The test also allows for detection of C cells (indicative of medullary thyroid carcinoma), parathyroid cells, and other non-thyroidal cells during this step.
  - Next, the ThyroSeq GC algorithm is used to process the generated NGS data.
  - It assesses each genetic alteration, mutation level, and combination of molecular alterations to estimate cancer probability in the nodule.
  - Test results are then reviewed, verified, and released by a board-certified pathologist. The ThyroSeq v3 GC. report provides probability of cancer in a given nodule, lists specific genetic alterations, and offers potential patient management, which is discussed later in this section.

Analytical and Clinical Validation

- The most recent version of the test, ThyroSeq v3 Genomic Classifier, was analytically validated in a study of 238 resected benign and malignant tissue samples, which included all major types of malignant and benign thyroid lesions, and 175 thyroid FNA samples with known surgical outcome [39]. The study established limits of detection of every type of genetic alteration assessed by ThyroSeq v3, including cancer-associated SNVs, indels, gene fusions, copy number alterations, and gene expression alterations. Because of the greater complexity of ThyroSeq v3, with the variety and number of alterations detected, a genomic classifier (GC) was established to categorize test results as negative (likely benign) or positive (likely malignant). Using the tissue training set, GC scores were calculated for each sample, and GC cutoffs were established that distinguished cancer from benign nodules with 94% sensitivity, 89% specificity, and 92% accuracy. The FNA validation set had a GC sensitivity of 98%, specificity of 82%, and 91% accuracy. The study established that the proportion of thyroid cells within a sample of 12% or higher was sufficient for reliable detection of all types of genetic alterations, whereas a proportion of 6% or lower was clearly insufficient for detection of such alterations. When the proportion of thyroid cells was between 6% and 12%, the sample had reliable detection of SNVs and gene fusions, but not other alteration types, and therefore was limited. Furthermore, the validation demonstrated that under variable stress conditions, ThyroSeq v3 GC generated reproducible and highly accurate results [39].

- ThyroSeq v3 Genomic Classifier was clinically validated in a prospective, double-blinded, multicenter clinical trial, with patient recruiting occurring at ten different study centers from January 2015 to December 2016 [40]. The primary outcomes of the clinical validation were the sensitivity, specificity, NPV, and PPV of ThyroSeq GC to predict the histopathological diagnosis of indeterminate thyroid nodules with Bethesda III and IV cytology. Because NIFTP is a surgically managed disease under current practice guidelines, it was included in the cancer group. Out of 782 enrolled patients with 1013 FNA samples, 257 samples had indeterminate cytology, informative ThyroSeq test results, and final surgical pathology diagnosis, and comprised the final informative study set. Central pathology review of histological slides was performed by a panel of expert thyroid pathologists who were blinded to the cytology and molecular results.
- Of the 257 samples with indeterminate cytology, 154 were Bethesda III, 93 were Bethesda IV, and 10 were Bethesda V. In Bethesda III and IV nodules combined, ThyroSeq GC demonstrated high sensitivity (94%) and reasonably high specificity (82%), as summarized in Table 14.4. In the same group, cancer/NIFTP prevalence was 28%, with a high NPV of 97%. The study found that 61% of nodules returned a negative ThyroSeq result, with a 3% residual cancer risk in those nodules. This 3% residual cancer risk is similar to that of benign cytology. Additionally, all false-negative nodules were

Table 14.4 Performance of ThyroSeq v3 Genomic Classifier in cytologically indeterminate thyroid nodules

Performance in Bethesda III nodules (n = 154; disease prevalence 23%)			
ThyroSeq result	**Cancer + NIFTP (n = 35)**	**Benign (n = 119)**	**Test performance, % (95% CI)**
Positive	32	18	Sensitivity, 91 (77–97)
			Specificity, 85 (77–90)
Negative	3	101	NPV, 97 (92–99)
			PPV, 64 (50–77)
Performance in Bethesda IV nodules (n = 93; disease prevalence 35%)			
ThyroSeq result	**Cancer + NIFTP (n = 33)**	**Benign (n = 60)**	**Test performance, % (95% CI)**
Positive	32	15	Sensitivity, 97 (85–100)
			Specificity, 75 (63–84)
Negative	1	45	NPV, 98 (89–100)
			PPV, 68 (54–80)
Performance in Bethesda III and IV nodules (n = 247; disease prevalence 28%)			
ThyroSeq result	**Cancer + NIFTP (n = 68)**	**Benign (n = 179)**	**Test performance, % (95% CI)**
Positive	64	33	Sensitivity, 94 (86–98)
			Specificity, 82 (75–87)
Negative	4	146	NPV, 97 (93–99)
			PPV, 66 (56–75)
Performance across the entire cohort (n = 257; disease prevalence 30%)			
ThyroSeq result	**Cancer + NIFTP (n = 76)**	**Benign (n = 181)**	**Test performance, % (95% CI)**
Positive	71	34	Sensitivity, 93 (86–97)
			Specificity, 81 (75–86)
Negative	5	147	NPV, 97 (93–99)
			PPV, 68 (58–76)

From Steward et al. [41]; with permission.
NIFTP noninvasive follicular thyroid neoplasm with papillary-like nuclear features, *NPV* negative predictive value, *PPV* positive predictive value

low-risk tumors that were intrathyroidal, without vascular invasion or clinical evidence of nodal or distant metastasis.

- The clinical trial found that ThyroSeq v3 GC demonstrated a PPV of 66% in a cohort of nodules with a cancer/NIFTP prevalence of 28%. The test correctly classified all (n = 10) Hürthle cell carcinoma and all (n = 5) hyperplastic Hürthle cell nodules. Of 34 Hürthle cell adenomas, 21 (62%) were correctly classified. Furthermore, ThyroSeq correctly classified one medullary thyroid carcinoma and one metastatic renal cell carcinoma, as well as all 11 NIFTP nodules as positive. There were 34 test-positive nodules that were pathologically benign as either adenomas or hyperplastic nodules. Among the test-positive nodules with benign surgical pathology, 94% (32 of 34) showed one or more clonal molecular alterations in a large proportion of cells, which could indicate neoplasia, not hyperplasia.
- ThyroSeq v3 GC also provided specific genetic alteration information to inform cancer probability in the 105 test-positive nodules. Depending on the specific genetic alteration, the probability of malignancy or NIFTP varied from 59% to 100% in these nodules.
- Overall, the study found that utilizing ThyroSeq testing may allow diagnostic surgery to be avoided in up to 61% of all Bethesda III/IV nodules and 82% of nodules with benign pathology. The study also concluded that when ThyroSeq results are positive, the additional detailed genetic alteration information may aid physicians in determining individualized treatment for patients, in correlation with imaging and other clinical information [40].

Patient Management Using ThyroSeq Results

- A feature unique of ThyroSeq is that, in addition to providing positive or negative test results, it reports the genetic profile of a given tumor, which allows refinement of the cancer probability in the tested nodule and provides cancer prognostication information, data that may help to inform the most appropriate management of patients. The refined cancer probability and potential patient management are shown in Fig. 14.4.
- There are three main categories of ThyroSeq results. A "negative" result is assigned when there are no genetic alterations detected in the sample. These nodules are expected to be non-clonal hyperplasias. As demonstrated in the ThyroSeq clinical validation study, the residual risk of malignancy in a ThyroSeq-negative, Bethesda III or IV nodule is about 3%, which is similar to that of benign cytology. According to the NCCN guidelines, observation can be considered when molecular testing, along with clinical and ultrasound features, predicts a risk of malignancy comparable to the risk in benign FNA cytology [20]. Therefore, in Bethesda III and IV nodules, a negative ThyroSeq result, in correlation with imaging and other relevant clinical information, may allow for patient observation.
- A "currently negative" ThyroSeq result is rendered when a low-risk gene mutation was detected, typically in a subpopulation of the cells in the sample. The mutation alone is not sufficient to cause full cancer development, but the cells carrying the mutation form a clone, or tumor, which is typically an adenoma. The mutant clone could undergo expansion and acquire additional mutations that could lead to cancer development. With this test result, patients may benefit from active surveillance with a repeat of the clinical exam and a potential FNA repeat with molecular testing in a year, if there is no suspicious imaging or other risk factors.
- A ThyroSeq "positive" result indicates that one or several genetic alterations associated with a significant cancer risk have been detected. As shown in Fig. 14.4, the specific alteration type correlates with level of risk and potential management. For example, a sample with multiple high-risk mutations is essentially diagnostic of cancer, with a patient likely requiring a total thyroidectomy and possibly regional lymph node dissection, depending on the specific molecular alterations present. Because an isolated *RAS* or *RAS*-like mutation has significant probability (40–80%) of low-risk cancer or NIFTP, patients are likely to benefit from therapeutic lobectomy. Also, as shown near the top of Fig. 14.3, ThyroSeq detects parathyroid disease, medullary thyroid carcinoma, and metastatic disease, which allows individualized management for these patients.

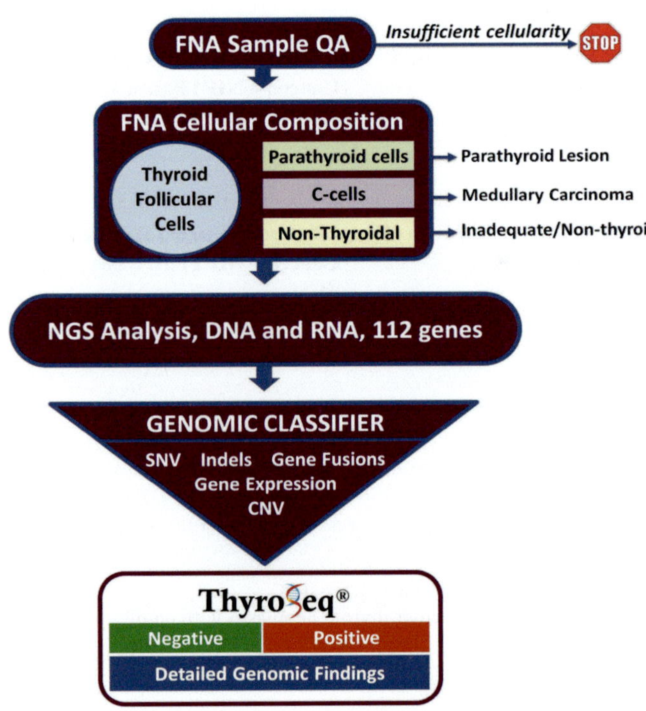

Fig. 14.3 Steps in ThyroSeq v3 Genomic Classifier testing. (*From* Nikiforova et al. [40]; with permission)

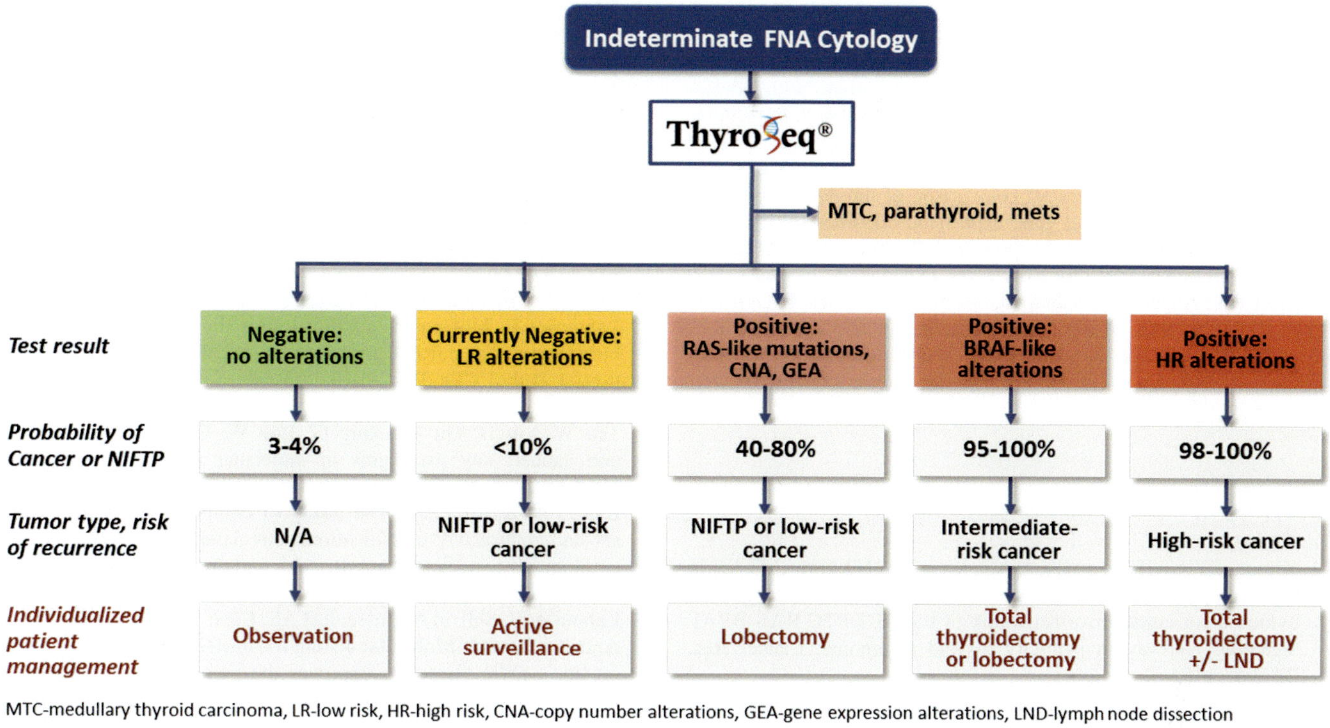

Fig. 14.4 Individualized patient management by ThyroSeq GC Test Results. *CNA* copy number alterations, *GEA* gene expression alterations, *HR* high-risk; *LND* lymph node dissection, *LR* low-risk, *MTC* medullary thyroid carcinoma

Summary

- ThyroSeq v3 Genomic Classifier has been validated in the largest clinical validation study of any commercial molecular test offered for thyroid FNA samples. Its use can prevent up to 61% of thyroid surgeries for nodules with Bethesda III and IV cytology and up to 82% of diagnostic surgeries for histologically benign nodules. It provides clinicians with specific molecular results, informing more individualized patient management. Ultimately, however, selection of the most appropriate patient management requires an integrated approach that includes imaging and other clinical information along with cytology and molecular results.

References

Introduction

1. Cancer Genome Atlas Research Network. Integrated genomic characterization of papillary thyroid carcinoma. Cell. 2014;159:676–90. https://doi.org/10.1016/j.cell.2014.09.050.
2. Patel KN, Angell TE, Babiarz J, Barth NM, Blevins T, Duh QY, et al. Performance of a genomic sequencing classifier for the preoperative diagnosis of cytologically indeterminate thyroid nodules. JAMA Surg. 2018a;153:817–24. https://doi.org/10.1001/jamasurg.2018.1153.
3. Haugen BR, Sawka AM, Alexander EK, Bible KC, Caturegli P, Doherty GM, et al. American Thyroid Association guidelines on the management of thyroid nodules and Differentiated Thyroid Cancer Task Force review and recommendation on the proposed renaming of encapsulated follicular variant papillary thyroid carcinoma without invasion to noninvasive follicular thyroid neoplasm with papillary-like nuclear features. Thyroid. 2017;27:481–3. https://doi.org/10.1089/thy.2016.0628.
4. Krane JF, Cibas ES, Alexander EK, Paschke R, Eszlinger M. Molecular analysis of residual ThinPrep material from thyroid FNAs increases diagnostic sensitivity. Cancer Cytopathol. 2015;123:356–61. https://doi.org/10.1002/cncy.21546.

Afirma

5. Alexander EK, Kennedy GC, Baloch ZW, Cibas ES, Chudova D, Diggans J, et al. Preoperative diagnosis of benign thyroid nodules with indeterminate cytology. N Engl J Med. 2012;367:705–15. https://doi.org/10.1056/NEJMoa1203208.
6. Alexander EK, Schorr M, Klopper J, Kim C, Sipos J, Nabhan F, et al. Multicenter clinical experience with the Afirma gene expression classifier. J Clin Endocrinol Metab. 2014;99:119–25. https://doi.org/10.1210/jc.2013-2482.
7. Lastra RR, Pramick MR, Crammer CJ, LiVolsi VA, Baloch ZW. Implications of a suspicious afirma test result in thyroid fine-needle aspiration cytology: an institutional experience. Cancer Cytopathol. 2014;122:737–44. https://doi.org/10.1002/cncy.21455.
8. Brauner E, Holmes BJ, Krane JF, Nishino M, Zurakowski D, Hennessey JV, et al. Performance of the Afirma Gene Expression Classifier in Hürthle cell thyroid nodules differs from other

indeterminate thyroid nodules. Thyroid. 2015;25:789–96. https://doi.org/10.1089/thy.2015.0049.
9. Harrell RM, Bimston DN. Surgical utility of Afirma: effects of high cancer prevalence and oncocytic cell types in patients with indeterminate thyroid cytology. Endocr Pract. 2014;20:364–9. https://doi.org/10.4158/EP13330.OR.
10. Angell TE, Heller HT, Cibas ES, Barletta JA, Kim MI, Krane JF, Marqusee E. Independent comparison of the Afirma genomic sequencing classifier and gene expression classifier for cytologically indeterminate thyroid nodules. Thyroid. 2019;29:650–6. https://doi.org/10.1089/thy.2018.0726.. [Epub ahead of print]
11. Patel KN, Angell TE, Babiarz J, Barth NM, Blevins T, Duh QY, et al. Performance of a genomic sequencing classifier for the preoperative diagnosis of cytologically indeterminate thyroid nodules. JAMA Surg. 2018b;153:817–24. https://doi.org/10.1001/jamasurg.2018.1153.

Interpace

12. Kimura ET, Nikiforova MN, Zhu Z, Knauf JA, Nikiforov YE, Fagin JA. High prevalence of BRAF mutations in thyroid cancer: genetic evidence for constitutive activation of the RET/PTC-RAS-BRAF signaling pathway in papillary thyroid carcinoma. Cancer Res. 2003;63:1454–7.
13. Nikiforova MN, Kimura ET, Gandhi M, Biddinger PW, Knauf JA, Basolo F, et al. BRAF mutations in thyroid tumors are restricted to papillary carcinomas and anaplastic or poorly differentiated carcinomas arising from papillary carcinomas. J Clin Endocrinol Metab. 2003;88:5399–404.
14. Nikiforov Y. Thyroid carcinoma: Molecular pathways and therapeutic targets. Mod Pathol. 2008;21:S37–43.
15. Zhao L, Dias-Santagata D, Sadow PM, Faquin WC. Cytological, molecular, and clinical features of non invasive follicular thyroid neoplasm with papillary-like nuclear features versus invasive forms of follicular variant of papillary thyroid carcinoma. Cancer Cytopathol. 2017;125:323–31. https://doi.org/10.1002/cncy.21839.
16. Howell GM, Hodak SP, Yip L. RAS mutations in thyroid cancer. Oncologist. 2013;18:926–32. https://doi.org/10.1634/theoncologist.2013-0072.
17. Placzkowski KA, Reddi HV, Grebe SK, Eberhardt NL, McIver B. The role of the PAX8/PPARgamma fusion oncogene in thyroid cancer. PPAR Res. 2008;2008:672829. https://doi.org/10.1155/2008/672829.
18. Xing M, Liu R, Liu X, Murugan AK, Zhu G, Zeiger MA, et al. BRAF V600E and TERT promoter mutations cooperatively identify the most aggressive papillary thyroid cancer with highest recurrence. J Clin Oncol. 2014;32:2718–26. https://doi.org/10.1200/JCO.2014.55.5094.
19. Liu R, Xing M. Diagnostic and prognostic TERT promoter mutations in thyroid fine needle aspiration biopsy. Endocr Relat Cancer. 2014;21:825–30. https://doi.org/10.1530/ERC-14-0359.
20. National Comprehensive Cancer Network. NCCN Clinical Practice Guidelines in Oncology Thyroid (version1.2018). 2018 May 22. https://www.nccn.org/professionals/physician_gls/default.aspx.
21. Gharib H, Papini E, Garber JR, Duick DS, Harrell RM, Hegedüs L, et al. American Association of Clinical Endocrinologists, American College of Endocrinology, and Associazione Medici Endocrinologi medical guidelines for clinical practice for the diagnosis and management of thyroid nodules – 2016 update. Endocr Pract. 2016;22(Suppl 1):1–60. https://doi.org/10.4158/EP161208.GL.
22. Nikiforov Y, Seethala RR, Tallini G, Baloch ZW, Basolo F, Thompson LD, et al. Nomenclature revision for encapsulated follicular variant of papillary thyroid carcinoma, a paradigm shift to reduce overtreatment of indolent tumors. JAMA Oncol. 2016;2:1023–9. https://doi.org/10.1001/jamaoncol.2016.0386.
23. Johnson DN, Furtado LV, Long BC, Zhen CJ, Wurst M, Mujacic I, et al. Noninvasive follicular thyroid neoplasms with papillary-like nuclear features are genetically and biologically similar to adenomatous nodules and distinct from papillary thyroid carcinomas with extensive follicular growth. Arch Pathol Lab Med. 2018;142:838–50. https://doi.org/10.5858/arpa.2017-0118-OA.
24. Oczko-Wojciechowska M, Pfeifer A, Rusinek D, Pawlaczek A, Zebracka-Gala J, Kowalska M, et al. The prevalence of somatic RAS mutations in medullary thyroid cancer – a Polish population study. Endocrinol Pol. 2015;66:121–5. https://doi.org/10.5603/EP.2015.0018.
25. Wylie D, Beaudenon-Huibregtse S, Haynes BC, Giordano TJ, Labourier E. Molecular classification of thyroid lesions by combined testing for miRNA gene expression and somatic gene alteration. J Pathol Clin Res. 2016;2:93–103. https://doi.org/10.1002/cjp2.38.
26. Tan W, Liu B, Qu S, Liang G, Luo W, Gong C. MicroRNAs and cancer: key paradigms in molecular therapy. Oncol Lett. 2018;15:2735–42. https://doi.org/10.3892/ol.2017.7638.
27. Banizs A, Silverman J. The utility of combined mutation analysis and microRNA classification in reclassifying cancer risk of cytologically indeterminant thyroid nodules. Diagn Cytopathol. 2019;47:268–74. https://doi.org/10.1002/dc.24087.
28. Labourier E, Shifrin A, Busseniers AE, Lupo MA, Manganelli ML, Andruss B, et al. Molecular testing for miRNA, mRNA, and DNA on fine needle aspiration improves the preoperative diagnosis of thyroid nodules with indeterminate cytology. J Clin Endocrinol Metab. 2015;100:2743–50. https://doi.org/10.1210/jc.2015-1158.
29. Kumar G, Ablordeppey K, Timmaraju VA, , Song-Yang JW, Yaqoob S, Repko B, et al. Comprehensive genotyping for somatic variation and microRNA expression accurately predicts malignancy risk of thyroid nodules (Poster). American Thyroid Association Annual Meeting, 2017.
30. Ablordeppey K, Timmaraju VA, Song-Yang JW, Yaqoob S, Mireskandari A, Narick C, et al. Overcoming challenges in expanding NGS based mutation panels to analyze indeterminate thyroid nodule aspirates. Thyroid. 2018;28(S1):A–23. https://doi.org/10.1089/thy.2018.29065.abstracts.
31. Kumar G, et al. The majority of non-diagnostic (insufficient) thyroid nodule cytology samples can effectively undergo molecular (combined mutational and microRNA classifier) analysis using a needle aspiration approach (Poster). American Thyroid Association Annual Meeting, Denver. 2016.
32. Kumar G, Timmaraju VA, Song-Yang JW, Repko B, Narick C, Mireskandari A, Finkelstein S. Utility of microdissected cytology smears for molecular analysis of thyroid malignancy. Diagn Cytopathol. 2019;47:289–96. https://doi.org/10.1002/dc.24100.

ThyroSeq

33. Nikiforov YE, Steward DL, Robinson-Smith TM, Haugen BR, Klopper JP, Zhu Z, et al. Molecular testing for mutations in improving the fine-needle aspiration diagnosis of thyroid nodules. J Clin Endocrinol Metab. 2009;94:2092–8. https://doi.org/10.1210/jc.2009-0247.
34. Cantara S, Capezzone M, Marchisotta S, Capuano S, Busonero G, Toti P, et al. Impact of proto-oncogene mutation detection in cytological specimens from thyroid nodules improves the diagnostic accuracy of cytology. J Clin Endocrinol Metab. 2010;95:1365–9. https://doi.org/10.1210/jc.2009-2103.
35. Nikiforov YE, Ohori NP, Hodak SP, Carty SE, LeBeau SO, Ferris RL, et al. Impact of mutational testing on the diagnosis and management of patients with cytologically indeterminate thyroid nodules: a prospective analysis of 1,056 FNA samples. J Clin Endocrinol Metab. 2011;96:3390–7. https://doi.org/10.1210/jc.2011-1469.

36. Nikiforov YE, Carty SE, Chiosea SI, Coyne C, Duvvuri U, Ferris RL, et al. Highly accurate diagnosis of cancer in thyroid nodules with follicular neoplasm/suspicious for a follicular neoplasm cytology by ThyroSeq v2 next-generation sequencing assay. Cancer. 2014;120:3627–34. https://doi.org/10.1002/cncr.29038.
37. Nikiforov YE, Carty SE, Chiosea SI, Coyne C, Duvvuri U, Ferris RL, et al. Impact of the multi-gene ThyroSeq next-generation sequencing assay on cancer diagnosis in thyroid nodules with atypia of undetermined significance/follicular lesion of undetermined significance cytology. Thyroid. 2015;25:1217–23. https://doi.org/10.1089/thy.2015.0305.
38. Shrestha RT, Evasovich MR, Amin K, Radulescu A, Sanghvi TS, Nelson AC, et al. Correlation between histological diagnosis and mutational panel testing of thyroid nodules: a two-year institutional experience. Thyroid. 2016;26:1068–76. https://doi.org/10.1089/thy.2016.0048.
39. Taye A, Gurciullo D, Miles BA, Gupta A, Owen RP, Inabnet WB 3rd, et al. Clinical performance of a next-generation sequencing assay (ThyroSeq v2) in the evaluation of indeterminate thyroid nodules. Surgery. 2018;163:97–103. https://doi.org/10.1016/j.surg.2017.07.032.
40. Nikiforova MN, Mercurio S, Wald AI, Barbi de Moura M, Callenberg K, Santana-Santos L, et al. Analytical performance of the ThyroSeq v3 Genomic Classifier for cancer diagnosis in thyroid nodules. Cancer. 2018;124:1682–90. https://doi.org/10.1002/cncr.31245.
41. Steward DL, Carty SE, Sippel RS, Yang SP, Sosa JA, Sipos JA, et al. Performance of a multigene genomic classifier in thyroid nodules with indeterminate cytology: a prospective blinded multicenter study. JAMA Oncol. 2018;5:204. https://doi.org/10.1001/jamaoncol.2018.4616. [Epub ahead of print].

Index

R. S. Hoda et al. (eds.), *Atlas of Thyroid Cytopathology on Liquid-Based Preparations*,
https://doi.org/10.1007/978-3-030-25066-9

MIX
Papier aus verantwortungsvollen Quellen
Paper from responsible sources
FSC® C105338

If you have any concerns about our products,
you can contact us on
ProductSafety@springernature.com

In case Publisher is established outside the EU,
the EU authorized representative is:
Springer Nature Customer Service Center GmbH
Europaplatz 3, 69115 Heidelberg, Germany

Printed by Libri Plureos GmbH
in Hamburg, Germany